Medications and Mathematics for the Nurse

8th Edition

Medications and Mathematics for the Nurse

Jane Rice

Delmar Publishers

an International Thomson Publishing company ITP®

Albany • Bonn • Boston • Cincinnati • Detroit • London • Madrid
Melbourne • Mexico City • New York • Pacific Grove • Paris • San Francisco
Singapore • Tokyo • Toronto • Washington

NOTICE TO THE READER

Publisher does not warrant or guarantee any of the products described herein or perform any independent analysis in connection with any of the product information contained herein. Publisher does not assume, and expressly disclaims, any obligation to obtain and include information other than that provided to it by the manufacturer.

The reader is expressly warned to consider and adopt all safety precautions that might be indicated by the activities described herein and to avoid all potential hazards. By following the instructions contained herein, the reader willingly assumes all risks in connection with such instructions.

The publisher makes no representations or warranties of any kind, including but not limited to, the warranties of fitness for particular purpose or merchantability, nor are any such representations implied with respect to the material set forth herein, and the publisher takes no responsibility with respect to such material. The publisher shall not be liable for any special, consequential or exemplary damages resulting, in whole or in part, from the readers' use of, or reliance upon, this material.

Cover Design: Charles Cummings Advertising

Publishing Team:
Publisher: Susan L. Simpfenderfer
Acquisitions Editor: Dawn F. Gerrain
Developmental Editor: Marjorie A. Bruce
Editorial Assistant: Donna Leto
Production Coordinator: Barbara A. Bullock
Art/Design Coordinator: Timothy J. Conners
Marketing Manager: Katherine M. Hans

Printed in the United States of America

For more information, contact:

Delmar Publishers
3 Columbia Circle, Box 15015
Albany, New York 12212-5015

International Thomson Publishing Europe
Berkshire House 168-173
High Holborn
London, WC1V7AA
England

Thomas Nelson Australia
102 Dodds Street
South Melbourne, 3205
Victoria, Australia

Nelson Canada
1120 Birchmount Road
Scarborough, Ontario
Canada M1K 5G4

International Thomson Editores
Campos Eliseos 385, Piso 7
Col Polanco
11560 Mexico D F Mexico

International Thomson Publishing Gmbh
Königswinterer Strasse 418
53227 Bonn
Germany

International Thomson Publishing Asia
221 Henderson Road #05-10
Henderson Building
Singapore 0315

International Thomson Publishing - Japan
Hirakawacho Kyowa Building, 3F
2-2-1 Hirakawacho
Chiyoda-ku, 102 Tokyo
Japan

1 2 3 4 5 6 7 8 9 10 XXX 99 98 97

Library of Congress Cataloging-in-Publication Data

Rice, Jane.
Medications and mathematics for the nurse.—8th ed. / Jane Rice.
p. cm.
Includes bibliographical references and indexes.
ISBN 0-8273-8328-2
1. Pharmacology. 2. Drugs—Administration. 3. Pharmaceutical arithmetic. 4. Nursing. I. Title.
[DNLM: 1. Drugs—administration & dosage—nurses' instruction. 2. Pharmacology—nurses' instruction. 3. Mathematics—nurses' instruction. QV 748 R496m 1998]
RM300.R53 1998
615.5′8—dc21
DNLM/DLC
for Library of Congress 97–13780
CIP

CONTENTS

- Emphasis is placed on legal implications and safety
- Drug administration procedures are presented in a step-by-step format with a competency checklist for each procedure. These checklists are stated with terminal performance objectives (TPOs) and the student is encouraged to use the checklists as guides during the practice of the given procedures. The instructor is encouraged to set a time limit for each procedure and to use the checklist for evaluation of student progress
- Self Assessment tests at the end of each chapter allow the student to assess his/her understanding of each chapter's content.

Section 4—Drugs and Related Substances presents essential information on antibiotics, anthelmintics, antiprotozoal agents, antiseptics, disinfectants, antifungal agents, antiviral agents, immunizing agents, antineoplastics, vitamins and minerals, psychotropic agents, and substance abuse.

Key Features

- Tables summarizing currently used drugs
- Each major drug classification includes:
  - —Description
  - —Action
  - —Uses
  - —Adverse Reactions
  - —Contraindications
  - —Warnings When Indicated
  - —Dosage and Route
  - —Implications for Patient Care
  - —Patient Teaching
  - —Special Considerations
- New Features for this section include:
  - —Spotlight
  - —Special Considerations: The Older Adult
  - —Special Considerations: The Child
  - —Critical Thinking Questions/Activities
  - —Spot Check
- Multiple choice and matching review questions are based upon the nursing process with numerous clinical situations described.

ACKNOWLEDGMENTS

I wish to express my deepest appreciation to those individuals who assisted me in this revision of MEDICATIONS AND MATHEMATICS FOR THE NURSE. Thank you for your time, knowledge, encouragement, expertise, and your valuable input.

—The staff at Delmar Publishers: Susan L. Simpfenderfer, Dawn F. Gerrain, Marjorie A. Bruce, Donna Leto, Barbara A. Bullock, Timothy J. Conners, Katherine M. Hans and Charles Cummings.

—The staff at Publishers' Design and Production Services: Gail Farrar, Arlene Kearns-Schofield, and Mary Mowrey.

—Husband and partner: Larry Rice

Reviewers

The author and staff at Delmar Publishers would like to thank the following individuals for their many suggestions for improvement in the manuscript. Their constructive evaluation contributed to an outstanding eighth edition of the text.

Mary Arnold
Blinn College
Bryan, TX 77801

LeVon Barrett, RN
McLennan Community College
Waco, TX 76712

Barbara C. Ellington, RN, MSN
Career Development Center
Newport News, VA 23608

Betty Facey, RN
Glendale Career college
Glendale, CA 91201

Kathy Gooch, RN
Gateway Technical Institute
Batesville, AR 72501

John H. Kuretich
Connelley Technical Institute
and Adult Learning Center
Pittsburgh, PA 15221

Mary S. Lewin, RN
Orleans Niagara BOCES
Medina, NY 14103

Rebecca S. Livigni, RN
Akron Medical Dental Institute
Cuyahoga Falls, OH 44223

Marion E. Monahan, RN
Jeff Technical
Reynoldsville, PA 15851

Janis C. Simpson, RN
Tennessee Technical Center
of Athens
Athens, TN 37303

I would like to thank those companies who responded to my request for photographs and permission to use their materials.

P R E F A C

MEDICATIONS AND MATHEMATICS FOR THE NURSE, 8th EDITION
for the nurse. Although directed at the nurse, this text can be used by any
fessional who needs essential information about mathematics and pharma

The text reflects current and commonly used practices, procedures,
and drug preparations. The content is explained in a clear and easy to un
guage. At all times, safety is emphasized—for the health professional adn
medications and for the patient receiving the medications.

The text is divided into five sections. Section 1—Basic Mathematics
to work each mathematical process correctly, using a step-by-step format
lems follow the mathematical presentation for immediate reinforcement.
tests at the end of each chapter allow the student to assess his/her unders
chapter's content.

Section 2—Calculations of Doses and Solutions builds the mathem
essary for the safe preparation and administration of medications to th
atric patient. Each mathematical process is presented in a clear, con
format with numerous solved problems as examples. Practice problem
actual clinical situations with the use of current drugs and dosages. Se
at the end of each chapter allow the student to assess his/her und
chapter's content.

Section 3—Administration of Medications provides a detailed e
essential to a thorough understanding of drug sources, legislation re
references, forms of drugs, drug classifications and actions, the me
principles for the equipment and supplies, and administration of pa

Key Features

- Stresses the "six rights" of proper drug administration
- Stresses proper documentation: the "sixth right"
- Drugs cited are current and commonly used
- Numerous photographs, drawings, tables and examples are provided
- Multiple choice and matching review questions are pr
- Basic principles for the administration of medications ing process

Section 5—Effects of Medications on Body Systems provides the learner with an explanation of the effects of specific medications on the circulatory, respiratory, gastrointestinal, urinary, musculoskeletal, nervous, and reproductive systems.

This section includes:

- Tables summarizing currently used drugs
- Each major drug classification includes:
  —Description
  —Action
  —Uses
  —Adverse Reactions
  —Contraindictions
  —Warnings when Indicated
  —Dosage and Route
  —Implications for Patient Care
  —Patient Teaching
  —Special Considerations
- New Features for this section include:
  —Spotlight
  —Special Considerations: The Older Adult
  —Special Considerations: The Child
  —Critical Thinking Questions/Activities
  —Spot Check
- Multiple choice and matching review questions are based upon the nursing process with numerous clinical situations described.

Appendix

The Appendix provides the answers to the practice problems, learning exercises, self assessment tests, and review questions.

Index

Two indexes are provided for ready reference to the learner. A drug reference allows the individual to locate any of the drugs described in the text and a general index covers all other topics.

Supplement

An Instructor's Guide accompanies the text and contains the following information:

1. Suggestions for utilization of *Medications and Mathematics*, 8th edition, in the classroom.
2. Suggested answers for the critical thinking questions/activities and the spot checks that appear in Chapters 18–31.
3. Answers to practice problems, self assessment tests, and review questions for Sections 1 and 2.
4. Comprehensive Examinations and answer keys for Sections 1–5.
5. Post Tests and answers keys for Chapters 11–31 (Sections 3–5).

SECTION 1

Basic Mathematics

CHAPTER 1

Introduction and Arithmetic Pretest

OBJECTIVES

Upon completion of this chapter, you should be able to:

- Explain why the knowledge of basic mathematics is so important to the safe preparation and administration of medications.
- Determine areas in which improvement in basic arithmetic is needed.

Introduction

The preparation and administration of medications is one of the most important and critical tasks that you can perform. Today, drugs are more potent and more likely to cause physiological changes in the body; therefore, anyone who administers medications must do so with extreme care.

Incorrectly calculated or measured dosages are the leading cause of error in the administration of medications. A drug error is a violation of a patient's rights. It is important that you develop a working knowledge of mathematics, so that you will be able to calculate or measure accurately a medication that is to be administered to a patient. As you progress through this textbook, you will acquire the knowledge and skill needed to administer medications safely, accurately, and efficiently.

In order to pinpoint individual weaknesses in arithmetic, the following pretest is recommended. Those areas that need improvement may be strengthened through study of the remaining chapters in this section.

ACKNOWLEDGMENTS

I wish to express my deepest appreciation to those individuals who assisted me in this revision of MEDICATIONS AND MATHEMATICS FOR THE NURSE. Thank you for your time, knowledge, encouragement, expertise, and your valuable input.

—The staff at Delmar Publishers: Susan L. Simpfenderfer, Dawn F. Gerrain, Marjorie A. Bruce, Donna Leto, Barbara A. Bullock, Timothy J. Conners, Katherine M. Hans and Charles Cummings.

—The staff at Publishers' Design and Production Services: Gail Farrar, Arlene Kearns-Schofield, and Mary Mowrey.

—Husband and partner: Larry Rice

Reviewers

The author and staff at Delmar Publishers would like to thank the following individuals for their many suggestions for improvement in the manuscript. Their constructive evaluation contributed to an outstanding eighth edition of the text.

Mary Arnold
Blinn College
Bryan, TX 77801

LeVon Barrett, RN
McLennan Community College
Waco, TX 76712

Barbara C. Ellington, RN, MSN
Career Development Center
Newport News, VA 23608

Betty Facey, RN
Glendale Career college
Glendale, CA 91201

Kathy Gooch, RN
Gateway Technical Institute
Batesville, AR 72501

John H. Kuretich
Connelley Technical Institute
and Adult Learning Center
Pittsburgh, PA 15221

Mary S. Lewin, RN
Orleans Niagara BOCES
Medina, NY 14103

Rebecca S. Livigni, RN
Akron Medical Dental Institute
Cuyahoga Falls, OH 44223

Marion E. Monahan, RN
Jeff Technical
Reynoldsville, PA 15851

Janis C. Simpson, RN
Tennessee Technical Center
of Athens
Athens, TN 37303

I would like to thank those companies who responded to my request for photographs and permission to use their materials.

P R E F A C E

MEDICATIONS AND MATHEMATICS FOR THE NURSE, 8th EDITION is designed for the nurse. Although directed at the nurse, this text can be used by any health professional who needs essential information about mathematics and pharmacology.

The text reflects current and commonly used practices, procedures, medications, and drug preparations. The content is explained in a clear and easy to understand language. At all times, safety is emphasized—for the health professional administering the medications and for the patient receiving the medications.

The text is divided into five sections. Section 1—Basic Mathematics explains how to work each mathematical process correctly, using a step-by-step format. Practice problems follow the mathematical presentation for immediate reinforcement. Self Assessment tests at the end of each chapter allow the student to assess his/her understanding of each chapter's content.

Section 2—Calculations of Doses and Solutions builds the mathematical skills necessary for the safe preparation and administration of medications to the adult and pediatric patient. Each mathematical process is presented in a clear, concise, step-by-step format with numerous solved problems as examples. Practice problems are based upon actual clinical situations with the use of current drugs and dosages. Self Assessment tests at the end of each chapter allow the student to assess his/her understanding of each chapter's content.

Section 3—Administration of Medications provides a detailed explanation of topics essential to a thorough understanding of drug sources, legislation relating to drugs, drug references, forms of drugs, drug classifications and actions, the medication order, basic principles for the equipment and supplies, and administration of parenteral medications.

Key Features

- Stresses the "six rights" of proper drug administration
- Stresses proper documentation: the "sixth right"
- Drugs cited are current and commonly used
- Numerous photographs, drawings, tables and examples of drugs and equipment are provided
- Multiple choice and matching review questions are provided for each chapter
- Basic principles for the administration of medications are based upon the nursing process

- Emphasis is placed on legal implications and safety
- Drug administration procedures are presented in a step-by-step format with a competency checklist for each procedure. These checklists are stated with terminal performance objectives (TPOs) and the student is encouraged to use the checklists as guides during the practice of the given procedures. The instructor is encouraged to set a time limit for each procedure and to use the checklist for evaluation of student progress
- Self Assessment tests at the end of each chapter allow the student to assess his/her understanding of each chapter's content.

Section 4—Drugs and Related Substances presents essential information on antibiotics, anthelmintics, antiprotozoal agents, antiseptics, disinfectants, antifungal agents, antiviral agents, immunizing agents, antineoplastics, vitamins and minerals, psychotropic agents, and substance abuse.

Key Features

- Tables summarizing currently used drugs
- Each major drug classification includes:

  —Description

  —Action

  —Uses

  —Adverse Reactions

  —Contraindications

  —Warnings When Indicated

  —Dosage and Route

  —Implications for Patient Care

  —Patient Teaching

  —Special Considerations
- New Features for this section include:

  —Spotlight

  —Special Considerations: The Older Adult

  —Special Considerations: The Child

  —Critical Thinking Questions/Activities

  —Spot Check
- Multiple choice and matching review questions are based upon the nursing process with numerous clinical situations described.

Section 5—Effects of Medications on Body Systems provides the learner with an explanation of the effects of specific medications on the circulatory, respiratory, gastrointestinal, urinary, musculoskeletal, nervous, and reproductive systems.

This section includes:

- Tables summarizing currently used drugs
- Each major drug classification includes:
  —Description
  —Action
  —Uses
  —Adverse Reactions
  —Contraindictions
  —Warnings when Indicated
  —Dosage and Route
  —Implications for Patient Care
  —Patient Teaching
  —Special Considerations
- New Features for this section include:
  —Spotlight
  —Special Considerations: The Older Adult
  —Special Considerations: The Child
  —Critical Thinking Questions/Activities
  —Spot Check
- Multiple choice and matching review questions are based upon the nursing process with numerous clinical situations described.

Appendix

The Appendix provides the answers to the practice problems, learning exercises, self assessment tests, and review questions.

Index

Two indexes are provided for ready reference to the learner. A drug reference allows the individual to locate any of the drugs described in the text and a general index covers all other topics.

Supplement

An Instructor's Guide accompanies the text and contains the following information:

1. Suggestions for utilization of *Medications and Mathematics*, 8th edition, in the classroom.
2. Suggested answers for the critical thinking questions/activities and the spot checks that appear in Chapters 18–31.
3. Answers to practice problems, self assessment tests, and review questions for Sections 1 and 2.
4. Comprehensive Examinations and answer keys for Sections 1–5.
5. Post Tests and answers keys for Chapters 11–31 (Sections 3–5).

CHAPTER 1

Introduction and Arithmetic Pretest

OBJECTIVES

Upon completion of this chapter, you should be able to:

- Explain why the knowledge of basic mathematics is so important to the safe preparation and administration of medications.
- Determine areas in which improvement in basic arithmetic is needed.

Introduction

The preparation and administration of medications is one of the most important and critical tasks that you can perform. Today, drugs are more potent and more likely to cause physiological changes in the body; therefore, anyone who administers medications must do so with extreme care.

Incorrectly calculated or measured dosages are the leading cause of error in the administration of medications. A drug error is a violation of a patient's rights. It is important that you develop a working knowledge of mathematics, so that you will be able to calculate or measure accurately a medication that is to be administered to a patient. As you progress through this textbook, you will acquire the knowledge and skill needed to administer medications safely, accurately, and efficiently.

In order to pinpoint individual weaknesses in arithmetic, the following pretest is recommended. Those areas that need improvement may be strengthened through study of the remaining chapters in this section.

SECTION 1

Basic Mathematics

Arithmetic Pretest

1. Express as Roman numerals.

   a. 15 ________ c. 5 ________ e. 20 ________ g. 8 ________

   b. 19 ________ d. 4 ________ f. 1 ________ h. 7 ________

2. Express as Arabic numerals.

   a. X ________ c. IX ________ e. III ________ g. XIV ________

   b. VI ________ d. XXVI ________ f. XXIV ________ h. XIII ________

3. Express in words.

   a. 1,005,221 ________________

   b. 125,936 ________________

   c. 48,224 ________________

   d. 2,001.5 ________________

   e. 1,200,000 ________________

4. Express as whole numbers of mixed numbers.

   a. $\frac{24}{12}$ = ________ c. $\frac{100}{25}$ = ________ e. $\frac{500}{25}$ = ________

   b. $\frac{9}{4}$ = ________ d. $\frac{16}{3}$ = ________ f. $\frac{67}{15}$ = ________

5. Round the following numbers to the next largest number.

   a. 498 to the nearest hundred ________________

   b. 2,597,500 to the nearest thousand ________________

   c. 1,997,855 to the nearest million ________________

6. Add the following decimals.

   a. 0.05, 0.010, 0.156 = ________________

   b. 1.005, 20.1, 400.5 = ________________

   c. 0.004, 42.015, 1,004.05 = ________________

7. Add the following fractions.

   a. $\frac{1}{5}$, $\frac{1}{2}$, $\frac{1}{4}$ = ________ c. $2\frac{3}{4}$, $4\frac{1}{8}$, $5\frac{1}{2}$ = ________

   b. $\frac{1}{6}$, $\frac{3}{8}$, $\frac{3}{4}$ = ________

8. Subtract the following fractions and mixed numbers.

   a. $\frac{2}{3} - \frac{1}{2}$ = ________ c. $4\frac{1}{2} - 2\frac{1}{3}$ = ________

   b. $\frac{4}{5} - \frac{1}{3}$ = ________ d. $10\frac{1}{4} - 6\frac{3}{8}$ = ________

9. Subtract the following.
   a. $2(5 + 3) - 4(2 + 1) =$ __________
   b. $4(3 - 2) - 3(4 - 3) =$ __________
   c. $4(3 - 1) - 2(2 - 2) =$ __________
   d. $5(5 + 5) - 3(5 + 3) =$ __________
10. Subtract the following decimals.
   a. $12.05 - 10.50 =$ __________
   b. $9.00 - 5.50 =$ __________
   c. $125.50 - 100.60 =$ __________
   d. $95.05 - 5.25 =$ __________
11. Multiply the following.
   a. $525 \times 0.51 =$ __________
   b. $550.10 \times 0.05 =$ __________
   c. $594.99 \times 0.99 =$ __________
   d. $841.08 \times 0.08 =$ __________
12. Divide the following.
   a. $\frac{3}{5} \div \frac{3}{10} =$ __________
   b. $\frac{4}{8} \div \frac{1}{16} =$ __________
   c. $14.25 \div 3.5 =$ __________
   d. $150.25 \div 0.25 =$ __________
13. Which is larger?
   a. $\frac{5}{6}$ or $\frac{5}{8}$ __________
   b. $\frac{3}{4}$ or $\frac{1}{3}$ __________
   c. 0.75 or 0.749 __________
   d. 0.25 or 0.255 __________
14. Express as decimals.
   a. Forty-five and five tenths __________
   b. Thirty-five and three hundredths __________
   c. Two and five ten thousandths __________
   d. One hundred sixty and three thousandths __________
15. Express the following fractions as decimals.
   a. $\frac{7}{10} =$ __________
   b. $5\frac{1}{4} =$ __________
   c. $2\frac{1}{2} =$ __________
   d. $\frac{1}{4} =$ __________
16. Express the following as percents.
   a. $\frac{1}{2}$ __________
   b. 0.007 __________
   c. $\frac{3}{4}$ __________
   d. 0.05 __________
   e. $\frac{1}{4}$ __________
   f. 0.50 __________
17. What is
   a. 5% of 75? __________
   b. 0.5% of 500? __________
   c. 6% of 400? __________
   d. 0.7% of 750? __________
   e. 10% of 500? __________
   f. 25% of 500? __________

18. Express as Arabic numerals.
    a. Four thousand two hundred and eighty ______
    b. Six hundred thousand ______
    c. Six million ______
    d. Forty thousand two hundred and eight ______
    e. Two hundred thousand and twenty ______
    f. Five hundred three and five tenths ______

CHAPTER 2

Numerals and Fractions

OBJECTIVES

Upon completion of this chapter, you should be able to:

- Define the terms listed in the vocabulary.
- Express Arabic numerals as Roman numerals.
- Express Roman numerals as Arabic numerals.
- Express a fraction as a simple, compound, complex, proper, or an improper fraction.
- Express fractions as equivalents.
- Determine the relative values of fractions.
- Express improper fractions as mixed numbers.
- Add, subtract, multiply, and divide fractions.
- Use the process of cancellation whenever possible.
- Work the practice problems correctly.
- Complete the Self Assessment Test.

Vocabulary

numerator (nu′me-ra″ter). The number *above* the line in a fraction. It is the number of parts into which a number may be divided. It is also known as the *dividend*.

Example: $\frac{1}{2}$ numerator — 1 of 2 parts or 1 divided by 2

denominator (de-nom″a-na′ter). The number *below* the line in a fraction. It indicates the number of equal parts into which the whole is divided. It is also known as the *divisor*.

Example: $\frac{1}{2}$ denominator — 2 divided into 1

horizontal (hor″i-zon′tl). Flat, even, or level. It is a line that separates the numerator from the denominator.

diagonal (di-ag′a-nl). Through an angle. It is a slanting line that is used to separate the numerator from the denominator.

unit (u′nit). The smallest whole number; one.

sum (sum). The total amount.

product (prod′ukt). The number found by multiplying two or more numbers.

quotient (kwo′shant). The number found when one number is divided by another number.

lowest common denominator (LCD). The least number into which the denominators of two or more fractions will go evenly.

mixed number. A whole number plus a fraction.

fraction (frak′shun). The result of dividing or breaking a whole number into parts.

minuend (min′yoo-end). The number from which another is to be subtracted.

subtrahend (sub′tra-hend). The number that is to be subtracted.

number (num′ber). A symbol # or word that designates the amount or quantity of a unit.

integer (in′ta-jer). Untouched, whole, entire. It is a whole number, such as 1, 4, 5, 10, and so forth.

addition (a-di′shun). The process of adding or totaling the numbers to arrive at a sum.

subtraction (sub-trak′shun). The process of subtracting or deducting an amount to find the difference between two numbers.

multiplication (mul″ta-pli-ka′shun). The process of finding the product by multiplying or increasing an amount a specified number of times.

division (da-vizh′an). The process of finding how many times a number (divisor) will go into another number (dividend) to obtain a quotient.

Arabic and Roman Numerals

Arabic numerals are those we use in our everyday calculations. They include the figures 0 through 9 or any combination of these figures.

Roman numerals make use of letters to represent numeric values. They are a part of the apothecaries' system of measurement. On occasion, you may see Roman numerals being used on prescriptions or medication orders. Table 2–1 shows some Arabic numbers and their Roman numeral equivalents.

Reading and Writing Roman Numerals

The following steps will guide you as you learn to read and write Roman numerals.

1. When using two Roman numerals of the same value that are repeated in sequence, you add their values. A Roman numeral may not be repeated more than three times.

   Example: XXX = 30

2. When a Roman numeral of a larger value is followed by one of a lesser value, you add the values.

   Example: XI = (10 + 1) = 11

Table 2–1 Arabic and Roman Numerals

Arabic Numerals	Roman Numerals	Arabic Numerals	Roman Numerals	Arabic Numerals	Roman Numerals
1	I	8	VII	60	LX
2	II	9	IX	70	LXX
3	III	10	X	80	LXXX
4	IV	20	XX	90	XC
5	V	30	XXX	100	C
6	VI	40	XL	500	D
7	VII	50	L	1,000	M

3. When a Roman numeral of a lesser value is followed by one of a larger value, you subtract the values.

   Example: IV = (5 – 1) = 4

4. When a Roman numeral is placed between two numerals of a larger value, you subtract the lesser value from the following numeral.

   Example: XIV = (10 + 5 – 1) = 14

5. Roman numerals over 100 are seldom used in medicine. The basic Roman numerals and their Arabic equivalents are:

Roman Numerals	Arabic Numerals	Roman Numerals	Arabic Numerals
I	1	C	100
V	5	D	500
X	10	M	1000
L	50		

◐ Practice Problems

1. Arabic and Roman Numerals: Express the following as Arabic or Roman numerals.

a. 3 ________	f. 7 ________	k. XVI ________
b. 5 ________	g. 50 ________	l. XIX ________
c. 8 ________	h. 60 ________	m. IX ________
d. 10 ________	i. XXIV ________	n. VIII ________
e. 100 ________	j. IV ________	o. XX ________

Fractions

The word *fraction* literally means the result of breaking; dividing. It is used to indicate a small part that is broken off, a small amount, degree, or fragment. In mathematics, a fraction is a quantity that is less than a whole. It may be written in either of the following ways and still have the same value: 0.2 (decimal fraction); $\frac{2}{10}$ common fraction).

A *common fraction* is a part of a whole number. It is obtained by dividing a number into a numerator separated from the denominator by a horizontal line ($\frac{2}{10}$) or by a diagonal line ($^2/_{10}$). In the fraction $\frac{2}{10}$, the 2 is the numerator, and the 10 is the denominator. The line separating the numerator from the denominator expresses the process of division: the numerator is divided by the denominator.

Example: denominator $10\overline{)2.0}$ numerator, quotient 0.2

$$\begin{array}{r} 0.2 \\ 10\overline{)2.0} \\ 2.0 \end{array}$$

Types of Common Fractions

Simple fractions are fractions that contain only one numerator and one denominator, such as $\frac{1}{3}$, $\frac{1}{4}$, and $\frac{2}{10}$.

Compound fractions are those in which an arithmetical process is necessary in either the numerator or denominator, as in $\frac{2 \times 4}{12} = \frac{8}{12}$ or $\frac{10}{6-4} = \frac{10}{2} = 5$.

Complex fractions may have simple fractions in either the numerator or the denominator, or both, as in

$\dfrac{1\frac{1}{2}}{6}$ numerator $\qquad \dfrac{6}{1\frac{1}{2}}$ denominator $\qquad \dfrac{1\frac{1}{2}}{6\frac{1}{2}}$ both.

Proper fractions have a numerator that is smaller than the denominator, as in $\frac{6}{8}$ or $\frac{4}{5}$.

Improper fractions have a numerator that is larger than the denominator, as in $\frac{16}{4}$ or $\frac{15}{3}$.

A *mixed number* contains a whole number and a fraction, as in $3\frac{1}{3}$ or $2\frac{1}{2}$.

Equivalent fractions are those that have the same value, as in $\frac{4}{8} = \frac{1}{2}$ or $\frac{5}{10} = \frac{1}{2}$.

Expressing Fractions as Equivalents

To express fractions as equivalents one must find the largest whole number that will divide evenly into both the numerator and the denominator. This is called reducing the fraction to *lowest terms*. It is easier and safer to work with smaller numbers than larger numbers.

Example: Reduce $\frac{27}{81}$ to lowest terms

Divide the numerator and the denominator by 27

$\frac{27}{81} = \frac{1}{3}$

Practice Problems

2. Reduce the following fractions to lowest terms.

a. $\frac{75}{100} =$ __________ c. $\frac{14}{56} =$ __________ e. $\frac{60}{1200} =$ __________

b. $\frac{34}{102} =$ __________ d. $\frac{33}{66} =$ __________ f. $\frac{21}{105} =$ __________

Expressing Improper Fractions as Mixed Numbers

To express improper fractions as mixed numbers, follow these steps:

1. Divide the numerator by the denominator.
2. Place the remainder as a fraction and reduce to lowest terms.

Example: $\frac{4}{3} = 3\overline{)4}$ with quotient $1\frac{3}{4}$; $4 - 3 = 1$ (remainder)

Practice Problems

3. Express the following improper fractions as mixed numbers. Reduce to lowest terms.

a. $\frac{16}{12} =$ __________ c. $\frac{9}{6} =$ __________ e. $\frac{10}{9} =$ __________

b. $\frac{24}{18} =$ __________ d. $\frac{8}{5} =$ __________ f. $\frac{15}{13} =$ __________

Expressing Mixed Numbers as Improper Fractions

To express mixed numbers as improper fractions, follow these steps:

1. Multiply the whole number by the denominator.
2. Add the numerator to the product of step 1.
3. Place the sum over the denominator.

Example: $2\frac{1}{2} = \frac{(2 \times 2) + 1}{2} = \frac{5}{2} = 2\frac{1}{2}$

◐ Practice Problems

4. Express the following mixed numbers as improper fractions. Check your work by changing the fractions back into mixed numbers.

a. $3\frac{1}{3} =$ __________ c. $5\frac{2}{3} =$ __________ e. $7\frac{1}{7} =$ __________

b. $4\frac{1}{4} =$ __________ d. $6\frac{7}{10} =$ __________ f. $9\frac{1}{9} =$ __________

Relative Values of Fractions

To determine the relative values of a series of fractions, you need to determine which fraction is the largest. Which is the largest, $\frac{1}{4}$, $\frac{1}{15}$, or $\frac{1}{3}$? To assist you in determining which fraction is the largest, follow these steps.

1. Make each fraction a whole number. The fraction with the smallest denominator is the largest, because it takes fewer parts to make a whole number.

Example: $\frac{1}{3}$ is the largest fraction in this series, because it takes 2 additional parts to make a whole.

$\frac{1}{4}$ is the next largest fraction, because it takes 3 additional parts to make a whole.

$\frac{1}{15}$ is the smallest fraction in this series, because it takes 14 additional parts to make a whole.

$\frac{1}{3} + \frac{2}{3} = \frac{3}{3} = 1$

$\frac{1}{4} + \frac{3}{4} = \frac{4}{4} = 1$

$\frac{1}{15} + \frac{14}{15} = \frac{15}{15} = 1$

2. When the fractions have the same denominators, the fraction with the largest numerator is the largest, because it takes fewer parts to make a whole. Which is the largest, $\frac{2}{8}$, $\frac{4}{8}$, or $\frac{7}{8}$?

Example: $\frac{7}{8}$ is the largest fraction in this series, because it takes 1 additional part to make a whole.

$\frac{4}{8}$ is the next largest fraction, because it takes 4 additional parts to make a whole.

$\frac{2}{8}$ is the smallest fraction, because it takes 6 additional parts to make a whole.

$\frac{7}{8} + \frac{1}{8} = \frac{8}{8} = 1$

$\frac{4}{8} + \frac{4}{8} = \frac{8}{8} = 1$

$\frac{2}{8} + \frac{6}{8} = \frac{8}{8} = 1$

Practice Problems

5. To determine the relative values of fractions, analyze each series of fractions that follows, and give the largest value on the first line, and the smallest value on the second line.

	Largest Value	Smallest Value
a. $\frac{1}{3}, \frac{1}{8}$	______	______
b. $\frac{1}{30}, \frac{1}{4}, \frac{1}{150}$	______	______
c. $\frac{1}{5}, \frac{3}{20}, \frac{1}{100}$	______	______
d. $\frac{2}{5}, \frac{4}{5}, \frac{3}{5}$	______	______
e. $\frac{2}{40}, \frac{8}{40}, \frac{10}{40}$	______	______
f. $\frac{1}{150}, \frac{1}{125}, \frac{1}{100}$	______	______
g. $\frac{1}{4}, \frac{3}{8}, \frac{3}{4}$	______	______
h. $\frac{1}{3}, \frac{1}{2}, \frac{1}{5}$	______	______
i. $\frac{25}{100}, \frac{75}{100}, \frac{50}{100}$	______	______
j. $\frac{3}{10}, \frac{5}{10}, \frac{8}{10},$	______	______

Addition of Fractions

Adding Common Fractions

When adding common fractions, the denominators must be the same. The following fractions can be added because their denominators are the same.

$$\frac{1}{4} + \frac{3}{4} = \frac{4}{4} = 1$$

To add fractions that have unlike denominators, follow these steps:

1. Express the fractions as equivalent fractions by finding the lowest common denominator (LCD).
2. Add the numerators and place the sum over the lowest common denominator.

Example: $\frac{1}{4} + \frac{1}{2} =$

4 (LCD)

$\frac{1}{4} = \frac{1}{4}$

$\frac{1}{2} = \frac{2}{4}$

$\frac{1}{4} + \frac{2}{4} = \frac{3}{4}$

Adding Mixed Numbers

When adding fractions and whole numbers, the denominators must be the same. When the denominators are the same, add the fractions, and then add the results to the whole numbers.

Example:

$$\begin{array}{r} 7\frac{1}{8} \\ +6\frac{2}{8} \\ \hline 13\frac{3}{8} \end{array}$$

To add fractions and whole numbers that have unlike denominators, follow these steps:

1. Express the fractions as equivalent fractions by finding the lowest common denominator (LCD).
2. Add the fractions and then add the whole numbers.

Example: $1\frac{1}{4} + 2\frac{5}{8} + 3\frac{1}{2} =$

Step 1. 8 (LCD)

$\frac{1}{4} = \frac{2}{8}$

$\frac{5}{8} = \frac{5}{8}$

$\frac{1}{2} = \frac{4}{8}$

Step 2.

$$\begin{array}{r} 1\frac{2}{8} \\ +2\frac{5}{8} \\ +3\frac{4}{8} \\ \hline 6\frac{11}{8} \end{array}$$

3. When addition of the fractions results in a numerator that is larger than the denominator, divide the numerator by the denominator and then add the results to the whole number.

Example: $6\frac{11}{8}$

$$\begin{array}{r} 1\frac{3}{8} \\ 8\overline{)11} \\ \underline{8} \\ 3 \end{array}$$ (remainder)

Step 3.

$$\begin{array}{r} 6 \\ +1\frac{3}{8} \\ \hline 7\frac{3}{8} \end{array}$$

Practice Problems

6. Addition of fractions: correctly add the following fractions. Reduce to lowest terms.

a. $\begin{array}{r} \frac{1}{6} \\ +\frac{3}{4} \\ \hline \end{array}$

c. $\begin{array}{r} \frac{6}{16} \\ \frac{7}{8} \\ +\frac{1}{4} \\ \hline \end{array}$

e. $\begin{array}{r} 22\frac{3}{4} \\ +76\frac{1}{4} \\ \hline \end{array}$

g. $\begin{array}{r} 9\frac{1}{3} \\ +33\frac{2}{3} \\ \hline \end{array}$

i. $\begin{array}{r} 13\frac{2}{5} \\ 16\frac{4}{10} \\ +\ 7\frac{5}{30} \\ \hline \end{array}$

k. $\begin{array}{r} \frac{1}{5} \\ \frac{14}{25} \\ +\frac{11}{50} \\ \hline \end{array}$

b. $\begin{array}{r} \frac{4}{7} \\ +\frac{1}{3} \\ \hline \end{array}$

d. $\begin{array}{r} \frac{2}{5} \\ \frac{6}{10} \\ +\frac{8}{20} \\ \hline \end{array}$

f. $\begin{array}{r} 49\frac{1}{7} \\ +106\frac{5}{7} \\ \hline \end{array}$

h. $\begin{array}{r} 18\frac{14}{12} \\ +\ 9\frac{20}{12} \\ \hline \end{array}$

j. $\begin{array}{r} 24\frac{3}{9} \\ 8\frac{16}{18} \\ +\ 3\frac{40}{36} \\ \hline \end{array}$

l. $\begin{array}{r} \frac{1}{4} \\ +\frac{3}{4} \\ \hline \end{array}$

Subtraction of Fractions

Subtracting Common Fractions

When subtracting common fractions, the denominators must be the same figure. The following fractions can be subtracted because their denominators are the same.

$$\frac{3}{4} - \frac{1}{4} = \frac{2}{4} = \frac{1}{2}$$

To subtract fractions that have unlike denominators, follow these steps:

1. Express the fractions as equivalent fractions by finding the lowest common denominator (LCD).
2. Subtract the numerators and place your answer over the lowest common denominator.

Example: $\frac{1}{2} - \frac{1}{4} =$

4 (LCD)

$\frac{1}{2} - \frac{2}{4}$

$\frac{1}{4} = \frac{1}{4}$

$\frac{2}{4} - \frac{1}{4} = \frac{1}{4}$

Subtracting Mixed Numbers

When subtracting fractions and whole numbers, the denominators must be the same figure. When the denominators are the same, subtract the fractions, and then subtract the whole numbers.

Example:

$$\begin{array}{r} 7\frac{9}{10} \\ -2\frac{6}{10} \\ \hline 5\frac{3}{10} \end{array}$$

To subtract fractions and whole numbers that have unlike denominators, follow these steps:

1. Express the fractions as equivalent fractions by finding the lowest common denominator (LCD).
2. Subtract the fractions and then subtract the whole numbers.
3. When subtracting fractions in which the subtrahend is larger than the minuend:
   a. borrow one whole unit from the whole number,
   b. add the borrowed unit (1) to the fraction of the minuend,
   c. subtract the fractions then subtract the whole numbers.

Example:

$$\begin{array}{r} 10\frac{1}{5} \\ -\ 8\frac{3}{5} \\ \hline \end{array} \qquad \begin{array}{r} 10\frac{1}{5} \\ -\ \ \frac{5}{5} \\ \hline 9\frac{6}{5} \end{array} \text{ (1) borrow} \qquad \frac{5}{5}+\frac{1}{5}=\frac{6}{5}$$

$$10\frac{1}{5} \text{ becomes } \begin{array}{r} 9\frac{6}{5} \\ -\ 8\frac{3}{5} \\ \hline 1\frac{3}{5} \end{array} \text{ now subtract}$$

4. Check the accuracy of your work by adding the answer and the subtrahend together. The sum will equal the minuend.

$$\begin{array}{rl} 8\frac{3}{5} & \text{(subtrahend)} \\ +\ 1\frac{3}{5} & \text{(answer)} \\ \hline 9\frac{6}{5} = 9\frac{6}{5} & \text{(minuend)} \end{array}$$

◐ Practice Problems

7. Subtraction of fractions: correctly subtract the following fractions. Reduce to lowest terms.

a. $\frac{7}{8} - \frac{2}{16}$

c. $\frac{16}{32} - \frac{9}{32}$

e. $21\frac{3}{9} - 5\frac{5}{9}$

g. $17\frac{9}{10} - 9\frac{12}{10}$

i. $91\frac{45}{25} - 42\frac{7}{25}$

k. $\frac{11}{12} - \frac{5}{6}$

b. $\frac{4}{15} - \frac{1}{45}$

d. $66\frac{2}{3} - 33\frac{1}{3}$

f. $14\frac{3}{15} - 5\frac{6}{30}$

h. $106\frac{7}{8} - 23\frac{3}{8}$

j. $\frac{25}{75} - \frac{16}{150}$

l. $16\frac{5}{6} - 14\frac{3}{8}$

The Process of Cancellation

When multiplying or dividing fractions, it is easier and more accurate to work with smaller numbers. To arrive at a smaller number, the process of cancellation is used.

Steps to Cancel

1. Divide the numerator and the denominator by the largest number contained in each.
2. After canceling, continue with the mathematical process of the problem.

Example: *Multiplication*

$$16 \times \frac{3}{8} = \frac{16}{1} \times \frac{3}{8}$$
$$= 16 \div 8 = 2$$
$$= 8 \div 8 = 1$$
$$= \frac{\overset{2}{\cancel{16}}}{1} \times \frac{3}{\underset{1}{\cancel{8}}} \qquad \frac{2 \times 3}{1 \times 1} = \frac{6}{1}$$
$$= 6$$

Multiplication of Fractions

Multiplying Common Fractions

To multiply common fractions, multiply the numerator by the numerator and the denominator by the denominator. Reduce to lowest terms when possible.

Example: $\frac{3}{7} \times \frac{4}{5} = \frac{12}{35} \quad \frac{(3 \times 4)}{(7 \times 5)}$

Reduce to lowest terms:

$$\frac{1}{6} \times \frac{3}{4} = \frac{3}{24} \quad \frac{(3 \times 1)}{(6 \times 4)}$$
$$= \frac{3}{24} \quad \frac{(3 \div 3)}{(24 \div 3)} = \frac{1}{8}$$

Multiplying a Fraction and a Whole Number

To multiply a fraction and a whole number, follow these steps:

1. Change the whole number to a fraction by placing the whole number over one (1).
2. Then multiply the numerator by the numerator and the denominator by the denominator.
3. Reduce to lowest terms when possible.

Example: $16 \times \frac{3}{8} =$

$$\frac{16}{1} \times \frac{3}{8} = \frac{48}{8} \quad \frac{(16 \times 3)}{(1 \times 8)}$$

$$= 48 \div 8 = 6$$

Multiplying Mixed Numbers

To multiply mixed numbers, follow these steps:

1. Change the mixed numbers to improper fractions.
2. Then multiply the numerator by the numerator and the denominator by the denominator.
3. Reduce to lowest terms when possible.

Example: $2\frac{7}{8} \times \frac{3}{5}$

$$8 \times 2 = 16 + 7 = \frac{23}{8} \times \frac{3}{5} = \frac{69\ (23 \times 3)}{40\ \ (8 \times 5)} = 69 \div 40 = 1\frac{29}{40}$$

◐ Practice Problems

8. Multiplication of fractions: correctly multiply the following fractions. Reduce to lowest terms.

   a. $\frac{23}{9} \times \frac{7}{16} =$ ______________________

   b. $\frac{2}{5} \times \frac{1}{3} =$ ______________________

   c. $\frac{14}{8} \times \frac{2}{4} =$ ______________________

   d. $6\frac{10}{12} \times \frac{15}{3} =$ ______________________

   e. $91\frac{2}{3} \times \frac{4}{6} =$ ______________________

   f. $\frac{18}{24} \times 5\frac{1}{10} =$ ______________________

   g. $42 \times \frac{1}{2} =$ ______________________

   h. $56 \times \frac{9}{20} =$ ______________________

   i. $365 \times \frac{12}{30} =$ ______________________

j. $18 \times \frac{2}{3} =$ ______

k. $\frac{2}{3} \times \frac{3}{4} =$ ______

l. $\frac{4}{5} \times \frac{1}{8} =$ ______

m. $\frac{4}{9} \times \frac{3}{8} =$ ______

n. $\frac{5}{7} \times 5\frac{1}{4} =$ ______

o. $\frac{5}{12} \times 4\frac{3}{4} =$ ______

Division of Fractions

Dividing Common Fractions

To divide common fractions, invert the divisor. *Inverting* a fraction means turning it upside down. It is most important that you invert the *divisor* and not the dividend. When $\frac{3}{4}$ is inverted, it becomes $\frac{4}{3}$.

To divide common fractions, follow these steps:

1. Invert the *divisor.*
2. Then multiply the numerator by the numerator and the denominator by the denominator.
3. Reduce to lowest terms when possible.

Example:

$$\frac{1}{6} \div \frac{3}{4} \text{ (divisor)}$$

$$\frac{1}{6} \times \frac{4}{3} = \frac{4}{18}\,\frac{(4 \times 1)}{(6 \times 3)}$$

$$= \frac{4}{18} = \frac{2}{9}$$

Dividing a Fraction and a Whole Number

To divide a fraction and a whole number, follow these steps:

1. Change the whole number to a fraction by placing the whole number over one (1).
2. Invert the *divisor.*
3. Then multiply the numerator by the numerator and the denominator by the denominator.
4. Reduce to lowest terms when possible.

Example:

$$16 \div \frac{3}{8} = \frac{16}{1} \div \frac{3}{8}$$

$$= \frac{16}{1} \times \frac{8}{3} = \frac{128}{3}\,\frac{(16 \times 8)}{(1 \times 3)} = 128 \div 3 = 42\frac{2}{3}$$

Dividing Mixed Numbers

To divide mixed numbers, follow these steps:

1. Change the mixed number to an improper fraction.
2. Invert the *divisor*.
3. Then multiply the numerator by the numerator and the denominator by the denominator.
4. Reduce to lowest terms when possible.

Example: $2\frac{7}{8} \div \frac{3}{5}$

$2 \times 8 = 16 + 7 = \frac{23}{8}$

$\frac{23}{8} \div \frac{3}{5}$

$\frac{23}{8} \times \frac{5}{3} = \frac{115}{24} = \frac{(23 \times 5)}{(8 \times 3)} = 115 \div 24 = 4\frac{19}{24}$

◐ Practice Problems

9. Division of fractions: correctly divide the following fractions. Reduce to lowest terms.

a. $\frac{23}{9} \div \frac{7}{16} =$ __________

b. $\frac{2}{5} \div \frac{1}{3} =$ __________

c. $\frac{14}{8} \div \frac{2}{4} =$ __________

d. $6\frac{10}{12} \div \frac{15}{3} =$ __________

e. $91\frac{2}{3} \div \frac{4}{6} =$ __________

f. $\frac{18}{24} \div 5\frac{1}{10} =$ __________

g. $42 \div \frac{1}{2} =$ __________

h. $56 \div \frac{9}{20} =$ __________

i. $\frac{7}{8} \div \frac{3}{4} =$ __________

j. $\frac{2}{3} \div \frac{1}{3} =$ __________

k. $\frac{1}{5} \div \frac{1}{10} =$ __________

l. $\frac{1}{150} \div \frac{1}{100} =$ __________

m. $\frac{2}{5} \div \frac{10}{15} =$ __________

n. $3 \div \frac{5}{3} =$ __________

o. $\frac{2}{3} \div 5\frac{1}{2} =$ __________

p. $\frac{3}{4} \div \frac{8}{9} =$ __________

◀▶ Self Assessment Test

This test is designed to assess your understanding of numerals and fractions. Please follow the directions for each question. After you have completed the test you may check your answers with those in the back of the text.

1. Express the following as Arabic or Roman numerals:

a. 15 __________

b. 25 __________

c. 50 __________

d. IV __________

e. XIX __________

f. XVI __________

2. Express the following mixed numbers as improper fractions:

   a. $5\frac{1}{2}$ ________
   b. $3\frac{1}{3}$ ________
   c. $8\frac{1}{6}$ ________
   d. $6\frac{7}{8}$ ________
   e. $4\frac{2}{3}$ ________
   f. $2\frac{1}{2}$ ________

3. Express the following improper fractions as mixed numbers:

   a. $\frac{9}{6}$ ________
   b. $\frac{7}{5}$ ________
   c. $\frac{6}{4}$ ________
   d. $\frac{15}{2}$ ________
   e. $\frac{8}{6}$ ________
   f. $\frac{3}{2}$ ________

4. Reduce the following fractions to lowest terms:

   a. $\frac{48}{96}$ ________
   b. $\frac{75}{100}$ ________
   c. $\frac{33}{66}$ ________
   d. $\frac{60}{100}$ ________
   e. $\frac{14}{56}$ ________
   f. $\frac{3}{15}$ ________

5. Add the following fractions:

   a. $\frac{1}{8} + \frac{3}{4}$ ________
   b. $22\frac{14}{12} + 2\frac{1}{6}$ ________
   c. $\frac{1}{7} + \frac{3}{21}$ ________
   d. $9\frac{1}{3} + 31\frac{2}{3}$ ________
   e. $\frac{1}{3} + \frac{1}{9}$ ________
   f. $102\frac{5}{6} + 98\frac{1}{3}$ ________

6. Subtract the following fractions:

   a. $\frac{3}{4} - \frac{1}{8}$ ________
   b. $21\frac{3}{9} - 5\frac{5}{9}$ ________
   c. $\frac{11}{12} - \frac{5}{6}$ ________
   d. $31\frac{2}{3} - 9\frac{1}{3}$ ________
   e. $\frac{25}{75} - \frac{16}{150}$ ________
   f. $14\frac{3}{5} - 5\frac{6}{10}$ ________

7. Multiply the following fractions:

   a. $\frac{4}{9} \times \frac{1}{8}$ ________
   b. $365 \times \frac{12}{30}$ ________
   c. $45 \times \frac{1}{5}$ ________
   d. $6\frac{11}{12} \times \frac{7}{3}$ ________

8. Divide the following fractions:

   a. $\frac{1}{150} \div \frac{1}{100}$ ________
   b. $\frac{3}{4} \div \frac{8}{9}$ ________
   c. $\frac{2}{3} \div 5\frac{1}{2}$ ________
   d. $56 \div \frac{9}{20}$ ________

CHAPTER 3

Decimal Fractions and Percents

OBJECTIVES

Upon completion of this chapter, you should be able to:

- Define the terms listed in the vocabulary.
- Read and write decimals correctly.
- Define and use the powers of ten.
- Express a common fraction as a decimal fraction.
- Express a decimal fraction as a common fraction.
- Add, subtract, multiply, and divide decimals.
- Express common fractions and decimal fractions as percents, and percents as common fractions and decimal fractions.
- Answer the questions in the learning exercise correctly.
- Work the practice problems correctly.
- Complete the Self Assessment Test.

Vocabulary

decimal (des′a-ml). A linear array of numbers based upon ten or any multiple of ten.

decimal place (des′a-ml plas). The position of a number to the right of a decimal point.

decimal point (des′a-ml point). The period placed to the left of a decimal fraction.

decimal fraction (des′a-ml frak′shun). A fraction with an unwritten denominator of 10 or a power of ten. It is expressed by placing a decimal point before the numerator.

decimal system (des′a-ml sis′tem). A number system based upon the number 10 or multiples of 10.

multiplier (mul″ta-pli′er). The number by which another number is multiplied. It is also known as the *multiplicand.*

multiplied (mul″ta-plid′). The process of finding the product of numbers by multiplication.

product (prod′ukt). The number found by multiplying two or more numbers.

dividend (div′a-dend). The number that is divided. It is also known as the *numerator.*

percent (per-sent′). Per hundred.

divisor (di-vi′zer). The number that is divided into another number or the number by which another can be divided. It is also known as the *denominator.*

quotient (kwo′shant). The number found when one number is divided by another number (the answer).

continuing number. A number that does not come out evenly, but continues indefinitely. It is good practice to carry a continuing number three decimal places and place a line over the last number.

Example:

$$\begin{array}{r} 0.33\overline{3} \\ 3\overline{)1.000} \\ \underline{9} \\ 10 \\ \underline{9} \\ 10 \\ \underline{9} \\ 1 \end{array}$$

Understanding Decimal Fractions

A decimal is a mathematical form that represents a straight line of units described as a fraction. The decimal point is in the center of the line. All the numbers to the left of the decimal point are *whole* numbers. All the numbers to the right of the decimal point are *decimals* or *decimal fractions.* The position of the number to the left or the right of the decimal point is its *place value.* The value of each place *left* of the decimal point is *ten* times that of the place to its right. The value of each place *right* of the decimal point is *one tenth* the value of the place to its left. See Figure 3–1.

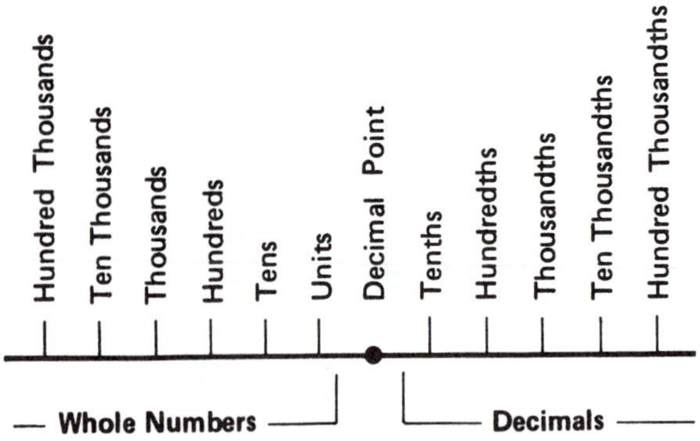

Figure 3–1

Reading and Writing Decimal Fractions

The following steps will guide you as you learn to read and write decimal fractions.

1. Note the place value of the decimal point.
2. Read the number to the right of the decimal point.
3. Use the name that applies to the decimal place of the last number.
4. Read using *th* or *ths* on the end of the denominator.
5. To read a whole number and a decimal fraction, the decimal point is read as *and* or *point.*
6. It is good practice to place a zero (0) before the decimal point. This is a safety measure that insures the reading of the number as a decimal and not as a whole number.
7. Study the following chart and the examples given.

Reading Decimals	
0.1	Read as one tenth
0.01	Read as one hundredth
0.001	Read as one thousandth
0.0001	Read as one ten-thousandth
0.00001	Read as one hundred-thousandth
0.000001	Read as one millionth

Examples:

1. Note that the number is directly to the right of the decimal point (0.1). Read as one tenth.
2. Note that the number is two places to the right of the decimal point (0.01). Read as one hundredth.
3. Note that the number is three places to the right of the decimal point (0.001). Read as one thousandth.
4. Note that the number is four places to the right of the decimal point (0.0001). Read as one ten-thousandth.
5. Note that the number is five places to the right of the decimal point (0.00001). Read as one hundred-thousandth.
6. Note that the number is six places to the right of the decimal point (0.000001). Read as one millionth.
7. The number 10.1 is a whole number and a decimal fraction. Read as ten and one tenth or ten point one.

Powers of Ten

The *power of ten* is the process of multiplying tens together. The number of tens multiplied determines the power. Remember that a decimal fraction is a fraction with an unwritten denominator of ten or any power of ten. Study the following chart for an understanding of the powers of ten.

Power	Number	Name or Value
1st	10	ten
2nd	100	hundred
3rd	1,000	thousand
4th	10,000	ten thousand
5th	100,000	hundred thousand
6th	1,000,000	million
7th	10,000,000	ten million
8th	100,000,000	hundred million
9th	1,000,000,000	billion
10th	10,000,000,000	ten billion

▶ Learning Exercise

Mastering decimals: answer the following questions that involve the use of decimals.

1. A __________ is a mathematical form that represents a straight line of units described as a fraction.
2. State the usage of a decimal.
3. All the numbers to the left of the decimal point are __________ numbers.
4. All the numbers to the right of the decimal point are __________ or __________ __________.
5. The position of the number to the left or right of the decimal point is its __________ __________.
6. The value of each place left of the decimal point is __________ times that of the place to its right.
7. The value of each place right of the decimal point is __________ of the value of the place to its left.
8. A __________ __________ is a fraction with an unwritten denominator of ten or a power of ten.
9. Why is it important to place a 0 before the decimal point?

10. The ______ ______ ______ is the process of multiplying tens together.

11. Read the following fractions. Write your answer on the space provided.

    a. $\frac{1}{10,000}$

    b. $\frac{2}{10}$

    c. $\frac{6}{100}$

    d. $\frac{10}{100,000}$

    e. $\frac{25}{1000}$

12. Read the following decimal fractions. Write your answer on the space provided.

    a. 0.25 ______

    b. 0.7 ______

    c. 0.150 ______

    d. 0.4200 ______

    e. 0.00006 ______

13. Read the following whole numbers and decimal fractions. Write your answer on the space provided.

    a. 2.5 ______

    ______

    b. 9.25 ______

    ______

    c. 125.040 ______

    ______

    d. 15.0150 ______

    ______

    e. 4.00005 ______

    ______

Expressing a Common Fraction as a Decimal Fraction

A *common fraction* is part of a whole number. It is the process of dividing a number into a numerator separated from the denominator by either a horizontal or diagonal line ($\frac{1}{2}$ or ½).

A *decimal fraction* is a fraction with an unwritten denominator of 10 or a power of ten ($0.5 = \frac{5}{10}$).

To express a common fraction as a decimal fraction follow these steps:

1. Divide the denominator of the fraction into the numerator.

$$\text{denominator} \quad 2\overline{)1} \quad \text{numerator}$$

2. Place a decimal point after the numerator.

$$2\overline{)1.} \quad \text{numerator}$$

3. Place a decimal point in the quotient (answer) directly over the decimal point of the numerator.

$$\begin{array}{rl} . & \text{quotient} \\ 2\overline{)1.} & \text{numerator} \end{array}$$

4. Place a 0 after the decimal point of the numerator.

$$\begin{array}{rl} . & \\ 2\overline{)1.0} & \text{numerator} \end{array}$$

5. Now divide.

$$\begin{array}{rl} .5 & \\ 2\overline{)1.0} & \text{numerator} \\ \underline{1\,0} & \end{array}$$

6. Place a 0 before the decimal point of the quotient.

$$\begin{array}{rl} 0.5 & \text{quotient} \\ 2\overline{)1.0} & \\ \underline{1\,0} & \end{array}$$

The common fraction $\frac{1}{2}$ is equal to the decimal fraction 0.5 ($\frac{5}{10}$). The number is 0.5 read as five tenths and can be reduced to $\frac{\cancel{5}^{1}}{\cancel{10}_{2}} = \frac{1}{2}$

7. To check the accuracy of your work, multiply the quotient by the denominator (divisor). This will give you the same number as the numerator (dividend).

$$\begin{array}{rl} 0.5 & \text{quotient} \\ \times\ \ 2 & \text{denominator (divisor)} \\ \hline 1.0 & \text{numerator (dividend)} \end{array}$$

Expressing a Decimal Fraction as a Common Fraction

To express a decimal fraction as a common fraction, follow these steps:

1. Read the decimal fraction.
2. The numerator is the number you get when you move the decimal point to the right past the last number.
3. The denominator is the number of spaces you moved the decimal point.
4. Remember that each space is represented by a factor of ten.
5. Reduce to lowest terms.

Example: 0.25 Read as twenty-five hundredths

0.25 Move the decimal point to the right of the last number; 0.25 becomes 25.

You moved two spaces to the right which is hundredths.

$$0.25 = \frac{25}{100} \quad \frac{\text{numerator}}{\text{denominator}}$$

Reduce to lowest terms. $\frac{\overset{1}{\cancel{25}}}{\underset{4}{\cancel{100}}} = \frac{1}{4}$

Practice Problems

1. Mastering decimals: express the following common fractions as decimal fractions.

a. $\frac{2}{3}$ = ___________ d. $\frac{1}{5}$ = ___________

b. $\frac{1}{4}$ = ___________ e. $\frac{7}{8}$ = ___________

c. $\frac{3}{4}$ = ___________

2. Express the following decimal fractions as common fractions.

a. 0.4 ___________ d. 0.0006 ___________

b. 0.05 ___________ e. 0.000002 ___________

c. 0.010 ___________

Addition of Decimals

To add decimals, follow these steps:

1. To add decimals, arrange the numbers in a column.
2. Line up the decimal points.
3. Make sure you form a straight line with the decimal points one under the other.
4. Add the numbers as in addition of whole numbers.

5. Now place the decimal point in your answer directly under the decimal points of the problem.

Examples:

```
   0.5            0.75
 + 0.50           0.125
 ------         + 0.1000
   0.10         --------
                  0.9750
```

Practice Problems

3. Mastering decimals: correctly add the following decimals.

a. 0.6 + 0.4 = __________ d. 0.25 + 0.001 + 0.100 = __________

b. 0.1 + 0.6 + 0.3 = __________ e. 10.5 + 123.75 + 0.010 = __________

c. 0.89 + 0.26 + 0.2 = __________

Subtraction of Decimals

To subtract decimals, follow these steps:

1. To subtract decimals, arrange the numbers in a column.
2. Line up the decimal points.
3. Make sure you form a straight line with the decimal points one under the other.
4. Subtract the numbers as in subtraction of whole numbers.
5. Now place the decimal point in your answer directly under the decimal points of the problem.

Examples:

```
  104.32          0.098
 - 76.21        - 0.010
 -------        -------
   28.11          0.088
```

6. To subtract a smaller number from a larger number, place a zero (0) after the larger number. A zero (0) placed after the number will *not* alter or change the decimal place or the decimal value.

Example:

```
   0.1            0.10
 - 0.03         - 0.03
 ------         ------
                  0.07
```

7. Check the accuracy of your work by adding the answer and the lower numbers (subtrahend) together. The sum will equal the upper numbers (minuend).

Examples:

```
   0.098  minuend          0.10  minuend
 - 0.010  subtrahend     - 0.03  subtrahend
 -------                 ------
 + 0.088  answer         + 0.07  answer
   0.098  minuend          0.10  minuend
 -------                 ------
```

◐ Practice Problems

4. Mastering decimals: correctly subtract the following decimals.

a. $0.1 - 0.04 =$ ________	f. $0.2 - 0.07 =$ ________
b. $2.25 - 1.75 =$ ________	g. $0.1 - 0.04 =$ ________
c. $304.65 - 264.26 =$ ________	h. $0.3 - 0.09 =$ ________
d. $9.123 - 6.055 =$ ________	i. $0.6 - 0.08 =$ ________
e. $1.000 - 0.556 =$ ________	j. $0.5 - 0.06 =$ ________

Multiplication of Decimals

To multiply decimals, follow these steps:

1. Multiply decimals just as you multiply whole numbers.
2. Count the number of decimal places in the multiplier and in the number to be multiplied. Total this amount.
3. Start on the right of your product and count off the number of decimal places you counted in the previous step.
4. Remember that you count off decimal places in the product from right to left.

Example:

```
          2.14   (2 decimal places)
        × 0.76   (2 decimal places)
        ------
         12 84
        149 8
        000
        ------
Product 1.6264   (count off 4 decimal places from right to left)
   left    ←——— right
```

Multiplying Decimals by Ten or Any Power of Ten

To multiply decimals by ten or any power of ten, follow these steps:

1. When you multiply by 10, you move the decimal point one place to the right.

$$0.6 \times 10 =$$
$$0.6. \times 10 = 6$$

2. When you multiply by 100, you move the decimal point two places to the right.

$$0.6 \times 100 =$$
$$0.60. \times 100 = 60$$

3. When you multiply by 1000, you move the decimal point three places to the right.

$$0.6 \times 1000 =$$
$$0.600. \times 1000 = 600$$

4. When you multiply by 10,000, you move the decimal point four places to the right.

$$0.6 \times 10{,}000 =$$
$$0.6000. \times 10{,}000 = 6{,}000$$

5. When you multiply by 100,000, you move the decimal point five places to the right.

$$0.6 \times 100{,}000 =$$
$$0.60000. \times 100{,}000 = 60{,}000$$

6. *RULE:* When you multiply decimals by 10 or any multiple of 10, you move the decimal point to the right in the product as many places as there are 0's in the multiplier.

$$3.6 \times 10 = 36$$
(1)
$$3.6 \times 100 = 360$$
(2)
$$3.6 \times 1000 = 3{,}600$$
(3)
$$3.6 \times 10{,}000 = 36{,}000$$
(4)
$$3.6 \times 100{,}000 = 360{,}000$$
(5)

◐ Practice Problems

5. Mastering decimals: correctly multiply the following decimals.

a. $4.25 \times 3.10 =$ ________	f. $2.5 \times 100{,}000 =$ ________
b. $3.75 \times 7.35 =$ ________	g. $10.4 \times 10{,}000 =$ ________
c. $83.126 \times 8.12 =$ ________	h. $5.2 \times 1{,}000 =$ ________
d. $66.66 \times 3.33 =$ ________	i. $1.1 \times 100 =$ ________
e. $0.0044 \times 72.16 =$ ________	j. $0.3 \times 10 =$ ________

Division of Decimals

The following methods of division of decimals are designed to guide you step by step through dividing decimals by whole numbers, dividing whole numbers by decimals, dividing decimals by decimals, and dividing decimals by 10 or any factor of 10. Master one step at a time and you will acquire a working understanding of division of decimals.

Dividing Decimals by Whole Numbers

To divide decimals by whole numbers, follow these steps:

1. To divide a decimal by a whole number, set up the division process as follows:

$$12.6 \div 2$$

$$2\overline{)12.6}$$

2. Place a decimal point on the answer line directly over the decimal point of the dividend.

$$\begin{array}{rl} . & \text{answer line} \\ 2\overline{)12.6} & \text{dividend} \end{array}$$

3. Now you divide the dividend by the divisor.

$$\begin{array}{rrl} & 6.3 & \text{quotient} \\ \text{divisor} & 2\overline{)12.6} & \text{dividend} \\ & \underline{12} & \\ & 6 & \\ & \underline{6} & \end{array}$$

4. $12.6 \div 2 = 6.3$
5. To check the accuracy of your work, multiply the quotient by the divisor. This will give you the same number as the dividend.

$$\begin{array}{rl} 6.3 & \text{quotient} \\ \times\ \ 2 & \text{divisor} \\ \hline 12.0 & \text{dividend} \end{array}$$

6. When you have a whole number (divisor) that will not go into the decimal (dividend), follow these steps:

   a. $0.016 \div 4 =$

$$4\overline{)0.016}$$

   b. Place a decimal point on the answer line directly over the decimal point of the dividend. To insure accuracy, place a 0 before the decimal point.

$$\begin{array}{rl} 0. & \text{answer line} \\ 4\overline{)0.016} & \text{dividend} \end{array}$$

c. Since 4 will not go into 0, you place a 0 on the answer line directly over the 0 of the dividend.

$$\begin{array}{rl} 0.0 & \text{answer line} \\ 4\overline{)0.016} & \text{dividend} \end{array}$$

d. Since 4 will not go into 1, you place a 0 on the answer line directly over the 1 of the dividend.

$$\begin{array}{rl} 0.00 & \text{answer line} \\ 4\overline{)0.016} & \text{dividend} \end{array}$$

e. Now 4 will go into 16, so divide.

$$\begin{array}{r} 0.004 \\ 4\overline{)0.016} \\ \underline{16} \end{array}$$

f. To check the accuracy of your work, multiply the quotient by the divisor. This will give you the same number as the dividend.

$$\begin{array}{rl} 0.004 & \text{quotient} \\ \times \quad 4 & \text{divisor} \\ \hline 0.016 & \text{dividend} \end{array}$$

Practice Problems

6. Mastering decimals: correctly divide the following decimals by whole numbers.

a. 28.8 ÷ 4 = __________

b. 36.12 ÷ 6 = __________

c. 100.40 ÷ 20 = __________

d. 56.14 ÷ 7 = __________

e. 86.86 ÷ 43 = __________

f. 0.018 ÷ 9 = __________

g. 0.025 ÷ 5 = __________

h. 0.035 ÷ 7 = __________

i. 0.04 ÷ 10 = __________

j. 10.33 ÷ 3 = __________

Dividing Whole Numbers by Decimals

To divide a whole number by a decimal, make the decimal (divisor) a whole number. There are two methods of making a decimal a whole number:

1. moving the decimal point to the right as many places as necessary to make a whole number or
2. multiplying the decimal by the place value of the decimal point.

Moving the Decimal Point to the Right. To move the decimal point to the right, follow these steps:

1. Place a decimal point at the end of the whole number of the dividend. $100 \div 0.1 =$

$$0.1\overline{)100.} \quad \text{dividend}$$

2. Place a 0 after the marked off decimal point.

$$0.1\overline{)100.0}$$

3. Move the decimal point one place to the right in the divisor, and one place to the right in the dividend.

divisor 0.1. 100.0. dividend

4. You have made the decimal (divisor) and the dividend whole numbers. Now you can divide.

$$\begin{array}{r} 1000 \\ 1\overline{)1000} \\ \underline{1} \\ 0 \\ \underline{0} \\ 0 \\ \underline{0} \\ 0 \\ \underline{0} \end{array}$$

5. To check the accuracy of your work, change the whole number and the decimal to fractions and then divide.

$$100 \div 0.1 = \frac{100}{1} \div \frac{1}{10} =$$
$$\frac{100}{1} \times \frac{10}{1} = \frac{1000}{1} = 1000$$

Multiplying the Decimal by the Place Value of the Decimal Point. To multiply the decimal by the place value, follow these steps:

1. Multiply the decimal (divisor) and the dividend by the same value of the decimal point.

   $100 \div 0.1 =$
   0.1 (decimal, divisor) has a place value of 10
   $0.1 \times 10 = 1$
   $100 \times 10 = 1000$

2. You have made the decimal (divisor) and the dividend whole numbers. Now you can divide.

$$\begin{array}{r} 1000 \\ 1\overline{)1000} \\ \underline{1} \\ 0 \\ \underline{0} \\ 0 \\ \underline{0} \\ 0 \\ \underline{0} \end{array}$$

Moving the decimal point to the right as many places as necessary to make a whole number, and multiplying the decimal by the place value of the decimal point to make a whole number, are two processes that will give you the same result.

0.1. = 1 $0.1 \times 10 = 1$	Moving the decimal one place to the right is the same as multiplying by the place value of 10.
0.01. = 1 $0.01 \times 100 = 1$	Moving the decimal two places to the right is the same as multiplying by the place value of 100.
0.001. = 1 $0.001 \times 1000 = 1$	Moving the decimal three places to the right is the same as multiplying by the place value of 1000.
0.0001. = 1 $0.0001 \times 10{,}000 = 1$	Moving the decimal four places to the right is the same as multiplying by the place value of 10,000.
0.00001. = 1 $0.00001 \times 100{,}000 = 1$	Moving the decimal five places to the right is the same as multiplying by the place value of 100,000.

◐ Practice Problems

7. Mastering decimals: correctly divide the following whole numbers by decimals.

a. $20 \div 0.2 =$ ________	f. $72 \div 0.009 =$ ________
b. $60 \div 0.03 =$ ________	g. $500 \div 0.0005 =$ ________
c. $150 \div 0.75 =$ ________	h. $86 \div 0.43 =$ ________
d. $100 \div 0.10 =$ ________	i. $60 \div 0.012 =$ ________
e. $1000 \div 0.01 =$ ________	j. $36 \div 0.4 =$ ________

Dividing Decimals by Decimals

To divide decimals by decimals, follow these steps:

1. To divide a decimal by a decimal, make the divisor a whole number by moving the decimal point to the right as many places as necessary or by multiplying the decimal by the place value of the decimal point.

$0.0016 \div 0.02 =$ divisor $0.02\overline{)0.0016}$

Moving the decimal 0.02. or multiplying 0.02 by the place value of 100 = 2.

$$
\begin{array}{r}
0.02 \\
\times\ 100 \\
\hline
0\ 00 \\
00\ 0 \\
002 \\
\hline
002.00
\end{array}
$$

2. Now you must do the same thing to the dividend that you did to the divisor.

$0.0016 \div 0.02 =$ $0.02\overline{)0.0016}$ dividend

Moving the decimal 0.00.16 or multiplying by the place value of 100 = .16.

$$
\begin{array}{r}
0.0016 \\
\times\ \ \ 100 \\
\hline
0\ 0000 \\
00\ 000 \\
000\ 16 \\
\hline
000.1600
\end{array}
$$

3. Now set up the problem as follows:

$$2\overline{).16}$$

To insure accuracy, place a 0 before the decimal point of the dividend.

$$2\overline{)0.16} \quad \text{dividend}$$

Place a decimal point on the answer line directly over the new decimal place of the dividend.

$$\begin{array}{rl} . & \text{answer line} \\ 2\overline{)0.16} & \text{dividend} \end{array}$$

Place a 0 before the marked off decimal point.

$$\begin{array}{r} 0. \\ 2\overline{)0.16} \end{array}$$

4. Now you have 0.16 ÷ 2. Divide.

$$\begin{array}{rl} 0. & \text{answer line} \\ 2\overline{)0.16} & \text{dividend} \end{array}$$

5. But, 2 will not go into 1, so you place a 0 on the answer line directly over the 1 of the dividend.

$$\begin{array}{rl} 0.0 & \text{answer line} \\ 2\overline{)0.16} & \text{dividend} \end{array}$$

6. Now 2 will go into 16.

$$\begin{array}{r} 0.08 \\ 2\overline{)0.16} \\ \underline{16} \end{array}$$

7. To check the accuracy of your work, multiply the quotient (answer) by the divisor. This will give you the same number as the dividend.

$$\begin{array}{rl} 0.08 & \text{quotient (answer)} \\ \times \quad 2 & \text{divisor} \\ \hline 0.16 & \text{dividend} \end{array}$$

◐ Practice Problems

8. Mastering decimals: correctly divide the following decimals.

a. $0.0024 \div 0.03 =$ ________

b. $0.054 \div 0.18 =$ ________

c. $0.02 \div 0.2 =$ ________

d. $0.86 \div 0.43 =$ ________

e. $0.2 \div 0.002 =$ ________

f. $7.5 \div 2.5 =$ ________

g. $0.49 \div 0.007 =$ ________

h. $0.81 \div 0.9 =$ ________

i. $0.0138 \div 0.46 =$ ________

j. $0.06 \div 0.6 =$ ________

Dividing Decimals by Ten or Any Power of Ten

To divide decimals by ten or any power of ten, follow these steps:

1. When you divide by 10, you move the decimal point one place to the left.

$$0.6 \div 10 =$$
$$.0.6 \div 10 = 0.06$$

2. When you divide by 100, you move the decimal point two places to the left.

$$0.6 \div 100 =$$
$$.00.6 \div 100 = 0.006$$

3. When you divide by 1000, you move the decimal point three places to the left.

$$0.6 \div 1000 =$$
$$.000.6 \div 1000 = 0.0006$$

4. When you divide by 10,000, you move the decimal point four places to the left.

$$0.6 \div 10{,}000 =$$
$$.0000.6 \div 10{,}000 = 0.00006$$

5. When you divide by 100,000, you move the decimal point five places to the left.

$$0.6 \div 100{,}000 =$$
$$.00000.6 \div 100{,}000 = 0.000006$$

6. *RULE:* When you divide by 10 or any multiple of 10, you move the decimal point to the left in the dividend as many places as there are 0's in the divisor.

$$3.6 \div 10 = 0.36$$
(1)
$$3.6 \div 100 = 0.036$$
(2)
$$3.6 \div 1000 = 0.0036$$
(3)
$$3.6 \div 10{,}000 = 0.00036$$
(4)
$$3.6 \div 100{,}000 = 0.000036$$
(5)

◐ Practice Problems

9. Mastering decimals: correctly divide the following decimals by the powers of ten.

a. 2.5 ÷ 100,000 = __________

b. 10.4 ÷ 10,000 = __________

c. 5.2 ÷ 1000 = __________

d. 1.1 ÷ 100 = __________

e. 0.3 ÷ 10 = __________

f. 88.8 ÷ 10 = __________

g. 0.150 ÷ 100 = __________

h. 0.66 ÷ 100,000 = __________

i. 0.7 ÷ 10,000 = __________

j. 0.100 ÷ 1000 = __________

In Review

Always remember that a *decimal fraction* is a fraction with an unwritten denominator of ten or any power of ten. The *product* is the number found by multiplying two or more numbers. The *multiplier* is the number by which another number is multiplied. The *dividend* is the number that is divided. The *divisor* is the number that is divided into another number.

To multiply decimals by 10 or any power of 10, move the decimal point to the RIGHT in the *product* as many places as there are 0's in the *multiplier*.

$$3.6 \times 10 = 36$$
(1)

To divide decimals by 10 or any power of 10, move the decimal point to the LEFT in the *dividend* as many places as there are 0's in the *divisor*.

$$3.6 \div 10 = 0.36$$
(1)

Percentage

The whole is expressed as 100 percent. Therefore, a certain percent indicates parts of 100. For example, 34% means $\frac{34}{100}$ or 0.34, or 340% means $\frac{340}{100}$ or 3.4 or $3\frac{2}{5}$. Since the strength of solutions is expressed in percentage, it is necessary for the nurse to be able to express percents as decimal fractions and common fractions. This is done by considering the percent sign as a denominator of 100, and then dividing the number by this 100.

- To express a percent as a fraction, remove the percent sign and write the percent as the numerator of a fraction. Write 100 as the denominator of the fraction and express in lowest terms.

Example: $50\% = \frac{50}{100} = \frac{1}{2}$

- If the percent is a mixed number or a fraction, the numerator of the complex fraction is divided by the denominator (100). The process may be simplified by merely multiplying the percent by $\frac{1}{100}$.

Examples: a. $5.5\% = 5\frac{1}{2}\% = \frac{5\frac{1}{2}}{100} = \frac{11}{2} \div 100 = \frac{11}{2} \times \frac{1}{100} = \frac{11}{200}$

b. $\frac{1}{4}\% = \frac{\frac{1}{4}}{100} = \frac{1}{4} \div 100 = \frac{1}{4} \times \frac{1}{100} = \frac{1}{400}$

- To express a fraction as a percent, multiply by 100 and add the percent sign.

Examples: a. $\frac{3}{4} = \frac{3}{\cancel{4}_1} \times \frac{\cancel{100}^{25}}{1} = 75\%$

b. $\frac{29}{400} = \frac{29}{400} \times \frac{100}{1} = \frac{2900}{400} = 7\frac{1}{4}\%$

- To express a percent as a decimal, simply remove the percent sign and move the decimal point two places to the left. This is the same as dividing by 100. If the percent has a fraction, the fraction must be expressed in decimal form before the decimal point may be moved.

Examples: $50\% = 0.5$ $5.5\% = 0.055$ $\frac{1}{4}\% = 0.25\% = 0.0025$

- To express a decimal as a percent, move the decimal point two places to the right and add the percent sign. You are actually multiplying by 100.

Examples: $0.3 = 30\%$ $0.35 = 35\%$ $0.355 = 35.5\%$ $0.0355 = 3.55\%$

Practice Problems

10. Express the following common fractions as percents.

a. $\frac{1}{4}$ = ___________ c. $\frac{2}{5}$ = ___________ e. $\frac{3}{25}$ = ___________

b. $\frac{1}{3}$ = ___________ d. $\frac{2}{3}$ = ___________

11. Express the *largest* decimal in each series as a percent.

a. 0.001	1.25	1.09	________
b. 0.07	0.69	0.349	________
c. 0.08	0.8	0.185	________
d. 0.495	4.95	0.049	________
e. 0.125	0.005	0.025	________

12. Change each of the following percents to a fraction *and* a decimal.

a. 2%	________	and	________
b. $4\frac{3}{4}$%	________	and	________
c. 40%	________	and	________
d. 19.3%	________	and	________
e. 64%	________	and	________

Determining Quantity if a Percent Is Given

- To find the percentage of a given number, express the percent as a decimal or fraction; multiply the whole number by the decimal or fraction.

Example: How much is 5% of 48?

(Conversion to decimal)	***(Conversion to fraction)***
$5\% = 0.05$	$5\% = \frac{5}{100}$ or $\frac{1}{20}$
$48 \times 0.05 = 2.4$	
Note: $2.4 = 2\frac{2}{5}$	$48 \times \frac{1}{20} = \frac{48}{20}$ or $2\frac{2}{5}$

◐ Practice Problems

13. Solve each of the following problems and give the answer as a decimal and as a fraction.

Problem	***Decimal***	***Fraction***
a. How much is 20% of 36?	______	______
b. How much is 8% of 60?	______	______
c. How much is $\frac{1}{2}$% of 750?	______	______
d. How much is 350% of 15?	______	______
e. How much is 2% of 10?	______	______

Self Assessment Test

This test is designed to assess your understanding of decimal fractions and percents. Please answer the questions and/or follow the directions as provided. After you have completed the test you may check your answers with those in the back of the text.

1. All the numbers to the left of the decimal point are __________ numbers.
2. All the numbers to the right of the decimal point are __________ or __________ __________.
3. The value of each place left of the decimal point is __________ times that of the place to its right.
4. The value of each place right of the decimal point is __________ of the value of the place to its left.
5. Read the following fractions, decimal fractions, whole numbers, and decimal fractions. Write your answers on the spaces provided.

   a. $\frac{5}{10}$ __________ d. 0.00005 __________

   b. $\frac{10}{1000}$ __________ e. 2.25 __________

   c. 0.50 __________ f. 8.75 __________
6. Express the following as decimal fractions:

   a. $\frac{1}{3}$ __________ b. $\frac{1}{4}$ __________
7. Express the following as common fractions:

   a. 0.5 __________ b. 0.00005 __________
8. Add the following:

   a. $0.5 + 0.5$ __________ b. $0.98 + 0.76$ __________
9. Subtract the following:

   a. $0.6 - 0.08$ __________ b. $9.123 - 6.055$ __________
10. Multiply the following:

    a. 66.66×3.33 __________ b. 1.1×100 __________
11. Divide the following:

    a. $0.018 \div 9$ __________ d. $60 \div 0.012$ __________

    b. $0.04 \div 10$ __________ e. $0.06 \div 0.6$ __________

    c. $86 \div 0.43$ __________ f. $0.49 \div 0.007$ __________
12. Express the following as percents:

    a. $\frac{1}{3}$ __________ b. $\frac{1}{4}$ __________ c. $\frac{2}{3}$ __________

CHAPTER 4

Ratio and Proportion

OBJECTIVES

Upon completion of this chapter, you should be able to:

- Define the terms listed in the vocabulary.
- Express a ratio as a quotient, as a fraction, and as a decimal.
- Name the four terms of a proportion.
- State why the proportion is a useful mathematical tool.
- Solve for *x*.
- Solve for *x* when only a part of the term is unknown.
- Solve for *x* when a fraction of the term is unknown.
- Solve for *x* when decimals are used in the proportion.
- Prove all of your answers.
- Work the practice problems correctly.
- Complete the Self Assessment Test.

Vocabulary

quotient (kwo′shant). The number found when one number is divided by another number.

fraction (frak′shun). A result of dividing or breaking a whole number into parts.

decimal (des′a-ml). A linear array of numbers based upon ten or any multiple of ten.

ratio (ra′she-oh). A way of expressing the relationship of a number, quantity, substance, or degree between two similar components.

proportion (pro-por′shun). A way of expressing comparative relationships of a part, share, or portion with regard to size, amount, or number.

proof (proof). The stages in resolving the accuracy of your work.

means (menz). The inner numbers or the second and third terms of the proportion.

extremes (eks-tremz′). The outer numbers or the first and fourth terms of the proportion.

positive (poz′a-tiv). A quantity greater than 0; plus.

negative (neg′a-tiv). A quantity less than 0; minus.

Understanding Ratio

Ratio is a way of expressing the relationship of a number, quantity, substance, or degree between two similar components. For example, the relationship of one to five is written 1:5. Note that the numbers are side by side and separated by a colon.

In mathematics a ratio may be expressed as a quotient, a fraction, or a decimal.

Ratio Expressed as a Quotient

Remember that a quotient is the number found when one number is divided by another number. One is to five written as a quotient is $1 \div 5$.

Ratio Expressed as a Fraction

Remember that a fraction is the result of dividing or breaking a whole number into parts. One is to five written as a fraction is $\frac{1}{5}$.

Ratio Expressed as a Decimal

Remember that a decimal is a linear array of numbers based upon ten or any multiple of ten. To express one is to five as a decimal you divide the denominator (5) into the numerator (1).

$$\text{denominator} \quad 5\overline{)1.0}^{\;0.2} \quad \text{numerator}$$

The RATIO 1:5 may be expressed as:

A QUOTIENT	A FRACTION	A DECIMAL
$1 \div 5$	$\frac{1}{5}$	0.2

◐ Practice Problems

Mastering ratios: express the following numbers as ratios, quotients, fractions, or decimals. Reduce to lowest terms when possible.

1. Express as a RATIO — Reduce to Lowest Terms

a. $\frac{1}{25}$ __________ __________

b. $\frac{2}{100}$ __________ __________

c. $\frac{10}{40}$ __________ __________

d. $\frac{25}{75}$ __________ __________

e. $\frac{8}{64}$ __________ __________

f. $\frac{1}{2}$ __________ __________

g. $\frac{1}{3}$ __________ __________

h. $\frac{1}{250}$ __________ __________

i. $\frac{6}{1000}$ __________ __________

j. $\frac{5}{2}$ __________ __________

2. Express as a QUOTIENT — Reduce to Lowest Terms
   a. 24:48 __________ __________
   b. 12:6 __________ __________
   c. 76:304 __________ __________
   d. 5:25 __________ __________
   e. 2:92 __________ __________
   f. 18:108 __________ __________
   g. 10:50 __________ __________
   h. 17:51 __________ __________
   i. 11:22 __________ __________
   j. 55:165 __________ __________

3. Express as a FRACTION — Reduce to Lowest Terms
   a. 33:66 __________ __________
   b. 4:10 __________ __________
   c. 75:100 __________ __________
   d. 22:88 __________ __________
   e. 43:86 __________ __________
   f. 2:13 __________ __________
   g. 7:49 __________ __________
   h. 4:100 __________ __________
   i. 1:150 __________ __________
   j. 12:36 __________ __________

4. Express as a DECIMAL — Reduce to Lowest Terms
   a. 1:50 __________ __________
   b. 8:100 __________ __________
   c. 6:1000 __________ __________
   d. 3:4 __________ __________
   e. 1:500 __________ __________

f. 2:25 __________ __________
g. 5:4 __________ __________
h. 1:1000 __________ __________
i. 1:200 __________ __________
j. 1:2 __________ __________

Understanding Proportion

Proportion is a way of expressing the comparative relationship between a part, share, or portion with regard to size, amount, or number. In mathematics, a proportion expresses the relationship between two ratios. In setting up a proportion, the ratios are separated by :: or an = sign. In this text, the equal sign (=) is used to separate ratios.

Example: $3:4 = 1:2$

Read: three is to four equals one is to two.

The four terms of a proportion are given special names. The *means* are the inner numbers or the second and third terms of the proportion.

Example: $3:4 = 1:2$
(2) (3)
means

The *extremes* are the outer numbers or the first and fourth terms of the proportion.

Example: $3:4 = 1:2$
(1) (4)
extremes

In a *true* proportion, the product of the means equals the product of the extremes.

Example: *means*
$8:16 = 1:2$
extremes
$16 \times 1 = 16$ (*means*)
$8 \times 2 = 16$ (*extremes*)

Solving for *x*

The proportion is a very useful mathematical tool. When a part, share, or portion of the problem is unknown, x represents the unknown factor. You can determine the unknown by solving for x. The unknown factor x may appear any place in the proportion.

Now solve for x in the problem: $3:4 = x:12$.

1. Multiply the terms that contain the x and place the product to the *left* of the equal sign ($4x$).

2. Multiply the other terms and place the product to the *right* of the equal sign (36).
3. To find x divide the product of x into the product of the other terms (36 ÷ 4).
4. Your answer will be equal to x (9).

Example: $3:4 = x:2$

$$4x = 36$$
$$x = 36 \div 4 = 9$$
$$x = 9$$

After finding the unknown factor, check your mathematical skills by determining if you have a *true* proportion. This technique is called *proof* or *proving* your answer. To prove your answer,

1. Place the answer you found for x back into the formula where you once had x.
2. Now multiply the *means* by the *means*, and the *extremes* by the *extremes*.
3. The results will equal each other.

Example: FORMULA: $3:4 = x:12$
PROOF: $3:4 = 9:12$
$36 = 36$

◐ Practice Problems

5. Solve for x and prove your answers.
   a. $4:5 = x:10$ __________
   b. $25:x = 5:10$ __________
   c. $50:x = 25:1000$ __________
   d. $8:10 = x:30$ __________
   e. $4:8 = x:16$ __________
   f. $9:15 = x:5$ __________
   g. $500:x = 5:25$ __________
   h. $4:28 = x:84$ __________
   i. $9:x = 5:300$ __________
   j. $x:600 = 4:120$ __________

Now solve for x when only a part of the term is unknown: $4:(x-2) = 6:3$.

1. Multiply the terms that contain the portion of x and place the product to the *left* of the equal sign.

2. Multiply the other terms and place the product to the *right* of the equal sign.
3. To find x when there is a negative (minus) or positive (plus) sign involved, change the sign as you transpose the number across the equal sign. A minus will become a plus, and a plus will become a minus.
4. To find x, divide the product of x into the product of the other terms.
5. Your answer will be equal to x.

Example: $4:(x-2) = 6:3$

$$6(x-2) = 6x - 12$$
$$6x - 12 = 4 \times 3 = 12$$
$$6x - 12 = 12$$
$$6x = 12 + 12 = 24$$
$$6x = 24$$
$$6x = 24 \div 6 = 4$$
$$x = 4$$

6. Now prove your answer. Remember to multiply *means* by *means*, and *extremes* by *extremes*.

Proof: $4:(4-2) = 6:3$

means $(4-2) = 2 \times 6 = 12$

extremes $4 \times 3 = 12$

means $12 =$ *extremes* 12

$12 = 12$

◐ Practice Problems

6. Solve for x and prove your answers.
   a. $6:(x-10) = 1:6$ ____________________
   b. $8:(x-4) = 2:6$ ____________________
   c. $5:(x+4) = 4:40$ ____________________
   d. $2:(x-2)\ 4:24$ ____________________
   e. $140:(x+10) = 1:100$ ____________________
   f. $4:(x-6) = 2:6$ ____________________
   g. $5:(x-32) = 5:9$ ____________________
   h. $(x+40):25 = 150:30$ ____________________
   i. $12:(x+3) = 6:9$ ____________________
   j. $7:(x-14) = 2:28$ ____________________

Now solve for x when a fraction of the term is unknown: $\frac{1}{2}x:1000 = 1:500$.

1. Multiply the fraction of the x by the appropriate term and place the product to the left of the equal sign.
2. Multiply the other terms and place the product to the *right* of the equal sign.
3. To find x, divide the product of x into the product of the other terms.
4. Your answer will be equal to x.
5. Prove your answer.

Example:

$$\frac{1}{2}x:1000 = 1:500$$

$$\frac{1}{2} \times \frac{500}{1} = 250$$

$$250x = 1000$$

$$x = 1000 \div 250 = 4$$

$$x = 4$$

Proof:

$$\frac{1}{2}\left(\times\frac{4}{1}\right) = 2$$

$$2:1000 = 1:500$$

$$1000 = 1000$$

◐ Practice Problems

7. Solve for x and prove your answers.

a. $\frac{1}{2}:x = 1:8$ ________________

b. $\frac{1}{4}:x = 20:400$ ________________

c. $\frac{1}{6}:\frac{5}{6} = 4:x$ ________________

d. $\frac{1}{2}:1000 = x:500$ ________________

e. $\frac{3}{4}:x = \frac{9}{10}:\frac{2}{3}$ ________________

f. $\frac{1}{0000}:\frac{1}{100} = x:60$ ________________

g. $\frac{1}{4}:500 = x:1000$ ________________

h. $\frac{1}{1000}:\frac{1}{50} = x:60$ ________________

i. $\frac{1}{10}:2000 = 1:100$ ________________

j. $\frac{1}{6}:1 = \frac{1}{8}:x$ ________________

Now solve for x when decimals are used in the formula: $0.6:0.4 = 9:x$.

1. Multiply the terms containing the x and place the product to the *left* of the equal sign. Remember your steps on multiplying decimals.
2. Multiply the other terms and place the product to the *right* of the equal sign.
3. To find x divide the product of x into the product of the other terms. Remember your steps on how to divide decimals.
4. Your answer will be equal to x.

5. Prove your answer.

Example: $0.6:0.4 = 9:x$

$0.6x = 3.6$

$x = 3.6 \div 0.6$

$x = 6$

$$0.6\overline{)3.6} = 0.6 \quad 36$$

Proof: $0.6:0.4 = 9:x$

$3.6 = 3.6$

Practice Problems

8. Solve for x and prove your answers.
   a. $0.4:0.2 = 6:x$ ____________
   b. $0.2:4 = 25:x$ ____________
   c. $0.7:x = 70:500$ ____________
   d. $0.5:15 = x:60$ ____________
   e. $0.3:30 = 10:x$ ____________
   f. $0.7:70 = x:1000$ ____________
   g. $0.002:x = 0.4:100$ ____________
   h. $0.6:24 = 0.75:x$ ____________
   i. $0.2:8 = 25:x$ ____________
   j. $0.25:5 = x:100$ ____________

Self Assessment Test

This test is designed to assess your understanding of ratio and proportion. Please follow the directions as provided. After you have completed the test you may check your answers with those in the back of the text.

1. Express the following numbers as a ratio, a quotient, a fraction, and a decimal:

	Ratio	*Quotient*	*Fraction*	*Decimal*
a. $\frac{1}{25}$	______	______	______	______
b. 12:6	______	______	______	______
c. 33:66	______	______	______	______
d. 1:50	______	______	______	______
e. $\frac{25}{75}$	______	______	______	______

2. Solve for x in each of the following:

a. $\frac{1}{2}:x = 1:8$ $x =$ ______

b. $9:x = 5:300$ $x =$ ______

c. $\frac{1}{100}:\frac{1}{10} = x:6$ $x =$ ______

d. $\frac{1}{4}:500 = x:1000$ $x =$ ______

e. $36:12 = \frac{1}{100}:x$ $x =$ ______

f. $6:24 = 0.75:x$ $x =$ ______

g. $x:600 = 4:120$ $x =$ ______

h. $0.7:70 = x:1000$ $x =$ ______

i. $4:(x - 6) = 2:6$ $x =$ ______

j. $6:12 = \frac{1}{4}:x$ $x =$ ______

CHAPTER 5

Temperature Equivalents

OBJECTIVES

Upon completion of this chapter, you should be able to:

- Define the terms listed in the vocabulary.
- Change a temperature reading from Celsius to Fahrenheit.
- Change a temperature reading from Fahrenheit to Celsius.
- Work the practice problems correctly.
- Complete the Self Assessment Test

Vocabulary

celsius (sel′se-us). A temperature scale with the freezing point of water at 0° and the boiling point at 100°. Celsius is the official scientific name for the centigrade scale.

fahrenheit (far′en-hit). A temperature scale with the freezing point of water at 32° and the boiling point at 212°.

centigrade (sen′ti-grad). Means having 100 degrees or steps.

thermometer (ther-mom′e-ter). An instrument used to measure degrees of heat.

temperature (tem′per-a-tur). The degree of heat of a living body; degree of hotness or coldness of a substance.

Introduction

The normal human body temperature range is 97° to 99° Fahrenheit (F) and 36.1° to 37.2° Celsius (C). The average human body temperature is 98.6° Fahrenheit or 37° Celsius.

Using a Fahrenheit, Celsius, or electronic thermometer, one may measure a patient's body temperature. In the United States, both the Fahrenheit and Celsius scales are used; in some countries the Celsius scale is preferred.

The mercury thermometer was developed by Gabriel Fahrenheit. Using a mixture of salt and ice, Fahrenheit experimented with temperature. The coldest mixture he could make he called "zero." He noted that water froze at 32° and it boiled at 212°.

Anders Celsius suggested a temperature scale based on the freezing point of water being 0° and its boiling point being 100°. The Celsius temperature scale is used in the metric system.

It is your responsibility to take and record a patient's body temperature accurately. It is to your advantage to understand both temperature scales. See Figure 5–1.

Five degrees on the Celsius scale corresponds to nine degrees on the Fahrenheit scale. Zero degrees on the Celsius scale corresponds to 32 degrees on the Fahrenheit scale. Several mathematical formulas are used to convert from one temperature scale to the other.

To convert a temperature from Fahrenheit to Celsius, subtract 32, multiply by 5, and divide by 9.

$$C = (F - 32) \times \frac{5}{9}$$

To convert a temperature from Celsius to Fahrenheit, multiply by 9, divide by 5, and add 32.

$$F = \frac{9 \times C}{5} + 32$$

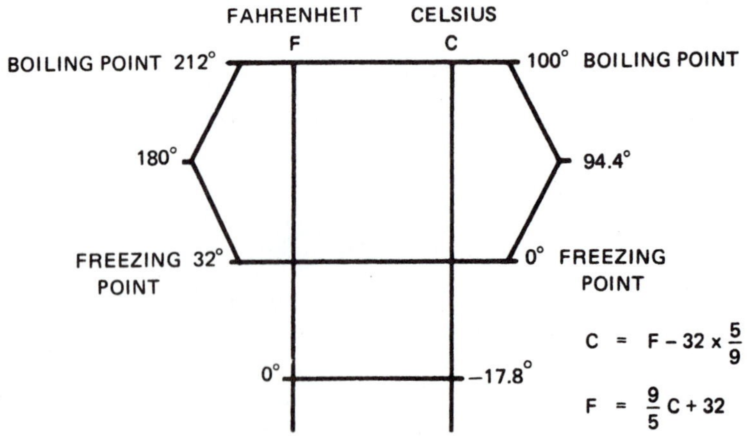

Figure 5–1 Fahrenheit and Celsius temperature equivalents

◐ Practice Problems

1. Conversion: using the foregoing formulas, convert each of the following temperatures.

a. 40°C = __________ F   c. 95°F = __________ C

b. 35°C = __________ F   d. 99°F = __________ C

Using the Proportional Method to Convert Temperature

Converting 37° Celsius to Fahrenheit

Formula: C:(F – 32) = 5:9

- Use the given formula for converting temperature.
- Substitute the known temperature in its proper place in the formula.
- Using the proportional method, solve for the unknown temperature.

Problem: 37:(F – 32) = 5:9

Step 1. Multiply the means by the means: $(F - 32) \times 5$.

$5\,F - 160$

Step 2. $5\,F - 160$ becomes the *left* side of the proportion: $5\,F - 160 =$

Step 3. Multiply the extremes by the extremes: $37 \times 9 = 333$.

Step 4. 333 becomes the *right* side of the proportion: $= 333$.

Step 5. Now, set up the proportion:

$5\,F - 160 = 333$

Step 6. Solve for the unknown:

$$5\,F - 160 = 333$$
$$5\,F = 333 + 160$$
$$5\,F = 493$$
$$F = \frac{493}{5}$$
$$F = 98.6°$$

- You have converted 37° Celsius to 98.6° Fahrenheit.

Converting 98.6° Fahrenheit to Celsius

Formula: C:(F – 32) = 5:9

- Use the given formula for converting temperature.
- Substitute the known temperature in its proper place in the formula.
- Using the proportional method, solve for the unknown temperature.

Problem: C:(98.6° – 32) = 5:9

Step 1. Subtract: 98.6° – 32 = 66.6

Step 2. Place 66.6 in the formula: C:66.6 = 5:9

Step 3. Multiply the means by the means: $66.6 \times 5 = 333$.

Step 4. = 333 becomes the *right* side of the proportion.

Step 5. Multiply the extremes by the extremes: $C \times 9 = 9\ C$

Step 6. 9 C becomes the *left* side of the proportion: 9 C =.

Step 7. Now, set up the proportion:

$9\ C = 333$

Step 8. Solve for the unknown:

$9\ C = 333$

$C = \frac{333}{9}$

$C = 37°$

- You have converted 98.6° Fahrenheit to 37° Celsius.
- Prove your answer using the same process as proving any proportional answer.

C:(F – 32) = 5:9

37:(98.6 – 32) = 5.9

333 = 333

Practice Problems

2. Conversion: using the proportional method, convert each of the following temperatures.

a. 102.2°F = __________ C

b. 97.8°F = __________ C

c. 99.6°F = __________ C

d. 103°F = __________ C

e. 104°F = __________ C

f. 36°C = __________ F

g. 37.2°C = __________ F

h. 37.8°C = __________ F

i. 38.3°C = __________ F

j. 39°C = __________ F

Self Assessment Test

This test is designed to assess your understanding of temperature equivalents. Please place the correct answer in the space provided. After you have completed the test you may check your answers with those in the back of the text.

1. The normal human body temperature range is __________ to __________ Fahrenheit and __________ to __________ Celsius.

2. Boiling point on the Fahrenheit scale is __________ degrees.
3. Freezing point on the Celsius scale is __________ degrees.
4. Convert the following temperatures to Fahrenheit or Celsius:

   a. 99°F = __________ C d. 39°C = __________ F

   b. 98.6°F = __________ C e. 36°C = __________ F

   c. 101°F = __________ C f. 41°C = __________ F

Table 5–1 Temperature Conversion Chart

Celsius to Fahrenheit									
C°	F°	C°	F°	C°	F°	C°	F°	C°	F°
0	32	11.1	52	22.2	72	33.3	92	44	111.2
0.6	33	11.7	53	22.8	73	33.9	93	44.4	112
1	33.8	12	53.6	23	73.4	34	93.2	45	113
1.1	34	12.2	54	23.3	74	34.4	94	45.6	114
1.7	35	12.8	55	23.9	75	35	95	46	114.8
2.1	35.6	13	55.4	24	75.2	35.6	96	46.1	115
2.2	36	13.3	56	24.4	76	36	96.8	46.7	116
2.8	37	13.9	57	25	77	36.1	97	47	116.6
3	37.4	14	57.2	25.6	78	36.7	98	47.2	117
3.3	38	14.4	58	26	78.8	37	98.6	47.8	118
3.9	39	15	59	26.1	79	37.2	99	48	118.4
4	39.2	15.6	60	26.7	80	37.5	99.6	48.3	119
4.4	40	16	60.8	27	80.6	37.8	100	48.9	120
5	41	16.1	61	27.2	81	38	100.4	49	120.2
5.6	42	16.7	62	27.8	82	38.3	101	49.4	121
6	42.8	17	62.2	28	82.4	38.9	102	50	122
6.1	43	17.2	63	28.3	83	39	102.2	50.6	123
6.7	44	17.8	64	28.9	84	39.4	103	51	123.8
7	44.6	18	64.4	29	84.2	40	104	51.1	124
7.2	45	18.3	65	29.4	85	40.6	105	51.7	125
7.8	46	18.9	66	30	86	41	105.8	52	125.6
8	46.4	19	66.2	30.6	87	41.1	106	52.2	126
8.3	47	19.4	67	31	87.8	41.7	107	52.8	127
8.9	48	20	68	31.1	88	42	107.6	53	127.4
9	48.2	20.6	69	31.7	89	42.2	108	53.3	128
9.4	49	21	69.8	32	89.6	42.8	109	53.9	129
10	50	21.1	70	32.2	90	43	109.4	54	129.2
10.6	51	21.7	71	32.8	91	43.3	110	54.4	130
11	51.8	22	71.6	33	91.4	43.9	111	55	131

(continued)

Table 5–1 Temperature Conversion Chart (*Continued*)

Celsius to Fahrenheit									
C°	F°	C°	F°	C°	F°	C°	F°	C°	F°
55.6	132	69.4	157	83.9	183	98	208.4	143.3	290
56	132.8	70	158	84	183.2	98.3	209	145	293
56.1	133	70.6	159	84.4	184	98.9	210	146.1	295
56.7	134	71	159.8	85	185	99	210.2	148.9	300
57	134.6	71.1	160	85.6	186	99.4	211	150	302
57.2	135	71.7	161	86	186.8	100	212	154.4	310
57.8	136	72	161.6	86.1	187	100.6	213	160	320
58	136.4	72.2	162	86.7	188	101	213.8	165.6	330
58.3	137	72.8	163	87	188.6	101.1	214	170	338
58.9	138	73	163.4	87.2	189	101.7	215	171.1	340
59	138.2	73.3	164	87.8	190	102	215.6	176.7	350
59.4	139	73.9	165	88	190.4	102.2	216	180	356
60	140	74	165.2	88.3	191	102.8	217	182.2	360
60.6	141	74.4	166	88.9	192	103	217.4	187.8	370
61	141.8	75	167	89	192.2	103.3	218	190	374
61.1	142	75.6	168	89.4	193	103.9	219	193.3	380
61.7	143	76	168.8	90	194	104	219.2	198.9	390
62	143.6	76.1	169	90.6	195	104.4	220	200	392
62.2	144	76.7	170	91	195.8	105	221	204.4	400
62.8	145	77	170.6	91.1	196	107.2	225	210	410
63	145.4	77.2	171	91.7	197	110	230	215.6	420
63.3	146	77.8	172	92	197.6	112.8	235	220	428
63.9	147	78	172.4	92.2	198	115	239	221.1	430
64	147.2	78.3	173	92.8	199	115.6	240	226.7	440
64.4	148	78.9	174	93	199.4	118.3	245	230	446
65	149	79	174.2	93.3	200	120	248	232.2	450
65.6	150	79.4	175	93.9	201	121.1	250	237.8	460
66	150.8	80	176	94	201.2	123.9	255	240	464
66.1	151	80.6	177	94.4	202	125	257	243.3	470
66.7	152	81	177.8	95	203	126.7	260	248.9	480
67	152.6	81.1	178	95.6	204	129.4	265	250	482
67.2	153	81.7	179	96	204.8	130	266	254.4	490
67.8	154	82	179.6	96.1	205	132.2	270	260	500
68	154.4	82.2	180	96.7	206	135	275	265.6	510
68.3	155	82.8	181	97	206.6	137.8	280	270	518
68.9	156	83	181.4	97.2	207	140	284		
69	156.2	83.3	182	97.8	208	140.6	285		

SECTION 2

Calculations of Doses and Solutions

CHAPTER 6

The Metric System

OBJECTIVES

Upon completion of this chapter, you should be able to:

- Define the terms listed in the vocabulary.
- State why the metric system is used as the universal system of measurement.
- List ten guidelines you will use as you work with the metric system.
- Name the seven common prefixes used in the metric system.
- Name the fundamental units of the metric system.
- State why you place a zero before the decimal point.
- Write the metric equivalents for length, volume, mass, and weight.
- Write the abbreviations for the metric equivalents of length, volume, mass, and weight.
- Name the metric equivalents that are most frequently used in the medical field.
- Use the proportional method to convert from one metric unit to another.
- Use moving the decimal method to convert from one metric unit to another.
- Answer the questions in the learning exercise correctly.
- Work the practice problems correctly.
- Complete the Self Assessment Test.

Vocabulary

SI units. The International System of Units, derived from the French name Le Système International d'Unités.

unit (u'nit). The smallest whole number; one.

equivalent (e-kwiv'a-lant). That which is equal in substance, degree, value, force, or meaning.

length (length). The state, quality, or fact of being long.

weight (wat). A measure of the heaviness or mass of an object.

volume (vol′um). The space occupied by a substance.

meter (me′ter). The fundamental unit of length in the metric system. It is derived from the Greek *metron*, which means to measure.

millimeter (mil′i-me″ter). One thousandth of a meter.

gram (gram). The metric unit of mass or weight.

microgram (mi′kro-gram). One thousandth of a milligram and one-millionth of a gram.

milligram (mil′i-gram). One thousandth of a gram.

kilogram (kil′o-gram). One thousand grams. A kilogram is equal to 2.2 pounds.

grain (gran). The smallest unit of weight used in the United States and Great Britain. It is equal to 0.0648 gram, which was originally the weight of a grain of wheat.

Introduction

The metric system was first proposed in France in 1670 by Gabriel Mouton, Vicar of Lyons. However, it was not officially adopted in France until the time of the French Revolution. During this time, a group of scientists met and established a universal system of measurement. This system, the metric system, offered a clear, concise mode for all physical measurement among the scientific, industrial, and educational communities. The metric system was adopted in France in April, 1795 by legislative action of the National Assembly.

In the United States, in the year 1866, Congress sanctioned the use of the metric system. However, it was not until 1975 that the United States made a real effort to convert to metrics. At that time, a U.S. Metric Board was established to help coordinate the shift of the United States to the metric system. Approximately 92 percent of the major countries of the world had already converted to the metric system, and the United States was being left behind in world trade, science and engineering. The SI units of measurement had become the official language of communication in the scientific and technical world. Therefore, the change to metrics had to occur in order for the United States to communicate and be competitive with the rest of the world.

The language of the metric system is a very simple, flexible, and accurate form of communication. It is based upon the decimal system; the number 10 or multiples of 10.

Metric System Guidelines

The following guidelines will help you as you learn basic facts about the metric system.

1. Arabic numbers are used to designate whole numbers: 1, 250, 500, 1000, and so forth.

2. Decimal fractions are used for quantities less than one: 0.1, 0.01, 0.001, 0.0001, and so forth.
3. To ensure accuracy, place a zero before the decimal point: 0.1, 0.001, 0.0001, and so forth.
4. The Arabic number precedes the metric unit of measurement: 10 grams, 2 milliliters, 5 liters, and so forth.
5. The abbreviation for gram should be capitalized (Gm) or written as (g) to distinguish it from grain (gr).
6. The abbreviation for liter is capitalized (L).
7. Prefixes are written in lowercase letters; milli, centi, deci, deka, and so forth.
8. Capitalize the measurement and symbol when it is named after a person: Celsius (C).
9. Periods are no longer used with most abbreviations or symbols.
10. Abbreviations for units are the same for singular and plural. An "s" is not added to indicate a plural.

The Language of the Metric System

In the metric system, 14 prefixes are used to denote the size of a metric unit. Each prefix is based upon a multiple or submultiple of 10. These prefixes are tera, giga, mega, kilo, hecto, deka, deci, centi, milli, micro, nano, pico, femto, and atto. You will not have to learn all 14 prefixes; however, you will need to know the seven common metric prefixes that are used in the medical field.

The Seven Common Metric Prefixes

Study the following list of prefixes. Once you know these prefixes, you will have a solid foundation for determining metric equivalents. When you combine a metric prefix with a root of physical quantity, you will know the multiples or submultiples of the metric system.

Example: milli (prefix) means one thousandth of a unit
meter (root) means to measure
millimeter is one thousandth of a meter
kilo (prefix) means one thousand units
liter (root) is a measure of volume
kiloliter is one thousand liters
micro (prefix) is one millionth of a unit
gram (root) is a measure of mass and/or weight
microgram is one millionth of a gram

Prefixes:	micro (mi′kro)	=	one millionth of a unit written as 0.000001
	milli (mil′i)	=	one thousandth of a unit written as 0.001
	centi (sen′ti)	=	one hundredth of a unit written as 0.01
	deci (des′i)	=	one tenth of a unit written as 0.1
	deka (dek′a)	=	ten units written as 10
	hecto (hek′to)	=	one hundred units written as 100
	kilo (kil′o)	=	one thousand units written as 1000

Fundamental Units

The following are the fundamental units of the metric system:

meter (m) – length
liter (L) – volume
gram (Gm, g) – mass and/or weight

The *meter* is the fundamental unit of length in the metric system and originally formed the foundation for the entire system. A meter is equal to 39.37 inches, which is slightly more than a yard or 3.28 feet.

Meter (m)	=	Length
1 millimeter (mm)	=	0.001 of a meter
1 centimeter (cm)	=	0.01 of a meter
1 decimeter (dm)	=	0.1 of a meter
1 *meter* (m)	=	1 *meter*
1 dekameter (dam)	=	10 meters
1 hectometer (hm)	=	100 meters
1 kilometer (km)	=	1000 meters

A millimeter is about the width of the head of a pin. It takes approximately $2\frac{1}{2}$ centimeters to make an inch; a decimeter is approximately 4 inches.

The *liter* is the metric unit of volume. A liter is equal to 1.056 quarts, which is 0.26 of a gallon or 2.1 pints.

Liter (L)	=	Volume
1 milliliter (ml)	=	0.001 of a liter
1 centiliter (cl)	=	0.01 of a liter
1 deciliter (dl)	=	0.1 of a liter
1 *liter* (L)	=	1 *liter*
1 dekaliter (dal)	=	10 liters
1 hectoliter (hl)	=	100 liters
1 kiloliter (kl)	=	1000 liters

A milliliter is equivalent to one cubic centimeter (cc), because the amount of space occupied by a milliliter is equal to one cubic centimeter. The weight of one milliliter of water equals approximately one gram. It takes approximately 15 milliliters to make one tablespoon. It takes 15 or 16 minims to make one milliliter.

The *gram* is the metric unit of mass and/or weight. It equals approximately the weight of one cubic centimeter or one milliliter of water. A gram is equal to approximately 15 grains or 0.035 of an ounce.

Gram (Gm, g)	=	Mass and/or Weight
1 microgram (mcg, µg)	=	0.000001 gram
1 milligram (mg)	=	0.001 of a gram
1 centigram (cg)	=	0.01 of a gram
1 decigram (dg)	=	0.1 of a gram
1 *gram* (Gm, g)	=	1 *gram*
1 dekagram (dag)	=	10 grams
1 hectogram (hg)	=	100 grams
1 kilogram (kg)	=	1000 grams

Metric Equivalents Most Frequently Used in the Medical Field

Length	Volume
$2\frac{1}{2}$ centimeters (cm) = 1 inch (in)	1000 milliliters (ml) or 1000 cubic centimeters (cc) = 1 liter (L)

Weight		
1000 micrograms (mcg)	=	1 milligram (mg)
1000 milligrams (mg)	=	1 gram (Gm, g)
1000 grams (Gm, g)	=	1 kilogram (kg)
1 kilogram	=	2.2 pounds (lb)

Learning Exercise

Mastering the metric system: place the correct answer in the space provided.

1. The fundamental units of the metric system are:

   a. __________ length b. __________ volume c. __________ weight

2. Write the name of the prefix for each of the following:

   a. __________ one thousand units e. __________ one thousandth of a unit
   b. __________ one tenth of a unit f. __________ ten units
   c. __________ one millionth of a unit g. __________ one hundredth of a unit
   d. __________ one hundred units

3. __________ __________ are used for quantities less than one.
4. To ensure accuracy, place a __________ before the decimal point.
5. A meter is equal to __________ inches.
6. Write in the correct equivalent for each of the following:

   a. 1 mm = __________ e. 1 dam = __________
   b. 1 cm = __________ f. 1 hm = __________
   c. 1 dm = __________ g. 1 km = __________
   d. 1 m = __________

7. It takes approximately __________ centimeters to make an inch.
8. A liter is equal to __________ quarts.
9. It takes __________ or __________ minims to make one milliliter.
10. A gram equals approximately the weight of __________ __________ __________ or __________ __________ of water.
11. Write in the correct equivalent for each of the following:

    a. 1 ml = __________ e. 1 dal = __________
    b. 1 cl = __________ f. 1 hl = __________
    c. 1 dl = __________ g. 1 kl = __________
    d. 1 L = __________

12. A gram is equal to approximately __________ grains or __________ of an ounce.
13. Write in the correct equivalent for each of the following:

    a. mcg, µg = __________ e. 1 Gm = __________
    b. 1 mg = __________ f. 1 dag = __________
    c. 1 cg = __________ g. 1 hg = __________
    d. 1 dg = __________ h. 1 kg = __________

14. Name the metric equivalents that are most frequently used in the medical field. Start with the smallest and go to the largest:

Volume

a. ________ b. ________

Weight

a. ________ c. ________

b. ________ d. ________

15. Write the correct abbreviation and unit of measurement for each of the following:
    a. one gram ________
    b. one fourth liter ________
    c. two hundred milligrams ________
    d. two tenths of a milliliter ________
    e. twelve kilograms ________
16. Write in the abbreviation for the unit that makes the equivalent correct:
    a. 1000 ml = 1 ________
    b. 2000 mg = 2 ________
    c. 1000 mcg, μg = 1 ________
    d. 2 kg = 4.4 ________
    e. 0.5 Gm, g = 500 ________

Conversion

The process of changing into another form, state, substance, or product is known as *conversion*. In the metric system, changing from one unit to another involves multiplying or dividing by 10, 100, 1000, and so forth. This can be done by the proportional method or by moving the decimal in the correct direction.

Proportional Method for Converting Metric Equivalents

There are six basic steps in the proportional method, plus an additional step to prove your answer. The following example will serve as a model for future applications of the proportional method of converting metric equivalents. Study this example and then proceed to the practice problems.

Converting 1500 milligrams to grams. 1500 mg = ________ Gm, g

Step 1. Since the unknown factor in the given formula is the number of grams contained in 1500 milligrams, you will substitute the symbol x for grams in the equation.

Step 2. Setting up the proportion requires that you know your metric equivalents. For example, in this problem you have to know that 1000 milligrams (mg) = 1 gram (Gm, g).

Step 3. Since you know that 1000 mg is equal to 1 Gm, you can create one-half of the equation. Write the equivalent that you know and place it on the *left* of the equal sign.

1000 mg : 1 Gm =

Step 4. Now that you have the *left* side of the equation, set up the right side by using the designated metric value 1500 mg : x Gm. Always write the smallest equivalent as to the largest equivalent: mg : Gm. By being consistent, you will be less likely to make errors.

1000 mg : 1 Gm = 1500 mg : x Gm

Step 5. Note that you have an equal equation: mg : Gm = mg : Gm. The *first* values on either side of the equal sign are *milligrams*, and the second values on either side are grams.

Step 6. Now solve for the unknown (x) by multiplication and division. Remember, multiply the means by the means and the extremes by the extremes.

Note: Once you have the proportion correctly set up, you may simply use the numbers as you multiply and divide.

$$1000:1 = 1500:x$$

$$1000x = 1500$$

$$x = 1500 \div 1000$$

$$x = 1.5$$

$$\begin{array}{r} 1.5 \\ 1000\overline{)1500.0} \\ \underline{1000} \\ 500\,0 \\ \underline{500\,0} \end{array}$$

Step 7. To make sure that you have a correct answer, *prove* your work: Place your answer 1.5 Gm into the formula where you once had x. Now multiply the means by the means and the extremes by the extremes.

1000 mg:1 Gm = 1500 mg : 1.5 Gm

1500 = 1500

◐ Practice Problems

1. Conversion: using the proportional method, convert each of the following metric equivalents.

a. 250 ml = __________ L

b. 0.5 L = __________ ml

c. 2 Gm = __________ mg

d. 500 mg = __________ Gm

e. 0.0300 Gm =	________	mg	h. 2 ml =	________	cc
f. 0.05 mg =	________	Gm	i. 1000 Gm =	________	kg
g. 1 mcg, μg =	________	mg	j. 2 kg =	________	lb

Moving the Decimal Method for Converting Metric Equivalents

Four basic steps are used to move the decimal in the correct direction. It is essential that you understand the following concepts. Study this example and then proceed to the practice problems.

Converting 2.5 grams to milligrams. 2.5 Gm = ________ mg

Step 1. Establish the placement of the decimal in the unit that is to be converted to another unit.

convert 2.5 Gm to mg

Step 2. Determine if you are converting a larger unit to a smaller unit or a smaller unit to a larger unit.

convert Gm (larger) unit to mg (smaller) unit

Step 3. When converting from a larger unit to a smaller unit, you multiply by 1000, which is the same as moving the decimal point three places to the *right.*

Larger unit	× multiply	to smaller unit
milligram		microgram
gram		milligram
liter		milliliter
kilogram		gram

Convert: 2.5 Gm to ________ mg

Multiply

$$\begin{array}{r} 2.5 \\ \times\ 1000 \\ \hline 2500.0 \end{array}$$

Moving the decimal point

2.500.

1,2,3 places to the right

Step 4. When converting a smaller unit to a larger unit, you divide by 1000, which is the same as moving the decimal point three places to the *left.*

Smaller unit	÷ divide	to larger unit
microgram		milligram
milligram		gram
milliliter		liter
gram		kilogram

Convert: 2500 mg to ________ Gm

Divide

$$\begin{array}{r} 2.5 \\ 1000\overline{)2500.0} \\ \underline{2000} \\ 500\ 0 \\ \underline{500\ 0} \end{array}$$

Moving the decimal point

2500. 2.500.

3,2,1 places to the left

◐ Practice Problems

2. Conversion: using the moving the decimal method, convert each of the following metric equivalents.

a. 60 mg = ________ Gm		f. 3.5 cc = ________ L	
b. 0.005 L = ________ ml		g. 4 kg = ________ Gm	
c. 200 ml = ________ L		h. 1 ml = ________ L	
d. 1 Gm = ________ kg		i. 0.1 L = ________ ml	
e. 0.0065 Gm = ________ mg		j. 0.05 mg = ________ Gm	

Calculating Dosage According to Kilogram of Body Weight

It may be your responsibility to calculate the amount of dosage ordered by the physician according to the patient's body weight. Today, many medications are ordered in this manner; therefore, it is essential that you learn how to calculate dosage according to this method. The following example will guide you step by step through the mathematical process of calculating dosage according to kilogram of body weight.

Remember there are 2.2 pounds in one kilogram.

Example: The physician ordered an antiepileptic agent, Depakene (valproic acid) 15 mg/kg/day capsules for Clark McGee, who weights 110 pounds. The medication is to be given in three divided doses.

Step 1. To express pounds in kilograms, divide the weight in pounds by 2.2.

Convert patient's weight to kilograms:

110 ÷ 2.2 = 50 kilograms

Step 2. Now, calculate the prescribed dosage by placing 50 in the appropriate place:

15 mg/50/day

15 × 50 = 750 mg/day

Step 3. To determine the amount of each dose, divide 750 by 3 (divided doses).

750 ÷ 3 = 250 mg per dose

> Depakene is available in 250 mg capsules and 250 mg/5 ml syrup. The physician ordered the medication in capsules, so Clark will receive a 250 mg capsule every 8 hours.

Using the Proportional Method to Calculate Kilogram of Body Weight

Example: The physician ordered an antiepileptic agent, Depakene (valproic acid) 15 mg/kg/day capsules for Clark McGee, who weights 110 pounds. The medication is to be given in three divided doses.

Step 1. To convert 110 pounds to kilograms, set up the proportion as follows:

2.2 lb : 1 kg = 110 lb : x kg

Step 2. Now, solve for x:

$$2.2 : 1 = 110 : x$$
$$2.2x = 110$$
$$x = 50$$

Step 3. Now, calculate the prescribed dosage by placing 50 in the appropriate place:

15 mg/50 kg/day

$15 \times 50 = 750$ mg/day

Step 4. To determine the amount of each dose, divide 750 by 3 (divided doses).

$750 \div 3 = 250$ mg per dose

> Depakene is available in 250 mg capsules and 250 mg/5 ml syrup. The physician ordered the medication in capsules, so Clark will receive a 250 mg capsule every 8 hours.

◐ Practice Problems

3. a. 184 lb = __________ kilograms c. 85 lb = __________ kilograms
   b. 210 lb = __________ kilograms d. 54 lb = __________ kilograms

- To express kilograms as pounds, multiply the kilogram weight by 2.2

Example: 25 kilograms × 2.2 = 55 lb

4. a. 30 kilograms = __________ lb c. 65 kilograms = __________ lb
   b. 45 kilograms = __________ lb d. 75 kilograms = __________ lb

5. The physician ordered Moxam (moxalactam disodium) 50 mg/kg every 6–8 hours, IM for a pediatric patient who weighs 88 pounds. Convert pounds to kilograms and then calculate the prescribed dosage.

Self Assessment Test

This test is designed to assess your understanding of the metric system. Please place the correct answer in the space provided. After you have completed the test you may check your answers with those in back of the text.

1. The fundamental units of the metric system are:

   a. __________ length b. __________ volume c. __________ weight

2. Write the prefix for each of the following:

   a. __________ one thousand units
   b. __________ one tenth of a unit
   c. __________ one millionth of a unit
   d. __________ one hundred units
   e. __________ one thousandth of a unit
   f. __________ ten units
   g. __________ one hundredth of a unit

3. It takes approximately __________ centimeters to make an inch.
4. A liter is equal to __________ quarts.
5. It takes __________ or __________ minims to make one milliliter.
6. Write in the abbreviation for the unit that makes the equivalent correct.

   a. 1000 ml = 1 __________
   b. 2000 mg = 2 __________
   c. 1000 mcg = 1 __________
   d. 2 kg = 4.4 __________
   e. 0.5 Gm = 500 __________

7. Correctly convert each of the following metric equivalents:

   a. 1 mcg = __________ mg
   b. 4 Gm = __________ kg
   c. 5 kg = __________ Gm
   d. 0.2 L = __________ ml
   e. 1 ml = __________ L
   f. 3.5 mg = __________ Gm

8. Correctly convert the following pounds to kilograms:

   a. 176 lb = __________ kg
   b. 100 lb = __________ kg
   c. 64 lb = __________ kg

CHAPTER 7

Household Measures and Apothecaries' Measurements

OBJECTIVES

Upon completion of this chapter, you should be able to:

- Define the terms listed in the vocabulary.
- Explain why you should have a working knowledge of household measures, and apothecaries' measurements.
- List five factors that may vary or alter the size of a drop.
- Write the abbreviations of the household measures and the apothecaries' measurements.
- State the household approximate equivalents and the apothecaries' measurements that are given in this unit.
- Use the proportional method to convert household and apothecaries' measurements.
- Answer the questions in the learning exercise correctly.
- Work the practice problems correctly.
- Complete the Self Assessment Test.

Vocabulary

Apothecaries' measurements (a-poth′e-ka-res mezh′ er-ments). A system of weights and measures based on 480 grains equal to 1 ounce, and 12 ounces equal to 1 pound.

household (hous′hold). A domestic dwelling including family and others living under the same roof.

measurement (mezh′er-ment). The act or process of being measured.

solution (sa-loo′shun). A homogeneous mixture; a medicine in a liquid form.

homogeneous (ho″ma-ja′ni-as). Same, similar, or identical in structure, quality or form.

dropper (drop′er). A small tube with a suction bulb at one end and a narrow opening at the other end used for dispensing a liquid by drops.

dispense (dis-pens). To give out; to prepare and give a medication to a patient.

viscosity (vis-kos′a-ti). The state of being thick and sticky.

bore (bor). To make a hole with a drill. The interior diameter of a tube; a hole.

minim (min′am). A small amount of liquid measure. It takes 15 to 16 minims to make one milliliter or one cubic centimeter. A minim is equal to $\frac{1}{60}$ fluidram or 0.00376 cubic inch.

dram (dram). A unit of weight in the apothecaries' system.

Household Measures

Household measures are more frequently used in the home than in the medical field. However, it may be your responsibility to instruct patients about preparing solutions for gargles, enemas, or douches, and your understanding of household equivalents will assist you in this matter.

Household measures are approximate measurements. Most household measuring devices lack standardization, and they are not accurate for measuring medications. For example, there are 3 or 4 teaspoons per tablespoon, depending upon the reference source and the size of each utensil. A teaspoon may vary in size from 4 to 5 milliliters or more. The American Standards Institute (ASI) has set the standards for an American teaspoon at 5 milliliters. In this text, the American standard is used.

When the physician orders a medication to be dispensed by drops, be sure to use the dropper that comes with the medicine. The size of a drop depends upon the following factors:

- The dropper size depends upon the diameter of the *bore;* therefore, the size of the drop may vary due to the smallness or largeness of the hole.
- The angle at which the dropper is held may vary the size of the drop. For example, when you hold the dropper at a 90° angle, you will have a more uniform drop than if you hold the dropper at a 60° angle.
- The pressure used to squeeze the dropper may alter the number and size of the drop.
- The type or viscosity of the liquid being dispensed may alter the size of the drop.
- The temperature of the liquid being dispensed may alter the size of the drop.

Household Abbreviations and Equivalents

The following household abbreviations and equivalents should be learned before you proceed to the learning exercise.

drop (drops)	gtt	pint	pt
teaspoon	t or tsp	quart	qt
tablespoon	T or tbsp	gallon	gal
teacup	tcp	ounce	oz
cup	C		

60 gtt	=	1 t or tsp		
3 t or tsp	=	1 T		
180 gtt	=	1 T	=	$\frac{1}{2}$ oz
2 T	=	1 oz	=	6 t or tsp
360 gtt	=	2 T		
1 oz	=	30 cc or 30 ml		
6 oz	=	1 tcp		
8 oz	=	1 C or 1 glass		
2 C	=	1 pt	=	1 6 oz
2 pt	=	1 qt	=	32 oz
4 C	=	1 qt	=	32 oz
4 qt	=	1 gal	=	128 oz

Table 7–1 Common Household Measures

Drop (gtt) = approximate liquid measure depending on kind of liquid measured and the size of the opening from which it is dropped.	
60 drops	1 teaspoon (t or tsp)
1 dash	Less than $\frac{1}{8}$ teaspoon
3 teaspoons	1 tablespoon (T or tbsp)
2 tablespoons	1 ounce (oz)
4 ounces	1 juice glass
6 ounces	1 tea cup
8 ounces	1 glass or cup
16 tablespoons or 8 ounces	1 measuring cup (c)
2 cups	1 pint (pt)
2 pints	1 quart (qt)
4 quarts	1 gallon (gal)

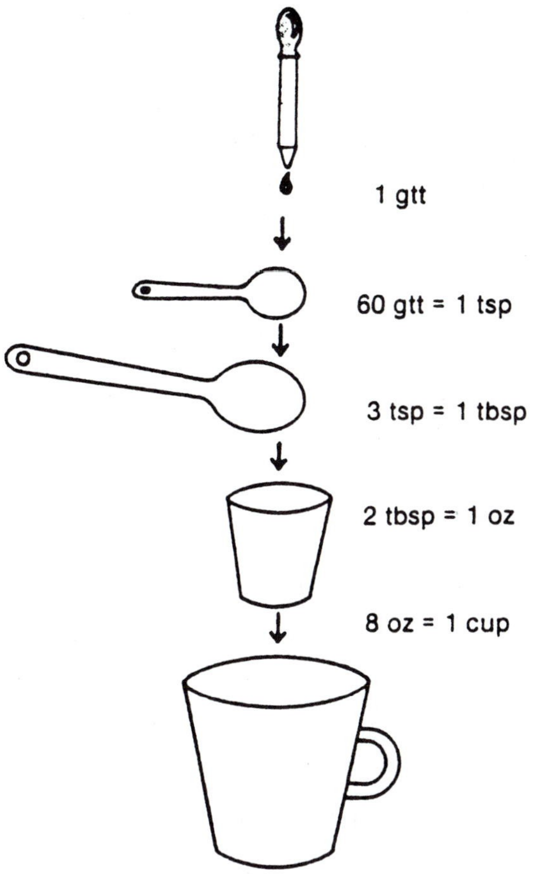

Figure 7–1

Comparing Household Units

Figure 7–1 illustrates the progression of the various units of volume in the household system of measurement.

Learning Exercise

Mastering household measures: place the correct answer in the space provided.

1. Write the correct abbreviation for each of the following:

a. ________ drops	d. ________ ounce	g. ________ pint
b. ________ teaspoon	e. ________ teacup	h. ________ quart
c. ________ tablespoon	f. ________ cup	i. ________ gallon

2. Indicate the smallest to the largest household measurement by placing a number from one to nine in the appropriate space. One will be placed in the space by the

smallest measurement, two will be placed by the measurement that is larger than one, and so on.

a. tablespoon ________	d. ounce ________	g. teacup ________
b. cup ________	e. quart ________	h. pint ________
c. drop ________	f. teaspoon ________	i. gallon ________

3. Write in the correct abbreviation for each of the following:

a. 180 ________ = 3 tsp	f. 16 ________ = 2 C
b. 1 ________ = $\frac{1}{60}$ tsp	g. 4 ________ = 2 pt
c. 2 ________ = 1 oz	h. 2 ________ = $\frac{1}{2}$ gal
d. 1 ________ = 6 tsp	i. 32 ________ = 1 qt
e. 6 ________ = 1 tcp	j. 1 ________ = 16 oz

Conversion

In the household system of measurements, changing (converting) from one measurement to another can be done by the proportional method.

Proportional Method

Converting 2 tablespoons to teaspoons. 2 T = ________ tsp

Step 1. Setting up the proportion requires that you know your household measurements. For example, in this problem you have to know that 3 teaspoons equal 1 tablespoon.

Step 2. Since you know that 3 tsp = 1 T, you can create one-half of the equation. Write the equivalent that you know and place it on the *left* of the equal sign.

3 tsp : 1 T =

Step 3. Now that you have the left side of the equation, set up the *right* side by using the designated household measures: x tsp : 2 T. Always write the smallest equivalent as to the largest equivalent: tsp : T. By being consistent, you will be less likely to make errors.

3 tsp : 1 T = x tsp : 2 T

Step 4. Note that you have an equal equation tsp : T = tsp : T. The *first* values on both sides of the equal sign are teaspoons, and the *second* values on both sides are tablespoons.

Step 5. Now solve for the unknown (x) by multiplication and division.

Remember, multiply the means by the means and the extremes by the extremes. Divide the number on the left of the equal sign into the number on the right.

$$3 \text{ tsp} : 1 \text{ T} = \text{x tsp} : 2 \text{ T}$$
$$1x = 6 \text{ tsp}$$
$$x = 6$$

Step 6. To make sure that you have a correct answer, prove your work: Place your answer, 6 tsp, into the formula where you once had x. Now multiply the means by the means and the extremes by the extremes.

$$3 \text{ tsp} : 1 \text{ T} = 6 \text{ tsp} : 2 \text{ T}$$
$$6 = 6$$

Two-Step Conversion

Converting 3 tablespoons to drops. 3 T = __________ gtt

Step 1. Setting up the proportion requires that you know your household measurements. For example, in this problem you need to know that 60 drops equal 1 teaspoon, and 3 teaspoons equal 1 tablespoon.

Step 2. In the two-step conversion, you will first find out how many drops are in 3 teaspoons. Since you know that 60 gtt = 1 tsp, set up the proportion as follows:

$$60 \text{ gtt} : 1 \text{ tsp} = x \text{ gtt} : 3 \text{ tsp}$$
$$1x = 180 \text{ gtt}$$
$$x = 180 \text{ gtt}$$
$$x = 180 \text{ gtt}$$

Step 3. Since 3 teaspoons are equal to 1 tablespoon, 180 gtt are equal to 1 T. Now use this measurement to set up the second proportion.

$$180 \text{ gtt} : 1 \text{ T} = x \text{ gtt} : 3 \text{ T}$$
$$1x = 540 \text{ gtt}$$
$$x = 540 \text{ gtt}$$

You have determined that there are 540 gtt in 3 T.

Step 4. Prove your answer:

$$180 \text{ gtt} : 1 \text{ T} = 540 \text{ gtt} : 3 \text{ T}$$
$$540 = 540$$

In Review

Remember the following guidelines as you set up any proportion:

- Write the measurement that you know and place it on the *left* of the equal sign.
- Always write the smallest measurement as to the largest measurement.
- Write the unknown factor (x) and place it on the *right* of the equal sign.
- Always check to see that you have an equal equation and that each part is correctly identified.
- Set up the proportion and solve for x.
- Always *prove* your answer.

◐ Practice Problems

1. Conversion: using the proportional method, convert each of the following household equivalents.

a. $2\frac{1}{2}$ tsp = ________ gtt

b. 10 oz = ________ pt

c. 12 T = ________ oz

d. $2\frac{1}{2}$ T = ________ tsp

e. 20 oz = ________ qt

f. 320 T = ________ oz

g. 1 oz = ________ gtt

h. $1\frac{1}{2}$ pt = ________ C

i. 4 tcp = ________ qt

j. $2\frac{1}{2}$ qt = ________ oz

Apothecaries' Measurements

Apothecaries' measurements are rarely used today, but they must be included in a textbook as a reference for anyone who has a need to understand this system of measurement. You will note that some of the apothecaries' measurements are also used as household measures. However, in the apothecaries' system, 12 ounces is equal to one pound, whereas in the household system 16 ounces is equal to one pound.

Units of Weight and Liquid Volume

The following are the units of weight and liquid measurements of the apothecaries' system.

Apothecaries' Units of Weight		
60 grains (gr)	=	1 dram (dr)
8 drams (dr)	=	1 ounce (oz)
12 ounces (oz)	=	1 pound (lb)

Apothecaries' Units of Liquid Volume	
60 minims (♏)	= 1 fluidram (fldr)
8 fluidrams (fldr)	= 1 fluidounce (floz)
16 fluidounces (floz)	= 1 pint (pt)
2 pints (pt)	= 1 quart (qt)
4 quarts (qt)	= 1 gallon (gal)

Conversion

Proportional Method for Converting Apothecaries' Equivalents

Converting 4 ounces to drams. 4 oz = __________ dr

Step 1. Setting up the proportion requires that you know the apothecaries' measurements. For example, in this problem you need to know that 8 drams is equal to 1 ounce.

Step 2. Since you know that 8 dr = 1 oz, you can create one-half of the equation. Write the equivalent that you know and place it on the *left* of the equal sign.

8 dr : 1 oz =

Step 3. Now that you have the left side of the equation, set up the *right* side by using the designated apothecaries' measures: x dr:4 oz. Always write the smallest equivalent as to the largest equivalent.

8 dr : 1 oz = x dr : 4 oz

Step 4. Note that you have an equal equation: dr:oz = dr:oz.

Step 5. Now solve for the unknown (x) by multiplication and division. Remember, multiply the means by the means and the extremes by the extremes. Divide the number on the left of the equal sign into the number on the right.

8 dr : 1 oz = x dr : 4 oz

$1x = 32$ oz

$x = 32$ oz

Step 6. Prove your answer.

8 dr : 1 oz = 32 dr : 4 oz

32 = 32

Practice Problems

2. Conversion: using the proportional method, convert each of the following apothecaries' equivalents.

a. 8 drams = __________ grains

b. $\frac{3}{4}$ dram = __________ grains

c. 3 ounces = __________ drams

d. 45 minims = __________ fluidrams

e. 3 pints = __________ quarts

f. 1 grain = __________ dram

g. 4 drams = __________ ounce(s)

h. $\frac{1}{2}$ pound = __________ ounces

i. $\frac{3}{4}$ pint = __________ quart

j. $\frac{1}{2}$ pint = __________ quart

Table 7–2 Approximate Equivalents among Metric, Apothecaries', and Household Systems

Metric		Apothecaries		Household
		Dry		
60 mg*	=	1 gr		
1 Gm	=	15 gr		
15 Gm	=	4 dr	=	1 tbsp (3 tsp)
30 Gm	=	1 oz (8 dr)	=	1 oz (2 tbsp)
		16 oz	=	1 lb (avoirdupois)
1 kg			=	2.2 lb
		Liquid		
		1 ♏	=	1 gtt
1 ml	=	15 ♏*	=	15 gtt
4 ml	=	1 dr		
5 ml*	=	75 ♏	=	1 tsp
15 ml	=	4 dr	=	1 tbsp (3 tsp)
30 ml	=	1 oz (8 dr)	=	1 fl oz (2 tbsp)
500 ml**	=	16 oz (1 pt)	=	16 oz (1 pt or 2 ocups)
1000 ml**	=	32 oz (1 qt)	=	32 oz (1 qt)
		Length		
2.5 cm			=	1 in
1 M			=	39.4 in

**Approximate equivalents sometimes fall within a range, eg., 60–65 mg = 1 gr, 4–5 ml = dr 1, 15–16 ♏ = 1 ml. For purposes of calculations in this text, the numbers in Table 7-2 will be used.*

***In common practice, these numbers are rounded up from 480 ml and 960 ml.*

Self Assessment Test

This test is designed to assess your understanding of household and apothecaries' measures. Please place the correct answer in the space provided. After you have completed the test you may check your answers with those in the back of the text.

1. Write the correct abbreviation for each of the following:

   a. __________ gallon d. __________ cup g. __________ tablespoon
   b. __________ quart e. __________ teacup h. __________ teaspoon
   c. __________ pint f. __________ ounce i. __________ drops

2. Write in the correct abbreviation for each of the following:

   a. 120 __________ = 2 tsp d. 1 __________ = 8 oz g. 6 __________ = 1 tcp
   b. 1 __________ = $\frac{1}{60}$ tsp e. 4 __________ = 2 oz h. 2 __________ = 1 pt
   c. 1 __________ = 8 tsp f. 1 __________ = 4 tsp i. 5 __________ = 10 C

3. Correctly convert each of the following household equivalents:

   a. $2\frac{1}{2}$ T = __________ tsp d. 540 gtt = __________ tsp
   b. 3 oz = __________ tsp e. 24 oz = __________ qt
   c. 60 tsp = __________ T

4. Write in the correct abbreviation for each of the following:

   a. 60 __________ = 1 dram c. 12 __________ = 1 pound
   b. 8 __________ = 1 ounce

5. Correctly convert each of the following apothecaries' equivalents:

   a. 4 drams = __________ ounce d. 3 ounces = __________ drams
   b. $\frac{3}{4}$ dram = __________ grains e. 45 minims = __________ fluidrams
   c. 1 grain = __________ dram f. $\frac{1}{2}$ pt = __________ quart

CHAPTER 8

Calculating Adult Dosages: Oral Forms

OBJECTIVES

Upon completion of this chapter, you should be able to:

- Define the terms listed in the vocabulary.
- Describe the oral route of drug administration.
- Name two measures used to determine the amount of medication to be administered and give an example of each measure.
- Define unit dose.
- Calculate oral dosages using the proportional method.
- Calculate oral dosages using a formula method.
- Work the practice problems correctly.
- Complete the Self Assessment Test.

Vocabulary

oral (or'al). Pertaining to the mouth.

unit dose. A premeasured amount of medication that is individually packaged on a per-dose basis.

multiple dose. More than one dose per container.

Introduction

The *oral route* of drug administration (by mouth, po) is the route most commonly used. It provides the safest, most convenient, and economical means of giving a medication. Drugs administered by mouth may be in a solid or a liquid form. Solid forms include tablets, capsules, caplets, powders, and lozenges. Liquid preparations include solutions, elixirs, and syrups.

Two measures are used to determine the amount of medication to be administered; these are by weight and by volume. The weight of a medication may be expressed as any of the following: milliequivalents (mEq), micrograms (mcg, μg), milligrams (mg), grams (Gm), grains (gr), and units (U). The volume of a medication may be expressed in milliliters (ml), cubic centimeters (cc), minims (♏), drams (dr), ounces (oz), and by a variety of household measures, such as the teaspoon (tsp).

The amount of medication in the *average dose* for an adult or a child is based upon the age and weight of an *average patient* in each category. The average patient is between 10 and 60 years of age, and weighs 150 pounds. In children, the dosage is determined by using any of several formulas described in Chapter 10 which compensate for the smaller size and weight of a pediatric patient according to age and body surface area.

Medications prepared for oral administration may be dispensed in multiple dose form (solid and liquid), or in unit dose form (solid and liquid). The physician orders the medication using one of the various types of medication orders described in Chapter 13. On the order, the physician designates the name of the drug, the dosage, the frequency and route of administration, and the purpose for which it is prescribed. It then becomes the nurse's responsibility to follow the physician's order and administer the medication correctly.

Today, most oral medications are prepared and dispensed in unit dose form. A unit dose is a premeasured amount of medication that is individually packaged on a per-dose basis. Occasionally, you may have to measure the dosage from a multiple dose supply. This usually occurs when the medication strength ordered is not available in unit dose. To measure medications from a multiple dose supply, you must be familiar with the systems of measure and the formulas used for calculating dosages.

Many different methods can be used when calculating the dosage to be administered. Two of the most useful methods, the proportional method and the formula method, are described in this chapter. Study each method and practice computing dosages. This will prepare you in the event that you are required to calculate a dosage of medication.

Conversion

Calculating Oral Dosages Using the Proportional Method

Example: The physician orders 0.2 Gm of Equanil tabs. The dose on hand is 400 mg tabs.

Step 1. Determine whether the medication ordered and the medication on hand are available in the same unit of measure.

Step 2. If the medication ordered and the medication on hand *are not* in the same unit of measure, *convert* so that both measures are expressed using the same unit of measure. (If you need to review this process, refer to Chapter 6.)

CONVERSION: To change 0.2 Gm to mg

$$1000 \text{ mg} : 1 \text{ Gm} = x \text{ mg} : 0.2 \text{ Gm}$$

$$x = 200 \text{ mg}$$

or

multiply $0.2 \times 1000 = 200$

Step 3. Now use the following proportion to calculate the dosage. Remember, you converted 0.2 Gm to 200 mg.

$$\frac{\text{Known unit on hand}}{400\text{ mg}} : \frac{\text{Known dosage form}}{1\text{ tab}} = \frac{\text{Dose Ordered}}{200\text{ mg}} : \frac{\text{Unknown amount to be given}}{x\text{ tab}}$$

$$400x = 200$$

$$x = \frac{\overset{1}{\cancel{200}}}{\underset{2}{\cancel{400}}} \quad \text{(Reduce fraction to lowest terms)}$$

$$x = \frac{1}{2}\text{ tab}$$

Step 4. Prove your answer. Remember to place your answer in the original formula in the x position.

$$400\text{ mg} : 1\text{ tab} = 200\text{ mg} : \tfrac{1}{2}\text{ tab}$$

$$200 = 200$$

> Scored tablets are those whose surfaces have been bisected by a groove, making it easier for the user to break the tablet into halves or quarters, thereby varying the dosage. See Figure 12–3A on page 135.

◐ Practice Problems

1. Using the proportional method, calculate the following dosages:
   a. The physician ordered Sorbitrate chewable tabs, 2.5 mg. Available are Sorbitrate chewable tabs, 5 mg. How many tablets will you give?

   b. The physician ordered Seconal Sodium CII caps, 200 mg. Available are Seconal Sodium CII caps, 100 mg ($1\frac{1}{2}$ gr). How many caps will you give?

c. The physician ordered Penicillin V Potassium tabs, 500 mg. On hand are Penicillin V Potassium tabs, 250 mg (400,000 U). How many tablets will you give?

d. The physician ordered Ampicillin liquid oral preparation, 250 mg. Available is Ampicillin liquid, 125 mg per 5 ml. How many milliliters will you give to the patient?

e. The physician ordered 0.5 Gm of Penicillin V Potassium tabs. Available are Penicillin V Potassium tabs, 250 mg (400,000 U). How many tablets will you give?

f. The physician ordered 0.250 mg of Lanoxin (digoxin) tabs. On hand are Lanoxin 0.125 mg tabs. How many tablets will you give?

g. The physician ordered 20 mg of Lasix (furosemide) tabs. On hand are Lasix 40 mg tabs. What is the correct dose?

h. The physician ordered 150 mg of Tagamet liquid. On hand is 300 mg/5 ml. How many milliliters will you give?

i. The physician ordered 500 mg of Ultracef. On hand are 1 gram tablets. The patient will receive __________ tabs.

j. The physician ordered 1 gram of chloral hydrate. On hand are 500 mg capsules. How many capsules will you give?

Calculating Oral Dosages Using the Formula Method

Example: The physician orders 0.2 Gm of Equanil tabs. The dose on hand is 400 mg tabs.

Step 1. Determine whether the medication ordered and the medication on hand are available in the same unit of measure.

Step 2. If the medication ordered and the medication on hand *are not* in the same unit of measure, *convert* so that both measures are expressed using the same unit of measure.

CONVERSION: To change 0.2 Gm to mg

$$1000 \text{ mg} : 1 \text{ Gm} = x \text{ mg} : 0.2 \text{ Gm}$$
$$x = 200 \text{ mg}$$

or

multiply $0.2 \times 1000 = 200$

Step 3. Now use the following formula to calculate the dosage.

$$\frac{\text{Dose ordered (desired)}}{\text{Dose on hand}} \times \text{Quantity (Q)} = \text{Amount to give (form of drug)}$$

or $\frac{\text{D}}{\text{H}} \times \text{Q} = \text{Amount to give}$

The physician ordered 0.2 Gm of Equanil tabs (0.2 Gm converts to 200 mg). The dose on hand is 400 mg tabs.

$$\frac{200 \text{ mg}}{400 \text{ mg}} \times 1 \text{ tab} = \frac{\overset{1}{\cancel{200}}}{\underset{2}{\cancel{400}}} \text{ or } \frac{1}{2} \text{ tab}$$

◐ Practice Problems

2. Using the formula method, calculate the following dosages:
   a. The physician ordered Mycostatin oral tabs, 1,000,000 units. Available are Mycostatin oral tabs, 500,000 units. How many tablets will you give?

   b. The physician ordered Pentids tabs, 200 mg. The dose on hand is Pentids tabs, 400 mg. How many tablets will you give?

   c. The physician ordered 3.75 mg of Coumadin tabs. Available are Coumadin, 7.5 mg tabs. How many tablets will you give?

   d. The physician ordered 600 mg of Equanil tabs. The dose on hand is Equanil, 400 mg tabs. How many tablets will you give?

   e. The physician ordered 62.5 mg of Diamox tabs. On hand are Diamox, 125 mg tabs. How many tablets will you give?

   f. The physician ordered 200 mg of Thorazine, bid, po. On hand are 100 mg tablets. How many tablets will you give?

   g. The physician ordered Amoxil 250 mg chewable tabs every 8 hours. On hand are 125 mg tabs. How many tablets will you give?

h. The physician ordered 0.25 mg of Lanoxin. On hand are Lanoxin tabs 0.125 mg. How many tablets will you give?

i. The physician ordered 1000 mg of Carafate. On hand are Carafate tabs 1 gram. How many tablets will you give?

j. The physician ordered 10 mg of Hydrocortisone. On hand are 20 mg tablets. How many tablets will you give?

Self Assessment Test

This test is designed to assess your understanding of calculating adult dosages. Please correctly calculate the following adult oral dosages. After you have completed the test you may check your answers with those in the back of the text.

1. The physician ordered Lanoxin tabs, 0.125 mg. Available are Lanoxin tabs, 0.25 mg. How many tablets will you give?

2. The physician ordered Coumadin tabs, 2.5 mg. Available are Coumadin tabs, 5 mg. How many tablets will you give?

3. The physician ordered Acetaminophen tabs, 650 mg. Available are Acetaminophen tabs, 325 mg. How many tablets will you give?

4. The physician ordered Carafate tabs, 500 mg. Available are Carafate 1 gram tabs. How many tablets will you give?

5. The physician ordered Duricef tabs, 1500 mg. Available are Duricef tabs, 1 gram. How many tablets will you give?

6. The physician ordered Diuril tabs, 250 mg. Available are Diuril tabs, 0.25 Gm. How many tablets will you give?

7. The physician ordered amoxicillin caps, 500 mg. Available are amoxicillin caps, 250 mg. How many capsules will you give?

8. The physician ordered Lasix oral solution, 30 mg to be given as a single dose. Available is Lasix oral solution, 60 ml bottle that contains 10 mg/ml. How many milliliters will you give?

CHAPTER 9

Calculating Adult Dosages: Parenteral Forms

OBJECTIVES

Upon completion of this chapter, you should be able to:

- Define the terms listed in the vocabulary.
- List the most frequently used parenteral routes.
- State an advantage to using the parenteral route of drug administration.
- Calculate parenteral dosages using the proportional method.
- Calculate parenteral dosages using the formula method.
- List six medications that are measured in units.
- Define insulin.
- List four categories of diabetes mellitus.
- Explain why the exact dosage of insulin is so important.
- List the precautions to be kept in mind when administering insulin.
- Recognize rapid-acting, intermediate-acting, and slow-acting insulins.
- Calculate unit dosages by the proportional or formula method.
- Calculate an IV drip rate.
- Work the practice problems correctly.
- Complete the Self Assessment Test.

Vocabulary

parenteral (pah-ren-teh′ral). Pertaining to the injection of a liquid substance into the body via a route other than the alimentary canal.

vial (vi′al). A small, sterile, prefilled glass bottle containing a hypodermic solution.

ampule (am′pul). A small, sterile, prefilled glass container that holds a hypodermic solution.

cartridge-needle unit. A disposable unit containing a premeasured amount of medication. This unit is designed for use in a nondisposable cartridge-holder syringe, such as the Tubex® and Carpuject®.

Introduction

The term *parenteral* is used to describe the injection of a liquid substance into the body via a route other than the alimentary canal. The most frequently used parenteral routes are:

Subcutaneous—Just below the surface of the skin. A subcutaneous injection is usually given at a 45° angle.

Intramuscular—Within the muscle. An intramuscular injection is given at a 90° angle, passing through the skin and subcutaneous tissue, and penetrating deep into muscle tissue.

Intradermal—Within the epidermal layer of the skin. An intradermal injection is given at an angle between 10° and 15°.

Intravenous—Within a vein. An intravenous injection is one where the needle is inserted (at less than a 15° angle) into the patient's vein.

Medications that have been prepared for use by injection are available in multiple dose form (vials), and in unit dose form (ampules and cartridge-needle units). Injectable medications are also packaged for use with intravenous solution systems.

Vial: A small, sterile, prefilled glass bottle containing a hypodermic solution. See Figure 9–1.

Ampule: A small, sterile, prefilled container that usually holds a single dose of a hypodermic solution. See Figure 9–2.

Cartridge-needle unit: A disposable unit containing a premeasured amount of medication. This unit is designed for use in a nondisposable cartridge-holder syringe such as the Tubex® or Carpuject®.

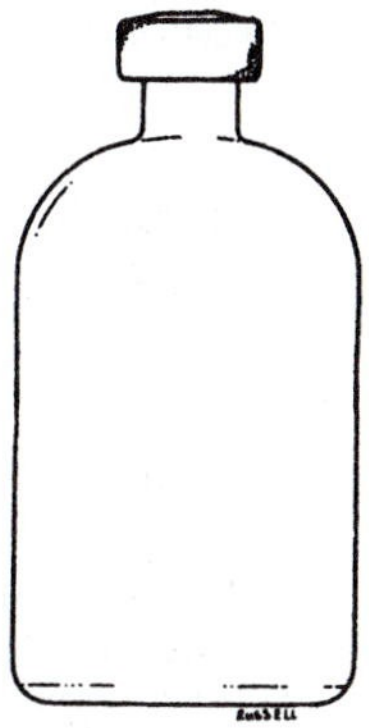

Figure 9–1 A vial
(Courtesy of James Russell, Jr.)

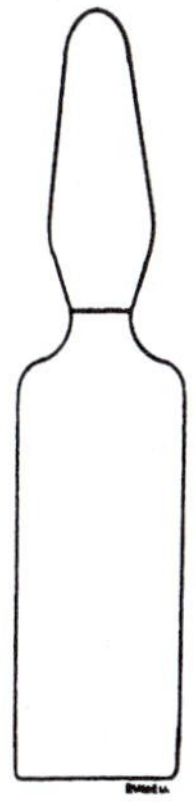

Figure 9–2 An ampule
(Courtesy of James Russell, Jr.)

Intravenous solutions: These medications are intended for intravenous use only and may be supplied in vials, ampules, and ready injectables (premeasured medicine packaged as a syringe-needle intravenous unit).

Because parenteral medications are intended for use by injection, they must be supplied as liquids. As such, the amount of medication is expressed in terms of volume (cubic centimeters, milliliters, or minims). The strength of the drug contained in the liquid is usually expressed in terms of its weight (milliequivalents, micrograms, milligrams, grams, grains, or units). Therefore, medications ordered for parenteral use are often ordered by both weight and volume. For example:

Atropine Sulfate Injection
0.4 mg ($\frac{1}{150}$ gr) per ml
(weight) (volume)

The parenteral route of drug administration offers an effective mode of delivering medication to a patient when a rapid and direct result is desired. Since the effect of a parenteral medication is faster than by the oral route, the accuracy of dosage calculation is very important.

Calculating Parenteral Dosages

Using the Proportional Method

Example: The physician orders Librium 50 mg IM. The dose on hand is Librium 100 mg per 2 ml.

Step 1. Determine if the medication ordered and the medication on hand are available in the same unit of measure.

Step 2. If the medication ordered and the medication on hand *are not* in the same unit of measure, *convert* so that both measures are expressed using the same unit of measure.

Step 3. Use the following proportion to calculate the dosage:

Known unit on hand	:	Known dosage form (volume)	=	Dose ordered	:	Unknown amount to give (volume)
100 mg	:	2 ml	=	50 mg	:	x ml

$$100x = 100$$
$$x = 1 \text{ ml}$$

Step 4. Prove your answer. Remember that you place your answer in the position occupied by x in the original formula.

$$100 \text{ mg} : 2 \text{ ml} = 50 \text{ mg} : 1 \text{ ml}$$
$$100 = 100$$

Practice Problems

1. Using the proportional method, calculate the following dosages:
   a. The physician ordered Demerol, 75 mg IM. On hand is Demerol 100 mg per 2 ml. How much Demerol will you administer?

   b. The physician ordered cyanocobalamin (vitamin B_{12}), 200 mcg IM or SQ. Available is cyanocobalamin, 1000 mcg per ml. What is the correct dosage to give to your patient?

   c. The physician ordered Seconal Sodium CII 75 mg IM. On hand is Seconal Sodium CII 50 mg ($\frac{3}{4}$ gr) per ml. What will you administer to your patient?

   d. The physician ordered Bicillin 600,000 units for deep IM injection. On hand is Bicillin 1,200,000 units per 2 ml. What is the correct dosage?

   e. The physician ordered Streptomycin 250 mg IM. Available is Streptomycin 0.5 Gm per 2 ml. How many ml will you give?

Using the Formula Method

Example: The physician ordered Librium 50 mg IM. The dose on hand is Librium 100 mg per 2 ml.

Step 1. Determine if the medication ordered and the medication on hand are available in the same unit of measure.

Step 2. If the medication ordered and the medication on hand *are not* in the same unit of measure, *convert* so that both measures are expressed using the same unit of measure.

Step 3. Now, use the following formula to calculate the dosage:

$$\frac{\text{Dose ordered (desired)}}{\text{Dose on hand}} \times \text{Quantity (Q)} = \text{Amount to givc}$$

$$\frac{D}{H} \times Q = \text{Amount to give}$$

$$\frac{50\text{ mg}}{100\text{ mg}} \times 2\text{ ml} = \frac{50}{100} \times \frac{2}{1} = \frac{\cancel{100}}{\cancel{100}} = 1\text{ ml}$$

◐ Practice Problems

2. Using the formula method, calculate the following dosages:

   a. The physician ordered Phenergan 75 mg IM. On hand is Phenergan 50 mg per ml. How many milliliters will you give?

   b. The physician ordered Kantrex 500 mg IM. Available is Kantrex 0.5 Gm per ml. How many milliliters will you give?

   c. The physician ordered Dramamine 35 mg IM. On hand is Dramamine 50 mg per ml. How many milliliters will you give?

d. The physician ordered Dilantin 25 mg IM. On hand is Dilantin 50 mg per ml. How many milliliters will you give?

e. The physician ordered Garamycin 60 mg IM. Available is Garamycin 40 mg per ml. How many milliliters will you givc?

f. The physician ordered Nubain, 10 mg IM. On hand is a 1 ml ampule that contains 20 mg/1 ml. What is the correct dosage?

g. The physician ordered Dilaudid, 25 mg IM. On hand is a 5 ml ampule that contains 50 mg/5 ml. What is the correct dosage?

h. The physician ordered Compazine, 10 mg IM. On hand is a 10 ml vial that contains 5 mg/ml. What is the correct dosage?

i. The physician ordered Depo-Medrol, 40 mg IM. On hand is a 5 ml vial that contains 80 mg/ml. What is the correct dosage?

j. The physician ordered Norflex, 30 mg IM. On hand is a 60 mg/2 ml ampule. What is the correct dosage?

Medications Measured in Units

Such medications as insulin, heparin, some antibiotics, hormones, vitamins, and vaccines are measured in units (U). These medications are standardized in units based on their strengths. The strength varies from one medicine to another, depending upon the source, condition, and method in which they are obtained.

Insulin

Insulin is a chemical substance (hormone) secreted by the beta cells of the islets of Langerhans. It is essential for the proper metabolism of carbohydrates, fats, and proteins. An inadequate secretion of insulin leads to a complex disorder known as diabetes mellitus. The National Diabetes Data Group of the National Institutes of Health organized the various forms of diabetes into the following categories:

TYPE I	Insulin-dependent diabetes mellitus (IDDM)
TYPE II	Noninsulin-dependent diabetes mellitus (NIDDM)
TYPE III	Women who develop glucose intolerance in association with pregnancy.
TYPE IV	Other types of diabetes associated with pancreatic disease, hormonal changes, adverse effects of drugs, or genetic or other anomalies.

Individuals with TYPE I insulin-dependent diabetes mellitus (IDDM) must take insulin injections on a regular basis to maintain life. The dosage of insulin is expressed in units, U-100, and is individualized by the physician for each patient. The amount of insulin that a person must take is based on blood glucose levels, diet, exercise, and the individual's needs.

Note: *It is extremely important that the exact dosage of insulin be taken by the patient.* Too little or too much insulin can cause serious problems, ranging from a blood sugar level too low or too high, to coma, and even death. It may be your responsibility to administer insulin, and/or to teach patients or their families how to administer insulin themselves.

When administering insulin, the U-100 syringe (1cc or LO-DOSE® 1/2cc) is preferred. U-100 means there are 100 units of insulin per milliliter or cubic centimeter. Insulin dosage should always be expressed in *units* rather than in milliliters or cubic centimeters. For example, if the physician orders 30 units of U-100 NPH insulin, you would use a U-100 syringe and draw up 30 units of U-100 NPH insulin.

Precautions to Keep in Mind When Administering Insulin

- Be sure to use the proper insulin, the one ordered by the physician.
- Do not substitute one insulin for another.

- Use the correct syringe U-100.
- Dosage of insulin is always measured in *units* and is *individualized* for each patient.
- Check the label for the name and type of insulin, strength, and expiration date.
- Make sure the insulin has the proper appearance. (See Tables 9–1 and 9–2.)
- When insulin is not in use, store it in a cool place and avoid freezing.
- Avoid shaking an insulin bottle. Roll gently in palms of hand to mix. This method prevents bubbles in the medication.

Table 9–1 Rapid-Acting Insulin

Insulin Preparations U-100				
Rapid-acting	**Onset of Action**	**Peak**	**Duration**	**Appearance**
Regular	$\frac{1}{2}$ hr	$2\frac{1}{2}$–5 hr	8 hr	Clear, colorless
Crystalline zinc	$\frac{1}{2}$ hr–1 hr	2–4 hr	8 hr	Clear, colorless
Semilente	$1\frac{1}{2}$ hr	5–10 hr	16 hr	Cloudy
Humulin R	15 min	1 hr	6–8 hr	Clear, colorless
Mixtard	$\frac{1}{2}$ hr	4–8 hr	24 hr	Cloudy
Velosulin	$\frac{1}{2}$ hr	1–3 hr	8 hr	Clear
Novolin	$\frac{1}{2}$ hr	$2\frac{1}{2}$–5 hr	8 hr	Clear

Table 9–2 Intermediate-Acting and Slow-Acting Insulin

Insulin Preparations U-100				
Intermediate-acting	**Onset of Action**	**Peak**	**Duration**	**Appearance**
NPH	$1\frac{1}{2}$ hr	4–12 hr	24 hr	Cloudy
Lente	$2\frac{1}{2}$ hr	7–15 hr	24 hr	Cloudy
Insulatard NPH	$1\frac{1}{2}$ hr	4–12 hr	24 hr	Cloudy
Novolin L	$2\frac{1}{2}$ hr	7–15 hr	22 hr	Cloudy
Novolin N	$1\frac{1}{2}$ hr	4–12 hr	24 hr	Cloudy
Humulin N	1 hr	4 hr	24 hr	Cloudy
Slow-acting				
Ultralente	4 hr	10–30 hr	36 hr	Cloudy
PZI (protamine zinc insulin)	4–8 hr	14–20 hr	36 hr	Cloudy

How to Calculate Unit Dosages

When calculating medications that are ordered in units, you may use either the proportional or formula method.

Example: The physician ordered 4000 USP units of heparin to be administered deep subcutaneously. On hand is heparin 5000 USP units per milliliter.

The Proportional Method

Step 1. Use the following proportion to calculate the dosage:

$$\frac{\text{Known unit on hand}}{5000\text{ U}} : \frac{\text{Known dosage form (volume)}}{1\text{ ml}} = \frac{\text{Dose ordered}}{4000\text{ U}} : \frac{\text{Unknown amount to give (volume)}}{x\text{ ml}}$$

$$5000x = 4000$$

$$x = \frac{\cancel{4000}}{\cancel{5000}} = \frac{4}{5}\text{ ml or }0.8\text{ ml}$$

You may use a tuberculin syringe to draw up 0.8 ml, or convert $\frac{4}{5}$ ml to minims. See step 2.

Step 2. If you choose to *convert* $\frac{4}{5}$ ml to minims, use the following example.

> There are 15 to 16 minims per milliliter. You will use 15 when the denominator of the fraction will go into 15 evenly. You will use 16 when the denominator of the fraction will go into 16 evenly.

To *convert* $\frac{4}{5}$ to minims, multiply

$$\frac{4}{5} \times \frac{15}{1} = \frac{4}{\cancelto{1}{5}} \times \frac{\cancelto{3}{15}}{1} = 12\text{ minims}$$

You will administer 12 minims (4000 U) to the patient.

The Formula Method

Example: The physician ordered 450,000 units of Bicillin for deep IM injection. Available is Bicillin 600,000 units per milliliter.

Step 1. Use the following formula to calculate the dosage:

$$\frac{\text{Dose ordered (desired)}}{\text{Dose on hand}} \times \text{Quantity (Q)} = \text{Amount to give}$$

$$\frac{450{,}000 \text{ U}}{600{,}000 \text{ U}} \times 1 \text{ ml} =$$

$$\frac{\overset{3}{\cancel{450{,}000}} \text{ U}}{\underset{4}{\cancel{600{,}000}} \text{ U}} \times 1 \text{ ml} = \frac{3}{4} \text{ ml}$$

Step 2. You may choose to convert to minims. If so, multiply $\frac{3}{4}$ by 16.

$$\frac{3}{\underset{1}{\cancel{4}}} \times \frac{\overset{4}{\cancel{16}}}{1} = 12 \text{ minims}$$

You will administer 12 minims (450,000 U) to the patient.

◐ Practice Problems

3. Use the proportional or formula method to calculate the following:
   a. The physician ordered 20 units of Acthar IM. Available is Acthar 40 units per milliliter. What is the correct dosage?

   b. The physician ordered 8000 USP units of heparin to be administered deep subcutaneously. On hand is heparin 10,000 USP units per ml. How much heparin will you administer?

   c. The physician ordered Bicillin 600,000 units for deep IM injection. The dose on hand is Bicillin 1,200,000 units per 2 milliliters. How many milliliters will you administer to your patient?

d. The physician ordered 32 units of U-100 regular insulin. Shade in the correct dosage on the U-100 syringe pictured below.

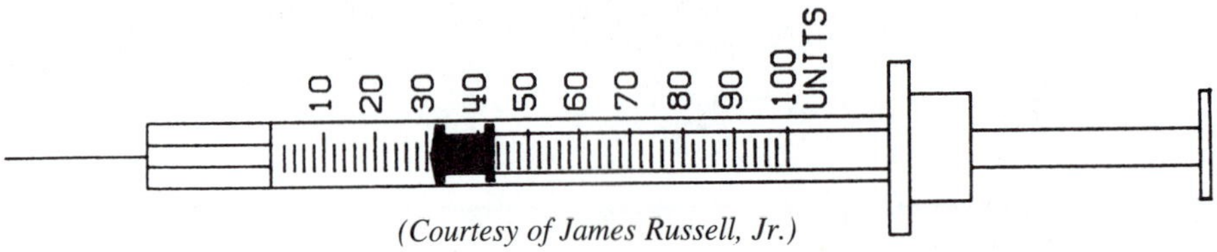

(Courtesy of James Russell, Jr.)

e. The physician ordered 64 units of U-100 Humulin R insulin. Shade in the correct dosage on the U-100 syringe pictured below.

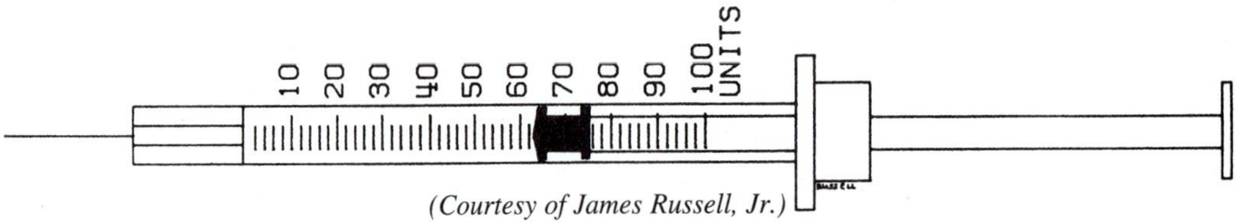

(Courtesy of James Russell, Jr.)

Calculating Intravenous Drip Rate

The type, amount, and flow rate of an intravenous fluid is determined by the physician. The physician assesses the patient's needs and physical condition. Intravenous fluids are used as replacements for fluids and electrolytes, and as a means to deliver routine or emergency medications. When the physician orders that a vein be kept open (KVO), a solution of 5% dextrose in water, D_5W, may be used. The drip rate may be 20 cc/hr (500 cc/24 hr) or 40 cc/hr (1000 cc/24 hr). It is very important to maintain the prescribed drip rate to prevent fluid and electrolyte imbalance.

Special preparation is required of those approved to start intravenous infusions and/or administer IV medications. A drug that is introduced directly into a patient's bloodstream produces an immediate effect. Therefore, those administering medications by this method should be well versed in the ethical and legal implications accompanying such responsibility.

An intravenous solution is ordered by the physician in milliliters per hour. When an infusion control device or a dosage calculator is not available, the nurse must mathematically determine the flow rate in drops (gtt) per minute. Various formulas are used to calculate intravenous drip rate. In this chapter, the following formula is used:

$$\frac{(\text{ml} \div \text{hr}) \times \text{calibrations (gtt/ml – drop factor)}}{\text{min}}$$

Before you calculate the drip rate, you need to know several important factors:

- You need to know the volume (amount) of solution that is to be infused.
- Next, you need to know the length of time (hours) that the fluid is to be infused.

- You need to know the calibrations (gtt/ml) of the infusion set that is to be used. The *drop factor* is identified on the package label. Be sure to read the label carefully. A *macro*drop may deliver 10 gtt/ml, 15 gtt/ml, or 20 gtt/ml, depending on the manufacturer. A *micro*drop delivers 60 gtt/ml, since this is standardized by all manufacturers. See Figure 9–3.

How to Calculate IV Drip Rate

Example: The physician ordered D_5W (5% dextrose in water) 1000 ml to be infused over 8 hours. The infusion set is calibrated to deliver 15 gtt/ml.

Step 1. Divide milliliters by hours (ml ÷ hr)

$$\frac{1000\text{ ml}}{8\text{ hr}} = 125\text{ ml/hr}$$

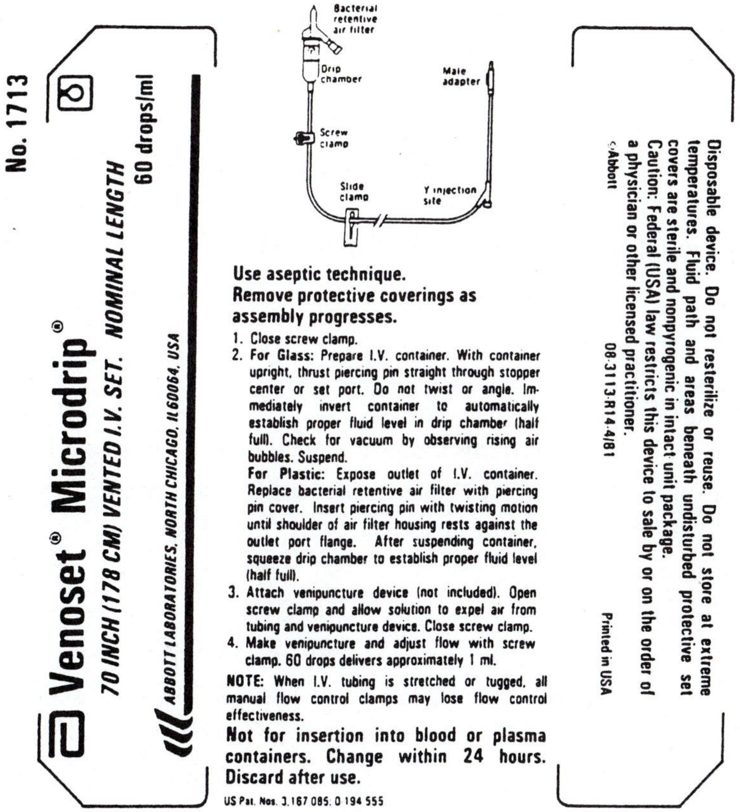

Figure 9–3 Venoset Microdrip IV set; 60 drops/ml *(Reprinted with permission from Abbott Laboratories, Pharmaceutical Products Division)*

Table 9–3 IV Flow Rates/1 L in gtt/Minute

Tubing Delivers	4 Hours	6 Hours	8 Hours	10 Hours	12 Hours
15 gtt/ml	62	42	31	25	21
10 gtt/ml	42	28	21	17	14
60 gtt/ml	250	167	125	100	83

Step 2. Multiply the answer you found by dividing milliliters by hours (125) by the calibrations (gtt/ml = 15).

$125 \times 15 = 1875$

Step 3. Divide the answer you found in step 2 by 60 min (1 hour).

$$\frac{1875}{60} = 31.25 \text{ gtt/min}$$

Now let's review the total process:

$$\frac{(\text{ml} \div \text{hr}) \times \text{calibrations (gtt/ml)}}{\text{min}}$$

$$\frac{125 \times 15}{60} = \frac{1875}{60} = 31.25 \text{ gtt/min (rate of flow)}$$

- Round number to nearest whole number 31 gtt/min. See Table 9–3.

Practice Problems

4. Using the formula given in this chapter, calculate the following IV drip rates:
   a. The physician ordered D_5W 1000 ml to be infused over 8 hours. The infusion set delivers 20 gtt/ml (drop factor).

   b. The physician ordered D_5R/L (5 percent dextrose Ringers/Lactate) 1000 ml to be infused over 12 hours. The infusion set delivers 60 gtt/ml (drop factor).

c. The physician ordered D_5NS (5 percent dextrose in normal saline) 1000 ml to be infused over 10 hours. The infusion set delivers 10 gtt/ml (drop factor).

d. The physician orders that 2500 ml be infused over 24 hours. The infusion set delivers 10 gtt/ml (drop factor).

e. The physician orders that 1200 ml be infused over 16 hours. The infusion set delivers 15 gtt/ml (drop factor).

Self Assessment Test

This test is designed to assess your understanding of calculating adult parenteral dosages. Please correctly calculate the following adult parenteral dosages. After you have completed the test you may check your answers with those in the back of the text.

1. The physician ordered Demerol, 50 mg IM. On hand is Demerol 100 mg per 2 ml. How many milliliters will you give?

2. The physician ordered Seconal Sodium CII, 75 mg IM. On hand is Seconal Sodium CII, 50 mg ($\frac{3}{4}$ gr) per ml. How many milliliters will you give?

3. The physician ordered Bicillin, 800,000 units for deep IM injection. On hand is Bicillin 1,200,000 units per 2 ml. How many minims will you give?

4. The physician ordered Phenergan, 100 mg IM. On hand is Phenergan 50 mg per ml. How many milliliters will you give?

5. The physician ordered 30 units of Acthar IM. Available is Acthar 40 units per milliliter. How many minims will you give?

6. The physician ordered D_5W 1000 ml to be infused over 8 hours. The infusion set delivers 20 gtt/ml (drop factor). Calculate the correct IV drip rate.

7. The physician ordered D_5NS (5 percent dextrose in normal saline) 1000 ml to be infused over 10 hours. The infusion set delivers 10 gtt/ml (drop factor). Calculate the correct IV drip rate.

CHAPTER 10

Calculating Children's Dosages

OBJECTIVES

Upon completion of this chapter, you should be able to:

- Define the terms listed in the vocabulary.
- Give the guidelines for administering pediatric medications.
- Calculate children's dosages according to kilogram of body weight and body surface area (BSA).
- Complete the practice problems correctly.
- Complete the Self Assessment Test.

Vocabulary

child (child). Any human between infancy and puberty.

infancy (in′fan-se). The stage of life from the time of birth through the completion of one year.

puberty (pyoo′bar-te). The stage of life when sexual reproduction becomes possible.

fetus (fet′us). The child in utero from the third month to birth.

embryo (em′bre-o). The human stage of development between the second and eighth week of life.

nomogram (nom′o-gram). A device-graph that shows the relationship among numerical values. One may estimate the body surface area (BSA) of a patient according to height and weight by using a nomogram. Note that there are separate nomograms for adults and children.

> ***Note:*** When determining the BSA of a child, make sure you use a nomogram designed for children.

Introduction

Each child is an individual, with differences in age, size, and weight. In the past, formulas such as Young's, Clark's, and Fried's rules were used to calculate pediatric dosages. These formulas determined what fraction of an adult dose was appropriate for a child. Since each child doesn't develop in the same way during a given time span, these formulas have been replaced by more exact methods of determining the correct dosage of medication for a child.

Today, there are two basic methods used to calculate children's dosages, these are: according to kilogram of body weight and body surface area (BSA). The body weight method is generally the method of choice, since most medications are ordered in this way and it is easier to calculate. The body surface area (BSA) is an exact method, but one must use a formula and a nomogram to determine a correct dosage. Both of these methods are described in this chapter along with numerous practice problems.

Guidelines for Administering Pediatric Medications

1. Follow the "6 Rights" of proper drug administration:
   - The Right Dose
   - The Right Drug
   - The Right Route
   - The Right Time
   - The Right Patient
   - The Right Documentation

> Correctly document the administration of a medication: Dose, Drug, Route, Time, Patient's name, and Documentation.

2. Carefully assess each pediatric patient:
   - Age
   - Weight
   - Body size
   - Physical state
   - Disease process
   - Mental and emotional state
   - Level of understanding
   - Allergies

3. Gain parental cooperation:
    - Identify yourself, call the parent and the child by name. Explain the procedure.
    - Whenever possible, allow the parent to assist you.
    - At times, it may be necessary to ask the parent to leave the room, as the parent's behavior may be upsetting to the child. When this is the case, explain to the parent and child that the procedure will only take a few minutes and you will ask another nurse to assist you.

4. Establish rapport with the child:
    - Use a positive straightforward approach. Do not waste time. The longer it takes to accomplish a procedure, the more apprehensive the child will become.
    - Explain the procedure at the level of the child's understanding.
    - Whenever possible, allow the child to assist you.
    - Show approval for positive behavior by the child. Clap, laugh, and reward with a "treat" if possible.

5. Route of administration: The route of administration will depend upon the child's age, weight, body size, physical, mental and emotional state, disease process, level of understanding, specific properties of the medication, and the physician's order.
    - **Oral Route:** Never force or give an oral medication to a crying child.

      —Liquid medications may be administered by dropper or an appropriate device such as an oral syringe or calibrated medication cup.

      —Solid medications are generally not ordered until the child is old enough to understand and cooperate by actually swallowing the medication. In the event a tablet is ordered, always check with the pharmacist to see if it can be crushed, and then mixed with an appropriate food or liquid (do not mix the medication in a baby's formula) for ease of administration. Certain medications should not be crushed or mixed with food.
    - **Parenteral Route:** Two people will be needed when administering an injection to a child. One to assist in maintaining a proper body position and the other to give the injection. Administer subcutaneous, intramuscular, and/or intravenous medications with extreme care.
    - **Rectal Route:** Consider the significance the child places on this part of his/her body. A toddler who is in the process of toilet training may resist this form of drug administration, while older children may feel as though this is an invasion of privacy and may react with embarrassment and resentment.

6. **Caution: When calculating children's dosages be extremely careful. It is advisable to have someone check your mathematical solutions.** Be sure to compare the normal dose range with the dosage you plan to administer. If there is any doubt, contact the physician and/or pharmacist.

Calculating Dosage per Kilogram of Body Weight

As a nurse, it may be your responsibility to calculate the amount of dosage ordered by the physician according to the child's body weight. The physician will usually order the medication dosage per kilogram of body weight.

There are two methods of calculating dosage according to kilogram of body weight.

- **Method One: Dividing pounds by 2.2 and multiplying dose ordered by kg of body weight**

Step 1. To convert pounds to kilograms, divide the pounds by 2.2 as (1 kg = 2.2 lb).

Step 2. Multiply the dose ordered by kilogram of body weight.

Step 3. If the dose is ordered in divided doses, divide the number of times into the answer you obtained in step two.

Example: The physician orders Ceftriaxone Sodium (Rocephin) 100 mg/kg of body weight, in divided doses every 12 hours (not to exceed 4 Gm), for Alice Potts who weighs 66 pounds. How many milligrams will Alice receive?

Step 1. Convert pounds to kilograms.

$$\frac{66 \text{ lb}}{2.2} = \text{X kg}$$

$$\begin{array}{r} 30 \\ 2.2\overline{)66.0} \\ \underline{66} \\ 0 \\ \underline{0} \end{array}$$

66 lb = 30 kg

Step 2. Multiply the dose ordered by kilogram of body weight.

100 mg/kg

$100 \times 30 = 3000$ mg = 3 Gm

Step 3. Ordered in divided doses.

Divide 3000 by 2 to arrive at the divided dose = 1500 mg.

Alice will receive 1500 mg of Rocephin every 12 hours, as ordered by the physician.

- **Method Two: Using the proportional method to calculate kilogram of body weight.**

Example: The physician orders Ceftriaxone Sodium (Rocephin) 100 mg/kg of body weight, in divided doses every 12 hours (not to exceed 4 Gm), for Alice Potts, who weighs 66 pounds. How many milligrams will Alice receive?

Step 1. To convert 66 pounds to kilograms, set up the proportion as follows:

$2.2 \text{ lb} : 1 \text{ kg} = 66 \text{ lb} : x \text{ kg}$

Step 2: Now solve for x:

$$2.2 : 1 = 66 : x$$
$$2.2x = 66$$
$$x = 30$$

Step 3. Now calculate the prescribed dosage by placing 30 in the appropriate place:

100 mg/30 kg

$100 \times 30 = 3000 \text{ mg} = 3 \text{ Gm}$

Step 4. To determine the amount of each dose, divide 3000 by 2 (every 12 hours).

$3000 \div 2 = 1500 \text{ mg}$

Alice Potts will receive 1500 mg of Rocephine every 12 hours, as ordered by the physician.

◐ Practice Problems

1. Calculate the following dosages according to kilogram of body weight.
   a. The physician orders Cefadroxil (Duricef), 30 mg/kg of body weight, for John Knight who weighs 44 pounds. The dose is to be divided and given every 12 hours. How many milligrams will you give?

   b. The physician orders codeine phosphate CII 0.5 mg/kg of body weight for pain. The patient weighs 50 pounds. The medication may be given every 4–6 hours. How many milligrams will the patient receive?

c. The physician orders cephapirin sodium (Cefadyl) 20 mg/kg every six hours, for a child who weighs 46 pounds. How many milligrams will you give?

d. The physician orders cefotaxime (Clarofan) 60 mg/kg divided into four equal doses for a child who weighs 42 pounds. What is the correct dosage and the amount to be given in four equal doses?

e. The physician orders gentamicin sulfate (Garamycin) 6 mg/kg/day for a child who weighs 52 pounds. How many milligrams will be given daily?

Body Surface Area (BSA)

The body surface area (BSA) is considered to be one of the most accurate methods of calculating medication dosages for *infants and children up to 12 years of age.* This method requires the use of a *nomogram* (a device-graph that shows the relationship among numerical values) that estimates the body surface area of the patient according to height and weight. Refer to Figure 10–1.

The body surface area is determined by drawing a straight line from the patient's height to the patient's weight. Intersection of the line with the surface area column is the estimated BSA. This figure is then placed in the following formula.

$$\frac{\text{BSA of child (m}^2\text{)}}{1.7\ (\text{m}^2)} \times \text{adult dose} = \text{child's dose}$$

This formula is based on the average adult who weighs 140 lb and has a body surface area of 1.7 square meters (1.7 m^2).

Example: Marion Green is a 4-year-old child who is 40 inches tall and weighs

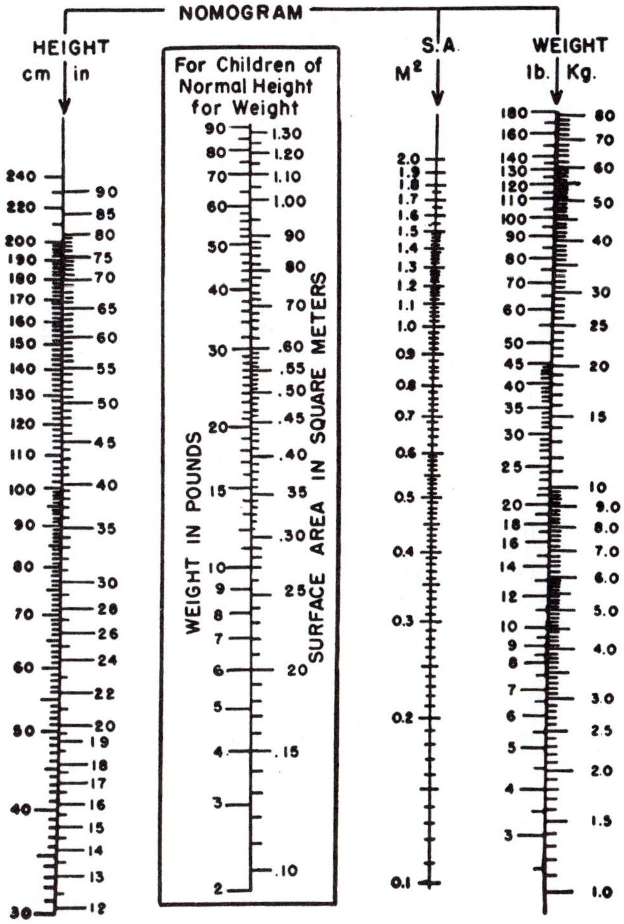

Figure 10–1 Body surface area (BSA) is determined by drawing a straight line from the patient's height in the left column to his or her weight in the far right column. Intersection of the line with the surface area (SA) column is the estimated BSA. For infants and children of normal height for weight, BSA may be estimated from weight alone by referring to the enclosed area. *(Reprinted from Behrman, R. E. and Vaughan, V. C.* Nelson Textbook of Pediatrics, *12th ed., 1983, W. B. Saunders Company, Philadelphia, PA 19105. Used with permission from W. B. Saunders Company and R. E. Behrman, MD, Case Western Reserve University, School of Medicine, Cleveland, OH 44106)*

38 lb (BSA 0.7). The physician has ordered Demerol for pain. The average adult dose of Demerol is 50 mg per ml. What dosage will be given to Marion according to the BSA Method?

$$\frac{0.7\ (\text{m}^2)}{1.7\ (\text{m}^2)} \times \frac{50\text{ mg}}{1} = \text{child's dose}$$

$$\frac{0.7\ (\text{m}^2)}{1.7\ (\text{m}^2)} \times \frac{50\text{ mg}}{1} = \frac{35}{1.7} = 20.5\text{ mg} = 21\text{ mg}$$

Now use the formula $\frac{\text{Desired}}{\text{Have}} \times$ Quantity to convert mg to ml.

$$\frac{21\text{ mg}}{50\text{ mg}} = x\text{ ml}$$

$$\frac{21}{50} = 0.42\text{ ml (administered with a tuberculin syringe)}$$

Practice Problems

2. Calculate the following dosages according to body surface area (BSA).
   a. If the adult dose of Sulfadiazine is 250 mg IM three times a day, what is the dosage for a 3-year-old child, 36 inches tall, weighing 30 pounds (BSA 0.6)?

   b. If the adult dose of Amoxicillin is 250 mg every 8 hours, what is the dosage for a $2\frac{1}{2}$-year-old child, 28 inches tall, weighing 25 pounds (BSA 0.5)?

   c. If the adult dose of an antibiotic is 250 mg, what is the dosage for a child with a BSA of 0.41?

   d. If the adult dose is 1000 units, what is the dosage for a child with a BSA of 0.56?

   e. If the adult dose is 500 units, what is the dosage for a child with a BSA of 0.5?

Self Assessment Test

This test is designed to assess your understanding of calculating children's dosages. Please correctly calculate the following children's dosages. After you have completed the test you may check your answers with those in the back of the text.

1. A 4-year-old child has a body surface area (BSA) of 0.7. The adult dose of medication is 50 mg per ml. What dosage will be given to the child?

2. The child weighs 66 pounds and the physician has ordered a medication to be given 30 mg/kg of body weight. What dosage will be given to the child?

3. The child weighs 44 pounds and the physician has ordered a medication to be given 30 mg/kg of body weight. What dosage will be given to the child?

4. If the adult dose of Sulfadiazine is 250 mg IM, what is the dosage for a 3-year-old child, 36 inches tall, weight 30 pounds (BSA 0.6)?

Young's Rule

$$\frac{\textit{Age of child}}{\textit{Age of child} + 12} \times \text{average adult dosage} = \text{child's dose}$$

Example: What dosage will be given to a 3-year-old child when the adult dose is 50 mg?

$$\frac{3}{3+12} \times 50$$

$$\frac{3}{15} \times 50 = \frac{150}{15} = 10 \text{ mg}$$

$$\frac{\overset{1}{\cancel{3}}}{\underset{1}{\underset{\cancel{5}}{\cancel{15}}}} \times \overset{10}{\cancel{50}} = 10 \text{ mg is the child's dose}$$

(The child's dose in this case is $\frac{1}{5}$ of the adult dose.)

Fried's Rule

Fried's Rule is used for calculation of infant dosage under two years of age. It may be used for older children.

$$\frac{\textit{Age in months}}{150} \times \text{adult dose} = \text{infant's dose}$$

Example: What dosage will be given to a 15-month-old infant when the adult dose is 50 mg?

$$\frac{15}{150} \times 50 \text{ mg}$$

$$\frac{1}{10} \times 50 = 5 \text{ mg is the child's dose}$$

(The child's dose in this case is $\frac{1}{10}$ of the adult dose.)

Clark's Rule

$$\frac{\textit{Child's weight in pounds}}{150} \times \text{adult dose} = \text{child's dose}$$

Example: Do the same problem using the child's weight instead of age. The adult dose is 50 mg. What dosage will be given to a 24-pound child?

$$\frac{24}{150} \times 50 \text{ mg} = 8 \text{ mg child's dosage}$$

SECTION 3

Administration of Medications

CHAPTER 11

Drug Sources, Standards, and Dosages

OBJECTIVES

Upon completion of this chapter, you should be able to:

- Define the terms listed in the vocabulary.
- Define pharmacology.
- Describe the five subdivisions of pharmacology.
- State the five medical uses for drugs.
- Give the three names assigned to a drug.
- List the five main sources for drugs, giving examples from each source.
- State the importance of the Federal Food, Drug and Cosmetic Act.
- Explain the significance of the Controlled Substances Act of 1970.
- Define the five controlled substances' schedules and give examples of drugs listed in each.
- Explain storage and record-keeping for controlled substances.
- List two reasons for the standardization of drugs.
- Define the terms used in describing various types of dosages.
- Differentiate between and correctly use the following drug reference books:
  - —*United States Pharmacopeia/ National Formulary (USP/NF)*
  - —*New Drugs*
  - —*Physician's Desk Reference (PDR)*
- Describe a drug package insert.
- Define dosage.
- List the factors that affect drug dosage.
- Define the terms used in describing dosage.
- Answer the review questions correctly.

Vocabulary

abuse (a-buse′). The excessive or improper use of a substance, person, or animal.

addictive (a-dik′tiv). Pertaining to habit-forming; a substance that may cause physical and/or psychological dependency.

administer (ad-min′is-ter). To give.

bioassay (bi″o-as′a). The process of determining the strength and quality of a drug by testing it on an animal or on an isolated organ.

biotechnology (bi″o-tek-nol′a-je). The biological and engineering study of the relationship between man and machines.

controlled substance (kon-tro′led sub′stans). A drug that has the potential for addiction and abuse.

Examples: opium and cocaine, and their derivatives; narcotics, stimulants, and depressants.

dispense (dis-pens′). To prepare and give out.

genetic engineering (jen-et′ik en″ja-ner′ing). The synthesis, alteration, or repair of genetic material through the application of engineering principles.

habit-forming (hab′it for″ming). Becoming addicted to a substance by the continued repetition of an act. After sufficient repetition, the activity is performed as a reflex action.

hybrid (hi′brid). Being of mixed origin. An offspring produced by breeding different varieties, species, or races of plants or animals.

narcotic (nar-kot′ik). Producing sleep or stupor. A narcotic drug is one that depresses the central nervous system and, in moderate dosages, relieves pain and produces sleep. Most narcotics are habit-forming.

practitioner (prak-tish′un-er). One who has met the professional and legal requirements of a certain occupation or profession.

prescribe (pre-skrib′). To order or recommend the use of a drug, diet, or other form of therapy.

Introduction

Pharmacology is the study of drugs; the science that is concerned with the history, origin, sources, physical and chemical properties, uses, and the effects of drugs upon living organisms. Because of the complexity of the subject, pharmacology has evolved into the following subdivisions:

- *Pharmacodynamics.* The study of drugs and their actions on living organisms. It involves the biochemical and physiological effects of drugs upon living organisms as well as their actions.
- *Pharmacognosy.* The science of natural drugs and their physical, botanical, and chemical properties.
- *Pharmacokinetics.* The study of the metabolism and action of drugs within the body. It involves the time required for absorption to take place, duration of action, distribution of the drug in the body, and the method of excretion.
- *Pharmcotherapeutics.* The study of drugs and their relationships to the treatment of disease. It involves determining which drug is most or least appropriate for a specific disease and the required dosage to achieve beneficial results.
- *Toxicology.* The study of poisons; the science concerned with toxic substances. It involves the study of the chemistry and pharmacological actions of substances and establishing antidotes, treatment, prevention, and methods for controlling exposure to harmful substances.

Drugs

A *drug* can be defined simply as a medicinal substance that may alter or modify the functions of a living organism. In general, there are five medical uses for drugs.

- *Therapeutic Use.* Certain drugs, such as antihistamines, may be used in the treatment of an allergy to relieve the symptoms or to sustain the patient until other measures are instituted.
- *Diagnostic Use.* Certain drugs such as Telepaque are used in conjunction with radiology to allow the physician to pinpoint the location of a disease process.
- *Curative Use.* Certain drugs such as antibiotics kill or remove the causative agent of a disease.
- *Replacement Use.* Certain drugs such as hormones and vitamins are used to replace substances normally found in the body.
- *Preventive or Prophylactic Use.* Certain drugs such as immunizing agents are used to ward off or lessen the severity of a disease.

Drug Names

Most drugs have the following three types of names: chemical, generic, and trade or brand name. The *chemical* name describes the drug's molecular structure and identifies its chemical structure. The *generic* name is the drug's *official* name and is assigned to the drug by the U.S. Adopted Names (USAN) Council.

A generic drug can be manufactured by more than one pharmaceutical company. When this is the case, each company markets the drug under its own unique *trade* or *brand* name. A trade or brand name is registered by the U.S. Patent Office as well as

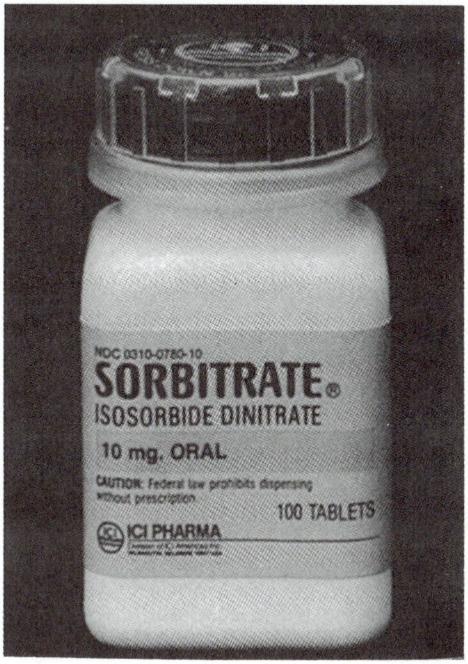

Figure 11–1 Sorbitrate® isosorbide dinitrate
(Courtesy of ICI Pharma, Division of ICI Americas, Inc., Wilmington, DE 19897)

approved by the U.S. Food and Drug Administration (FDA). The ® symbol that follows the drug's trade name denotes the fact that this name is the registered trademark used by the manufacturer. Some trade (brand) names are followed by the letters™ which also indicate that the name is registered and protected by laws that govern the use of trademarks.

Example: *Chemical* name: 1,4,3,6-dianhydrosorbitol-2, 5-dinitrate

Generic name: isosorbide dinitrate

Trade or *Brand* name: Sorbitrate® (first letter capitalized). See Figure 11–1.

Sources of Drugs

Drugs prepared from roots, herbs, bark, and other forms of plant life are among the earliest known pharmaceuticals. Their origin can be traced back to primitive cultures where they were first used to evoke magical powers and drive out evil spirits. In South America, the Carib Indians coated the tips of their arrows with a poisonous substance obtained from trees; thereby improving their chances of success in hunting. The pharmacologically active ingredients of this substance (Curare) facilitates muscle relaxation and, like many of the compounds discovered by primitive groups, is still used by drug manufacturers as a component of modern day medications.

Having discovered that certain plants were pharmacologically useful, early man began a search for other potential sources of drugs that continues to this day. In addition to plants, drugs are now derived from animals, and minerals, and are produced in laboratories utilizing chemical and biochemical processes.

Plants

As previously mentioned, the leaves, roots, stems, or fruit of certain plants may contain medicinal properties. The dried leaf of the purple foxglove plant is a source for *digitalis*, a cardiac glycoside used in the treatment of congestive heart failure.

The kelp plant is a rich source of iodine, a nonmetallic element. *Iodine* is not only used as a disinfectant, but is essential for the proper development and functioning of the thyroid gland. See Figure 11–2.

Animals

A number of essential extracts are obtained from such tissues as the pancreas and adrenal glands of animals. Refer again to Figure 11–2.

Insulin is a hormone extracted from the pancreas of cows (bovine) and hogs (porcine). It is also produced synthetically by pharmaceutical companies. This hormone is instrumental in controlling the level of blood sugar within the body, and is commonly

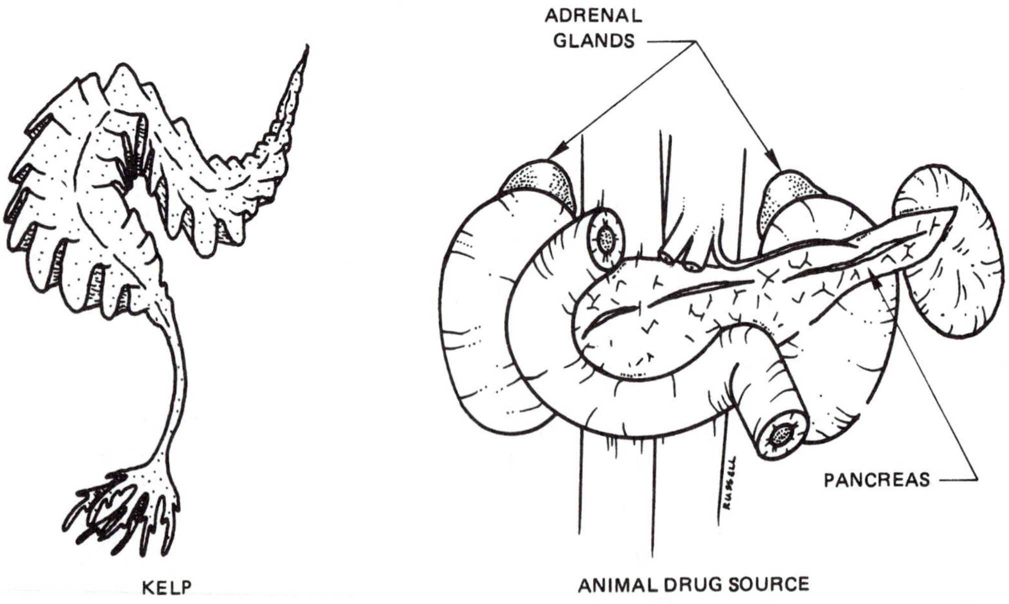

Figure 11–2 Sources of drugs *(Courtesy of James Russell, Jr.)*

associated with the treatment of a condition known as diabetes mellitus. Some diabetic patients can control their condition with oral hypoglycemic agents, diet, and exercise. However, many diabetic patients rely upon insulin as a part of their life.

Adrenalin and *cortisone* are two commonly used compounds that can be extracted from the adrenal glands of animals. Adrenalin is a sympathomimetic drug used to relieve respiratory distress, hypersensitivity reactions, and to prolong the action of infiltration anesthetics. Cortisone is an anti-inflammatory agent used in the treatment of rheumatoid arthritis and certain skin conditions.

Minerals

Some naturally occurring mineral substances are used in medicine in a highly purified form. One such mineral is *sulfur*, a nonmetallic element, that has been used for many years as a key ingredient in certain bacteriostatic drugs. Now prepared synthetically, sulfa drugs have widespread use in the treatment of urinary and intestinal tract infections.

Synthetic Drugs

A more recent source for drugs has been found in pharmaceutical labs in the form of synthetic drugs. These drugs are artificially prepared medications. By combining various chemicals, scientists can produce compounds that are identical to a natural drug, or create entirely new substances.

For example, *Chloromycetin* may be produced naturally by organic means, or it may be created synthetically from ingredients that make up its chemical formula. Other drugs, such as *Sulfathiazole*, cannot be produced by organic means, and are available only as a result of synthetic processes. Two advantages of synthetically prepared drugs are that they can be produced in great volume and, consequently, are usually less expensive than organically derived medications.

Genetically Engineered Pharmaceuticals

Genetic engineering is a *biotechnology* that has revolutionized agriculture, industry, health, and medicine. Scientists are now capable of creating new strains of bacteria using a technique known as *gene splicing*. Through this process, *hybrid* forms of life have been created that benefit mankind by providing an alternate source of drugs, such as insulin (Humulin®) for the diabetic patient, and interferon for use in the treatment of cancer.

Genetic engineering has proved to be one of the most extraordinary sources of drugs ever known to man. Like synthetic drugs, these medications can be produced in significant quantities, making them far less expensive than naturally occurring substances.

Drug Legislation

Qualified medical *practitioners* who *prescribe, dispense*, or *administer* drugs must comply with federal and state laws governing the manufacture, sale, possession, administration, and dispensing and prescribing of drugs. All drugs available for legal use are controlled by the Federal Food, Drug and Cosmetic Act. This law protects the public by insuring the purity, strength, and composition of food, drugs, and cosmetics. It also prohibits the movement, in interstate commerce, of adulterated and misbranded food, drugs, devices, and cosmetics. Enforcement of the Federal Food, Drug and Cosmetic Act is the responsibility of the Food and Drug Administration (FDA), which is a part of the Department of Health and Human Services (HHS) of the U.S. Government.

Controlled Substances Act of 1970

The Controlled Substances Act of 1970 controls the manufacture, importation, compounding, selling, dealing in, and giving away of drugs that have the potential for *addiction* and *abuse*. These drugs, known as *controlled substances*, include opium and cocaine, and their derivatives; *narcotics*, stimulants, and depressants. The Drug Enforcement Administration (DEA) of the U.S. Justice Department enforces the act, which is also known as the Comprehensive Drug Abuse Prevention and Control Act. Under federal law, medical practitioners who prescribe, administer, or dispense controlled substances must register with the DEA, and physicians are required to renew their registration annually.

Drug Schedules

Controlled substances are classified according to five drug schedules. Table 11–1 lists the five drug schedules and gives examples of the controlled substances in each classification.

Table 11–1 Drug Schedules with Examples of Controlled Substances

SCHEDULE I	Heroin, lysergic acid diethylamide (LSD), marijuana, mescaline, peyote, and psilocybin are some examples.
SCHEDULE II	Amobarbital, amphetamine, cocaine, codeine, hydromorphone, opium, meperidine, methadone, morphine, nembutal, pentobarbital, percodan, quaalude, secobarbital, and Marinol are some examples.
SCHEDULE III	Barbituates, various drug combinations containing codeine and paregoric, glutethimide, mazindol, methyprylon, phenmetrazine, and amphetamine-like compounds are included in this schedule.
SCHEDULE IV	Chloral hydrate, diazepam, meprobamate, paraldehyde, phenobarbital, Librium, Valium, and Darvon are some of the drugs listed.
SCHEDULE V	Lomotil, Donnagel, and drugs containing low-strength codeine, such as Actifed with codeine, are typical of the medications listed.

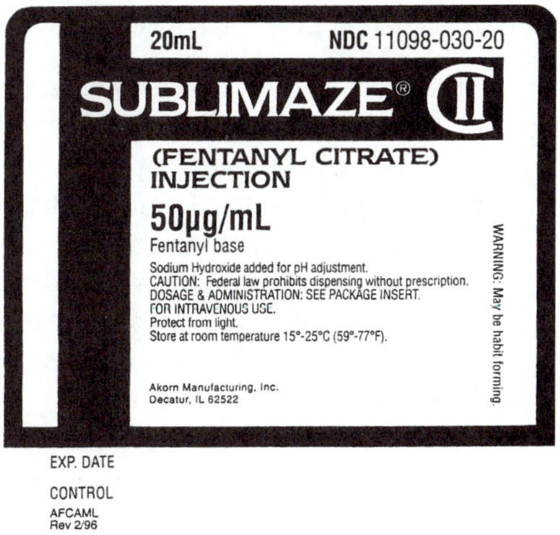

Figure 11–3 An example of a Schedule II drug
(Courtesy of Akorn Manufacturing, Inc., Decatur, IL)

Schedule I specifies drugs that have a high potential for abuse and are not accepted for medical use within the United States. *Schedule II* includes drugs that also have a high potential for abuse, but do have an accepted medical use within the United States. It has been determined that abuse of a drug included in this schedule may lead to psychological or physical dependency. See Figure 11–3. *Schedule III* drugs have a low to moderate potential for physical dependency, yet they have a high potential for psychological dependency. *Schedule IV* includes drugs that have a low potential for abuse relative to Schedule II drugs. Abuse of Schedule IV drugs may lead to limited physical or psychological dependency. *Schedule V* drugs have the lowest abuse potential of the controlled substances. They consist of preparations containing limited quantities of certain narcotic drugs generally used as antitussives and antidiarrheals in combination products.

Federal law requires that all controlled substances be kept separate from other drugs. They are to be stored in a substantially constructed metal box or compartment that is equipped with a double lock. Narcotics may be kept in a double-locked medication cabinet or a double-locked section of a medication cart. A nurse who is responsible for administering narcotics must keep the narcotics key protected from possible misuse. The key should be in the nurse's possession during the hours of duty.

A separate record book is required for information concerning the dispensing or administration of controlled substances. This data system must be maintained on a daily basis and kept for a minimum of two years (three years in some states). Narcotics are counted at the end of each shift by an oncoming and offgoing nurse. The nurse in charge of administering medications may be a primary care or medication nurse. The inventory of the controlled drugs must be recorded on an audit sheet and signed for correctness of count by an oncoming and an offgoing nurse.

Drug References/Standards

The *United States Pharmacopeia/National Formulary* (USP/NF) is recognized by the U.S. Government as the official list of standardized drugs. Published every five years by the United States Pharmacopeial Convention, this reference book includes only those drugs that have been tested and certified as having met established standards of quality, purity, and potency. Such testing may involve *assay* whereby the ingredients of the drug are identified and measured, and/or *bioassay* wherein the dosage necessary to produce a therapeutic effect is established utilizing animal studies. Each revision of the USP/NF includes new drugs and drops those older products that have been replaced by safer or more effective drugs.

Upon release by the FDA, the drug may be listed in *New Drugs* until it has been proved to be of sufficient value to be included in the *United States Pharmacopeia/ National Formulary*. The Federal Food, Drug and Cosmetic Act specifies that a drug is official when it is listed in the USP/NF.

New Drugs, published annually by the Council on Pharmacy of the American Medical Association, lists all drugs having reached a certain frequency of use. Listing does not imply endorsement of any drug by the AMA. This publication provides health professionals with an up-to-date listing of drugs new to the market.

The *Physician's Desk Reference* (PDR) is a useful drug information book for physicians and health professionals. Published annually by Medical Economics Company, Inc., in cooperation with pharmaceutical companies, it is an excellent drug reference book, see Figure 11–4. Supplements to the PDR are provided to purchasers of the book as they become available throughout the year, thereby keeping this reference current.

What's in the PDR?

Contents

Manufacturers' Index (white pages) Section 1: Alphabetical arrangement of all pharmaceutical manufacturers participating in the PDR. Includes addresses, phone numbers, and emergency contacts. Shows each manufacturer's products and the page number of those described in the PDR.

Brand and Generic Name Index (pink pages) Section 2: Gives the page number of each product by brand and generic name.

Product Category Index (blue pages) Section 3: Lists all fully described products by prescribing category.

Product Identification Guide (gray pages) Section 4: Presents full-color, actual-size photos of tablets and capsules, plus pictures of a variety of other dosage forms and packages. Arranged alphabetically by manufacturer.

Product Information (white pages) Section 5: Provides prescribing information. This section includes an alphabetical arrangement by manufacturer of over 2,500

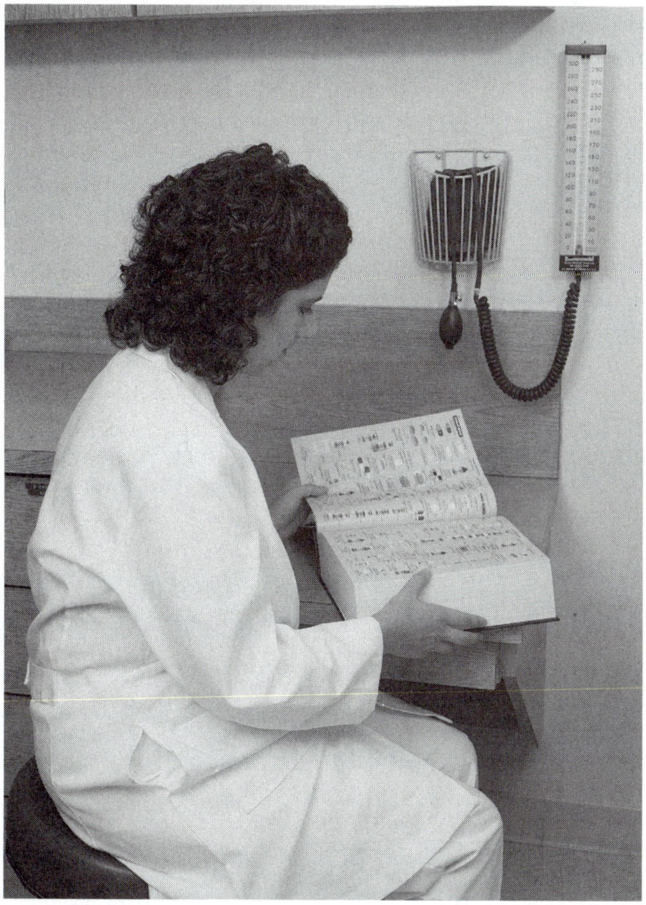

Figure 11–4 The *Physicians' Desk Reference* is a useful drug information source

products. The general format of this section is as follows:

Brand Name	Contraindications
[phonetic spelling]	Warnings
Generic Name	Precautions
Description	Adverse Reactions
Clinical Pharmacology	Dosage and Administration
Indications and Usage	How supplied

Diagnostic Product Information (green pages) Section 6: Gives usage guidelines for a variety of common diagnostic agents. Included in this section you will find:

Certified Poison Control Centers
Discontinued Products
U.S. Food and Drug Administration Telephone Directory
Key to Controlled Substances Categories
Key to FDA Use-In-Pregnancy Ratings
Drug Information Centers

Note: All controlled substances listed in the PDR are indicated with the symbol C, with the Roman numeral II, III, IV, or V printed inside the C to designate the schedule in which the substance is classified.

Example: DURAMORPH® Ⓒ
morphine sulfate injection, USP

How to Use the PDR

Drugs contained in the *Physicians' Desk Reference* are listed according to

- Brand name and generic name (PINK section)
- Classification or category (BLUE section)
- Alphabetical arrangement by manufacturers (WHITE section)

The following guidelines will assist you as you learn to use a PDR:

1. If you know the brand name of the drug, turn to the pink section and locate the drug in the alphabetical listing. The manufacturer's name will be in parentheses, followed by a page number, or two page numbers. The first number is the product identification page number. The second number is the product information section (WHITE).

Example: Look up Achromycin V capsules in a current PDR. (This example is based on the 1996 edition.)

Achromycin® V
[a-kro-mi-cin]
tetracycline HCL
for ORAL USE

Turn to page 1367-1368 and note all the information provided about the drug.

Description. Gives the origin and chemical composition of the drug.

Clinical Pharmacology. Indicates the effect of the drug upon the body and the process by which the drug exerts this effect.

Indications. States the various conditions, diseases, types of microorganisms, etc. that the drug is used for.

Contraindications. This drug is contraindicated in persons who have shown hypersensitivity to any of the tetracyclines.

Warnings. Gives the potential dangers of the drug.

Precautions. States the possible unfavorable effects that the drug may have upon a patient.

Adverse Reactions. Lists the side effects of the drug.

Dosage and Administration. States the amount (usual daily dose for adults and children) and time sequence of administration.

How supplied. Lists the various forms of the drug and their dosages.

2. If you know the classification of the drug turn to the BLUE section and locate the category of the drug.

Example: Antibiotics, Systemic
Tetracyclines
Achromycin V capsules (Lederle) p. 1367

3. On occasion you may not find the drug that you are looking for listed in the PDR; when this happens
   a. Refer to another drug reference book.
   b. Refer to the product information insert that comes in the drug package.
   c. Ask a pharmacist about the drug.

An important source of information about a particular drug is the *product information insert* that most manufacturers provide with their product. This is a brief description of the drug, its clinical pharmacology, indications and usage, contraindications, warnings, precautions, drug interactions, adverse reactions, overdosage, dosage, and administration. The package insert can be a valuable source of information about new drugs that might not be listed elsewhere. See Figure 11–5.

Drug Dosage

The *dosage* is the amount of medicine that is prescribed for administration. It is determined by the physician or a qualified practitioner who considers the following factors in the decision:

- Weight, sex, and age of the patient

  Age. The usual adult dose is usually suitable for the 20–60 age group. Infants, young children, adolescents, and the aged require individualized dosage.

  Pediatric patients are usually divided into three age groups:

  Newborn—0 to 4 weeks.
  Infant—5 to 52 weeks.
  Child—1 to 16 years. Adolescent 12 to 16 years.

Wyeth®
Omnipen®-N
(ampicillin sodium)
for **IM** or **IV** injection

A.H.F.S. Category 8:12.16

Description
Omnipen-N (ampicillin sodium) for Injection is a semisynthetic penicillin derived from the basic penicillin nucleus, 6-amino penicillanic acid.

NOTE: Omnipen-N contains 3.1 milliequivalents of sodium per gram of ampicillin as the sodium salt.

Actions
MICROBIOLOGY
In vitro studies have shown sensitivity of the following microorganisms to ampicillin:

Gram-Positive: Alpha- and beta-hemolytic streptococci, *Diplococcus pneumoniae*, staphylococci (nonpenicillinase-producing), *Bacillus anthracis*, clostridia spp., *Corynebacterium xerosis*, and most strains of enterococci.

The drug does not resist destruction by penicillinase; hence, it is not effective against penicillin-G-resistant staphylococci.

Gram-Negative: Hemophilus influenzae, Neisseria gonorrhoeae, Neisseria meningitidis, Proteus mirabilis, and many strains of Salmonella (including *Salmonella typhosa*), Shigella, and *Escherichia coli*.

Testing for Susceptibility: The invading organism should be cultured and its sensitivity demonstrated as a guide to therapy. If the Kirby-Bauer method of disc sensitivity is used, a 10-mcg ampicillin disc should be used to determine the relative *in vitro* susceptibility.

HUMAN PHARMACOLOGY
Ampicillin is stable in the presence of gastric acid and is well absorbed from the gastrointestinal tract. It diffuses readily into most body tissues and fluids. However, penetration into the cerebrospinal fluid and brain occurs only with meningeal inflammation. Ampicillin is excreted largely unchanged in the urine. Its excretion can be delayed by concurrent administration of probenecid.

Ampicillin is the least serum-bound of all the penicillins, averaging 20% compared to 60-90% for other penicillins.

Blood serum levels obtained on IM injection are proportionate to the dose administered. Levels of approximately 40 mcg/mL per 1-gram IM dose are attained at one-half hour. Higher levels are attainable with IV injection, depending on the dose and rate of administration.

Indications
Ampicillin is indicated primarily in the treatment of infections caused by susceptible strains of the following microorganisms: Shigella, Salmonella (including *S. typhosa*), *E. coli, H. influenzae, P. mirabilis, N. gonorrhoeae*, and enterococci. It is also effective in the treatment of meningitis due to *N. meningitidis*. Since it is effective against the commonest pathogens causing meningitis, it may be used intravenously as initial therapy before the results of bacteriology are available. Ampicillin is also indicated in certain infections caused by susceptible gram-positive organisms: penicillin-G-sensitive staphylococci, streptococci, and pneumococci. Bacteriologic studies to determine the causative organisms and their sensitivity to ampicillin should be performed. Therapy may be instituted prior to the results of culture and sensitivity testing.

It is advisable to reserve the parenteral form of this drug for moderately severe and severe infections and for patients who are unable to take the oral forms (capsules, oral suspension, or pediatric drops). A change to oral Omnipen (ampicillin) may be made as soon as appropriate.

In patients at particularly high risk for bacterial endocarditis (e.g., those with prosthetic heart valves), the American Heart Association recommends the use of parenteral prophylactic antibiotics prior to dental procedures and surgery of the upper respiratory tract and before genitourinary- or gastrointestinal-tract surgery and instrumentation.[1] (See "Dosage.")

Contraindications
Ampicillin is contraindicated in patients with a history of a hypersensitivity reaction to the penicillins.

Warnings
Serious and occasionally fatal hypersensitivity (anaphylactoid) reactions have been reported in patients on penicillin therapy. Although anaphylaxis is more frequent following parenteral therapy, it has occurred in patients on oral penicillins. These reactions are more apt to occur in individuals with a history of sensitivity to multiple allergens.

There have been reports of individuals with a history of penicillin hypersensitivity who experienced severe reactions when treated with cephalosporins. Before therapy with any penicillin, careful inquiry should be made concerning previous hypersensitivity reactions to penicillins, cephalosporins, or other allergens. If an allergic reaction occurs, appropriate therapy should be instituted and discontinuation of ampicillin therapy considered. **Serious anaphylactoid reactions require immediate emergency treatment with epinephrine. Oxygen, intravenous steroids, and airway management, including intubation, should be administered as indicated.**

USAGE IN PREGNANCY
Safety for use in pregnancy has not been established.

Precautions
As with any potent drug, periodic assessment of renal, hepatic, and hematopoietic function should be made during prolonged therapy.

The possibility of superinfections with mycotic or bacterial pathogens should be kept in mind during therapy. If superinfections occur, appropriate therapy should be instituted.

Adverse Reactions
As with other penicillins, it may be expected that untoward reactions will be essentially limited to sensitivity phenomena. They are more likely to occur in individuals who have previously demonstrated hypersensitivity to penicillins and in those with a history of allergy, asthma, hay fever, or urticaria.

The following adverse reactions have been reported in association with ampicillin uses:

GASTROINTESTINAL: Glossitis, stomatitis, nausea, vomiting, diarrhea. (These reactions are usually associated with oral dosage forms.)

HYPERSENSITIVITY: Erythematous maculopapular rashes have been reported fairly frequently. Urticaria, erythema multiforme, and an occasional case of exfoliative dermatitis have been reported. Anaphylaxis is the most serious reaction experienced and has usually been associated with the parenteral dosage form.

NOTE: Urticaria, other skin rashes, and serum-sicknesslike reactions may be controlled with antihistamines and, if necessary, systemic corticosteroids. Whenever such reactions occur, ampicillin should be discontinued, unless, in the opinion of the physician, the condition being treated is life-threatening and amenable only to ampicillin therapy. Serious anaphylactoid reactions require the immediate use of epinephrine, oxygen, and intravenous steroids.

HEPATIC: A moderate rise in serum glutamic-oxaloacetic transaminase (SGOT) has been noted, particularly in infants, but the significance of this finding is unknown.

HEMIC AND LYMPHATIC: Anemia, thrombocytopenia, thrombocytopenic purpura, eosinophilia, leukopenia, and agranulocytosis have been reported during therapy with the penicillins. These reactions are usually reversible on discontinuation of therapy and are believed to be hypersensitivity phenomena.

Dosage (IM or IV)

Infection	Organisms	Adults	Children*
Respiratory tract	streptococci, pneumococci, nonpenicillinase-producing staphylococci, *H. influenzae*	250-500 mg q. 6 h.	25-50 mg/kg/day in equal doses q. 6 h.
Gastrointestinal tract	susceptible pathogens	500 mg q. 6 h.	50 mg/kg/day in equal doses q. 6 h.
Genitourinary tract	susceptible gram-negative or gram-positive pathogens	500 mg q. 6 h.	50 mg/kg/day in equal doses q. 6 h.
Urethritis (acute) in adult males	N. gonorrhoeae	500 mg b.i.d. for 1 day (IM)	
	(In complications such as prostatitis and epididymitis, prolonged and intensive therapy is recommended. Gonorrhea cases with suspected primary lesion of syphilis should have dark-field examinations before treatment. In any case suspected of concomitant syphilis, monthly serologic tests for at least 4 months are necessary.)		
Bacterial meningitis	*N. meningitidis, H. influenzae*	8-14 gram/day	100-200 mg/kg/day
	(Initial treatment is usually by IV drip, followed by frequent [q. 3-4 h.] IM injections.)		
Bacterial endocarditis prophylaxis (See "Indications.")	*S. viridans*	Omnipen-N 1-2 gram PLUS Gentamicin 1.5 mg/kg (Both IM or IV 30 minutes before procedure)	Omnipen-N 50 mg/kg PLUS Gentamicin 2 mg/kg
	(Initial treatment is followed by either: one full parenteral dose 8 hours later; or oral penicillin V, 1 gram, 6 hours later.)		

***Children's dosage recommendations are intended for those whose weight will not result in a dosage higher than for the adult.**

Smaller doses than those recommended in the table above should not be used. In stubborn or severe infections, therapy may be required for several weeks, and even higher doses may be needed. In treatment of chronic urinary or intestinal infections, frequent bacteriological and clinical appraisal is necessary, with follow-up for several months after cessation of therapy.

Figure 11–5 An example of a package insert *(Courtesy of Wyeth Laboratories, Inc., Philadelphia, PA)*

Pediatric patients require a smaller amount of a medication because of differences in gastrointestinal function, body composition, metabolism and reduced renal function. The dosage is often determined by the size of the child rather than age. See Chapter 10.

Geriatric patients are not necessarily divided into a specific age group because of the wide variance in the aging process. A person who is 60 years old or older may or may not be considered a geriatric patient. Therefore, the physician will consider all factors, including the mental and physical state of the individual to determine an appropriate dosage regimen. The geriatric patient requires special considerations because of the following factors:

—Decreased gastrointestinal function that may cause poor absorption. Geriatric patients often suffer from constipation.

—Impaired or reduced metabolism.

—Changes in body composition; limitations, deformities.

—Alterations in circulation, liver and kidney function.

—Changes in body functioning; systems, eyes, ears, and speech.

—Sensitivity to drugs.

—Number of medications the patient is taking; drug interactions.

—Psychosocial changes:

Alertness	*Forgetfulness*
Confusion	*Misunderstanding of directions*
Attitude	*Memory loss*

—Disease process; multiple conditions.

—Self medication; over-the-counter (OTC) drugs.

—Cost.

—Living conditions; alone, with mate, nursing home or other care facility.

—Poor water intake.

- Pregnancy and lactation.
- The physical and emotional condition of the patient.
- The disease process.
- The presence of another disease process.
- The causative microorganism and the severity of the infection.
- The patient's past medical history, allergies, idiosyncrasies, and so forth.
- The safest method, route, time, and amount to effect the desired maximum result.

Terms Used to Describe Dosages

- An *initial dose* is the first dose.
- An *average dose* is the amount of medication proven most effective with minimum toxic effect.
- A *maintenance dose* is the amount that will keep concentrations of the drug at a therapeutic level in the patient's bloodstream.

- A *maximum dose* is the largest amount of a medication that can be given safely to a patient.
- A *therapeutic dose* is the amount needed to produce the desired effect.
- A *divided dose* is a fractional portion administered at short intervals.
- A *unit dose* is a premeasured amount of the medication, individually packaged on a per dose basis.
- A *cumulative dose* is the summation of the drug present in the body after repeated medication.
- A *lethal dose* is the amount of the medication that could kill a patient.
- A *toxic dose* is the amount of a drug that causes signs and symptoms of drug toxicity.
- A *minimum dose* is the smallest dose that will be effective.

◆ Review Questions

Directions: Select the best answer to each multiple choice question. Circle the letter of your choice.

1. The action to order or recommend the use of a drug, diet, or other form of therapy is known as ________.

   a. administer   b. dispense   c. prescribe   d. bioassay

2. The ________ name of a drug is its official name.

   a. chemical   b. generic   c. trade or brand   d. medical

3. Drugs are obtained from several sources. These include plants, animals, ________.

   a. and minerals
   b. minerals, and synthetics
   c. minerals, synthetics, and genetically engineered
   d. none of these

4. The Federal Food, Drug and Cosmetic Act ________.

   a. protects the public
   b. prohibits the movement, in interstate commerce, of adulterated and misbranded food, drugs, devices, and cosmetics
   c. both a and b
   d. none of these

5. ________ includes drugs that have an accepted medical use with certain restrictions.

   a. Schedule I
   b. Schedule II
   c. Schedule III
   d. Schedule IV
   e. Schedule V

6. Federal law requires that all controlled substances be ________.
   a. kept with other drugs
   b. stored in a substantially constructed metal box or compartment that is equipped with a double lock
   c. kept separate from other drugs
   d. both b and c
7. When preparing controlled substances for administration you must ________.
   a. be sure that the order sheet has been signed by two physicians
   b. have a witness during the preparation and administration process
   c. correctly record appropriate information concerning the preparation and administration of the controlled substance in a separate record book
   d. all of these
8. An average dose is the ________.
   a. first dose
   b. amount needed to produce the desired effect
   c. amount of medicine that could be lethal
   d. amount of medicine proven most effective with minimum toxic effect
9. The Federal Food, Drug and Cosmetic Act specifies that a drug is official when it is listed in the ________.
   a. *National Formulary*
   b. *Physicians' Desk Reference*
   c. *United States Pharmacopeia/National Formulary*
   d. all of these
10. The ________ is published annually by Medical Economics Company, Inc.
    a. *National Formulary*
    b. *Physician's Desk Reference*
    c. *United States Pharmacopeia*
    d. all of the above
11. If you know the brand name of a drug you would turn to the __________ section of a *Physician's Desk Reference.*
    a. Gray b. White c. Blue d. Pink
12. The amount of medicine that is prescribed for administration is known as ________.
    a. schedule b. dosage c. medication d. route
13. Factors that affect drug dosage are ________.
    a. weight, sex, and age
    b. pregnancy and lactation
    c. disease process
    d. none of the above

14. Pediatric patients require a ________ amount of a medication than adults.

    a. smaller b. larger c. greater d. none of the above

15. The geriatric patient requires special considerations because of ________.

    a. decreased gastrointestinal function

    b. changes in body compositions

    c. changes in body functioning

    d. all of the above

16. ________ is the summation of a drug present in the body after repeated medication.

    a. Maximum dose c. Cumulative dose

    b. Maintenance dose d. Average dose

Matching: Place the correct letter from Column II on the appropriate line of Column 1.

	Column I	Column II
17. ________	Abuse	A. To give.
18. ________	Toxicology	B. Pertaining to habit-forming.
19. ________	Pharmacodynamics	C. Being of mixed origin.
20. ________	Pharmacokinetics	D. To order or recommend the use of a drug, diet, or other form of therapy.
21. ________	Addictive	E. Producing sleep or stupor.
22. ________	Administer	F. The excessive or improper use of a substance, person, or animal.
23. ________	Hybrid	G. The study of drugs and their actions on living organisms.
24. ________	Narcotic	H. The study of the metabolism and actions of drugs within the body.
25. ________	Prescribe	I. The study of poisons.
		J. The study of drugs and their relationships to the treatment of disease.

CHAPTER 12

Forms of Drugs and How They Act

OBJECTIVES

Upon completion of this chapter, you should be able to:

- Define the terms listed in the vocabulary.
- List the forms in which drugs are prepared, and give examples of these preparations.
- List the routes used for drug administration.
- Classify drugs according to preparation and therapeutic action.
- Define selected classifications of drugs and give examples of each.
- List the three general ways that drugs may be grouped.
- Define the actions of drugs according to the descriptive terms listed in this chapter.
- Describe the factors that affect drug action.
- Describe the undesirable actions of drugs.
- Answer the review questions correctly.

Vocabulary

form (form). The shape, structure, and size of anything that distinguishes it from another object.

homogeneous (ho″mow-ge′ne-us). Similar or same in structure, composition or nature.

potency (po′ten-se). The power or strength of a substance.

solute (sol′ut). The substance that is dissolved to form a solution.

solvent (sol′vent). That in which a substance is dissolved.

suspended (sus-pend′ed). Large particles of a drug are dispersed or scattered in a liquid.

Introduction

Drugs are compounded in three basic types of preparations: liquids, solids, and semisolids. The ease with which a drug's ingredients can be dissolved largely determines the variety of *forms* manufactured. Some drug agents are soluble in water, others in alcohol, and yet others in a mixture of several *solvents.*

The method for administering a drug depends upon its form, its properties, and the effects desired. See Figure 12–1. When given orally, a drug may be in the form of a liquid, powder, tablet, capsule, or caplet. If it is to be injected, it must be in the form of a liquid. For topical use, the drug may be in the form of a liquid, a powder, or a semisolid. Oral and injectable medications are examples of preparations designed for *internal use.*

Forms of Drugs

Liquid Preparations

Liquid preparations are those containing a drug that has been dissolved or suspended. Depending upon the solvent used, the drug may be further classified as an aqueous (water) or alcohol preparation. When prescribed for internal use, liquid preparations other than emulsions are rapidly absorbed through the stomach or intestinal walls. The following are types of liquid preparations.

- *Emulsions.* Emulsions consist of fine droplets of an oil in water or water in oil. They separate into layers after standing for long periods of time and must be shaken vigorously before they are ready for use. An example of an emulsion is castor oil.
- *Solutions.* One or more drugs can be dissolved in an appropriate solvent to make a solution. The solution will appear to be clear and homogeneous. An example of a solution is normal saline.
- *Mixtures and suspensions.* Drugs that have been mixed with a liquid, but not dissolved, are called mixtures or suspensions. These preparations must be shaken before being administered to the patient. Milk of magnesia is an example of a mixture or suspension.

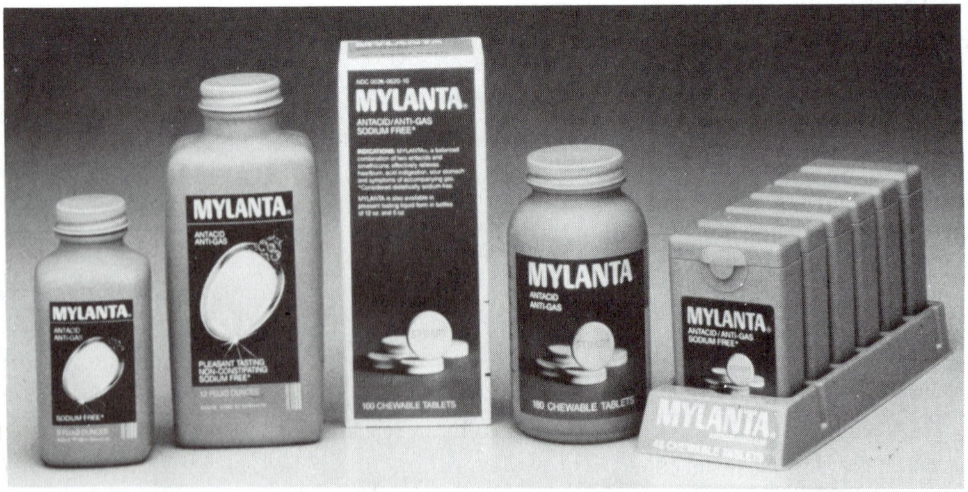

Figure 12–1 Mylanta liquid and tablets *(Courtesy of Stuart Pharmaceuticals)*

- *Syrups.* Drugs dissolved in a solution of sugar and water and then flavored are called syrups. An example is Benylin DM cough syrup.
- *Elixirs.* Drugs dissolved in a solution of alcohol and water that has been sweetened and flavored are elixirs. When prepared in this manner, the bitter or salty taste of the drug is disguised. For this reason, elixirs are frequently used for children's medications. An example of an elixir is Donnatal® (phenobarbital, hyoscyamine sulfate, atropine sulfate, and scopolamine hydrobromide). Donnatal is also available in tablets and capsules. See Figure 12–2.
- *Tinctures.* Tinctures are drugs dissolved in alcohol or alcohol and water. For the most part, they are made to represent 10 percent of the drug agent. An example is tincture of digitalis. Another example, tincture of iodine, is an exception to the 10 percent rule. It may be found as a 7 percent or 2 percent tincture.
- *Spirits.* Alcoholic solutions of volatile (easily vaporized) drugs are called spirits. A spirit is also called an essence. Examples are spirits of peppermint and aromatic spirits of ammonia.
- *Fluidextracts.* Drugs that have been processed to a concentrated strength using alcohol as the solvent are called fluidextracts. Examples include fluidextract of ergot, fluidextract of ipecac, and cascara sagrada fluidextract.

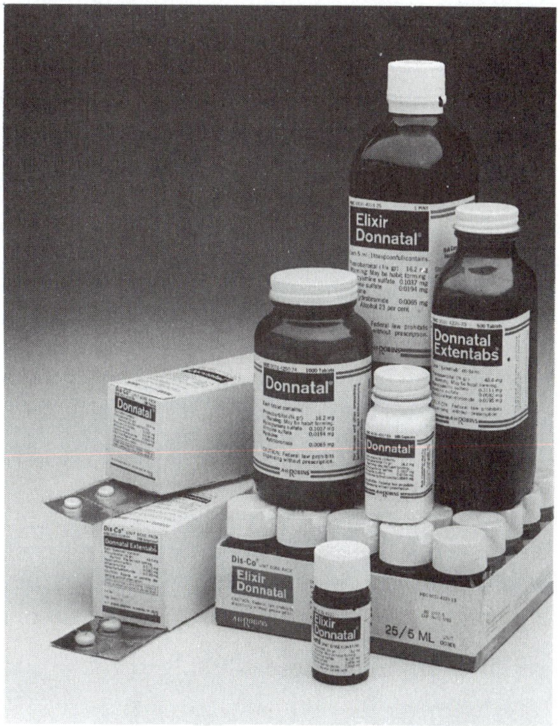

Figure 12–2 Donnatal Elixir, tablets, Extentabs, and capsules *(Courtesy of A. H. Robins Company)*

- *Lotions.* Aqueous preparations of suspended ingredients used externally (without massage) to treat skin conditions are lotions. They may be a clear solution, suspension, or emulsion. Examples are Calamine lotion, and Caladryl.
- *Liniments.* Liniments are drugs that are used externally, with massage, to produce a feeling of heat to the area. An example is methyl salicylate.
- *Sprays.* As the name implies, sprays are drugs prepared to such a consistency that they may be administered by an atomizer. They are used primarily to treat nose and throat conditions. Some drugs administered by this method function as astringents and produce a shrinking or contracting effect. Others function as antiseptics and inhibit the growth of bacteria. Oil is usually used as a solvent. An example of a spray is Neo-synephrine®.
- *Aerosols.* These preparations may contain medications, ointments, creams, lotions, powders, or liquids. They utilize a propellant, such as butane and are packaged in pressurized units. An example is Azmacort™ inhaler in a metered-dose aerosol unit. Azmacort is an anti-inflammatory steroid. (See Figure 15–20 in Chapter 15, page 214.)

Solid and Semisolid Preparations

Tablets, capsules, caplets, troches or lozenges, suppositories, and ointments are examples of solid and semisolid preparations. These products offer great flexibility as a means of dispensing different dosages of drugs. See Figure 12–3. The following describes these products in detail.

- *Capsules* are small, two-part containers (hard or soft shell) which are usually made of a gelatin substance that is designed to dissolve in the stomach or gastrointestinal tract. Some capsules contain drug-impregnated beads (sustained-action) that are designed to release the medication at different rates.
- *Caplets* have the size and shape of a capsule, but the consistency of a tablet. They are coated, solid preparations for oral administration.
- *Tablets* are medication in the form of a powder that has been compressed into a small, disklike shape. Tablets come in various sizes, shapes, colors, and compositions. The following are some of the descriptive names for certain tablets.

  —*Enteric-coated* tablets are designed to pass through the stomach without dissolving. Their special coating will dissolve in the small intestine.

  —*Buccal* tablets are formulated to be dissolved and absorbed when placed between the cheek and gum.

  —*Sublingual* tablets are designed to be placed under the tongue where they dissolve and are absorbed.

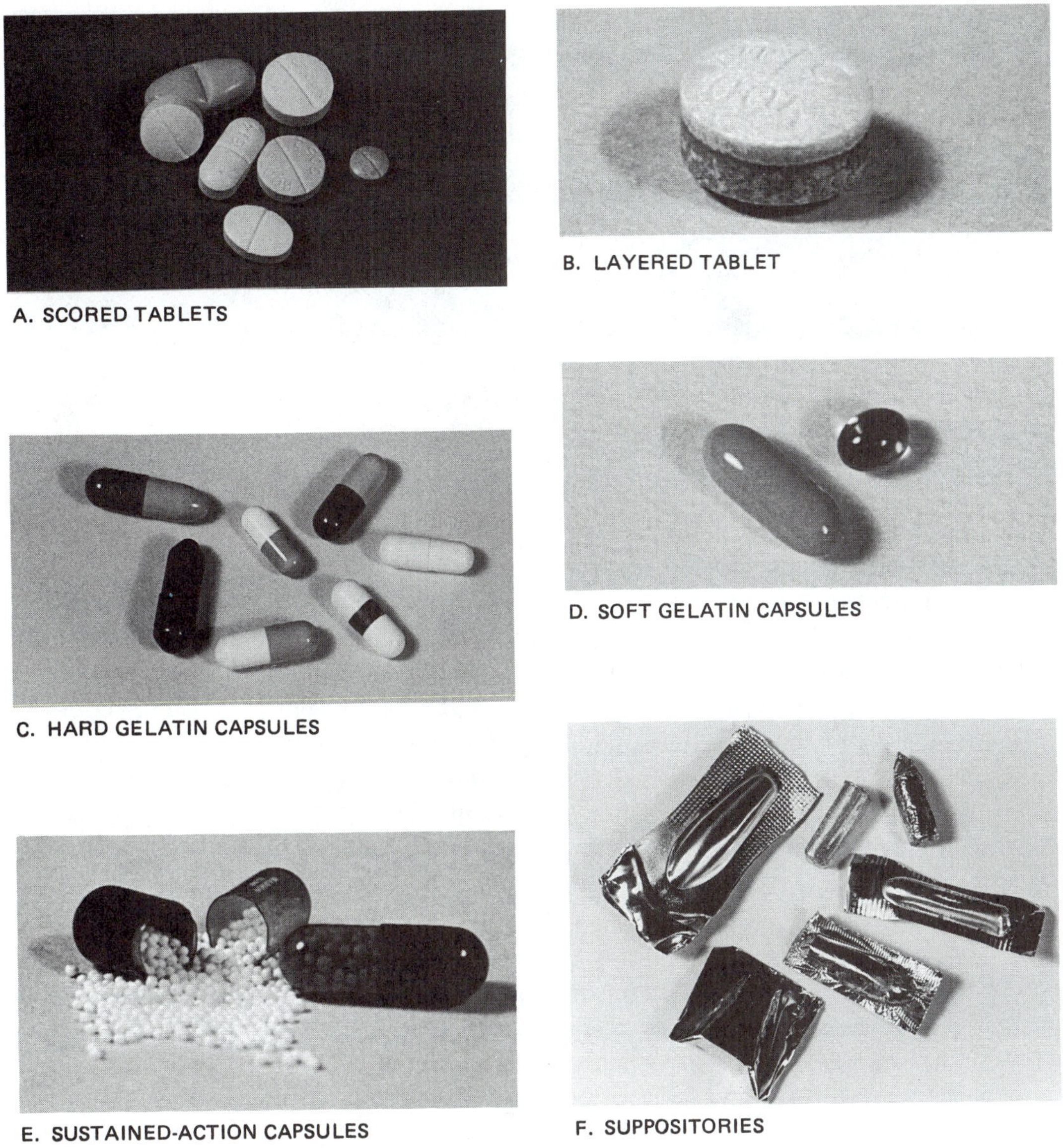

Figure 12–3 Examples of solid and semisolid preparations

—*Layered* tablets contain two or more layers of ingredients, or the same ingredient that has been treated to provide a different absorption rate.

—*Scored* tablets are those whose surfaces have been bisected by a groove to make it easy for the user to break them into halves or quarters in order to vary the dosage. See Figure 12–4.

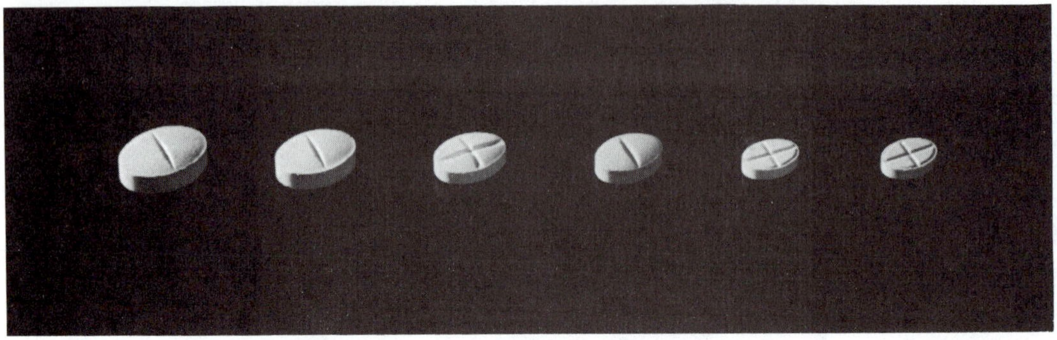

Figure 12–4 Medrol scored tablets (2, 4, 8, 16, 24, and 32 mg) *(Courtesy of The Upjohn Company)*

- *Troches* or *lozenges* are hard, circular or oblong discs that consist of a medication in a candy-like base. They dissolve in the mouth and are commonly used to treat a sore throat. The effectiveness of this medication is destroyed by drinking liquids too soon after use.
- *Suppositories* are semisolid preparations designed for insertion into the rectum, vagina, or urethra. A suppository consists of a drug agent or agents combined with a base of soap, glycerinated gelatin, or cocoa butter oil. These bases are selected because they are readily fusible (will melt) when subjected to body heat. Suppositories are usually shaped like a cylinder or cone and are classified as drugs for external use. Often supplied in a foil or other wrapper that must be removed before insertion, suppositories are usually lubricated with a water soluble jelly.
- *Topical* preparations are designed for use on the skin. They exert either a local or systemic effect. Their mode of action depends upon the composition of the drug or drugs contained within the preparation. They may be compounded with an oily base (ointments) or a water base (lotions, creams). See Figure 12–5 for an example of a cream. Other topical preparations may be in the form of a liniment, oil, gel, foam, soap, or powder.

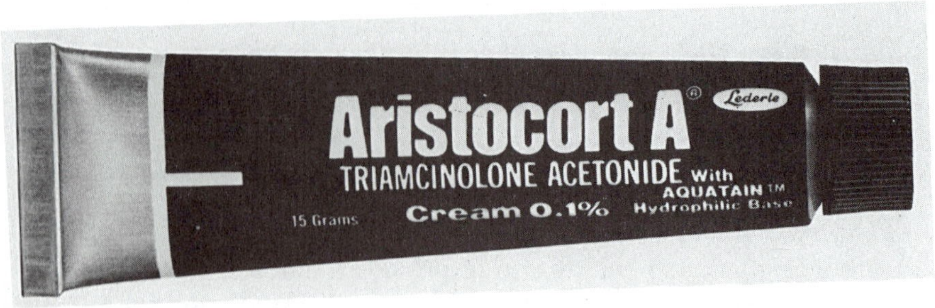

Figure 12–5 Aristocort A® cream 0.1% *(Courtesy of Lederle Laboratories Division of American Cyanamid Company)*

Other Drug Delivery Systems

Technological advances have introduced new ways by which drugs can be introduced into the patient. In addition to the conventional preparations already covered, the following miniature therapeutic systems offer "special delivery" of medication to targeted areas.

Transdermal System. A small adhesive patch that may be applied to intact skin near the treatment site. For example, Transderm Scop® used for preventing motion sickness may be applied behind the ear; Transderm-Nitro® used for preventing angina pectoris may be applied to the chest; Estraderm used to treat menopausal symptoms may be applied to the trunk and Nicoderm® used to relieve the body's craving for nicotine may be applied to any area above the waist. A transdermal system generally consists of four layers (see Figure 12–6):

1. An impermeable backing that keeps the drug from leaking out of the system.
2. A reservoir containing the drug.
3. A membrane with tiny holes in it that controls the rate of drug release.
4. An adhesive layer or gel that keeps the device in place.

Eye-curing Lens. Another innovative drug delivery system in which a drug contained between two ultrathin plastic membranes is placed inside the lower eyelid. It appears to cause little or no discomfort and provides a controlled release of the medication for an extended period of time. Pilocarpine, a miotic that causes contraction of the pupil, is being used in this method for the treatment of glaucoma.

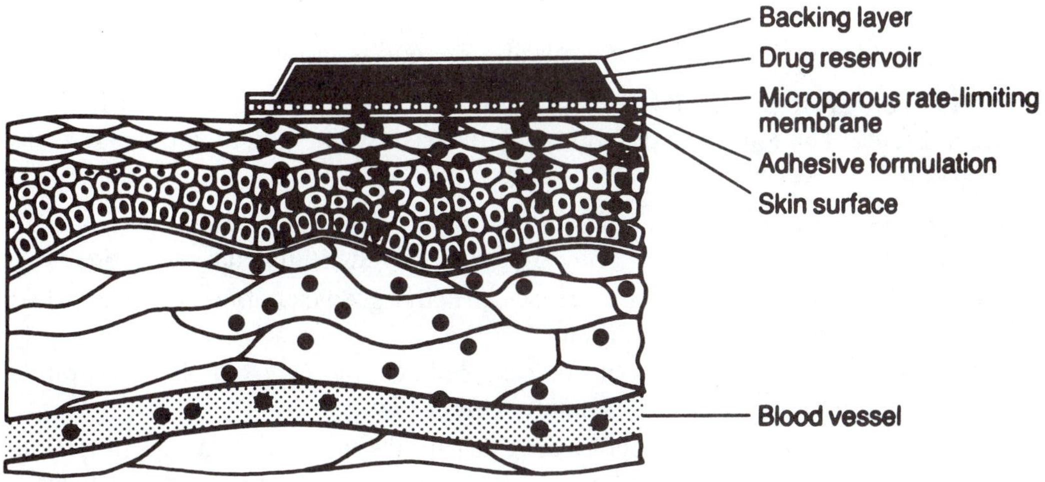

Figure 12–6 The multilayer unit comprising Transderm-Nitro® delivers nitroglycerin into the bloodstream in a consistent controlled manner for 24 hours. The very thin unit contains a backing layer, a reservoir of nitroglycerin, a unique rate-limiting membrane, and an adhesive layer that has a priming dose of nitroglycerin. *(Courtesy of CIBA Pharmaceutical Company)*

Implantable Devices. These devices come in several shapes and sizes and are positioned just beneath the skin, near blood vessels that lead directly to an area to be medicated. For example, an infusion pump that is about the size of a hockey puck can be implanted below the skin, near the waist to provide continuous delivery of chemotherapy to patients with liver cancer. This device, which has a refillable drug reservoir, is connected by an outlet catheter to the patient's blood vessel. In addition to providing a continuous supply of medication, these devices have the advantage of delivering higher doses with fewer side effects than can be realized through the systemic route.

Classification of Drugs/Therapeutic Action

There are many ways that drugs are classified. Two of these ways are by preparation and by therapeutic action. The therapeutic action of the drug involves the process of treating, rclicving, or obtaining results through the action of the medication upon the body. Table 12–1 includes selected classifications, pronunciation guide, action, and examples.

Principle Actions of Drugs

Drugs may be used as a cure for disease. They may also be used to restore a disturbed or diseased physical state to one that is normal or improved. In the latter case, drugs assist the body to overcome its own difficulties by causing a change in cell activity without altering basic cell functions. In general, drugs may be grouped as follows:

- Those that act directly upon one or more tissues of the body.
- Those that act upon microorganisms invading the body (chemotherapy and antibiotics).
- Those that replace body chemicals and secretions (hormones).

Certain drugs are prescribed because of the selective actions that result when they are administered. The following descriptive terms have been applied to drugs because of the action that takes place:

- *Selective action* is a term applied to drugs that act upon certain tissues or on specific organs of the body. They are principally the stimulants and depressants.
  —*Stimulants* are drugs that increase cell activity. An example is caffeine, which acts to stimulate the cerebrum.
  —*Depressants* are drugs that decrease cell activity. An example is morphine, that acts to depress the respiratory center in the brain.
- *Agonist action* is that in which a drug has affinity for the cellular receptors (specific sites in certain cells) of another drug or natural substance and initiates/produces a drug response.
- *Antagonist action* is that in which a drug binds to a cellular receptor for a hormone, neurotransmitter, or another drug blocking the action of that substance without producing any drug effect itself.

Table 12–1 Selected Drug Classification

Classification	Action	Examples
Analgesic (an″al-je′sik)	An agent that relieves pain without causing loss of consciousness.	acetaminophen (Tylenol) aspirin ibuprofen (Advil, Motrin)
Anesthetic (an″es-thet′ik)	An agent that produces a lack of feeling. May be local or general depending upon the type and how administered.	lidocaine HCL (Xylocaine) procaine HCL (Novocain)
Antacid (ant-as′id)	An agent that neutralizes acid.	Amphojel, Gelusil, Mylanta, Aludrox, Milk of Magnesia
Antianxiety (an″ti-ang-zi′e-te)	An agent that relieves anxiety and muscle tension.	benzodiazepines: diazepam (Valium) and chlordiazepoxide HCL (Librium)
Antiarrhythmic (an″te-a-rith′mik)	An agent that controls cardiac arrhythmias.	lidocaine HCL (Xylocaine) propranolol HCL (Inderal)
Antibiotic (an″ti-bi-ot′ik)	An agent that is destructive to or inhibits growth of microorganisms.	penicillins (Pentids, Duracillin, Polycillin, Pipracil, Augmentin) cephalosporins (Keflin, Mandol, Rocephin)
Anticholinergic (an″ti-ko″lin-er′jik)	An agent that blocks parasympathetic nerve impulses.	atropine, scopolamine, trihexyphenidyl HCL (Artane)
Anticoagulant (an″ti-ko-ag′u-lant)	An agent that prevents or delays blood clotting.	heparin sodium, Dicumarol, warfarin sodium (Coumadin)
Anticonvulsant (an″ti-kon-vul′sant)	An agent that prevents or relieves convulsions.	carbamazepine (Tegretol) phenytoin (Dilantin) ethosuximide (Zarontin)
Antidepressant (an″ti-dep-res′ant)	An agent that prevents or relieves the symptoms of depression.	monoamine oxidase (MAO) inhibitors: isocarboxazid (Marplan), phenelzine sulfate (Nardil), amitriptyline HCL (Elavil), imipramine HCL (Tofranil)
Antidiarrheal (an″ti-di-a-re′al)	An agent that prevents or relieves diarrhea.	Lomotil, Pepto-Bismol, Kaopectate
Antidote (an-ti′dot)	An agent that counteracts poisons and their effects.	naloxone (Narcan)
Antiemetic (an″ti-e-met′ik)	An agent that prevents or relieves nausea and vomiting.	Tigan, Dramamine, Phenergan, Reglan, Marinol
Antihistamine (an″ti-his′ta-min)	An agent that acts to prevent the action of histamine.	Dimetane, Benadryl, Seldane
Antihypertensive (an″ti-hi″per-ten′siv)	An agent that prevents or controls high blood pressure.	methyldopa (Aldomet) clonidine HCL (Catapres) metoprolol tartrate (Lopressor)
Anti-inflammatory (an″ti-in-flam′a-to-re)	An agent that prevents inflammation.	naproxen (Naprosyn), aspirin, ibuprofen (Advil, Motrin)
Antimanic (an″ti-man′ik)	An agent used for the treatment of the manic episode of manic-depressive disorder.	lithium

(continued)

Table 12–1 Selected Drug Classification (*Continued*)

Classification	Action	Examples
Antineoplastic (an″ti-ne″o-plas′tik)	An agent that prevents the replication of neoplastic cells.	busulfan (Myleran) cyclophosphamide (Cytoxan)
Antipyretic (an″ti-pi-ret′ik)	An agent that reduces fever.	aspirin, acetaminophen (Tylenol)
Antitussive (an″ti-tus′iv)	An agent that prevents or relieves cough.	codeine, dextrometorphan
Bronchodilator (brong″ko-dil-a′tor)	An agent that dilates the bronchi.	isoproterenol HCL (Isuprel) albuterol (Proventil)
Contraceptive (kon″tra-sep′tiv)	Any device, method, or agent that prevents conception.	Enovid-E 21, Ortho-Novum 10/11-21; 10/11-28 Triphasil-21
Decongestant (de″con-gest′ant)	An agent that reduces nasal congestion and/or swelling.	oxymetazoline (Afrin) phenylephrine HCL (Neo-Synephrine) pseudoephedrine HCL (Sudafed)
Diuretic (di″u-ret′ik)	An agent that increases the excretion of urine.	chlorothiazide (Diuril) furosemide (Lasix) mannitol (Osmitrol)
Expectorant (ek-spek′to-rant)	An agent that facilitates removal of secretion from broncho-pulmonary mucous membrane.	guaifenesin (Robitussin)
Hemostatic (he″mo-stat′ik)	An agent that controls or stops bleeding.	Humafac, Amicar, vitamin K
Hypnotic (hip-not′ik)	An agent that produces sleep or hypnosis.	secobarbital (Seconal); chloral hydrate; ethchlorvynol (Placidyl)
Hypoglycemic (hi″po-gli-se′mik)	An agent that lowers blood glucose level.	insulin; chlorpropamide (Diabinese)
Laxative (lak′sa-tiv)	An agent that loosens and promotes normal bowel elimination.	Metamucil powder, Dulcolax
Muscle relaxant (mus′el re-lak′sant)	An agent that produces relaxation of skeletal muscle.	Robaxin, Norflex, Paraflex, Skelaxin, Valium
Sedative (sed′a-tiv)	An agent that produces a calming effect without causing sleep.	amobarbital (Amytal) Butabarbital sodium (Buticaps) phenobarbital
Tranquilizer (tran″kwi-liz′er)	An agent that reduces mental tension and anxiety.	Thorazine, Mellaril, Haldol
Vasodilator (vas″o-di-la′tor)	An agent that produces relaxation of blood vessels; lowers blood pressure.	isorbide dinitrate (Isordil) nitroglycerin
Vasopressor (vas″o-pres′or)	An agent that produces contraction of muscles, of capillaries and arteries; elevates blood pressure.	metaraminol (Aramine) norepinephrine (Levophed)

Note: A receptor is a receiver, a cell component that combines with a hormone, neurotransmitter, or drug to alter the function of the cell.

- *Local action* is the term applied to an external drug designed to act on the area to which it is administered. An example is methyl salicylate, a medication that is often applied to sore muscles or painful joints by rubbing it into the affected area.
- *Remote action* is the term applied to a drug affecting a part of the body that is distant from the site of administration. An example is an apomorphine injection into the arm to stimulate the vomiting center in the brain.
- *Specific action* is the term applied to a drug that has a particular effect on a certain pathogenic organism. An example is the action of primaquine on the malarial parasite.
- *Systemic action* is the term applied to a drug that, when in the bloodstream as a result of injection or absorption, is carried throughout the body.

Factors That Affect Drug Action

The principal factors that affect drug action are: absorption, distribution, biotransformation, and elimination. These factors depend upon the individual patient, the form and chemical composition of the drug, and the method of administration.

- *Absorption* is the process whereby the drug passes into body fluids and tissues. The rate of absorption depends on the route of administration, the drug, differences in gastrointestinal function (pediatrics and geriatrics), and individual differences.
- *Distribution* is the process whereby the drug is transported from the blood to the intended site of action, site of biotransformation, site of storage, and site of elimination. The rate and extent of distribution depends upon the physical and chemical properites of the drug, the ability of the drug to bind to plasma proteins, and individual differences (such as cardiovascular function).
- *Biotransformation* is the chemical alteration that a substance (drug) undergoes in the body. Through this process enzymes may be activated to break down the drug and prepare it for elimination. Most biotransformation occurs in the liver.
- *Elimination* is the process whereby a substance is excreted from the body. Many drugs are eliminated via the kidneys, while others may be eliminated via the gastrointestinal tract, respiratory tract, the skin, mucous membranes, and mammary glands (breast feeding).

Undesirable Actions of Drugs

Most drugs have the potential for causing an action other than their intended action. For example certain antibiotics that are administered orally may disrupt the normal bacterial flora of the gastrointestinal tract and cause gastric discomfort. This type of reaction is known as a side effect. A *side effect* is an undesirable action of the drug and may limit the usefulness of the drug.

An *adverse reaction* is an unfavorable or harmful unintended action of a drug. Using a recent edition of the Physician's Desk Reference look up Demerol® and note the adverse reactions. Lightheadedness, dizziness, sedation, nausea, and sweating are the most frequent adverse reactions to Demerol. To report an adverse reaction to a drug, you may call 1-800-FDA-1088.

A drug *interaction* may occur when one drug potentiates or diminishes the action of another drug. These actions may be desirable or undesirable. Drugs may also interact with various foods, alcohol, tobacco, and other substances. It is recommended that a pharmacist be consulted any time there is the possibility of a drug interaction.

Loss of Drug Potency

The factors that determine the life of a drug include date of manufacture, the type of container in which it is packaged, the method of storage, and the drug's unique properties. Drugs, such as antibiotics, have an expiration date imprinted on their packages. Beyond this date, the product should not be used due to its gradual deterioration or change in potency.

Glass and/or plastic containers are often used to package medications because they allow the contents to be seen without exposure to air. Most unit dose medications are packaged within individual clear plastic envelopes that have a foil backing. Other medications require dark (opaque) containers to prevent deterioration due to exposure to light. Certain medications, such as reconstituted antibiotics, have to be refrigerated to prevent deterioration. Other drugs require the presence of an absorbent material to remove moisture from the air within the container; otherwise, the moisture would be absorbed by the drug, affecting its potency.

◆ Review Questions

Directions: Select the best answer to each multiple choice question. Circle the letter of your choice.

1. Tablets that are designed to dissolve in the intestines and not in the stomach are known as __________.

   a. buccal b. layered c. sublingual d. enteric-coated

2. The term solvent means __________.

   a. similar or same structure
   b. strength of a substance
   c. that in which a substance is dissolved
   d. the substance that is dissolved to form a solution

3. Drugs are compounded in three basic types of preparations. These types are __________.
   a. hypodermic, oral, sublingual
   b. oral, parenteral, topical
   c. liquids, solids, and semisolids
   d. intradermal, intramuscular, intravenous
4. The correct definition of an elixir is a/an __________.
   a. drug dissolved in a solution of alcohol and water which has been sweetened and flavored
   b. drug dissolved in a solution of sugar and water and then flavored
   c. drug made to represent 10 percent of the drug agent
   d. alcoholic solution that is easily vaporized
5. __________ tablets are designed to be placed under the tongue where they dissolve and are absorbed.
   a. Scored b. Layered c. Sublingual d. Enteric-coated
6. The following are all true statements about suppositories except:
   a. semisolid preparations
   b. usually lubricated with a water soluble jelly before insertion
   c. will not melt when subjected to body heat
   d. classification as drugs for external use
7. __________ is a small adhesive patch or disc that may be attached to the body near the treatment site.
   a. Eye-curing lens
   b. Implanted device
   c. Transdermal system
   d. all of these
8. Drugs that increase cell activity are known as __________.
   a. depressants b. stimulants c. antibiotics d. hormones
9. An unfavorable or harmful action induced by resistance to another action is known as __________.
   a. addiction
   b. local action
   c. adverse reaction
   d. specific action
10. The factors that determine the life of a drug are __________.
    a. date of manufacture
    b. type of container in which it is packaged
    c. method of storage
    d. all of these
11. Xylocaine and Novocain are examples of __________.
    a. analgesics b. anesthetics c. hypnotics d. sedatives

12. An agent that blocks parasympathetic nerve impulses is known as __________.
    a. anticonvulsant c. antidepressant
    b. anticholinergic d. antidiarrheal
13. Dicumarol and Coumadin are examples of __________.
    a. antiarrhythmics c. anticoagulants
    b. anticholinergics d. anticonvulsants
14. Dimetane, Benadryl, and Seldane are examples of__________.
    a. antihistamines c. antihypertensives
    b. antiemetics d. antitussives
15. An agent that prevents the replication of neoplastic cells is called an __________.
    a. antipyretic c. antineoplastic
    b. anti-inflammatory d. antimanic
16. Aspirin and acetaminophen are examples of __________.
    a. analgesics and antipyretics
    b. antitussives and decongestants
    c. antihistamines and antiemetics
    d. antidotes and antibiotics
17. The most frequently utilized routes of administering medications to a patient are __________.
    a. sublingual and buccal c. rectal and vaginal
    b. oral and parenteral d. inhalation and instillation
18. Medications applied directly to the skin may be in the form of __________.
    a. lotions, creams c. transdermal systems
    b. liniments, ointments d. all of the above
19. An agent that lowers blood glucose level is known as __________.
    a. hyperglycemic c. hypoglycemic
    b. hypnotic d. hypertensive
20. Diuril and Lasix are examples of __________.
    a. muscle relaxants b. diuretics c. antidiuretics d. antiemetics
21. An agent that reduces mental tension and anxiety is known as a __________.
    a. sedative b. hypnotic c. muscle relaxant d. tranquilizer
22. __________ action occurs when the drug is absorbed into the bloodstream.
    a. Local b. Remote c. Systemic d. Antagonist
23. A __________ is a receiver, a cell component that combines with a hormone, neurotransmitter, or a drug to alter the function of the cell.
    a. receptor b. stimulant c. depressant d. none of the above

24. __________ is the process whereby the drug passes into body fluids and tissues.
    a. Absorption
    b. Distribution
    c. Biotransformation
    d. Elimination

25. A (An) __________ is an unfavorable or harmful unintended action of a drug.
    a. interaction
    b. side effect
    c. adverse reaction
    d. specific action

Matching: Place the correct letter from Column II on the appropriate line of Column I.

Column I

26. __________ Form
27. __________ Homogeneous
28. __________ Potency
29. __________ Solute
30. __________ Solvent

Column II

A. That in which a substance is dissolved.
B. The substance that is dissolved to form a solution.
C. Similar or same in structure, composition, or nature.
D. The shape, structure, and size of anything that distinguishes it from another.
E. The power or strength of a substance.
F. The color and consistency of a substance.

CHAPTER 13

The Medication Order

OBJECTIVES

Upon completion of this chapter, you should be able to:

- Define the terms listed in the vocabulary.
- Describe the following types of medication orders: PRN, routine, single, standing, stat, written, verbal, telephone, and prescription.
- State the essential information that is included on a medication order.
- Define the following prescription terms: superscription, inscription, subscription, and signature.
- List seven guidelines for understanding the medication order.
- Describe the medication record forms given in this chapter.
- Understand medication labels (prescription and nonprescription).
- Give the time schedule that may be used for routine medications.
- Read and write the common medical abbreviations given in this chapter.
- Answer the review questions correctly.

Vocabulary

compounding (kom-pound′ing). The process of combining and mixing.

pharmacist (far′ma-sist). One who is licensed to prepare and dispense drugs.

How Medication Orders Are Given

It is the physician's responsibility to diagnose the cause of an illness and to prescribe a medication. The drug prescribed is generally referred to as a *medication* or *medicine order.* Once prescribed, it is the responsibility of any legally approved health professional to carry out the physician's medication order. Thus, it is essential that those whose duties include giving medications be familiar with the methods used to give such orders.

The medicine order, written by the physician, is for a specific patient. The order designates the drug to be used, the dosage, the form of the drug, the time or frequency for administration, and the method or route by which it is to be given.

Types of Medication Orders

- *PRN Order.* With this type of order, medication is given "as necessary" or "when needed." The physician orders the drug, dosage, frequency, and route, and may give the purpose for the administration.

Example: Demerol (meperidine hydrochloride) 75 mg IM q̄ 4h PRN for severe pain.

A PRN order for a narcotic is permissible, but *must be rewritten* every 3 to 5 days, depending upon the policy of the health care facility.

- *Routine Order.* This is a prescribed, detailed course of action that is to be followed regularly. The physician orders the medication, dosage, route, and frequency, and gives the purpose for the administration.

Example: Tylenol 1–2 tabs by mouth q̄ 4–6h for a temperature above 100°F or 37.8°C.

This type of order is not permissible for narcotic drugs or barbiturates.

- *Single Order.* This type is given *one time only.* The physician orders the medication, dosage, route, and time for administration, and gives the purpose for the administration.

Example: Demerol (meperidine hydrochloride) 100 mg IM 1h before surgery.

- *Standing Order.* A type of protocol that is predetermined by a physician (or group of physicians) that sets forth specific instructions, guidelines, procedures, treatments, and/or medications for various patient care situations.

Example: Dulcolax suppository i̇ q̄ am for constipation.

- *Stat Order.* An order for *immediate* administration of a medication. The physician may write it as NOW rather than *stat* to guarantee that the medication is given at once. The physician gives the name of the drug, dosage, route, and time for administration (NOW).

Example: Hyperstat (diazoxide) 100 mg IV NOW.

- *Written Order.* One that is inscribed by a physician (or other qualified practitioner) onto one of the following: the physician's order sheet, or a prescription for a patient. Legally, this is the best type of medication order. Courts usually do not question the legality of a drug order that was written and signed by a physician; nor do they usually question an order written by another health professional and countersigned by a physician. (As long as such order is a safe drug, safe dose, and so forth.) Any order that is illegible or questionable must be verified with the physician before the medication is administered.
- *Verbal Order (VO).* One expressed by speech and not written out. Student nurses should *never* take a verbal or telephone order. Licensed or certified health care providers should protect themselves by:

1. Writing down the order exactly as heard.
2. Repeating the order back to the physician.
3. Following the "Six Rights" of proper drug administration. (See Chapter 14.)
4. Carefully documenting all appropriate information about the administration.
5. Having the physician *cosign the order* within twenty-four hours.

- *Telephone Order (TO).* A type of verbal order that is transmitted via a telecommunication system. Telephone and verbal narcotic orders are approved, with reluctance, by the Narcotics Bureau. The Bureau has made this major concession to hospitals for use in a true emergency situation. Whenever possible, it is a good idea to have another person listen on an extension phone when verbal orders are transmitted via the telephone.
- *Prescription.* A prescription is a separate written order that is not a part of the patient's chart. Its purpose is to control the sale and use of drugs that can be used safely or effectively only under the supervision of a physician. A prescription is not needed for over-the-counter (OTC) drugs.

Parts of a Prescription (Refer to Figure 13–1)

1. The physician's name, address, telephone number, and registration number.
2. The patient's name, address, and the date on which the prescription is written.

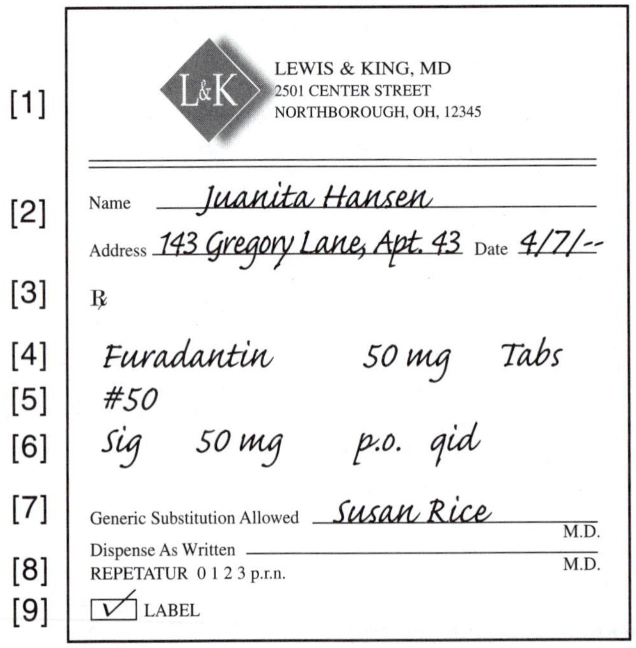
[1] L&K LEWIS & KING, MD
2501 CENTER STREET
NORTHBOROUGH, OH, 12345
[2] Name Juanita Hansen
Address 143 Gregory Lane, Apt. 43 Date 4/7/--
[3] ℞
[4] Furadantin 50 mg Tabs
[5] #50
[6] Sig 50 mg p.o. qid
[7] Generic Substitution Allowed Susan Rice M.D.
Dispense As Written M.D.
[8] REPETATUR 0 1 2 3 p.r.n.
[9] ☑ LABEL

Figure 13–1 Parts of a prescription

3. The *superscription* that includes the symbol ℞ ("take thou").
4. The *inscription* that states the names and quantities of ingredients to be included in the medication.
5. The *subscription* that gives directions to the pharmacist for filling the prescription.
6. The *signature* (Sig) that gives the directions for the patient.
7. The physician's signature blanks. Where signed, indicates if a generic substitute is allowed or if the medication is to be dispensed as written.
8. REPETATUR 0 1 2 3 PRN. This is where the physician indicates whether or not the prescription can be refilled.
9. ☐ LABEL Direction to the pharmacist to label the medication appropriately.

Guidelines for Understanding the Medication Order

1. Become knowledgeable about the medications that the physician prescribes.
   - Make a list of the drugs.
   - Make a drug card for each drug.
   - File each drug card (in alphabetical order or according to classification) in a small metal box.
2. Write down each verbal order exactly as heard.
3. Repeat the order back to the physician.
4. Make sure you understand the medication order before administering any drug.
5. If there are any questions, ask before giving.
6. If you are ever in doubt, seek the assistance of the physician.
7. Be knowledgeable of new drugs on the market, especially any new drugs that the physician may order for specific disease processes.

Medication Record Forms

The medication record may consist of a physician's order sheet or a prescription, a medication sheet, a pharmacy patient profile, a medication administration form (Kardex, Medex), a controlled substance record book and audit form, the nurse's notes, and/or a computerized medication administration record.

Selected examples of typical medication record forms, with accompanying illustrations, have been included to acquaint you with these important documents.

The *Physician's Order Sheet* is a triplicate document containing a place for the date, time, medication order, and a patient's drug sensitivity. The physician, using one order form per patient, writes on the form the medications to be administered, and signs the order. The original is maintained on the patient's chart, a copy goes to the pharmacy, and a copy goes to the medication nurse. See Figure 13–2 for an example of a physician's order sheet.

ALBANY MEDICAL CENTER HOSPITAL

Physician's Order Sheet

INSTRUCTIONS:
1. Imprint patient's plate before placing in chart.
2. After each set of orders are written, remove first yellow copy and send to PHARMACY.
3. "X" out remaining unused lines after last copy is used.
4. Imprint new set and place in chart.

ALLERGIES:

Date Ordered	Time Ordered	Time Executed	Time Posted	USE BALL POINT PEN ONLY
				Present Weight lbs. kg. Present Height in. cm.

"ALL ORDERS SHOULD BE PRECEDED BY THE NUMBER AND TITLE OF THE PROBLEM TO WHICH THEY REFER. NUMBER ONE (# 1) IS RESERVED FOR ROUTINE ADMISSION AND MAINTENANCE ORDERS."

Figure 13–2 Example of a physician's order sheet. Always remember to imprint the patient's identification plate in the space provided in the upper right-hand corner. *(Courtesy of Albany Medical Center, Albany, NY)*

The physician's order is then transcribed onto a medical administration form (Kardex, Medex). The transcribed order is initialed by the transcriber who may be the charge nurse, the medication nurse, a ward secretary, or other person authorized by the employer to perform this task. The nurse giving the medication is ultimately responsible for the proper transcription of the medication order. If there is any reason for doubt, the order and transcription are checked for accuracy and completeness.

Medex is the name given to a medication record system used by some hospitals, nursing homes, and personal care facilities. The Medex is a large, one-piece card of stiff paper. Its format divides it into several sections, each devoted to a specific type of medication order. The first section usually is used for recording PRN medications. The inside section of the folded Medex card is for *routine* medications. This part of the form contains the greatest number of spaces for medication entries, and has a section for signatures of those who administered the medicines. The third and final section is where *changes* are recorded. These may include tubing changes, op-site changes, filter changes, or set-up changes.

A Medex card is prepared for each patient. Along its lower edge are spaces for the room number, patient's name, diagnosis, and the physician's name. The format of this record allows the nurse to document the administration of various types of medications for a period of eight days.

Kardex is a trade name for a large, one-piece record form printed on stiff paper. When folded, the Kardex becomes an $8\frac{1}{2} \times 11$ inch, three or four page patient record. Typically a Kardex provides for patient identification, diagnosis, the attending physician's name, the patient's room number, and the admission data. The form may be divided into parts, with one part devoted to lab work and/or diagnostic tests, another part to the *patient care plan* and, in some cases, a section for medication orders.

A *computerized Medication Administration Record* (MAR) may be used by hospitals and other health care facilities that are furnished with the proper equipment. There are various medication administration computerized programs and record forms. The drug order is written by the physician on a physician's order sheet, then this data is transmitted to the pharmacy or entered into the computer, depending upon the system used for medication administration. Information from the medication administration record can also be used by the business office for the posting of charges. A hard copy of the medication administration record (MAR) is posted in the patient's chart.

Patient data and drug information that has been previously entered into the computer system such as drug allergies, drug incompatibilities, usual dosage range, recommended administration time, recommended route of administration, and injection sites can be assessed by the pharmacist and nurse. This provides a valuable means of assuring that the correct drug, dosage, time, and route of administration is provided for the correct patient.

Hospitals that provide computers at each nurse's station allow the nurse to access the data and evaluate the drug order before administration. It also allows for direct documentation of the administration of the drug after it has been given to the patient.

The Medication Label

The medication label can be a source of valuable information to the nurse and the patient. Regardless of whether one is administering a prescription drug or taking a nonprescription drug product, an understanding of the information provided on the label

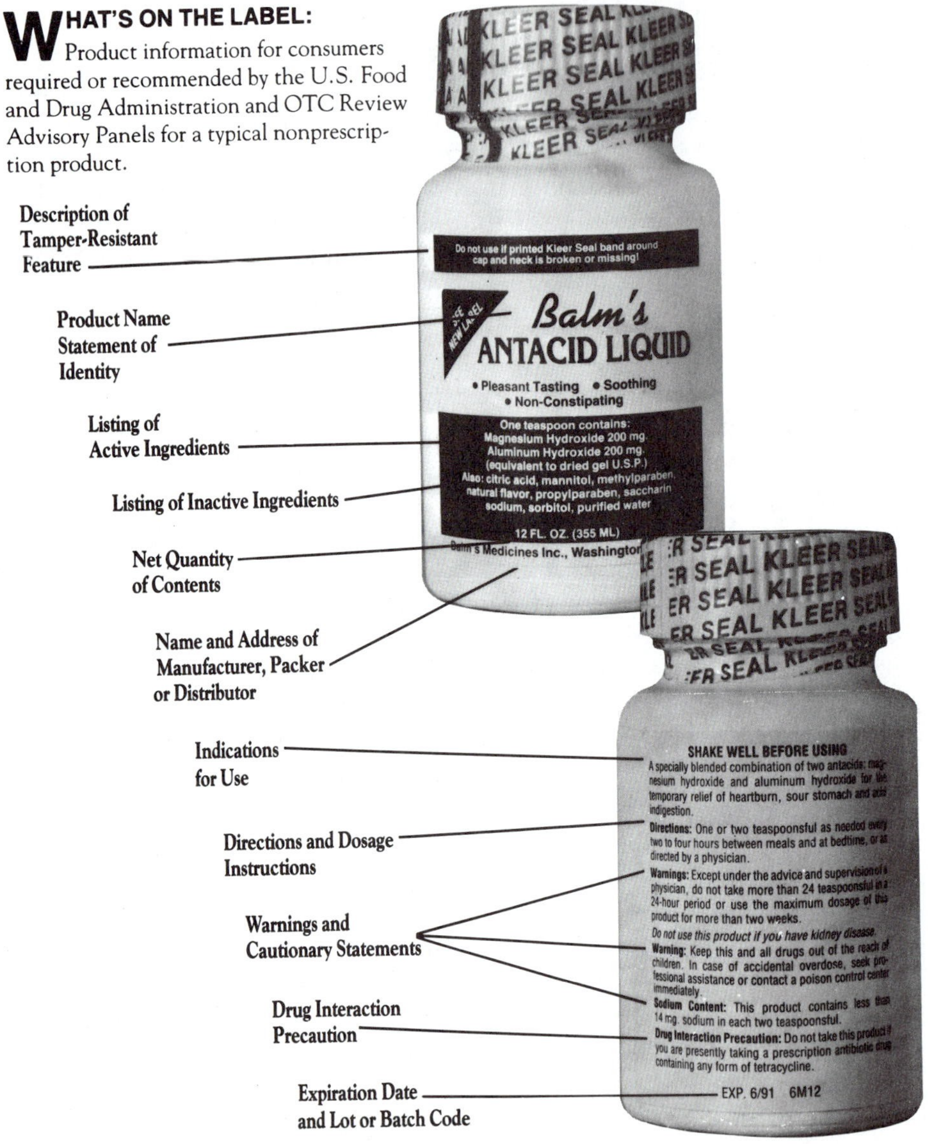
WHAT'S ON THE LABEL:
Product information for consumers required or recommended by the U.S. Food and Drug Administration and OTC Review Advisory Panels for a typical nonprescription product.
Description of Tamper-Resistant Feature
Product Name Statement of Identity
Listing of Active Ingredients
Listing of Inactive Ingredients
Net Quantity of Contents
Name and Address of Manufacturer, Packer or Distributor
Indications for Use
Directions and Dosage Instructions
Warnings and Cautionary Statements
Drug Interaction Precaution
Expiration Date and Lot or Batch Code
KLEER SEAL
Do not use if printed Kleer Seal band around cap and neck is broken or missing!
NEW LABEL
Balm's
ANTACID LIQUID
• Pleasant Tasting • Soothing
• Non-Constipating
One teaspoon contains:
Magnesium Hydroxide 200 mg.
Aluminum Hydroxide 200 mg.
(equivalent to dried gel U.S.P.)
Also: citric acid, mannitol, methylparaben, natural flavor, propylparaben, saccharin sodium, sorbitol, purified water
12 FL. OZ. (355 ML)
Medicines Inc., Washington
SHAKE WELL BEFORE USING
A specially blended combination of two antacids: magnesium hydroxide and aluminum hydroxide for the temporary relief of heartburn, sour stomach and acid indigestion.
Directions: One or two teaspoonsful as needed every two to four hours between meals and at bedtime, or as directed by a physician.
Warnings: Except under the advice and supervision of a physician, do not take more than 24 teaspoonsful in a 24-hour period or use the maximum dosage of this product for more than two weeks.
Do not use this product if you have kidney disease.
Warning: Keep this and all drugs out of the reach of children. In case of accidental overdose, seek professional assistance or contact a poison control center immediately.
Sodium Content: This product contains less than 14 mg. sodium in each two teaspoonsful.
Drug Interaction Precaution: Do not take this product if you are presently taking a prescription antibiotic drug containing any form of tetracycline.
EXP. 6/91 6M12

Figure 13–3 What's on the label? *(Courtesy of The Proprietary Association)*

is essential to the safe and effective use of any medicine. In addition to the name and address of the manufacturer, the following are the most important items of information that may be on a medication label. See Figure 13–3.

- The trade or brand name for the medication.
- The generic name (or listing of active and inactive ingredients).

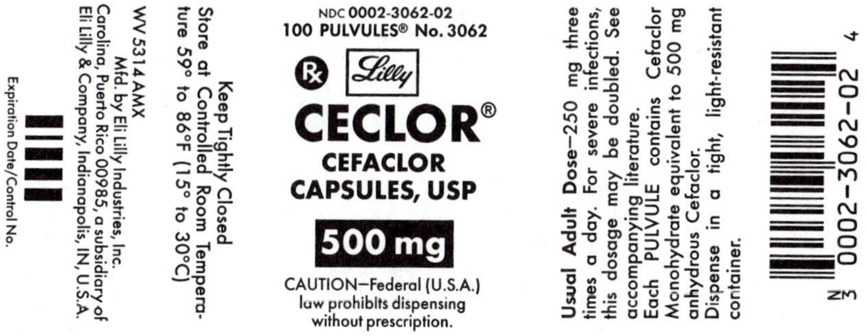

Figure 13–4 Sample of a medication label: Ceclor® *(Courtesy of Eli Lilly & Company, Indianapolis, IN 46285)*

- The National Drug Code (NDC) numbers that can be used to identify the manufacturer, the product, and the size of the container.
- The dosage strength in a given amount of the medication.
- The usual dosage and frequency of administration.
- The form in which the drug is supplied.
- CAUTION.
- The expiration date for the medication and the lot or batch code.
- The manufacturer's name.
- The total number and/or volume of the drug contained.

Other information that may be on a prescription label are the directions for storage and the directions for mixing or reconstituting a powdered form of the drug. Prescription medications that are listed in the Federal Controlled Substances Act are so identified on the label by the symbols CI, CII, CIII, CIV, CV.

Understanding the Medication Label

Refer to Figure 13–4: Sample of a medication label: Ceclor, and note the following information as it relates to this label.

1. The trade or brand name for the medication: **Ceclor**.
2. The generic name: **cefaclor**.
3. The National Drug Code (NDC) numbers that can be used to identify the manufacturer, the product, and the size of the container: **0002-3062-02**.
4. The dosage strength in a given amount of the medication: **500 mg**.
5. The usual dosage and frequency of administration: **Usual Adult Dose—250 mg three times a day. For severe infections, this dosage may be doubled**.

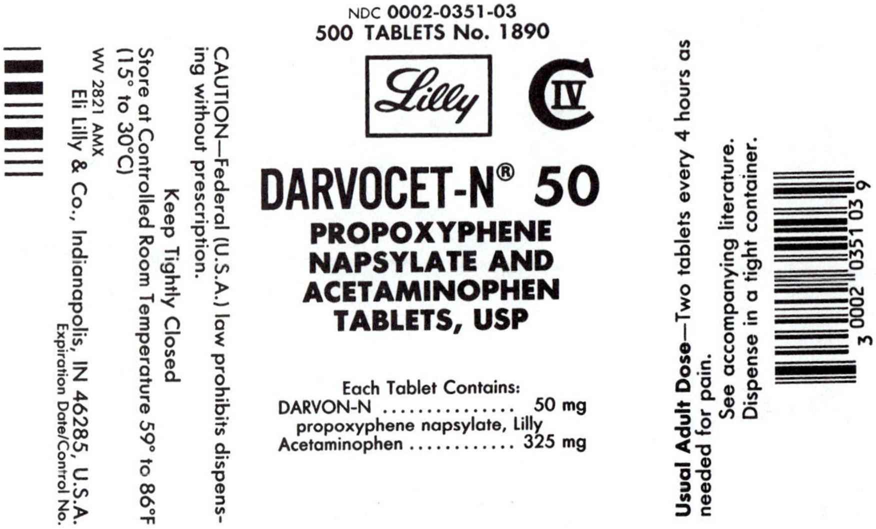

Figure 13–5 Sample of a medication label: Darvocet-N® 50 *(Courtesy of Eli Lilly & Company, Indianapolis, IN 46285)*

6. The form in which the drug is supplied: **Capsules, USP**.
7. CAUTION: **Federal (USA) law prohibits dispensing without prescription**.
8. The expiration date for the medication and the lot or batch code: **Expiration date not given on the sample label. Lot or batch code No. 3062**.
9. The manufacturer's name: **Lilly**.
10. The total number and/or volume of the drug contained: **100 Pulvules**.

Refer to Figure 13–5: Sample of a medication label: Darvocet-N 50 ©, and note the following information as it relates to this label.

1. The trade or brand name for the medication: **Darvocet-N 50**.
2. The generic name: **propoxyphene napsylate and acetaminophen**.
3. The National Drug Code (NDC) numbers that can be used to identify the manufacturer, the product, and the size of the container: **0002-0351-03**.
4. The dosage strength in a given amount of the medication: **Darvon-N® 50 mg propoxyphene napsylate and acetaminophen 325 mg**.
5. The usual dosage and frequency of administration: **Usual Adult Dose: two tablets every 4 hr PRN**.
6. The form in which the drug is supplied: **Tablets, USP**.
7. CAUTION: **Federal (USA) law prohibits dispensing without prescription**.

Table 13–1 An Example Time Schedule

qd	daily 10 am	q2h	2, 4, 6, 8, etc. or 1, 3, 5, 7, etc.
bid	10 am/6 pm	q3h	3, 6, 9, 12
tid	10 am/2 pm/6 pm	q4h	8, 12, 4, 8
qid	10 am/2 pm/6 pm/10 pm or 9 am, 1 pm, 5 pm, 9pm	q6h	12, 6, 12, 6
		q8h	8, 4, 12, 8

8. The expiration date for the medication and the lot or batch code: **Expiration date not given on the sample label. Lot or batch code No. 1890**.
9. The manufacturer's name: **Lilly ©**.
10. The total number and/or volume of the drug contained: **500 Tablets**.

Nonprescription medications, also known as over-the-counter (OTC) products, are intended for use without medical supervision. As such, the labeling of these products is very important to their safe and proper use by the consumer. Figure 13–3, on page 152, illustrates the required or recommended label information contained on a typical nonprescription product.

Time Schedule for Routine Medicines

Table 13–1 gives an example time schedule that may be helpful in the administration of *routine medications*. Bear in mind that schedule times vary. For example, every 6 hours may be 12–6, 12–6 or it could 2–8, 2–8, depending upon the time the medication was initiated. When possible, times are scheduled to allow a patient to sleep with as few interruptions as necessary. Nursing units may also vary; for example, cardiac units often put tid drugs on an every-8-hour schedule.

Note that some medications may require administration with the patient's meals, whereas other medications may require that they be given on an empty stomach. It is very important that you administer the medication as ordered and at the right time. Hypoglycemic agents that are ordered daily are given early in the morning after the patient's blood sugar level has been checked.

Abbreviations

Abbreviations are the shorthand of the medical field. They are a clear and concise means for writing orders. This medical shorthand is an international language used by professional and nonprofessional people who are concerned with patient care. All of the abbreviations listed in Table 13–2 should be learned in order to properly fulfill your role in the administration of medications.

Table 13–2 Abbreviations and Their Meanings

Abbreviation	Meaning
$\overline{aa}$	of each
ac	before meals
ad lib	as desired, as much as needed
agit	shake, stir
alt dieb	alternating days
am	morning
amp	ampule
aq	water
bid	two times a day, twice daily
c̄	with
cap	capsule
chem	chemotherapy
DEA	Drug Enforcement Administration
dil	dilute
disp	dispense
D/NS	dextrose in normal saline
D/S	dextrose and saline
DW	distilled water
D/W	dextrose in water
Eq	equivalent
FDA	Food and Drug Administration
fl	fluid
FM	flowmeter
garg	gargle
(H)	hypodermic
h, hr	hour
hs	hour of sleep
H_2O	water
IM	intramuscular
inf	infusion
IU	immunizing unit
IV	intravenous
L/min	liters per minute
med	medicine
mEq	milliequivalent
MLD	minimum lethal dose
mn	midnight
MO	mineral oil
MOM	milk of magnesia
MOPP	nitrogen mustard, oncovin, prednisone, procarbazine
MOPV	monovalent oral poliovirus vaccine
MS	morphine sulfate
MTD	maximum tolerated dose
MTX	methotrexate
noct	at night
N/S	normal saline
O_2	oxygen
OD	overdose
OD	right eye
OS	left eye
OU	both eyes
OTC	over the counter (drugs)
pc	after meals
PL	placebo
pm	afternoon
PMI	patient medication instruction
POMP	prednisone, oncovin, methotrexate, 6-mercaptopurine
pr	per rectum
pwd	powder
q	every
qd	every day
qh	every hour
q2h	every two hours
q3h	every three hours
q4h	every four hours
qid	four times a day
qm	every morning
qn	every night
qod	every other day
qs	quantity sufficient
R	rectal
Rx	"take thou"
S, Sig	give the following directions
s̄	without
SC	subcutaneous
subq	subcutaneous
$\overline{ss}$	one-half
stat	immediately
tid	three times a day
tinct	tincture
TO	telephone order
tus	cough
U	unit
vag	vagina
ves	bladder
VO	verbal order
W/O	water in oil
cm	centimeter
mcg, µg	microgram
mg	milligram
Gm, g	gram
kg	kilogram
cc	cubic centimeter
mL, ml	milliliter
L	liter
gr	grain
dr	dram
oz	ounce
lb	pound
♏	minim
gtt	drops
t, tsp	teaspoon
T, tbs	tablespoon
C	cup, Celsius
pt	pint
qt	quart
gal	gallon
F	Fahrenheit

◆ Review Questions

Directions: Select the best answer to each multiple choice question. Circle the letter of your choice.

1. A type of medication order that is given "as necessary" or "when needed" is known as a __________.
   a. routine order
   b. single order
   c. standing order
   d. PRN order
2. Legally, the best type of medication order is a __________.
   a. verbal order
   b. telephone order
   c. written order
   d. stat order
3. All of the following are true statements about prescriptions except:
   a. it is a written order that is not a part of a patient's chart
   b. it includes a superscription, inscription, and subscription
   c. it is used for all types of drugs
   d. it includes physician's signature blanks
4. A standing order is a type of protocol that includes all of the following except:
   a. it is written by a physician or group of physicians
   b. it sets forth specific instructions for various patient-care situations
   c. it is given one time only
   d. a Dulcolax suppository (one every am for constipation) is an example
5. The abbreviation that means *of each* is __________.
   a. ac b. ad lib c. $\overline{aa}$ d. aq
6. The abbreviation that means *with* is __________.
   a. $\bar{c}$ b. $\bar{s}$ c. ac d. pc
7. The abbreviation that means *after meals* is __________.
   a. ac b. pc c. $\bar{c}$ d. am
8. Hypoglycemic agents that are ordered daily are given __________.
   a. early in the morning
   b. after the patient's blood sugar level is checked
   c. late in the morning
   d. a and b

9. When taking verbal orders, you may protect yourself by all of the following except:
   a. remembering the order without writing it down
   b. repeating the order back to the physician
   c. following the "Six Rights" of proper drug administration
   d. having the physician cosign the order within twenty-four hours

10. A medication order includes all of the following except:
    a. drug to be used
    b. dosage
    c. color of the drug
    d. time of administration

11. The abbreviation OS means __________.
    a. left eye
    b. right eye
    c. both eyes
    d. none of the above

12. The abbreviation for *before meals* is __________.
    a. pc
    b. ac
    c. c̄
    d. am

13. The abbreviation Sig means __________.
    a. one-half
    b. take thou
    c. give the following directions
    d. signature

14. An understanding of the information provided on a label is essential to safe and __________.
    a. uneffective use of any medicine
    b. effective use of any medicine
    c. ineffective use of any medicine
    d. none of these

15. The National Drug Code numbers on a label identify the __________.
    a. manufacturer
    b. product
    c. size of the container
    d. all of these

16. Prescription medications that are listed in the Federal Controlled Substances Act are identified by the symbols and/or abbreviations __________.
    a. FCSA
    b. NDC
    c. C-I, C-II, C-III, C-IV, and C-V
    d. All of these

17. Nonprescription medication labels contain certain information that is recommended or required by __________.
    a. the U.S. Food and Drug Administration
    b. the Federal Controlled Substances Act
    c. OTC Review Advisory Panels
    d. a and c

Matching: Place the correct letter from Column II on the appropriate line of Column I.

Column I

18. ________ Stat order
19. ________ Compounding
20. ________ Pharmacist
21. ________ Prescription
22. ________ Inscription
23. ________ Subscription
24. ________ Signature
25. ________ REPETATUR

Column II

A. A written legal document that gives directions for compounding, dispensing, and administering a medication to a patient.

B. States the names and quantities of ingredients to be included in the medication.

C. Includes the symbol ℞ (“take thou”).

D. Gives the directions for a patient.

E. Indicates whether or not the prescription can be refilled.

F. Immediate administration.

G. One who is licensed to prepare and dispense drugs.

H. The process of combining and mixing.

I. Gives directions to the pharmacist for filling the prescription.

CHAPTER 14

Basic Principles for the Administration of Medications

OBJECTIVES

Upon completion of this chapter, you should be able to:

- Define the terms listed in the vocabulary.
- Describe the five steps of the nursing process.
- Give the legal implications of administering medications.
- State the "Six Rights" of proper drug administration.
- List the basic medication guidelines.
- List safety measures for drug administration.
- Describe safe storage of medications.
- Describe a general procedure for reporting an adverse drug reaction.
- List signs of drug hypersensitivity according to body system affected.
- List ten types of medication errors.
- Explain the proper steps to take if a medication error occurs.
- Answer the review questions correctly.

Vocabulary

buccal (buh'kal). Pertaining to the cheek.

inhalation (in"ha-la'shun). The process of breathing air, vapor, gas, or other substance into the lungs.

meniscus (men-is'kus). A term used to describe the convex or concave upper surface of a column of liquid in a container. Crescent shaped.

precipitate (pre-sip'i-tat). A substance, in the form of fine particles, that separates from a solution if allowed to stand for a period of time.

The Nursing Process

Basic principles for the administration of medications are based upon the nursing process. This process is the framework of nursing practice and involves the patient, family, and community. The five steps of the nursing process are: assessment, diagnosis, planning, implementation, and evaluation. For this text, only the pharmacological aspects of the nursing process will be considered.

Step 1: Assessment

The systematic gathering, organizing, and interpretation of data to determine a patient's nursing needs is called assessment. This process begins upon a patient's admission to a hospital and continues until the patient is discharged. When a patient is discharged from a hospital setting and placed in an extended-care facility or when home-health care is given, the nursing process continues. In a physician's office or clinic this same process is used, as each patient is treated as an individual, with individual needs.

Medication History. It is essential that you know the person who is your patient. Besides the person's name, occupation, diagnosis, age and weight, you need to be familiar with the patient's medication history. The following are some of the questions that may be asked to determine a patient's medication history.

1. Do you have any allergies?
   a. to medicines (list)
   b. to food (list)
   c. to insects (list)
2. What medicines are you currently taking?
   a. prescription
   b. over-the-counter
   c. home remedies
3. What condition(s) are you taking these medications for?
   Examples: headache, hypertension, chest pain, etc.
4. Do they work for you?
5. How long have you been taking these medicines?
6. What other medicines have you taken in the past month, six months, year?
7. Have you experienced any problems when taking medications?
   Examples: skin rash, nausea/vomiting, drowsiness, constipation, diarrhea, dry mouth, blurred vision, ringing in the ear, loss of hair, tremors, etc.
8. Do you have any difficulty taking medications?
   a. can't swallow pills
   b. forget to take medicine
   c. forget which medicine you took
   d. have to crush medicine
   e. have to take with food
9. Do you ever give your medicine to others?
10. Do you ever take medicine that is not yours?

11. Do you follow the prescription order?
    a. dosage
    b. time
    c. duration
12. Do you use tobacco, alcohol?
    a. how often?
    b. amount?

Step 2: Diagnosis

The term, diagnosis means "through knowledge." A nursing diagnosis is a clinical judgment about individual, family, or community responses to actual and potential health problems/life processes. Nursing diagnoses provide the basis for selection of nursing interventions to achieve outcomes for which the nurse is accountable (NANDA, 1990).

Four steps are involved in the formulation of a nursing diagnosis:

1. Data base is established by acquiring information about the patient from all available sources. This data base is continually updated.
2. Analysis of patient's needs, problems, concerns, and human responses.
3. Organization of data to make a diagnostic statement that summarizes the patient information obtained.
4. Evaluation of the sufficiency and accuracy of the data base.

Examples of appropriate diagnoses are as follows:

Elimination	Possible Cause
bowel incontinence	excessive use of laxatives
constipation	adverse reaction to Basaljel
diarrhea	adverse reaction to Milk of Magnesia

Step 3: Planning

Planning involves the development of nursing actions designed to enhance the patient's responses to treatment or to prevent drug-related problems. The planning segment of the nursing process involves:

1. Set goals.
2. Develop outcomes that the patient will be able to do as a result of nursing actions.
3. Develop nursing interventions that describe how the nurse can assist the patient to achieve outcomes.
4. Document the plan.

Nursing Actions for Problems Related to Drug Therapy if Not Contraindicated	
Constipation	Encourage fluids Encourage a diet rich in fiber Encourage regular exercise Encourage regular pattern of elimination
Diarrhea	Monitor intake and output Maintain hydration (clear fluids) Encourage nonirritating foods Reduce stress Encourage proper handwashing and body hygiene Apply ointment to rectal area

Step 4: Implementation

Implementation is the process of putting into effect, fulfillment, or carrying through with the plan of action. In the nursing process this step involves all aspects of actual caring for the patient and requires full knowledge of the assessment and planning steps. Included in this step are patient-care areas such as hygiene, physical and mental comfort, assistance in daily living habits such as feeding and elimination, maintaining and controlling the patient's physical environment, and teaching the patient about factors that are important to his/her care and what actions to take to help facilitate recovery.

In drug therapy, implementation may involve psychological and physical care measures to help enhance the effectiveness of the medication(s), to reduce the need for certain medications, to consult with the physician or pharmacist regarding changes in the drug regimen, and patient teaching.

Example: Patient Teaching

Jane Rice June 3, 1998

Cephalexin 250 mg cap 20 capsules

Take one (1) cap 4 times daily till all used

About Your Medicine

Cephalexin is an antibiotic that is used to treat bacterial infections. It does not work for colds, flu, or other viral infections.

Before Using This Medicine

Inform your doctor, nurse, and pharmacist if you:

- are allergic to any medicine.
- are pregnant.

- are breast-feeding.
- are taking medication, especially probenecid (Benemid—used for gout).
- have a history of stomach or intestinal disease.

Proper Use of This Medicine

Cephalexin may be taken on a full or empty stomach. It may be taken with food or crushed and mixed with food. You must take the medicine 4 times daily (9 am, 1 pm, 5 pm, 9 pm) and take all of the medicine.

Precautions

If your symptoms do not improve within a few days, or if they become worse, inform your physician.

> **Diabetics:** This medicine may cause false test results with some urine sugar tests.

If diarrhea occurs inform your physician. Do not take any diarrhea medicine without checking with your physician.

Do not give this medicine to other people.

Possible Side Effects—Report to Your Physician Immediately

Abdominal or stomach cramps, pain, and bloating (severe); convulsions (seizures); diarrhea (watery, severe, bloody); fever; increased thirst; joint pain; loss of appetite; nausea or vomiting; skin rash, itching, redness, or swelling; unusual tiredness or weakness; weight loss (unusual)

Step 5: Evaluation

Evaluation is an integral part of each step of the nursing process. It ascertains the quality and effectiveness of the plan of care for the patient and allows you to reflect upon the worth of the process. Some questions you may ask are:

1. Did the prescribed medication(s) alleviate the signs and symptoms of disease? How effective was the medication?
2. Were there any adverse reactions to the medication? If so, did you take appropriate action?

3. Did the patient understand the prescribed medication regimen? Did the patient understand the purpose, effects, precautions, and any bodily changes that could occur as a result of a medicine?
4. Did you consult with the physician or pharmacist to approve the patient's drug regimen?
5. Did you follow the "Six Rights" of proper drug administration?

Legal Implications

Members of the health-care profession who prepare and administer medications are ethically and legally responsible for their own actions. Under the law, these individuals are required to be licensed, registered, or otherwise authorized by a physician.

Each state has enacted laws governing the practice of medicine, nursing, and pharmacy. These laws vary from state to state; therefore, it is essential that one become familiar with the laws of the state in which one is employed before giving any medication. In some states, the only health professional authorized to give injections, other than a physician, is the registered nurse. On the other hand, legislation in some states gives physicians broad authority to delegate responsibility for giving medications. Other states have passed laws that specify which qualified and properly trained persons may perform certain medical acts.

Regardless of the differences in state authorization laws, the courts will not permit the careless actions of health-care workers to go unpunished, especially when such actions result in harm to or the death of the patient. Under the law, those administering medications are expected to be familiar with the drugs administered and the effects they might have on a patient. In that there are thousands of drugs on the market, the task of keeping up with current information on each medication is overwhelming. Therefore, it is necessary to keep reference books handy and to refer to them every time there is any question about a drug. The following precautions should guide the administration of any medication:

P Patients are individuals who depend upon the nurse for proper care.
R Right Patient, Right Dose, Right Drug, Right Route, Right Time, Right Documentation.
E Explain to the patients the effects the drug should (or could) have on the body.
C Check for contraindications before giving a medication.
A Always check for drug *allergies* to the medication being given.
U Understand the drug, its uses and actions.
T Toxic effects; know the symptoms to look for.
I Information on unfamiliar medications should be obtained before its administration.
O Observe the patient for signs of superinfection when administering antibiotics.
N Never administer medications without the proper authorization
S Side effects; be alert for signs of drug hypersensitivity.

The "Six Rights" of Proper Drug Administration

The "Six Rights" have been developed as a checklist of activities to be followed by those who give medications. This easy-to-remember list should always be followed to insure the proper administration of any drug. See Figure 14–1.

- *Right Drug* (Figure 14–1A): To be sure that the correct drug has been selected, compare the medication order with the label on the medication. A frequent check of the medication label is a good way to avoid a medication error. One should make a practice of reading the label on each of the following three occasions:
  1. When the medication is taken from the storage area.
  2. Just before removing it from its container.
  3. Upon returning the medication container to storage or prior to discarding the empty container.
- *Right Dose* (Figure 14–1B): It is essential that the patient receive the right dose. If the dose ordered and the dose on hand are *not the same*, carefully determine the correct dose through mathematical calculation. When calculating dosage, it is advisable to have another qualified person verify the accuracy of your calculations *before the medication is administered.*
- *Right Route* (Figure 14–1C): Check the medication order to be sure that you have the right route of administration.
- *Right Time* (Figure 14–1D): You are responsible for medicating the patient at the proper time. Check the medication order to insure that a drug is administered according to the time interval prescribed. For a drug to be maintained at the proper blood level, care must be taken to administer it at the right time.
- *Right Patient* (Figure 14–1E): Before administering any medication, always be sure that you have the right patient. A good safety practice is to correctly identify the patient on each occasion when you administer a medication. In a hospital, always check the patient's identification bracelet. In a physician's office or other health-care facility, call the patient by name or ask the patient to state his or her name.
- *Right Documentation* (Figure 14–1F): A patient's chart (Figure 14–2) is a legal document. It is essential that the following data about drug administration be entered correctly:

  —The patient's name

  —The date and time of administration

  —The name of the medication and the amount (dosage) administered

  —The route by which the medication was administered

  —Any adverse reactions experienced by the patient

  —Any complications in administering the drug (patient refusing to take the medication, difficulty in swallowing, and so forth)

  —If the medication was *not given*, state why, dispose of the medication according to agency policy.

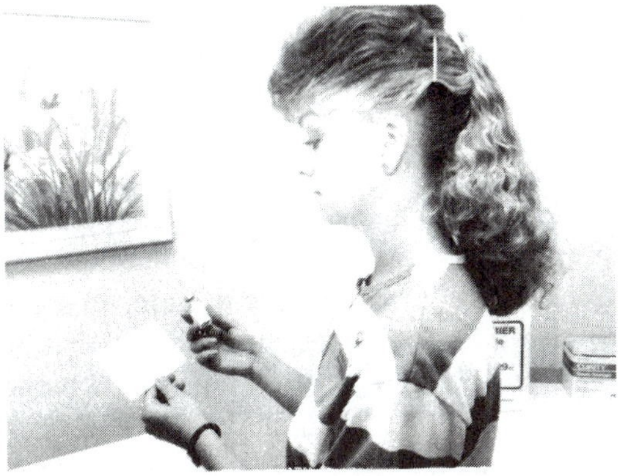

(A) *The Right Drug.* The nurse compares the medication label with the physician's order.

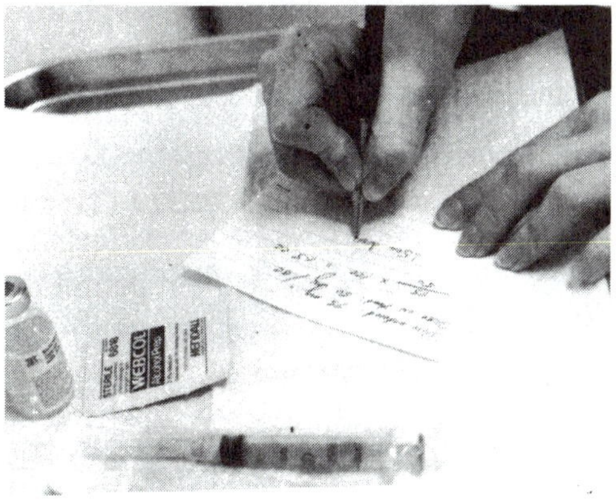

(B) *The Right Dose.* The nurse calculates the correct dose of medication.

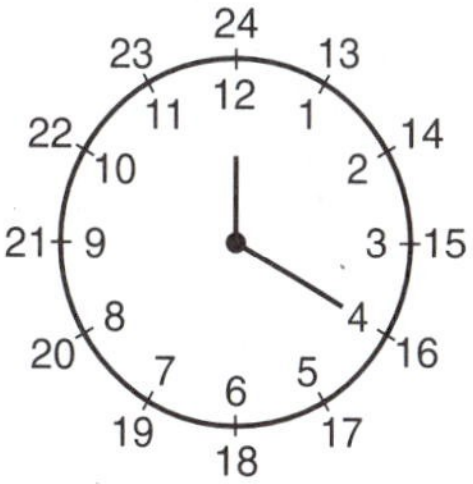

From midnight to noon the 12-hour clock and the 24-hour clock are identical. From noon to midnight, add 12 to each hour to arrive at the 24-hour clock.

12 M/N	2400	12:00 N	1200
1:00 am	0100	1:00 pm	1300
2:00 am	0200	2:00 pm	1400
3:00 am	0300	3:00 pm	1500
4:00 am	0400	4:00 pm	1600
5:00 am	0500	5:00 pm	1700
6:00 am	0600	6:00 pm	1800
7:00 am	0700	7:00 pm	1900
8:00 am	0800	8:00 pm	2000
9:00 am	0900	9:00 pm	2100
10:00 am	1000	10:00 pm	2200
11:00 am	1100	11:00 pm	2300

(D) *The Right Time.* You are responsible for administering medication to a patient at the proper time. Check the medication order to ensure that a drug is given at the prescribed interval. For a drug to be maintained at the proper blood level, it must be administered on time.

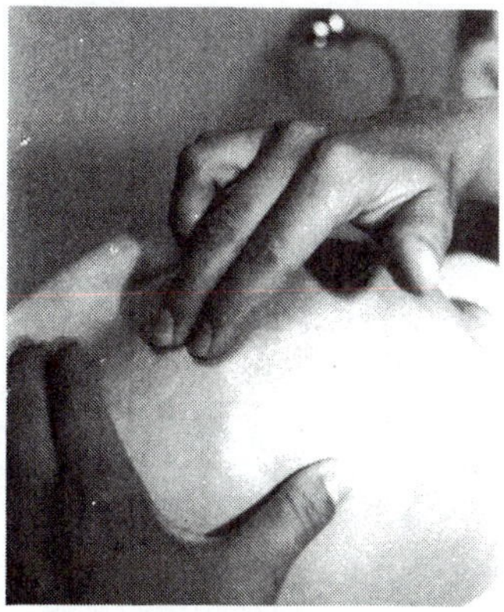

(C) *The Right Route.* The nurse uses a practice model to locate the right route for an IM injection.

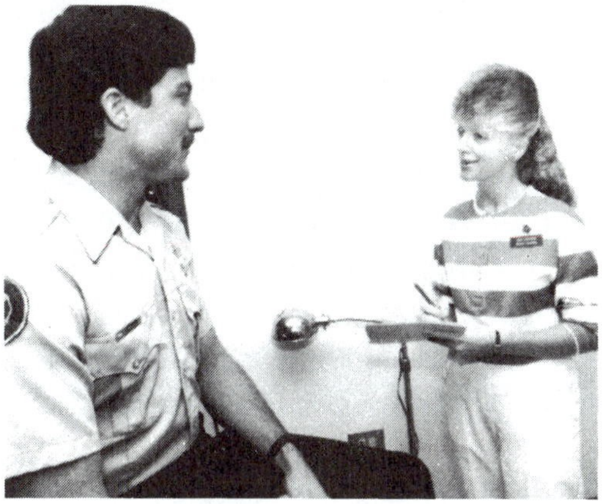

(E) *The Right Patient.* The nurse identifies the patient.

Figure 14–1 The "Six Rights" of proper drug administration

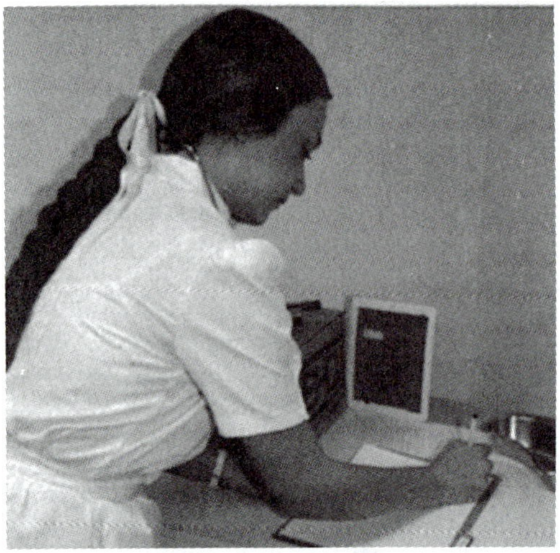

Figure 14–1 (*Continued*) (F) *The Right Documentation.* The nurse enters drug administration data into a patient's chart.

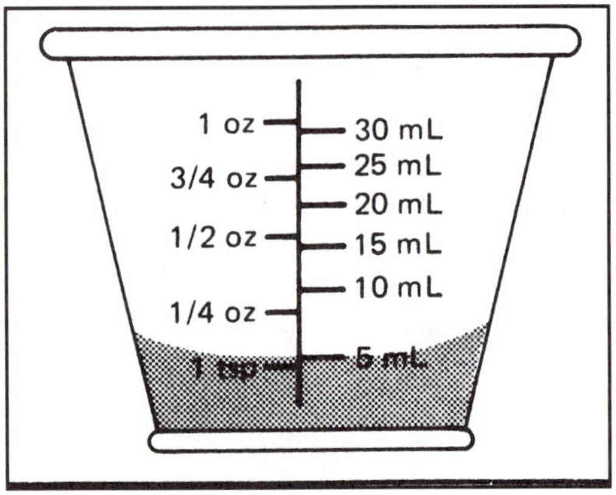

Figure 14–2 Always measure the volume of a liquid medication at the *lowest point* of the meniscus. This medicine cup contains 5ml of liquid.

Basic Medication Guidelines

Regardless of a medication's form or the route by which it is administered, certain basic guidelines must be followed. These guidelines are:

- Know the system for medication distribution. Cards, Kardex, Medex, MediAide, computer printout, unit dose, and multiple dose are some of the different systems that may be encountered.
- Check each medication order carefully.
- Be familiar with the following types of medication orders: routine, PRN, single, stat, and standing.
- It is advisable to always have a written order from a physician or other authorized practitioner before giving any medication.
- Give only drugs that are ordered by a licensed physician or practitioner authorized to prescribe medications.
- *Never* give a medication if there is any question about the order.
- Be completely familiar with the drug that you are administering before giving it to your patient. You are expected to know the following about any drug that you are to administer:

Safe dosage limit	Route of administration
Side effects	Time of administration
Contraindications	Action of the drug
Route of excretion	Clinical nursing implications

- Know the circumstances in which you may be allowed to withhold a drug and not give it to a patient. These could occur in conjunction with diagnostic tests, laboratory tests, and/or with surgery.
- Always check the expiration date on the medication label.
- Never give a drug if its normal appearance has been altered in any way (color, structure, consistency, or odor).
- Practice medical asepsis. Wash your hands before and after administering a medication.
- When administering oral medications, stay with the patient until you are certain that the medication has been taken.
- Always check for allergies before administering any medication.

Standard Precautions

The Centers for Disease Control and Prevention (CDC) recommends a set of infection control guidelines to help protect health-care providers, patients, and their visitors from infectious diseases. Standard precautions for infection control should be utilized by all health-care professionals for all patients.

Standard precautions combine many of the basic principles of universal precautions with techniques known as body substance isolation (BSI), a system that maintains that personal protective equipment should be worn for contact with all body fluids whether or not blood is visible. Advantages of the new standard precautions are that they include all of the major recommendations of universal precautions and body substance isolation, while incorporating new information intended to protect all patients, all health-care providers, and all visitors.

According to the CDC, standard precautions are "designed to reduce the risk of transmission of microorganisms, from both recognized and unrecognized sources of infection in hospitals (CDC, 1994)." Standard precautions apply to:

1. blood;
2. all body fluids, secretions, and excretions regardless of whether or not they contain visible blood;
3. nonintact skin;
4. mucous membranes.

To be effective, standard precautions must be practiced conscientiously at all times. Table 14–1 provides a comprehensive review of the standard precautions.

Table 14–1 Standard Precautions for Infection Control Issued by the CDC in 1996

Standard Precautions for Infection Control

Wash Hands (Plain soap)
Wash after touching **blood, body fluids, secretions, excretions**, and **contaminated items**.
Wash immediately **after gloves are removed** and **between patient contacts**.
Avoid transfer of microorganisms to other patients or environments.

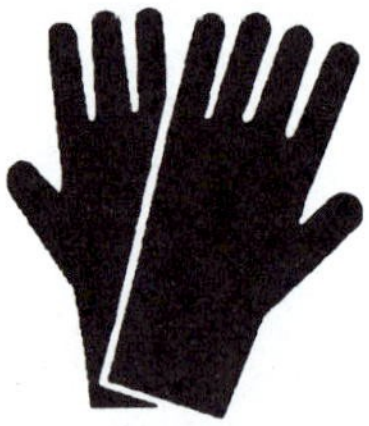

Wear Gloves
Wear when touching **blood, body fluids, secretions, excretions**, and **contaminated items**.
Put on **clean** gloves just **before touching mucous membranes** and **nonintact skin**.
Change gloves between tasks and procedures on the same patient after contact with material that may contain high concentrations of microorganisms. Remove gloves promptly after use, before touching noncontaminated items and environmental surfaces, and before going to another patient, and wash hands immediately to avoid transfer of microorganisms to other patients or environments.

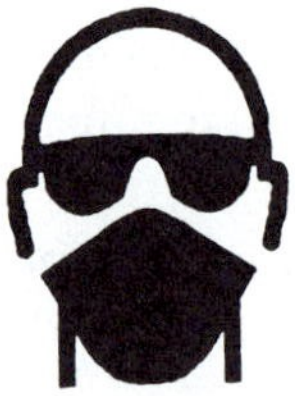

Wear Mask and Eye Protection or Face Shield
Protect mucous membranes of the eyes, nose and mouth during procedures and patient-care activities that are likely to generate **splashes** or **sprays** of **blood, body fluids, secretions**, or **excretions**.

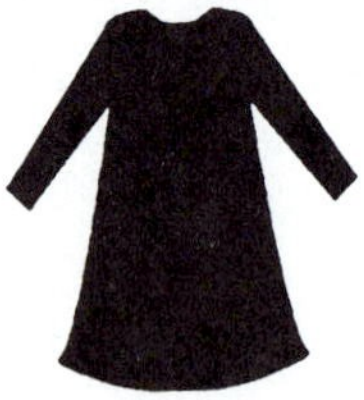

Wear Gown
Protect skin and prevent soiling of clothing during procedures that are likely to generate **splashes** or **sprays** of **blood, body fluids, secretions**, or **excretions**. Remove a soiled gown as promptly as possible and wash hands to avoid transfer of microorganisms to other patients or environments.

Patient-Care Equipment
Handle used patient-care equipment soiled with **blood, body fluids, secretions**, or **excretions** in a manner that prevents skin and mucous membrane exposures, contamination of clothing, and transfer of microorganisms to other patients and environments. Ensure that reusable equipment is not used for the care of another patient until it has been appropriately cleaned and reprocessed and single use items are properly discarded.

Table 14–1 (*Continued*)

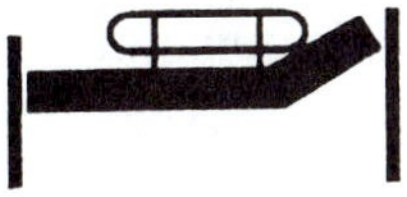

Environmental Control
Follow hospital procedures for routine care, cleaning, and disinfection of environmental surfaces, beds, bedrails, bedside equipment and other frequently touched surfaces.

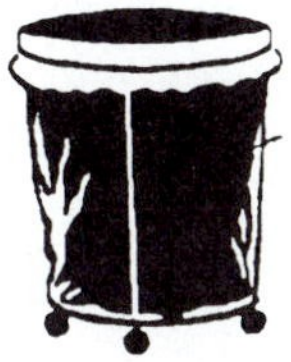

Linen
Handle, transport, and process used linen soiled with **blood, body fluids, secretions**, or **excretions** in a manner that prevents exposures and contamination of clothing, and avoids transfer of microorganisms to other patients and environments.

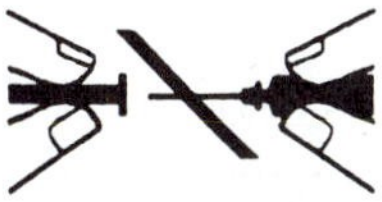

Occupational Health and Bloodborne Pathogens
Prevent injuries when using needles, scalpels, and other sharp instruments or devices; when handling sharp instruments after procedures; when cleaning used instruments; and when disposing of used needles.

Never recap used needles using both hands or any other technique that involves directing the point of a needle toward any part of the body; rather, use either a one-handed "scoop" technique or a mechanical device designed for holding the needle sheath.

Do not remove used needles from disposable syringes by hand, and do not bend, break, or otherwise manipulate used needles by hand. Place used disposable syringes and needles, scalpel blades, and other sharp items in puncture-resistant sharps containers located as close as practical to the area in which the items were used, and place reusable syringes and needles in a puncture-resistant container for transport to the reprocessing area.

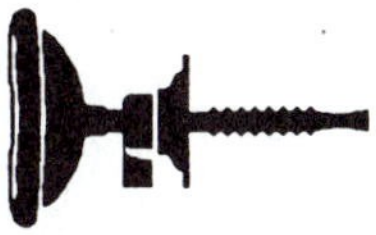

Use **resuscitation devices** as an alternative to mouth-to-mouth resuscitation.

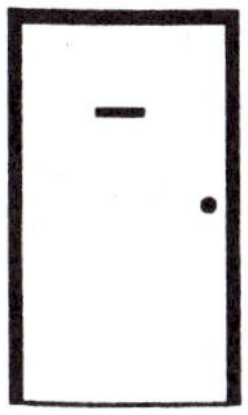

Patient Placement
Use a **private room** for a patient who contaminates the environment or who does not (or cannot be expected to) assist in maintaining appropriate hygiene or environmental control. Consult Infection Control if a private room is not available.

(Courtesy Brevis Corp.)

Safety Measures for Drug Administration

The following are important measures to follow for safety in drug administration:

- Always wash your hands before preparing and administering medications.
- When preparing medications, work in a well-lighted area that is quiet and free of distractions.
- Always observe the "Six Rights."
- Carefully follow the correct procedure for administering controlled substances.
- Give only those medications that you have actually prepared for administration.
- Do not allow someone else to give a medication that you prepared.
- Once you have prepared a medication for administration, do not leave it unattended.
- Be careful in transporting the medication to the patient.
- Keep all drugs not being administered in a locked storage area (such as the medication cart, medication cabinet, and so forth).
- If the dosage ordered is greater than the safe dosage limit, check the order again. Contact the prescribing physician for verification.
- Do not open unit dose medications until you are at the patient's bedside. In this way, if the patient refuses the medicine, you have not wasted the medicine, and the patient will not be charged for the medicine.
- A product that contains a precipitate should be shaken thoroughly before it is poured. If the product is discolored or contains an unusual precipitate, it should be returned to the pharmacy for replacement.
- When pouring a liquid medicine, hold the measuring device at eye level, and read the correct amount at the lowest point of the meniscus. See Figure 14–2.
- Do not contaminate the cap of a bottle while pouring a medication. Place the cap with the rim pointed upward to prevent contamination of that portion that comes into contact with the medication.
- Do not crush or alter any medication unless you have made sure that you can do so. (See Table 14–2 for some medications that should not to be crushed or altered.)
- In the event of a medication error, appropriate action should be taken immediately to safeguard the patient. Report the error to the proper authority.
- *Always* keep safety precautions in mind. The U.S. Department of Health and Human Services, Public Health Service, Centers for Disease Control and Prevention recommends the following universal precautions for prevention of HIV and other blood-borne disease transmission in health-care settings.

  1. All health-care workers should routinely use appropriate barrier precautions to prevent skin and mucous-membrane exposure when contact with blood or other body fluids of any patient is anticipated. Gloves should be worn for

Table 14–2 Tablets That Cannot Be Crushed or Altered

TABLE 1: CHECK OUT THIS LIST BEFORE ALTERING A DRUG.

A. Don't crush or alter these common sustained-release, enteric-coated, and sublingual tablets.

Afrinol Repetabs
Asbron G Inlay-Tabs
Avazyme
Azulfidine EN-tabs

Belladenal-S
Bellergal-S
bisacodyl
Bronkodyl S-R

Chlor-Trimeton Repetabs
Choledyl SA
Constant-T

Diamox Sequels
Dimetane Extentabs
Dimetapp Extentabs
Donnatal Extentabs
Donnazyme
Drixoral
Dulcolax

Easprin
Ecotrin
E-Mycin
Eskalith CR

Fero-Grad-500
Fero-Gradumet
Festal II

Hydergine (Sublingual)

Iberet Filmtabs
Iberet-500 Filmtabs

Ilotycin
Indocin SR
Isordil (Sublingual)
Isuprel Glossets

Kaon-Cl
Kaon-Cl-10
K-Dur
Klor-Con
Klotrix
K-Tab

Lithobid

Mestinon Timespan
Micro-K Extencaps
MS Contin

Nico-Span
Nitro-Bid
Nitrostat
Norflex

Pabalate
Pancrease
Peritrate SA
Permitil Chronotab
Phazyme-PB
Phyllocontin
Polaramine Repetab
Preludin Repetab
Preludin Enduret
Procan SR
Pronestyl-SR

Quibron-T/SR
Quinaglute Dura-Tabs

Quinidex Extentabs

Ritalin SR
Roxanol SR

Slow-K
Sorbitrate SA
Sustaire

Tedral SA
Theo-Dur
Theolair-SR
Trilafon Repetabs

Sudafed SA
Temaril Spansules
Theobid
Theo-Dur Sprinkle
Thorazine Spansules
Tuss-Ornade Spansules

Valrelease

B. You can open these sustained-release capsules and carefully mix the contents in a liquid or with a soft food, such as applesauce. Vigorous mixing, however, could alter the rate of release.

Artane Sequels

Combid Spansules
Compazine Spansules

Dexedrine Spansules

Feosol Spansules

Inderal LA
Inderide LA
Isordil Tembids (capsules)

Nicobid
Nitrostat SR
Ornade Spansules

Pavabid

Slo-bid Gyrocaps
Slo-Phyllin Gyrocaps

C. Because of the makeup of these miscellaneous drugs, do not crush or alter them.

- *Accutane* (liquid-filled capsule). Liquid can irritate mucous membrane.
- *Chymoral.* Crushing may interfere with enzymatic activity.
- *Depakene* (liquid-filled capsule). Liquid can irritate mucous membrane.
- *Feldene.* Powder from this capsule can irritate mucous membrane.
- *Klorvess* (effervescent tablet). If this tablet isn't dissolved before it's given, gastrointestinal upset will occur, and gastrointestinal damage may occur.

(continued)

Table 14–2 Tablets That Cannot Be Crushed or Altered (*Continued*)

TABLE 2: WATCH FOR THESE NAMES AS A TIP-OFF.			
A. These drug manufacturers' names indicate a sustained-release or an enteric-coated form of a drug.	Duracap	Lontab	**B.** When attached to a drug name, these terms indicate a sustained-release form of a drug.
	Dura-tab	Repetab	
	Enduret	Sequel	
	Enseal	Spansule	
	EN-tab	Tab-in	
	Extencap	Tembid	Bid
BidCap	Extentab	Tempule	Dur
Cenule	Gradumet	Tentab	Plateau Cap
Chronosule	Granucap	TimeCap	SA
Chronotab	Gyrocap	Timecelle	Span
D-Lay	Kronocap	Timespan	SR
Dospan	Lanacap		

(Courtesy of Springhouse Corporation)

touching blood and body fluids, mucous membranes, or nonintact skin of all patients, for handling items or surfaces soiled with blood or body fluids, and for performing venipuncture and other vascular access procedures. Gloves should be changed after contact with each patient. Masks and protective eyewear or face shields should be worn during procedures that are likely to generate droplets of blood or other body fluids to prevent exposure of mucous membranes of the mouth, nose, and eyes. Gowns or aprons should be worn during procedures that are likely to generate splashed of blood or other body fluids.

2. Hands and other skin surfaces should be washed immediately and thoroughly if contaminated with blood or other body fluids. Hands should be washed immediately after gloves are removed.
3. All health-care workers should take precautions to prevent injuries caused by needles, scalpels, and other sharp instruments or devices during procedures; when cleaning used instruments; during disposal of used needles; and when handling sharp instruments after procedures. To *prevent needlestick injuries, needles should not be recapped, purposely bent or broken by hand, removed from disposable syringes, or otherwise manipulated by hand.* After they are used, disposable syringes and needles, scalpel blades, and other sharp items should be placed in puncture-resistant containers for disposal; the puncture-resistant containers should be located as close as practical to the use area. Large-bore reusable needles should be placed in a puncture-resistant container for transport to the reprocessing area.
4. Mouth-to-mouth resuscitation mouthpieces, resuscitation bags, or other ventilation devices should be available for use in areas in which the need for resuscitation is predictable.

Adverse Reactions. Phlebitis/thrombophlebitis following IV administration, and discomfort/swelling at the injection site following IM administration. Diarrhea, nausea and/or vomiting, skin rash, anaphylaxis, pancytopenia, abdominal cramps, purpura, hypotension, weakness, headache, fever, and malaise.

Dosage and Route. Dosage and route of administration should be determined by susceptibility of the causitive organisms, severity and site of infection, and the condition of the patient. For urinary tract infection IM, IV: 500 mg or 1 Gm every 8–12 hours; IM, IV: moderately severe systemic infection 1 Gm or 2 Gm every 8–12 hours; IM, IV: severe systemic or life-threatening infections 2 Gm every 6–8 hours.

Implications for Patient Care. The nurse should obtain a history of hypersensitivity to any antibiotic or other drug. It is important to relay this information to the physician. Antibiotics should be given with caution to any patient who has had some form of allergy to drugs.

Additional Antibiotics

Table 18–6 lists additional antibiotics. Only the basic drug information is provided. Before administering any of these drugs, you should refer to the *Physicians' Desk Reference* or some other drug reference book for more detailed information.

Table 18–6 Additional Antibiotics/Antibacterials

Medication	Usual Dosage			Adverse Reactions
polymyxin B bacitracin neomycin (Neosporin)	*Ointment or Cream:*		Apply a thin layer to the area 2–5 times a day.	Ototoxicity, nephrotoxicity, hypersensitivity to neomycin.
chloramphenicol (Chloromycetin)	*Oral and IV:*		50 mg/kg/day every 6 hours in divided doses.	Bone marrow depression, blood dyscrasias, headache, confusion, nausea, vomiting, diarrhea, stomatitis, hypersensitivity, superinfection.
lincomycin HCl (Lincocin)	*Oral:*	*Adults:*	500 mg every 6–8 hours.	Nausea, vomiting, diarrhea, hypersensitivity, superinfection, hematopoietic changes.
		Children:	Over 1 month old 30–60 mg/kg/day in 3–4 divided doses.	
	IM:	*Adults:*	600 mg once or twice daily.	
		Children:	Over 1 month old, 10 mg/kg once or twice daily.	

(continued)

Table 18–6 Additional Antibiotics/Antibacterials *(Continued)*

Medication	Usual Dosage	Adverse Reactions
	IV: *Adults:* 600–1000 mg every 8–12 hours. *Children:* Over 1 month old, 10–20 mg/kg/day.	
metronidazole HCl (Flagyl)	*Oral:* 7.5 mg/kg every 6 hours. *IV:* Initially 15 mg/kg infused over 1 hour as a loading dose; thereafter 7.5–mg/kg infused over 1 hour every 6 hours.	Nausea, vomiting, diarrhea, skin rash, seizures, peripheral neuropathy.
troleandomycin (TAO)	*Oral:* *Adults:* 250–500 mg qid *Children:* 125–250 mg qid	Hypersensitivity, nausea, vomiting, diarrhea, abdominal cramps, superinfection.
vancomycin HCl (Vancocin HCl)	*Oral:* *Adults:* 500 mg every 6 hours or 1000 mg every 12 hours. *Children:* 44 mg/kg/day in divided doses. *IV:* *Adults:* 500 mg every 6 hours or 1000 mg every 12 hours. *Children:* 44 mg/kg/day in divided doses.	Nausea, chills, fever, urticaria, macular rashes, eosinophilia, hypersensitivity.
ciprofloxacin HCl (Cipro)	*Oral:* *Adults:* Infectious diarrhea: 500 mg every 12 hours. Other: 250–750 mg every 12 hours. *IV:* *Adults:* 200–400 mg twice daily infused slowly over 60 minutes.	Nausea, diarrhea, vomiting, rash headache, tremors, abdominal pain.
imipenemcilastatin sodium (Primaxin)	*IV:* *Adults:* 250–1 Gm every 6–8 hours not to exceed 50 mg/kg/day or 4 Gm day.	Nausea, diarrhea, confusion, myoclonia, seizures, superinfection.
spectinomycin HCl (Trobicin)	*IM:* *Adults:* 2 Gm	Urticaria, dizziness, nausea, chills fever, insomnia.
clindamycin HCl (Cleocin)	*Oral:* *Adults:* 150–450 mg every 6 hours with 8 ounces of water. *Children:* 8–20 mg/kg/day in 3–4 divided doses. *IM, IV:Adults:* 1.2–2.7 Gm/day in 2–4 equal divided doses. *Children:* 20–40 mg/kg/day in 3–4 equal divided doses.	Diarrhea, rash, GI upset, jaundice, renal dysfunction.

Anthelmintics

Helminthiasis is a condition in which there is an intestinal infestation by parasitic worms. Infections of this type are a major cause of disease in many areas of the world and have been associated with unsanitary living conditions. Although most commonly found in the developing countries, worm infestations can occur in any society. The helminths that infest humans belong to two groups: *Nemathelminthes* (roundworms) and *Platyhelminthes* (flatworms). The roundworms, pinworms, hookworms, and other *Nemathelminthes* of class *Nematoda* are the organisms responsible for the most common helminthic diseases worldwide and in the United States. The flatworms causing parasitic diseases are tapeworms and flukes. Most of these intestinal parasites can be eliminated by therapy with the appropriate anthelmintic. See Table 18–7.

Table 18–7 Anthelmintics

Medication	Infected by	Usual Dosage	Adverse Reactions
mebendazole (Vermox)	Roundworm, hookworm, whipworm, pinworm	Oral: 100 mg twice/day (morning and evening) for 3 consecutive days. Oral: 100 mg as a single dose.	diarrhea, fever, dizziness, transient abdominal pain
niclosamide (Niclocide)	Beef tapeworm, fish tapeworm. Dwarf tapeworm	Oral, (Adult): 4 tablets (2 Gm) as a single dose. (Child): 2–3 tablets (dosage based on kg of body weight). Oral, (Adult): 4 tablets/day for 7 days. (Child): 2–3 tablets/day for 6 days (based on kg of body weight).	drowsiness, dizziness, headache, irritability, skin rash, sweating, nausea, abdominal discomfort, edema of an arm, rectal bleeding, diarrhea
oxaminiquine (Vansil)	Blood fluke	Oral, (Adult): 12–15 mg/kg as a single dose. (Child): 20 mg/kg in 2 doses of 10 mg/kg each at 2–8 hr intervals.	drowsiness, headache, insomnia, malaise, fever, anorexia, abdominal pain, nausea, urticaria
piperazine citrate (Antepar)	Roundworm Pinworm	Oral, (Adult): 3.5 Gm 1 time/day for 2 consecutive days. (Child): 75 mg/kg. Oral, (Adult, Child): 65 mg/kg once daily for 7–8 consecutive days.	low toxicity. With higher doses: headache, vertigo, blurred vision, nausea, abdominal cramps, diarrhea, urticaria, bronchospasm
praziquantel (Biltricide)	Blood fluke Other flukes Tapeworms	Oral: 60 mg/kg in 3 divided doses at 4–6 hour intervals per day. Oral: 75 mg/kg in 3 doses/same day. Oral: 10–20 mg/kg as a single dose.	abdominal pain, nausea, anorexia, dizziness, headache, malaise, giddiness, pruritus, urticaria, fever
pyrantel pamoate (Antiminth)	Pinworm, roundworm	Oral: 11 mg/kg (5 mg/lb) in a single dose, (maximum total dose 1 Gm).	dizziness, drowsiness headache, anorexia, nausea, abdominal distention, rash

(continued)

Table 18–7 Anthelmintics *(Continued)*

Medication	Infected by	Usual Dosage	Adverse Reactions
pyrvinium pamoate (Povan)	Pinworm	Oral: 5 mg/kg as a single dose, may be repeated in 2–3 weeks, (maximum adult dose: 350 mg).	nausea, vomiting, diarrhea, cramps, photosensitivity, rash, dizziness
quinacrine HCl (Atabrine)	Beef, pork, or fish tapeworm,	Oral: 200 mg 10 minutes apart for 4 doses together with 600 mg of sodium bicarbonate for each dose.	restlessness, irritability, insomnia, nightmares, psychotic reactions, yellow pigmentation, urticaria, contact dermatitis, nausea, vomiting, anorexia, vertigo, dizziness, headache
	dwarf tapeworm	Oral, (Adult): 900 mg in 3 portions 20 minutes apart; then 100 mg 3 times daily for 3 days. (Child): initial dose 200–400 mg based on age; then 100 mg 3 times daily for 3 days.	
thiabendazole (Mintezol)	Roundworm, pinworm, hookworm, threadworm	Oral, (Patient less than 150 lb): 10–25 mg/kg in 2 doses per day; (patient over 150 lb): 1.5 Gm in 2 doses per day.	hypotension, bradycardia, anorexia, nausea, vomiting, jaundice, cholestasis, liver damage, headache, blurred vision, malodor of urine

Special Considerations

- An accurate body weight is taken before drug therapy is initiated.
- Antiminth and Vermox may be taken with food. Mintezol is usually given after meals.
- The patient's close contacts are examined and treated when necessary.
- Patient education includes ways to avoid reinfestation. Beef and pork should be thoroughly cooked to prevent the possibility of tapeworms. Avoid walking barefoot in areas where hookworms are endemic. Thoroughly wash fruits and vegetables before eating to prevent the possibility of roundworms. Instruct patient in proper hygienic measures especially handwashing procedure before meals and after using the bathroom.

Antiprotozoal Agents

Protozoa rival worms as the world's leading cause of disease and although there has been great improvement in worldwide sanitation, developing countries continue to have a high incidence of parasitic disease. Travel and military service often expose Americans to such protozoal diseases as malaria, giardiasis, trichomoniasis, and amebiasis. Worldwide, malaria is the most common cause of infectious disease. Although not widespread in the United States, the organisms that cause this disease are becoming increasingly resistant to the drugs used in treating the disease. Antiprotozoal agents are listed in Table 18–8.

Table 18–8 Antiprotozoal Agents

Medication	Disease	Usual Dosage	Adverse Reactions
chloroquine HCl (Aralen HCl)	Malaria	IM, (Adult): 160–200 mg of base repeated in 6 hours if necessary (maximum, 800 mg [base] in the first 24 hours). IM, (Child): 5 mg base/kg repeated in 6 hours (maximum, 10 mg base/kg/24 hours).	fatigue, irritability, psychoses, nightmares, heart block, hypotension, eczema, vomiting, abdominal cramps, visual disturbances
chloroquine phosphate (Aralen Phosphate)	Malaria	Oral, (Adult): 600 mg of base, then 300 mg of base at 6, 24, and 48 hours.	same as above
	Amebiasis (hepatic)	Oral, (Adult): 600 mg of base daily for 2 days, then 300 mg base/day for 2–3 weeks.	
diloxanide furoate (Entamide)	Amebiasis	Oral, (Adult): 500 mg 3 times/day for 10 days, repeated if necessary. (Child): 20 mg/kg/day in 3 divided doses for 10 days, repeated if necessary.	infrequent reactions: flatulence, nausea, diarrhea, esophagitis, pruritus
furazolidone (Furoxone)	Giardiasis	Oral, (Adult): 100 mg 4 times daily. (Child): 25–50 mg 4 times daily.	anorexia, nausea, vomiting, fever, hypotension, malaise
hydroxychloroquine sulfate (Plaquenil)	Malaria	Oral, (Adult): 800 mg followed by 400 mg after 6–8 hours, then 400 mg on each of the next 2 days for a total of 2 Gm.	GI distress, visual disturbances, retinopathy, vertigo, nerve deafness, tinnitus
iodoquinol (Yodoxin)	Amebiasis, trichomoniasis	Oral, (Adult): 650 mg 3 times/day for 20 days, to be taken after meals. (Child): 30–40 mg/kg in 2–3 doses for 20 days, not to exceed 2 Gm per day.	headache, vertigo, muscle pain, paresthesias, blurred vision, optic atrophy, discoloration of hair and nails
metronidazole (Flagyl)	Amebiasis, trichomoniasis, giardiasis	Oral, (Trichomoniasis): 2 Gm in a single or divided dose (one day therapy). Oral, (Amebiasis): (Adult): 500–750 mg 3 times/day for 5–10 days. (Child): 35–50 mg/kg/day in 3 doses for 10 days.	rash, flushing, headache, vertigo, confusion, insomnia, depression polyuria, cystitis, nausea, vomiting, anorexia, abdominal cramps, dry mouth, bitter taste, leukopenia
paromomycin sulfate (Humatin)	Amebiasis	Oral: 25–35 mg/kg divided in 3 doses, for 5–10 days.	headache, vertigo, abdominal cramps, diarrhea, nausea, ototoxicity, nephrotoxicity
primaquine phosphate	Malaria	Oral: 15 mg of base daily for 14 days.	hemolytic anemia in patients with G6PD deficiency, nausea
pyrimethamine (Daraprim)	Malaria	Oral: 25 mg once weekly.	anorexia, vomiting, skin rash, folic acid deficiency

Trichomoniasis is primarily a disease of the vagina, although it can be present in the male urethra and the rectum of either sex. Infection by *Trichomonas vaginalis* is characterized by a thin, yellow, malodorous discharge and pruritus. Giardiasis is caused by the flagellate *Giardia lamblia* which inhabit the small intestine. Many hosts are asymptomatic to the organism which is increasingly found in the United States as a result of travel to and from other countries. Amebiasis is caused by *Entamoeba histolytica* and is transmitted by ingestion of mature cysts. Colonies develop in the intestinal tract, causing diarrhea and abdominal pain in many infected by the organism.

Special Considerations

- Patients on long-term drug therapy for malaria should have periodic blood cell counts, liver function tests, and vision and hearing tests.
- Hemolytic reactions may occur in dark-skinned persons taking primaquine phosphate. Patients should be instructed to report any evidence of bleeding (blood in urine; nosebleed).
- Most anti-malarial drugs are given before or after meals to prevent gastrointestinal distress.
- Patients with amebiasis and trichomonal infections need to know the nature of their condition and its mode of transmission. Education should include proper hygienic methods.
- For treatment of trichomoniasis to be effective both male and female sexual partners must be treated simultaneously.
- Patients taking metronidazole should be instructed to avoid the use of alcohol as it may cause nausea, vomiting, headache, and abdominal cramps. Also, that the urine may change color and turn reddish-brown.

Antiseptics and Disinfectants

Antiseptics are substances that prevent or inhibit the growth of microorganisms. The process by which growth is inhibited is called *bacteriostatic* action. Antiseptics are generally applied to the surface of living tissue. Due to their lack of potency, they do little or no damage to surrounding tissue.

Disinfectants are substances, usually of chemical origin, that kill vegetative forms of microorganisms. They are described as having a *bactericidal* action due to their destruction of bacteria. Sometimes referred to as *germicides*, these agents are of sufficient strength to cause harm to living tissue; therefore, they are usually applied to inanimate objects. Disinfectants rapidly kill microorganisms on the surfaces to which they are applied, and are used on walls, floors, bed linens, furniture, and bathroom fixtures. *Fungicides* are closely related agents with the ability to kill fungi and their spores.

Phenol was the first antiseptic. Other antiseptics are compared with phenol to measure their effectiveness; this measure is known as the phenol coefficient (P/C). Many antiseptics contain phenol and related compounds (see Table 18–9).

Table 18–9 Antiseptics and Disinfectants

Substance	Strength	Action	Comments
alcohol Ethyl Isopropyl (rubbing)	 70% solution full strength	antiseptic germicide	For external use only. Used to prepare the skin for injections, venipuncture, and IV therapy. Flammable.
benzalkonium chloride (Zephiran)	1:750 1:2000–1:5000 1:5000 1:5000–1:10,000 1:2000–1:20,000	antiseptic	On intact skin, mucous membranes, superficial injury. Vaginal douching. Wet dressings. Irrigations of the eye, body cavities. Infected wounds.
phenolics (Cresol) (Lysol) (Amphyl)	2%–5%	disinfectant	On contaminated objects: linens, basins, bedpans. Action not affected by organic material.
(Staphene)	$\frac{1}{2}$% $2\frac{1}{2}$%	antiseptic disinfectant	As a footbath for athlete's foot; prolonged use may be injurious to tissues.
gentian violet	1:100–1:1000	antiseptic fungicide dye	Used on skin and mucous membrane for fungus infections (thrush, impetigo).
iodine (solution or tincture)	2%	antiseptic fungicide	Used on small wounds and abrasions. *Check for allergies.*
(Wescodyne) (Betadine)	$1–1\frac{1}{2}$% iodine and detergent	germicide	Used as a surgical prep to reduce number of organisms on the skin and reduce the chance of infection. Hand rinse.
hydrogen peroxide	3% (diluted with 1–4 parts water)	antiseptic	Cleans wounds of pus, dead tissue. Deteriorates upon standing. Store in a cool, dark place.
hexachlorophene (pHisoHex) (WescoHex) (Septi-Soft) (Septisol)	3% topical emulsion, liquid soap, lotions, ointments, and shampoos	bacteriostatic against gram + bacteria on the skin	Not used for bathing infants. Rinse skin after use. May produce erythema, dryness, and scaling on patients with sensitive skin.
formalin (Cidex)	0.5–0.9% 6–12 hours	disinfectant	Effective against viruses, spores; irritates tissues.
green soap (solution or tincture)	1:10	antiseptic	Handwash; used to wash thermometers.
silver nitrate	1% (ophthalmic solution) 1:1000 1:10,000	antiseptic antiseptic antiseptic	Prevents gonorrheal conjunctivitis in newborns. Astringent. Bladder irrigations.
sodium hypochlorite (household bleach)	1:10 1:100	germicide germicide	HIV (AIDS) inactivator. Use on contaminated surfaces.

Alcohol may be used as an antiseptic or as a germicide depending upon the type used and its strength. Ethyl alcohol (70 percent solution) is often used as an antiseptic for minor injuries, and to prepare the skin for injections. Used full strength, isopropyl alcohol is a germicide for the disinfection of instruments. It may also be used in a 70 percent solution for the disinfection of oral thermometers.

Tincture of iodine contains 2 percent iodine and 2.4 percent sodium iodide diluted in 50 percent ethyl alcohol. It may be used as a disinfectant for the skin, and as a germicide. Adding three drops of tincture of iodine to a quart of water will kill amebas and bacteria within 30 minutes, and the water will still be palatable (see Table 18–9).

The effectiveness of an antiseptic or a disinfectant depends upon the following factors:

- the strength of the solution,
- the temperature of the solution,
- the time of exposure,
- the ionization rate of the substance used.

Table 18–9 lists antiseptics and disinfectants that are in general use. Note that the brand or trade name for these products is shown in parenthesis.

◆ Review Questions

Directions: Select the best answer to each multiple choice question. Circle the letter of your choice.

1. An individual hypersensitivity to a substance, usually an antibody-antigen reaction is known as __________.

   a. anaphylaxis b. allergy c. superinfection d. toxicity

2. __________ is the process whereby a pathogenic agent invades the body, multiplies, and produces injury.

   a. Inflammation b. Allergy c. Infection d. Disease

3. __________ may be natural or synthetic substances that inhibit growth of or destroy microorganisms.

   a. Disinfectants
   b. Antiseptics
   c. Antibiotics
   d. Antineoplastics

4. __________ may occur when there is overgrowth of a resistant strain of bacteria, fungi, or yeast.

   a. Hypersensitivity
   b. Organ toxicity
   c. Superinfection
   d. Renal impairment

5. The most common adverse reaction to penicillins is __________.
   a. an allergic one b. nausea c. fever d. diarrhea
6. The usual adult oral dose of ampicillin is __________.
   a. 200,000 to 500,000 units every 6–8 hours
   b. 125 to 500 mg every 6–8 hours
   c. 250 to 500 mg every 6 hours
   d. 382 mg to 764 mg qid
7. The cephalosporins are chemically and pharmacologically related to __________.
   a. tetracyclines
   b. penicillins
   c. aminoglycosides
   d. erythromycin
8. The usual adult parenteral dose of Mandol is __________.
   a. 1 to 2 Gm every 4–6 hours
   b. 250 mg to 2 Gm every 8–12 hours
   c. 1 Gm once a day every 24 hours
   d. 500 mg to 1 Gm every 4–8 hours
9. Tetracyclines are contraindicated in __________.
   a. patients with renal and liver impairment
   b. pregnant and lactating patients
   c. children eight years of age and younger
   d. all of these
10. __________ can cause irreversible damage to the auditory branch of the 8th cranial nerve (acoustic).
    a. Penicillins
    b. Aminoglycosides
    c. Tetracyclines
    d. Cephalosporins
11. Signs of ototoxicity are __________.
    a. diarrhea, fever, and sweating
    b. nausea, vomiting, and vertigo
    c. pruritus, stomatitis, and headache
    d. oliguria and proteinuria
12. A broad-spectrum antibiotic, similar to penicillins, and one which is often used against penicillin-resistant microorganisms is __________.
    a. erythromycin
    b. neosporin
    c. chloromycetin
    d. TAO (troleandomycin)

13. Before administering any drug you should __________.
    a. check the drug's expiration date
    b. verify the order
    c. refer to a drug reference book for detailed information
    d. all of these

14. The usual oral adult dose of E.E.S. is __________.
    a. 500 mg every 6 hours
    b. 300 mg every 6 hours
    c. 250 mg every 6 hours
    d. 400 mg every 6 hours

15. Emergency medications that should be readily available when administering any drug should include __________.
    a. epinephrine
    b. diphenhydramine
    c. dopamine and corticosteroids
    d. all of these

16. Cefotetan (Cefotan) is classified as a __________.
    a. penicillin
    b. tetracycline
    c. cephalosporin
    d. erythromycin

17. Signs of nephrotoxicity are __________.
    a. jaundice, headache, dizziness
    b. jaundice, diarrhea, constipation
    c. oliguria and proteinuria
    d. nausea, vomiting, diarrhea

18. A condition in which there is an intestinal infestation by parasitic worms is known as __________.
    a. giardiasis
    b. amebiasis
    c. helminthiasis
    d. trichomonas

19. Diarrhea, fever, dizziness, and transient abdominal pain are adverse reactions of __________.
    a. Atabrine
    b. Mintezol
    c. Vermox
    d. Vansil

20. When a person is infected by tapeworms, Biltricide may be prescribed. The usual oral dose is __________.
    a. 11 mg/kg
    b. 5 mg/kg
    c. 10–20 mg/kg
    d. 12–15 mg/kg

21. The following are all protozoal diseases except __________.
    a. malaria
    b. giardiasis
    c. amebiasis
    d. monilia

22. Zithromax is indicated in the treatment of certain infections that are caused by susceptible bacteria and should not be used in patients who are __________ years of age or younger.

    a. 21 b. 15 c. 17 d. 22

23. Anorexia, vomiting, skin rash, and folic acid deficiency are adverse reactions of __________.

    a. Aralen HCl b. Entamide c. Flagyl d. Daraprim

24. A patient asks why bathing with Betadine before surgery is necessary. The nurse's reply is based on the understanding that Betadine (iodine solution) is used to __________.

    a. sterilize the skin
    b. reduce the number of microorganisms, which will help prevent infection
    c. improve circulation
    d. relieve itching

Case Study: John James, 13 years old, is admitted to the hospital with a possible ruptured appendix. An emergency appendectomy is performed and a drain is inserted in the incision. He is placed on antibiotics and medication for pain. (Questions 25–28 relate to this.)

25. In monitoring John for hypersensitivity to antibiotics, the nurse should observe for __________.

    a. hypertension b. anorexia c. urticaria d. constipation

26. The physician orders that epinephrine and diphenhydramine be kept at the bedside. The nurse should know that the trade names for these medications are __________.

    a. Amoxil and Depo-Medrol
    b. Adrenalin and Benadryl
    c. Hydrocortisone and Valium
    d. Dilaudid and Norflex

27. John is to receive Ceftin 20 mg/kg every 12 hours. John weighs 88 pounds. What is the correct dosage?

    a. 500 mg b. 600 mg c. 800 mg d. 1000 mg

28. John is to receive Demerol 50 mg every 4 hours for pain. On hand is Demerol 100 mg/ml. What is the correct dosage?

    a. 1 ml b. $\frac{1}{2}$ ml c. $\frac{3}{4}$ ml d. 2 ml

Matching: Place the correct letter from Column II on the appropriate line of Column I.

Column I

29. __________ Bactericidal
30. __________ Bacteriostatic
31. __________ Disinfectant
32. __________ Infection
33. __________ Pathogen
34. __________ Antiseptic
35. __________ Bacteria
36. __________ Microorganism

Column II

A. A microorganism or substance that is capable of producing disease.

B. A minute living body that is not visible to the naked eye.

C. A substance that prevents or inhibits the growth of microorganisms, especially bacteria.

D. Pertaining to the killing or destruction of bacteria.

E. Pertaining to inhibiting or retarding bacterial growth.

F. A chemical agent that kills vegetative forms of bacteria.

G. The process or state whereby a pathogenic agent invades the body or a body part, multiplies, and produces injury.

H. Any microorganism of the *Schizomycetes* class.

I. A chemical substance that destroys fungi.

CHAPTER 19

Antifungal, Antiviral, and Immunizing Agents

OBJECTIVES

Upon completion of this chapter, you should be able to:

- Define the terms listed in the vocabulary.
- State the actions, uses, contraindications, adverse reactions, dosages, routes, and implications for patient care of selected antifungal and antiviral agents.
- Define acquired immune deficiency syndrome (AIDS).
- List the groups of people who make up 98 percent of all AIDS cases.
- Describe symptoms that become apparent as AIDS progresses.
- Become familiar with the CDC's 1993 Revised Classification of HIV infection and AIDS.
- List nine facts about HIV in babies and children.
- Describe zidovudine's role in the reduction of perinatal transmission of HIV.
- Explain how HIV infection and AIDS can be contracted by a child.
- List the signs and symptoms of AIDS in the older adult.
- Explain how AIDS is diagnosed in the older adult.
- Describe the treatment regimen for AIDS in the older adult.
- Complete the critical thinking questions/activities presented in this chapter.
- Differentiate between active and passive immunization.
- State the general recommendations of immunization.
- Describe the conditions when a live, attenuated-virus vaccine should not be given.
- Define *vaccine, toxoid, immune globulin, specific immune globulin*, and *antitoxin*.
- State who should be immunized against vaccine-preventable diseases.

- List the emergency supplies and medications that must be readily available when administering any drug to a patient.
- Describe the Standards for Pediatric Immunization Practices.
- Become familiar with the immunization schedules given in this chapter.
- Complete the Spot Check on childhood immunizations.
- Answer the review questions correctly.

Vocabulary

adenovirus (ad″e-no-vi′rus). One of a group of closely related viruses that can cause infections of the upper respiratory tract.

antibody (an′ti-bod″e). A protein substance that is developed in response to an antigen.

antigen (an′ti-jen). Substances such as bacteria, toxins, certain allergens, that induce the formation of antibodies that specifically interact with the antigen.

antigenic (an-ti-jen′ik). Capable of causing the production of an antibody.

Candida (kan′di-da). A genus of yeastlike fungi. It is a part of the normal flora of the mouth, skin, intestinal tract, and vagina. *Candida* is one of the most common causes of vaginitis in women during the reproductive years. Formerly called Monilia.

cryptococcosis (krip″to-kok-o′sis). A systemic fungus infection that may involve any organ of the body, especially the lungs, skin, brain and its meninges.

cytomegalovirus (si″to-meg″a-lo-vi′rus). One of a group of species-specific herpesvirus.

epidemiological (ep″i-de-me-ol′o-ji-cal). Pertaining to the science concerned with defining and explaining the interrelationship of factors that determine the frequency and distribution of disease.

herpes simplex virus (her′pez sim′pleks vi′rus). Type 1 (HSV-1) causes cold sores or fever blisters. Type 2 (HSV-2) causes genital herpes.

histoplasmosis (his-to-plaz-mo′sis). A systemic, fungal respiratory disease.

human immunodeficiency virus (HIV). The appropriate name for the retrovirus that has been implied as the causative agent of AIDS (acquired immune deficiency syndrome). Accepted by a subcommittee of the International Committee for the Taxonomy of Viruses, 1986. The AIDS virus has been variously termed human T-lymphotropic virus type III (HTLV-III/LAV), lymphadenopathy-associated virus (LAV), AIDS-associated retrovirus (ARV), or human immunodeficiency virus (HIV).

immunocompetence (im″u-no-kom′pe-tens). Being capable of developing an antibody (antigenic response) to stimulation by an antigen.

immunodeficiency (im″u-no-de-fish′en-se). A decreased or lack of ability to respond to antigenic stimuli, thus suppressing or altering the body's natural immune response.

phagocytosis (fag″o-si-to′sis). The ingestion and digestion of bacteria and particles by cells of the reticuloendothelial system and white blood cells.

retrovirus (ret′ro-vi″rus). Ribonucleic acid (RNA)-containing virus.

varicella (var″i-sel′a). A benign, highly contagious disease caused by varicella-zoster (V-Z) virus. Chickenpox.

volar (vo′lar). Refers to the palm of the hand or the palmar surface.

Introduction

Viruses are parasites, minute organisms that may invade normal cells and cause disease. They depend upon the invaded cells for nutrition, metabolism, and reproduction. To date, over 300 viruses have been isolated from animal hosts. Many of these viruses are considered to be harmless, but others are the cause of approximately half of all infectious diseases. The common cold (coryza), smallpox, yellow fever, most childhood diseases, herpes, influenza, Epstein-Barr syndrome, rabies, hepatitis-B, and AIDS (acquired *immune deficiency* syndrome) are virus-related infections.

Fungi are plant-like organisms that also depend upon a host for their existence. These organisms, which include molds and yeasts, may be parasitic, or grow in dead and decaying organic matter. Many forms of fungi are pathogenic to plants and animals, causing such diseases as histoplasmosis, *Candida* infections, cryptococcosis, athlete's foot, and tinea.

As mentioned in Chapter 18, the immune system is the body's defense mechanism against viruses, fungi, bacteria, and other foreign substances. Known collectively as *antigens*, these foreign substances, when detected, are the targets of a number of specialized cells that are activated in response to their presence. Simply stated, there are four general phases associated with the body's immune response to a foreign substance.

1. The recognition of the enemy or foreign substance
2. Amplification of the body's defenses—white blood cells
   - *Phagocytes:* the "cell eater," especially macrophages
   - *Lymphocytes:* T-Cells and B-cells

     —*Helper T-cell* is the commander in chief. It identifies the enemy and rushes to the spleen and lymph nodes, where it stimulates the production of other cells to aid in the fight of the infection.

     —*Killer T-cell* specializes in killing cells of the body that have been invaded by foreign substances. It also fights cells that have turned cancerous.

     —*B-cell* is the biologic arms factory. It resides in the spleen or lymph nodes and produces antibodies.

3. The attack phase, during which these defenders of the body seek to kill and remove the foreign invader.
4. The slowdown phase, during which the number of defenders return to normal following victory over the foreign invader.

Antifungal Agents

Antifungal agents are synthetic drugs that destroy or inhibit the growth of fungi. They are also effective against yeast.

Characteristics and Uses

Actions. Antifungal agents act by exerting *fungistatic* or *fungicidal* action on both resting and growing cells. They bind to certain sterols of thc cell membrane, thus allowing leakage of essential intracellular compounds which results in death of the cell. They are not effective against bacteria, *rickettsiae*, or viruses.

Uses. Antifungal agents are used for systemic, skin, and mucous membrane fungal infections. Some diseases for which a physician may prescribe an antifungal agent are: *histoplasmosis, Candida* infections of the skin, mucous membrane, intestines, and vagina; *cryptococcosis*, athlete's foot, and tinea (ringworm) infections.

Contraindications. Hypersensitivity to antifungal agents. Contraindicated in patients with bone marrow depression or renal function impairment. Safe use of some agents during pregnancy and lactation has not been established.

Adverse Reactions. Nausea, vomiting, diarrhea, headache, vertigo, muscle pain, tinnitus, anemia, leukopenia, and hypersensitive reactions such as pruritus, urticaria, rash, fever, and anaphylaxis.

Dosage and Route. The dosage and route of administration is determined by the physician. See Table 19–1 for selected antifungal agents.

Implications for Patient Care. Observe the patient for any signs of hypersensitivity. Care should be exercised when inserting an antifungal agent intravaginally. To prevent possible spread of the disease, one must wear latex gloves. When applying a cream, lotion or ointment to the candidal lesions, one must wear latex gloves, use an appropriate applicator, and not contaminate the medication container.

Patient Teaching. Instruct the patient in the importance of following the prescribed medication regimen. Patients with vaginal infections should be advised that fungus or yeast infections are easily spread. Some physicians prefer that the patient refrain from sexual intercourse while the infection is being treated. Inform the patient that her infection can be spread through sexual intercourse and that her partner could become infected, and then possibly reinfect her. It is highly recommended that a protective device, such as a condom, be utilized during sexual intercourse.

Table 19–1 Selected Antifungal Agents

Medication	Usual Dosage	Adverse Reactions
nystatin (Mycostatin)	*Oral:* 500,000–1,000,000 units (1–2 tabs) tid *Suspension:* *Adults and Children:* 4–6 ml qid (400,000–600,000 units). *Infants:* 2 ml qid (200,000 units). *Vaginal Tabs:* 100,000 units (1 tab) daily for 2 weeks.	Virtually nontoxic—large oral doses have occasionally produced diarrhea, nausea, vomiting.
flucytosine (Ancobon)	*Oral:* 50–150 mg/kg/day at 6 hour intervals.	Nausea, vomiting, diarrhea, rash, anemia, leukopenia, thrombopenia, elevated hepatic enzymes.
miconazole nitrate (Monistat) (See Figure 19–1)	*Vaginal Suppository:* one 100 mg suppository is inserted intravaginally once daily at bedtime for 7 nights. *Vaginal Cream:* 1 applicatorful intravaginally once daily at bedtime for 7 days.	Vulvovaginal burning, itching or irritation, cramping, headache, hives, skin rash.
amphotericin B (Fungizone)	*Cream, lotion, ointment:* applied liberally to the Candidal lesions 2–4 times a day.	No evidence of systemic toxicity; may have a "drying" effect on some skin, local irritation, erythema, pruritus or burning.
ketoconazole (Nizoral)	*Oral: Adults:* 200 mg (1 tab); 400 mg (2 tab) once daily. *Children:* Over 2 years of age: 3.3–6.6 mg/kg daily dose.	Anaphylaxis (rare cases), hypersensitivity, nausea vomiting, abdominal pain, pruritus, headache, fever, diarrhea, gynecomastia, impotence, oligospermia.
griseofulvin (Grifulvin V)	*Oral: Adults:* 500 mg daily dose. *Children:* 5 mg/lb body weight, per day: 30–50 lbs 125–250 mg, over 50 lbs 250–500 mg.	Hypersensitivity, skin rashes, urticaria, oral thrush, nausea, vomiting, epigastric distress, diarrhea, headache, fatigue, dizziness.
clotrimazole (Lotrimin)	*Cream, lotion, solution:* Gently massage sufficient Lotrimin into the affected and surrounding skin areas twice a day, in the morning and evening.	Erythema, stinging, blistering, peeling, edema, pruritus, urticaria, burning and general irritation of the skin.
fluconazole (Diflucan)	*Oral:* 200 mg on the first day, then 100 mg once a day for 2–4 weeks. *IV:* maximum rate of 200 mg/hour given as a continuous infusion.	Nausea, headache, skin rash, vomiting, abdominal pain, diarrhea.

Patients with Candida infections should be instructed in correct handwashing procedure, proper personal hygiene (drying the genital area after bathing, showering, or swimming; wiping from front to back after a bowel movement, so that the organisms from the rectum will not be spread to the vagina), and wearing natural (cotton) underclothes. They should also avoid using heavily fragranced products such as soaps, bubble baths,

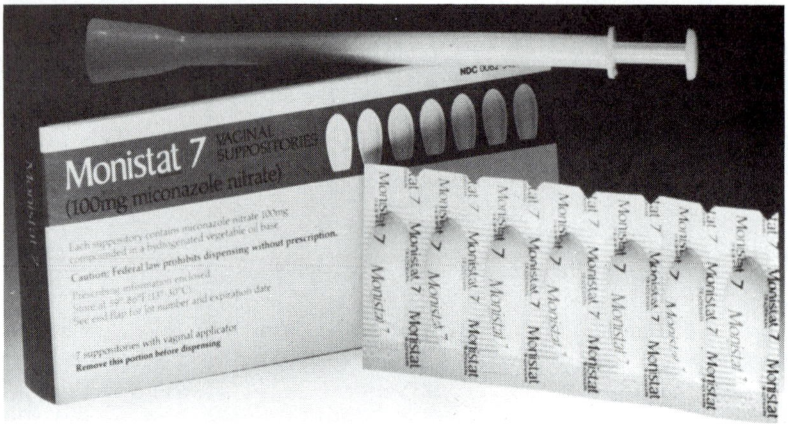

Figure 19–1 Monistat™ 7 *(Courtesy of Ortho Pharmaceutical Corporation)*

toilet paper and feminine hygiene sprays, as these products contain ingredients that can worsen any local irritation.

To improve safety and effectiveness of over-the-counter antifungal products the Federal Food and Drug Administration (FDA) has released guidelines on topical products used to treat tinea infections, athlete's foot, jock itch, and ringworm. These guidelines include the following:

- Product may contain only one active ingredient—limited to clioquinol, halprogin, miconazole nitrate, povidone-iodine, tolnaftate, or undecylenic acid and its salts.
- Ingredients banned because of their ineffectiveness as antifungal agents are: alcloxa, aluminum sulfate, basic fuchsin, boric acid, camphor, chloroxylenol, menthol, and salicylic acid.
- Antifungal products must carry a label that reads, "This product is not effective on the scalp or nails" and a warning against use in children under 2 unless directed by a physician and then, only using the product externally.

Antiviral Agents

Antiviral agents are synthetic drugs that have been developed to combat specific viral diseases. Viruses are responsible for many diseases, such as the common cold (coryza), influenza, genital herpes, herpes zoster, and acquired immune deficiency syndrome (AIDS). In the United States, only a few antiviral drugs are employed in the treatment of specific viral diseases. Details on these drugs follow. (Note: The generic drug name is listed first, followed by the trade name in parenthesis.)

acyclovir (Zovirax)

Actions. In vitro inhibitory activity against *herpes simplex virus* types 1 and 2 (HSV-1 and HSV-2), *varicella-zoster*, Epstein-Barr and *cytomegalovirus.*

Uses. Treatment for initial episodes and the management of recurrent episodes of genital herpes in certain patients. *It is not a cure for genital herpes.*

Contraindications. In patients who develop hypersensitivity or intolerance to the components of the formulation. Not used during pregnancy. Cautious use during lactation.

Adverse Reactions. Nausea, vomiting, diarrhea, dizziness, anorexia, fatigue, edema, skin rash, leg pain, inguinal adenopathy, confusion, and headache.

Dosage and Route

Oral: Initial: 200 mg cap every 4 hours for total of 5 caps daily for 10 days (total of 50 caps)
Recurrent disease: one 200 mg cap tid for up to 6 months

Ointment: apply sufficient quantity to adequately cover all lesions every 3 hours, 6 times a day for 7 days

> **CAUTION:** A finger cot or latex glove should be used when applying Zovirax to prevent autoinoculation of other body sites and transmission of infection to other persons.

Implications for Patient Care. The nurse should observe the patient for any signs of hypersensitivity, nausea, and vomiting. Care should be exercised when applying Zovirax to lesions. To prevent possible spread of the disease one *must* wear a finger cot or latex gloves.

Patient Teaching. The patient should be informed that genital herpes is a sexually transmitted disease, and that intercourse should be avoided when lesions are visible because of the risk of infecting one's sexual partner. Advise the patient to contact her physician if sufficient relief is not obtained, if there are any adverse reactions, if she becomes pregnant or plans to become pregnant, or if she has any questions.

famciclovir (Famvir)

Actions. In vitro and in vivo antiviral activity against herpes simplex virus types 1 (HSV-1) and 2 (HSV-2) and varicella-zoster virus (VZV).

Uses. Indicated for the management of acute herpes zoster (shingles).

Contraindications. In patients with known hypersensitivity to the product.

Adverse Reactions. Headache, nausea, diarrhea, and fatigue.

Dosage and Route. 500 mg every 8 hours for seven days

Implications for Patient Care. For best results treatment should begin as soon as herpes zoster is diagnosed. Treatment is most effective if started within 48 hours of rash onset. In patients with reduced renal function, dosage reduction is recommended.

Patient Teaching. Famvir may be taken without regard to meals. Advise patient to report any adverse reactions to his/her physician.

amantadine hydrochloride (Symmetrel)

Actions. Antiviral activity against influenza A is not completely understood. The mode of action appears to be prevention of the release of infectious viral nucleic acid into the host cell.

Uses. Influenza A virus respiratory tract illness-prevention and treatment. Also used in Parkinson's disease/syndrome and drug-induced extrapyramidal reactions.

Contraindications. In patients with known hypersensitivity to the drug. Not used during pregnancy. Cautious use during lactation.

Adverse Reactions. Depression, congestive heart failure, orthostatic hypotensive episodes, psychosis, urinary retention, drowsiness, and dizziness.

Dosage and Route

Oral: Adults: 200 mg daily dose (two 100 mg caps) or 4 tsp of syrup.

Children: 1–9 years of age: 100 mg twice a day (one 100 mg cap) or 2 tsp bid.

Implications for Patient Care. Medication should be taken after meals. Patient assessment includes observing for signs of hypersensitivity and adverse reactions.

Patient Teaching. Instruct the patient not to stand or change positions too quickly, as orthostatic hypotensive episodes may occur. With these episodes the patient would feel faint as the blood pressure drops suddenly.

vidarabine (Vira-A)

Actions. Antiviral activity against herpes simplex virus types 1 and 2, and in vitro activity against varicella-zoster virus.

Uses. Herpes simplex virus encephalitis and herpes zoster.

Contraindications. In patients who develop a hypersensitivity to the drug. Not used during pregnancy or lactation.

Adverse Reactions. Anorexia, nausea, vomiting, diarrhea, tremor, dizziness, headache, confusion, psychosis, and ataxia.

Dosage and Route

IV Infusion by the physician or a registered nurse:

Herpes simplex virus encephalitis: 15 mg/kg/day for 10 days.
Herpes zoster: 10 mg/kg/day for 5 days.

Ophthalmic Ointment: keratoconjunctivitis: approximately $\frac{1}{2}$ inch into lower conjunctival sac 5 times a day at 3 hour intervals.

Implications for Patient Care. Patient assessment includes observing the patient for signs of gastrointestinal upset, central nervous symptoms, and hypersensitivity.

IV Infusion: The medication is slowly infused and the patient is carefully monitored during the process.

Patient Teaching. Instruct the patient in the proper technique of applying an ophthalmic ointment.

rimantadine (Flumadine)

Actions. Antiviral activity against influenza A virus.

Uses. In adults, rimantadine is indicated for the prevention and treatment of illness caused by various strains of influenza A virus. In children, it is only approved for prevention.

Contraindications. Known hypersensitivity to rimantadine or other drugs of the adamantane class such as amatadine (Symadine, Symmetrel).

Adverse Reactions. Nausea, vomiting, nervousness, insomnia, and dizziness.

Dosage and Route

Oral: Adults: 100 mg twice a day.

Geriatric patients or anyone with kidney failure or severe liver problems, the dose is reduced to 100 mg once a day.

Children: 10 years or older 100 mg twice a day.
1–9 years 5 mg/kg, but not exceeding 150 mg.

Implications for Patient Care. For prevention, one should start on medication as early as possible after a community outbreak of influenza A. For additional prophylaxis after one has been vaccinated, medication may be taken for two to four weeks.

Patient Teaching. Advise patient to report any adverse reactions to his/her physician. Inform the geriatric patient that he/she may experience gastrointestinal problems, insomnia, and nervousness.

trifluridine (Viroptic ophthalmic solution 1%)

Actions. Antiviral activity against herpes simplex virus, types 1 and 2 and vacciniavirus. Some strains of *Adenovirus* are also inhibited in vitro.

Uses. Topical treatment of epithelial keratitis caused by herpes simplex virus, types 1 and 2. Treatment of primary keratoconjunctivitis.

Contraindications. In patients who develop hypersensitivity reactions or chemical intolerance to trifluridine. Not used during pregnancy or lactation.

Adverse Reactions. Mild burning or stinging upon instillation; hypersensitivity.

Dosage and Route

Ophthalmic: Instill 1 drop onto cornea of affected eye every 2 hours. Maximum daily dose 9 drops until corneal ulcer has completely re-epithelialized.

Implications for Patient Care. Use aseptic technique when instilling eye drops.

Patient Teaching. Instruct the patient to follow the recommended dosage and not to exceed the number of drops prescribed. Aseptic technique should be used when instilling eye drops. Instruct the patient in the proper instillation of eye drops.

ribavirin (Virazole)

Actions. Antiviral inhibitory activity in vitro against respiratory syncytial virus, influenza virus, and herpes simplex virus. The mechanism of action is unknown.

Uses. Ribavirin aerosol is indicated in the treatment of carefully selected hospitalized infants and young children with severe lower respiratory tract infections due to respiratory syncytial virus (RSV).

Contraindications. In women or girls who are or may become pregnant during exposure to the drug. Ribavirin may cause fetal harm.

Adverse Reactions. Chronic obstructive lung disease, dyspnea, chest soreness, worsening of respiratory status, bacterial pneumonia, pneumothorax, apnea, ventilator dependence, cardiac arrest, hypotension, and digitalis toxicity.

Dosage and Route. Ribavirin is lyophilized for aerosol administration. Before use one must read thoroughly the Viratek Small Particle Aerosol Generator (SPAG) Model APAG-2 Operations Manual for small particle aerosol generator operating instructions.

Acquired Immune Deficiency Syndrome (AIDS)

The following information is adapted from the American Red Cross, "What Everyone Needs to Know About AIDS," and the Centers for Disease Control and Prevention

VISUAL IDENTIFICATION GUIDE

Use this section to quickly verify the identity of a capsule, tablet, or other solid oral medication. More than 200 leading products are shown in actual size and color, organized alphabetically by generic name. Each product is labeled with its brand name, if applicable, as well as its strength and the name of its supplier.

ACARBOSE TABLETS

PRECOSE
BAYER

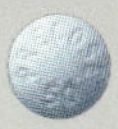

50 mg

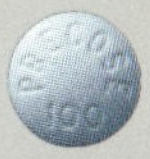

100 mg

ACYCLOVIR (ACYCLOGUANOSINE)

ZOVIRAX
GLAXO WELLCOME

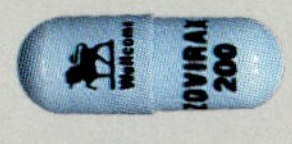

200 mg

ALENDRONATE SODIUM

FOSAMAX
MERCK

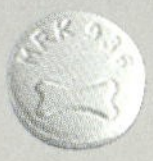

10 mg

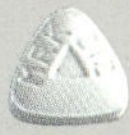

40 mg

ALPRAZOLAM

XANAX
UPJOHN

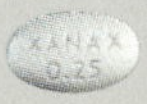

0.25 mg

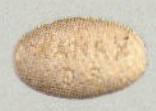

0.5 mg

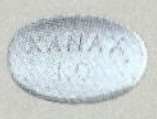

1 mg

AMLODIPINE

NORVASC
PFIZER LABS

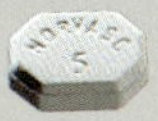

5 mg

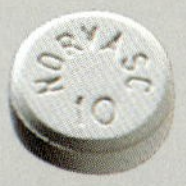

10 mg

AMOXICILLIN (AMOXYCILLIN)

AMOXIL
SMITHKLINE BEECHAM

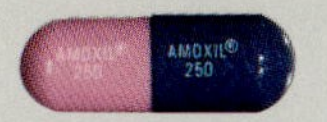

250 mg

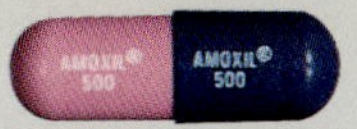

500 mg

AMOXICILLIN AND POTASSIUM CLAVULANATE

AUGMENTIN
SMITHKLINE BEECHAM

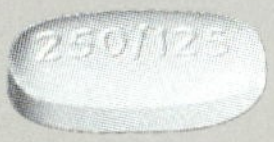

250 mg / 125 mg

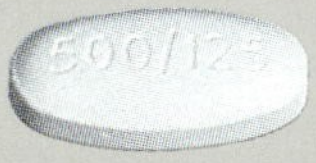

500 mg / 125 mg

ASTEMIZOLE

HISMANAL
JANSSEN

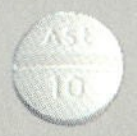

10 mg

ATENOLOL

TENORMIN
ZENECA

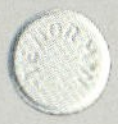

50 mg

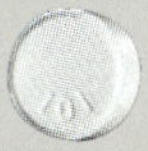

100 mg

AZITHROMYCIN

ZITHROMAX
PFIZER LABS

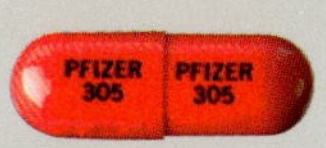

250 mg

BENAZEPRIL HCL

LOTENSIN
CIBAGENEVA

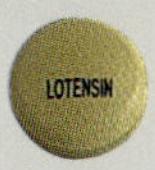

10 mg

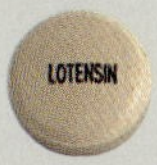

20 mg

BUMETANIDE

BUMEX
ROCHE

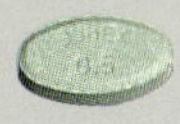

0.5 mg

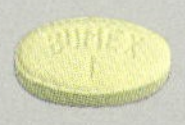

1 mg

BUSPIRONE HCL

BUSPAR
BRISTOL-MYERS SQUIBB

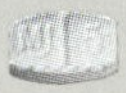

5 mg

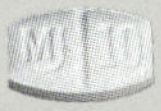

10 mg

CAPTOPRIL

CAPOTEN
BRISTOL-MYERS SQUIBB

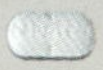

12.5 mg

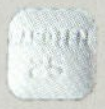

25 mg

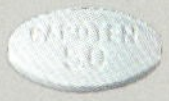

50 mg

CARBAMAZEPINE

TEGRETOL
CIBAGENEVA

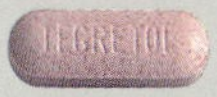

200 mg

CEFACLOR

CECLOR
ELI LILLY

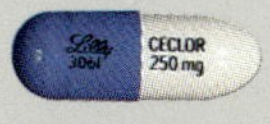

250 mg

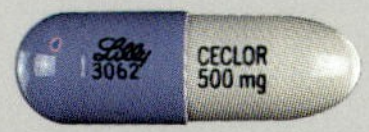

500 mg

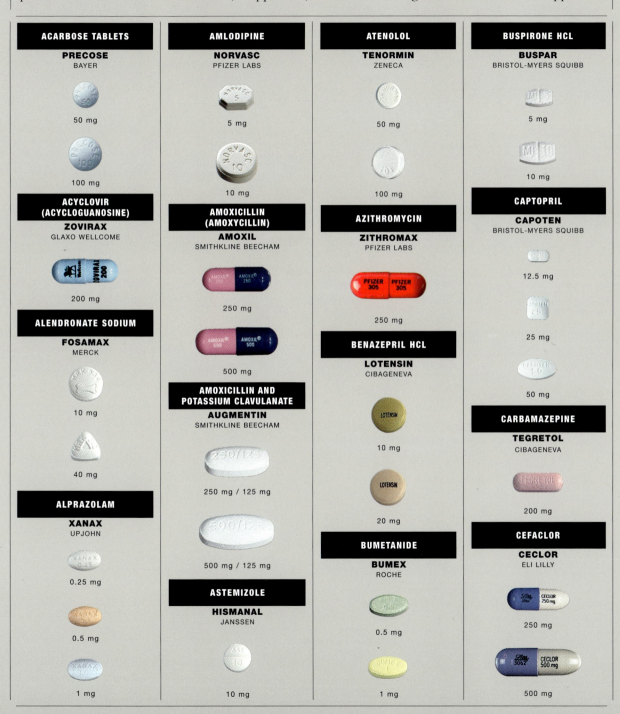

CEFADROXIL MONOHYDRATE

DURICEF
BRISTOL-MYERS SQUIBB

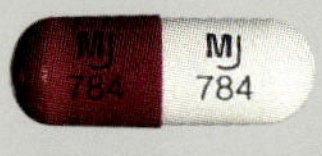

500 mg

CEFIXIME

SUPRAX
LEDERLE

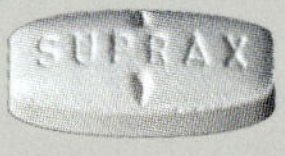

400 mg

CEFPROZIL

CEFZIL
BRISTOL-MYERS SQUIBB

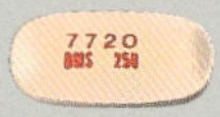

250 mg

CEFUROXIME AXETIL

CEFTIN
GLAXO

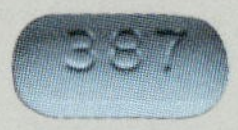

250 mg

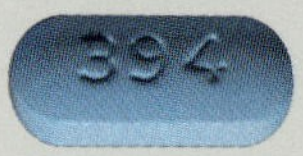

500 mg

CIMETIDINE

TAGAMET
SMITHKLINE BEECHAM

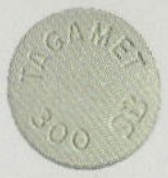

300 mg

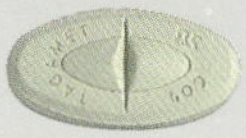

400 mg

CIPROFLOXACIN HCL

CIPRO
BAYER

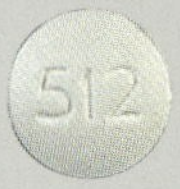

250 mg

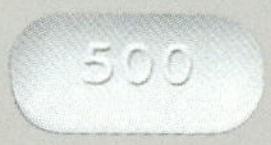

500 mg

CLARITHROMYCIN

BIAXIN
ABBOTT

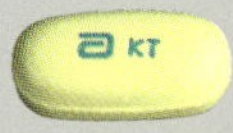

250 mg

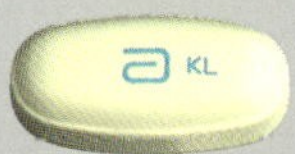

500 mg

CLONAZEPAM

KLONOPIN
ROCHE

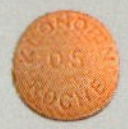

0.5 mg

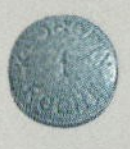

1 mg

CYCLOBENZAPRINE HCL

FLEXERIL
MERCK

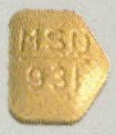

10 mg

DARVOCET-N 100

ACETAMINOPHEN AND PROPOXYPHENE NAPSYLATE
ELI LILLY

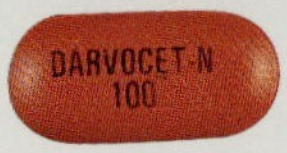

650 mg / 100 mg

DIAZEPAM

VALIUM
ROCHE

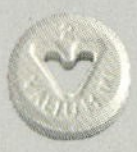

2 mg

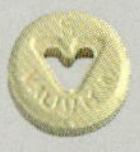

5 mg

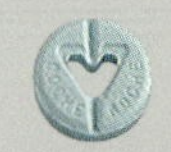

10 mg

DICLOFENAC SODIUM

VOLTAREN
CIBAGENEVA

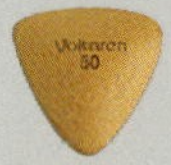

50 mg

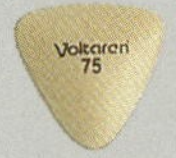

75 mg

DICYCLOMINE HCL

BENTYL
HOECHST MARION ROUSSEL

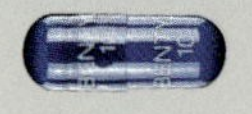

10 mg

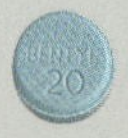

20 mg

DIGOXIN

LANOXIN
BURROUGHS WELLCOME

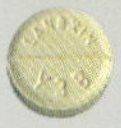

0.125 mg

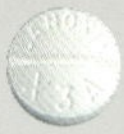

0.25 mg

DILTIAZEM HCL

CARDIZEM CD
HOECHST MARION ROUSSEL

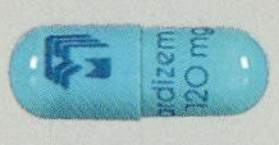

120 mg

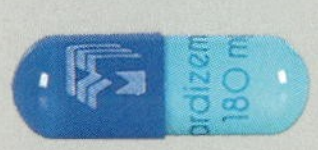

180 mg

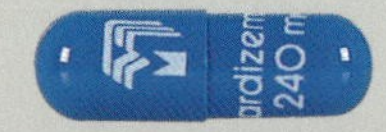

240 mg

DIVALPROEX SODIUM

DEPAKOTE
ABBOTT

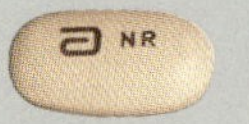

250 mg

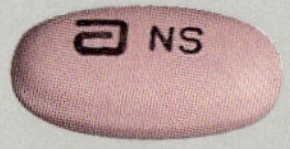

500 mg

DOXAZOSIN MESYLATE

CARDURA
ROERIG

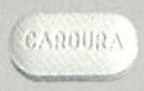

1 mg

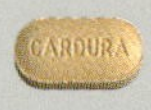

2 mg

ENALAPRIL MALEATE

VASOTEC
MERCK

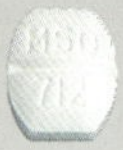

5 mg

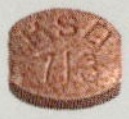

10 mg

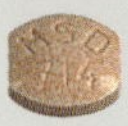

20 mg

ERYTHROMYCIN BASE

ERY-TAB
ABBOTT

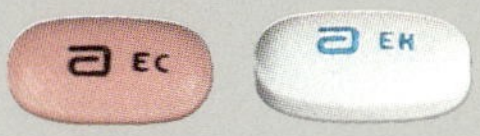

250 mg 333 mg

ERYTHROMYCIN
ABBOTT

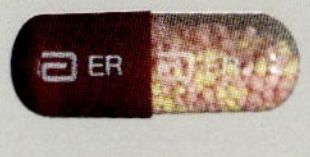

250 mg

PCE
ABBOTT

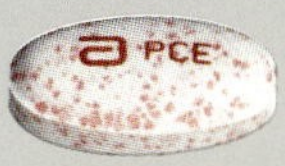

333 mg

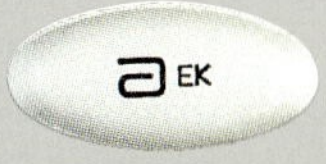

500 mg

ERYTHROMYCIN STEARATE

ERYTHROCIN STEARATE FILMTAB
ABBOTT

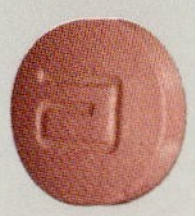

250 mg

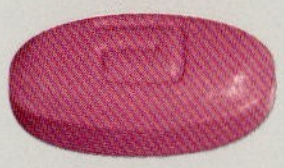

500 mg

ESTROGENS CONJUGATED

PREMARIN
WYETH-AYERST

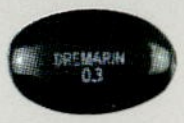

0.3 mg

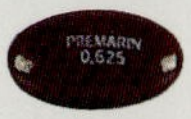

0.625 mg

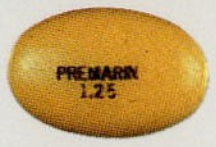

1.25 mg

ESTROPIPATE (PIPERAZINE ESTRONE SULFATE)

OGEN
UPJOHN

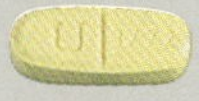

0.625 mg

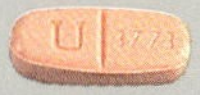

1.25 mg

ETODOLAC

LODINE
WYETH-AYERST

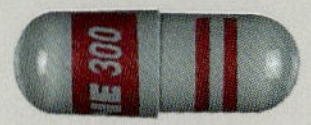

300 mg

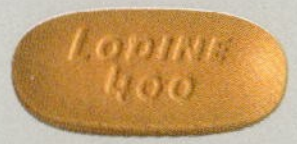

400 mg

FAMOTIDINE

PEPCID
MERCK

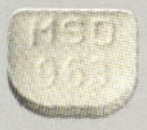

20 mg

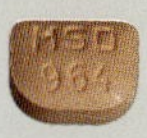

40 mg

FINASTERIDE

PROSCAR
MERCK

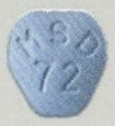

5 mg

FIORINAL

BUTALBITAL AND ASPIRIN AND CAFFEINE
SANDOZ

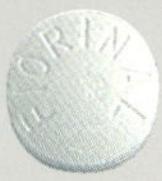

50 mg / 325 mg / 40 mg

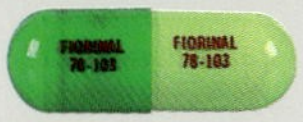

50 mg / 325 mg / 40 mg

FLUOXETINE HCL

PROZAC
DISTA

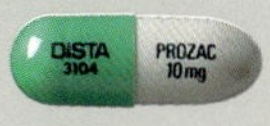

10 mg

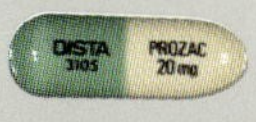

20 mg

FLURBIPROFEN

ANSAID
UPJOHN

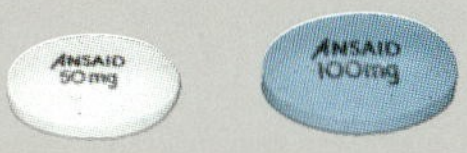

50 mg 100 mg

FOSINOPRIL SODIUM

MONOPRIL
BRISTOL-MYERS SQUIBB

10 mg 20 mg

FUROSEMIDE

LASIX
HOECHS MARION ROUSSEL

20 mg 40 mg

GEMFIBROZIL

LOPID
PARKE-DAVIS

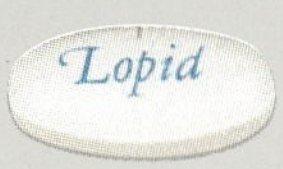

600 mg

GLIPIZIDE

GLUCOTROL
PRATT

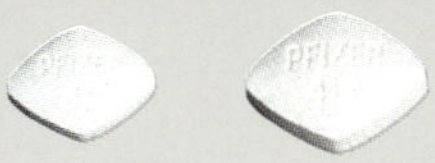

5 mg 10 mg

GLYBURIDE

DIABETA
HOECHS MARION ROUSSEL

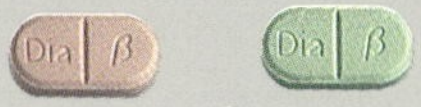

2.5 mg 5 mg

GLYNASE PRESTAB
UPJOHN

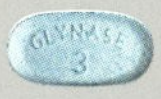

3 mg

MICRONASE
UPJOHN

2.5 mg 5 mg

GUANFACINE HCL

TENEX
A. H. ROBINS

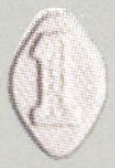

1 mg

HYDROCODONE BITARTRATE AND ACETAMINOPHEN

VICODIN
KNOLL

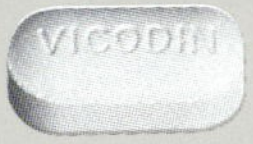

5 mg / 500 mg

IBUPROFEN

MOTRIN
UPJOHN

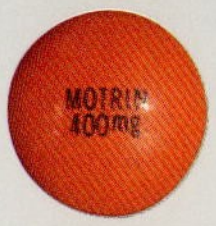

400 mg

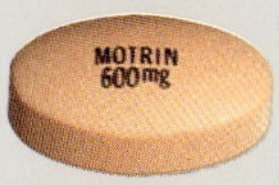

600 mg

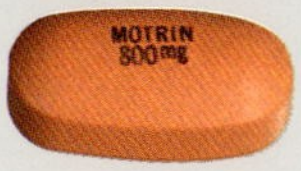

800 mg

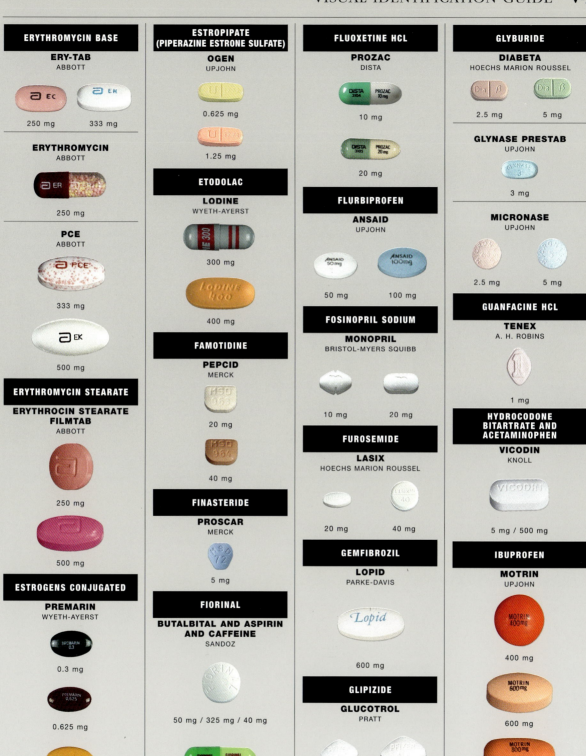

INDAPAMIDE

LOZOL
RHONE-POULENC RORER

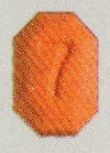

1.25 mg

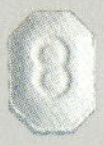

2.5 mg

ISOSORBIDE DINITRATE TABLETS

ISORDIL TITRADOSE
WYETH-AYERST

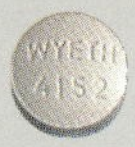

5 mg

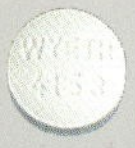

10 mg

ISRADIPINE

DYNACIRC
SANDOZ

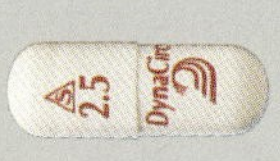

2.5 mg

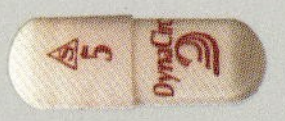

5 mg

KETOCONAZOLE

NIZORAL
JANSSEN

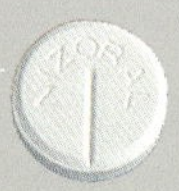

200 mg

KETOROLAC TROMETHAMINE

TORADOL
SYNTEX

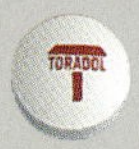

10 mg

LEVOTHYROXINE SODIUM

SYNTHROID
KNOLL

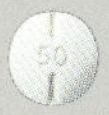

0.05 mg

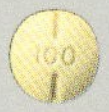

0.1 mg

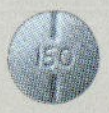

0.15 mg

LISINOPRIL

PRINIVIL
MERCK

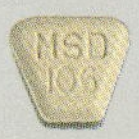

10 mg

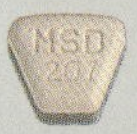

20 mg

LISINOPRIL

ZESTRIL
STUART

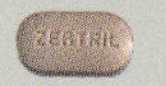

5 mg

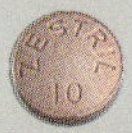

10 mg

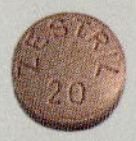

20 mg

LORACARBEF

LORABID
ELI LILLY

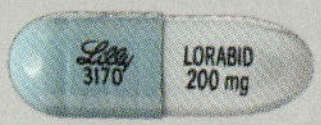

200 mg

LORATADINE

CLARITIN
SCHERING

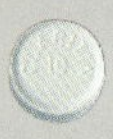

10 mg

LORAZEPAM

ATIVAN
WYETH-AYERST

0.5 mg

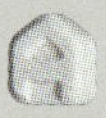

1 mg

LOSARTAN POTASSIUM

COZAAR
MERCK

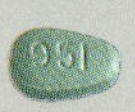

25 mg

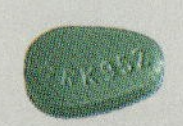

50 mg

LOVASTATIN (MEVINOLIN)

MEVACOR
MERCK

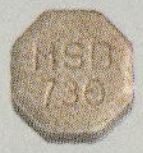

10 mg

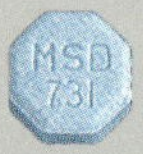

20 mg

MEDROXYPROGESTERONE ACETATE

PROVERA
UPJOHN

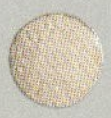

2.5 mg

10 mg

METFORMIN HCL

GLUCOPHAGE
BRISTOL-MYERS SQUIBB

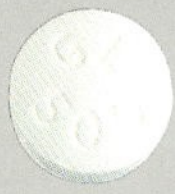

500 mg

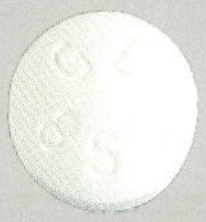

850 mg

METHYLPHENIDATE HCL

RITALIN
CIBAGENEVA

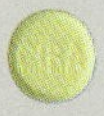

5 mg

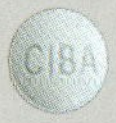

10 mg

METHYLPREDNISOLONE

MEDROL
UPJOHN

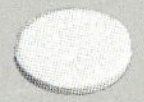

4 mg

METOPROLOL TARTRATE

LOPRESSOR
CIBAGENEVA

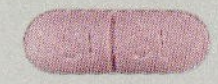

50 mg

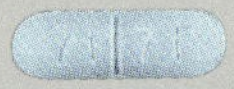

100 mg

MISOPROSTOL

CYTOTEC
G. D. SEARLE

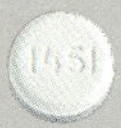

100 mcg

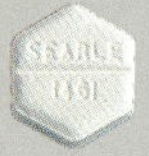

200 mcg

NABUMETONE

RELAFEN
SMITHKLINE BEECHAM

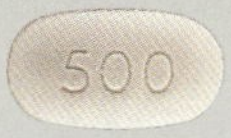

500 mg

NADOLOL

CORGARD
BRISTOL-MYERS SQUIBB

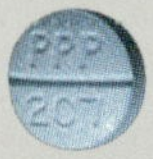

40 mg

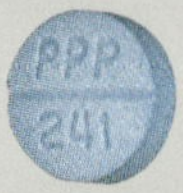

80 mg

NAPROXEN

NAPROSYN
ROCHE

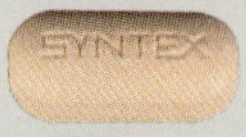

375 mg

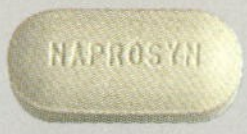

500 mg

NAPROXEN SODIUM

ANAPROX
ROCHE

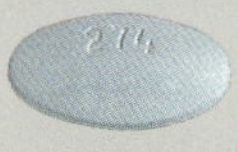

275 mg

ANAPROX DS
ROCHE

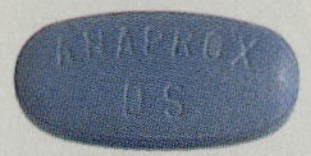

550 mg

NEFAZODONE HCL

SERZONE
BRISTOL-MYERS SQUIBB

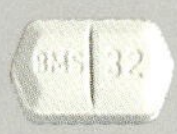

100 mg

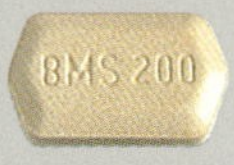

200 mg

NIFEDIPINE

PROCARDIA XL
PRATT

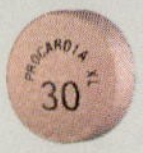

30 mg

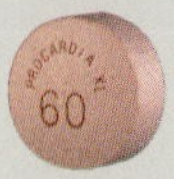

60 mg

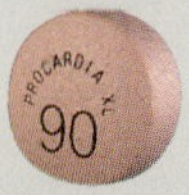

90 mg

NIZATIDINE

AXID
ELI LILLY

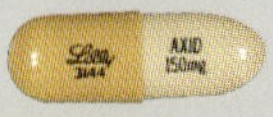

150 mg

NORTRIPTYLINE HCL

PAMELOR
SANDOZ

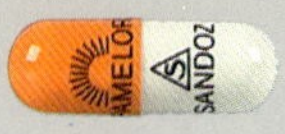

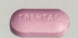

25 mg

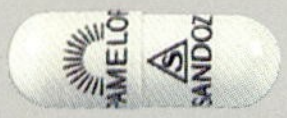

50 mg

OFLOXACIN

FLOXIN
MCNEIL

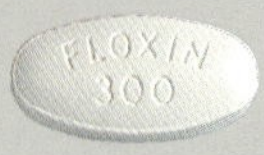

300 mg

OMEPRAZOLE

PRILOSEC
ASTRA MERCK

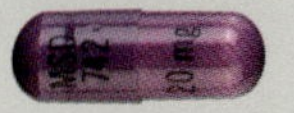

20 mg

OXAPROZIN

DAYPRO
G. D. SEARLE

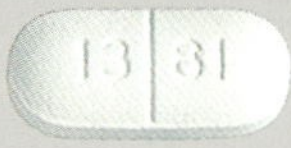

600 mg

OXYCODONE AND ACETAMINOPHEN

PERCOCET
DUPONT

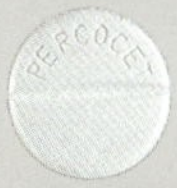

5 mg / 325 mg

PAROXETINE HCL

PAXIL
SMITHKLINE BEECHAM

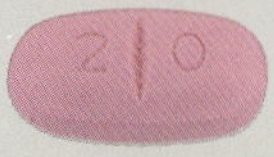

20 mg

PENICILLIN V POTASSIUM (PHENOXYMETHYL PENICILLIN POTASSIUM)

PEN-VEE K
WYETH-AYERST

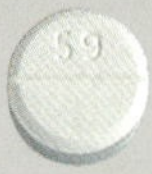

250 mg

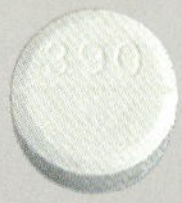

500 mg

PENTOXIFYLLINE

TRENTAL
HOECHST MARION ROUSSEL

400 mg

PHENYTOIN SODIUM, EXTENDED

DILANTIN KAPSEALS
PARKE-DAVIS

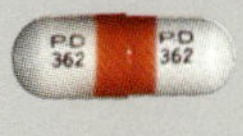

100 mg

POTASSIUM CHLORIDE

K-DUR
KEY

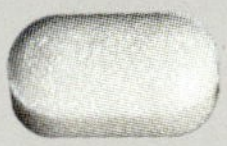

10 mEq

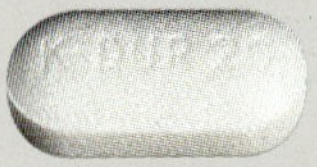

20 mEq

KLOR-CON 10
UPSHER-SMITH

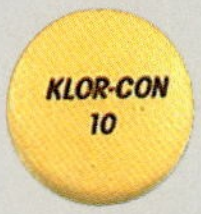

10 mEq

MICRO-K 10 EXTENCAPS
A. H. ROBINS

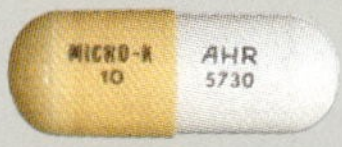

10 mEq

PRAVASTATIN SODIUM

PRAVACHOL
BRISTOL-MYERS SQUIBB

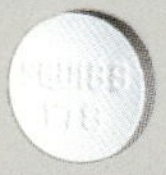

20 mg

PREDNISONE

DELTASONE
UPJOHN

5 mg

10 mg

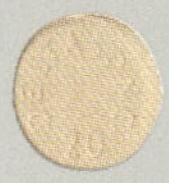

20 mg

PROPRANOLOL HCL

INDERAL
WYETH-AYERST

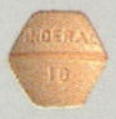
10 mg

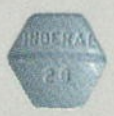
20 mg

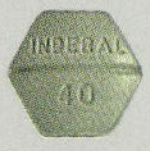

40 mg

INDERAL LA
WYETH-AYERST

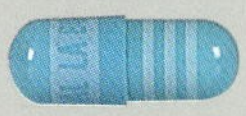
80 mg

QUINAPRIL HCL

ACCUPRIL
PARKE-DAVIS

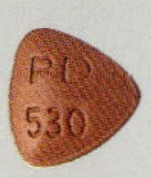

10 mg

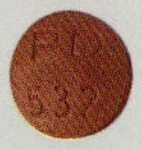
20 mg

RAMIPRIL

ALTACE
HOECHST MARION ROUSSEL

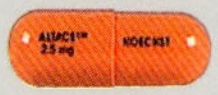
2.5 mg

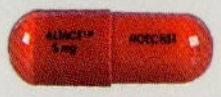
5 mg

RANITIDINE HCL

ZANTAC
GLAXO

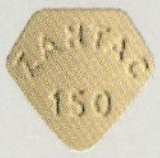

150 mg

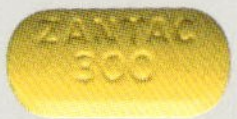

300 mg

SERTRALINE HCL

ZOLOFT
ROERIG

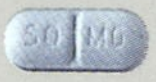
50 mg

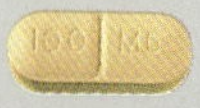
100 mg

SIMVASTATIN

ZOCOR
MERCK

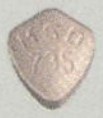
10 mg

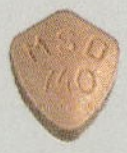
20 mg

SUCRALFATE

CARAFATE
HOECHST MARION ROUSSEL

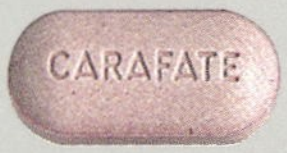

1 gm

TAMOXIFEN

NOLVADEX
ZENECA

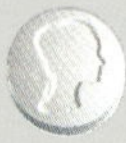
10 mg

TEMAZEPAM

RESTORIL
SANDOZ

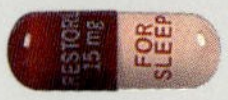
15 mg

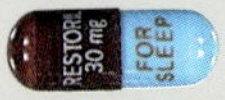

30 mg

TERAZOSIN

HYTRIN
ABBOTT

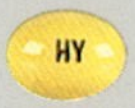

2 mg

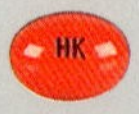

5 mg

TERFENADINE

SELDANE
HOECHST MARION ROUSSEL

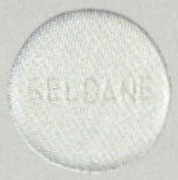
60 mg

TERFENADINE AND PSEUDOEPHEDRINE HCL

SELDANE-D
HOECHST MARION ROUSSEL

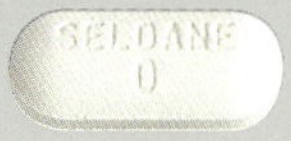

60 mg / 120 mg

THEOPHYLLINE

THEO-DUR
KEY

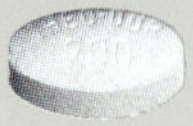
200 mg

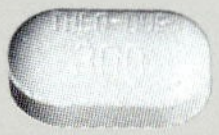
300 mg

TRIAMTERENE AND HYDROCHLOROTHIAZIDE TABLETS

MAXZIDE
LEDERLE

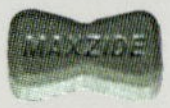

37.5 mg/25 mg

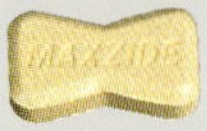

75 mg/50 mg

TRIAMTERENE AND HYDROCHLOROTHIAZIDE CAPSULES

DYAZIDE
SMITHKLINE BEECHAM

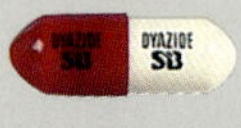
37.5 mg / 25 mg

TRIAZOLAM

HALCION
UPJOHN

0.125 mg

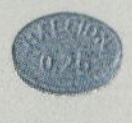
0.25 mg

TRIMETHOPRIM AND SULFAMETHOXAZOLE

BACTRIM DS
ROCHE

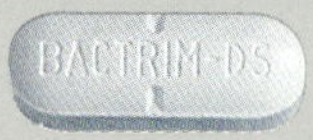

160 mg / 800 mg

TYLENOL WITH CODEINE TABLETS

ACETAMINOPHEN AND CODEINE PHOSPHATE
MCNEIL

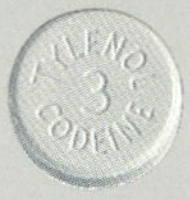

300 mg / 30 mg

VERAPAMIL

CALAN SR
G. D. SEARLE

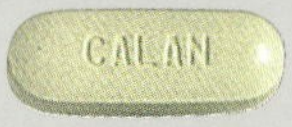

240 mg

WARFARIN SODIUM

COUMADIN
DUPONT PHARMA

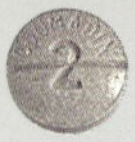
2 mg

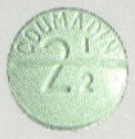
2.5 mg

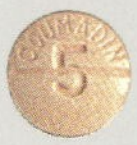
5 mg

A GUIDE TO DRUG COMPATIBILITY

	Acyclovir Sodium	Amiodarone HCl	Amikacin Sulfate	Aminophylline	Amphotericin B	Ampicillin Sodium	Ampicillin Sodium-Sulbactam Sodium	Amrinone Lactate	Atracurium Besylate	Atropine Sulfate	Aztreonam	Bretylium Tosylate	Calcium Chloride	Calcium Gluconate	Cefazolin Sodium	Cefoperazone Sodium	Cefotaxime Sodium	Cefotetan Disodium	Cefoxitin Sodium	Ceftazidime	Ceftizoxime Sodium	Ceftriaxone Sodium	Cefuroxime Sodium	Cimetidine HCl	Ciprofloxacin	Clindamycin Phosphate	Dexamethasone Sodium Phosphate	Digoxin	Diltiazem HCl	Diphenhydramine HCl	Dobutamine HCl	Dopamine HCl	Droperidol	Enalaprilat	Epinephrine HCl	Erythromycin Lactobionate	Esmolol HCl	Famotidine	Fentanyl Citrate	Filgrastim	Fluconazole	Foscarnet Sodium	Furosemide	Gentamicin Sulfate	Heparin Sodium	Hydrocortisone Sodium Succinate	Hydromorphone HCl	Imipenem-Cilastatin Sodium	Isoproterenol HCl	Labetalol HCl	Lidocaine HCl	Magnesium Sulfate	Meperidine HCl	Methylprednisolone Sodium Succinate	Metoclopramide HCl	Metronidazole	Mezlocillin Sodium	Midazolam HCl	Milrinone Lactate	Morphine Sulfate	Nafcillin Sodium	Nitroglycerin	Nitroprusside Sodium	Norepinephrine Bitartrate	Ondansetron HCl	Oxacillin Sodium	Pancuronium Bromide	Penicillin G Potassium	Phenylephrine HCl	Piperacillin Sodium	Piperacillin Sodium-Tazobactam Sodium	Potassium Chloride	Procainamide HCl	Ranitidine HCl	Sargramostim	Sodium Bicarbonate	Tacrolimus	Theophylline	Ticarcillin Disodium	Ticarcillin Disodium-Clavulanate Potassium	Tobramycin Sulfate	Trimethoprim-Sulfamethoxazole	Vancomycin HCl	Vecuronium Bromide	Verapamil HCl	Zidovudine
Acyclovir Sodium																																																																																								
Amiodarone HCl																																																																																								
Amikacin Sulfate																																																																																								
Aminophylline																																																																																								
Amphotericin B																																																																																								
Ampicillin Sodium																																																																																								
Ampicillin Sodium-Sulbactam Sodium																																																																																								
Amrinone Lactate																																																																																								
Atracurium Besylate																																																																																								
Atropine Sulfate																																																																																								
Aztreonam																																																																																									
Bretylium Tosylate																																																																																									
Calcium Chloride																																																																																									
Calcium Gluconate																																																																																									
Cefazolin Sodium																																																																																								
Cefoperazone Sodium																																																																																								
Cefotaxime Sodium																																																																																								
Cefotetan Disodium																																																																																								
Cefoxitin Sodium																																																																																								
Ceftazidime																																																																																								
Ceftizoxime Sodium																																																																																								
Ceftriaxone Sodium																																																																																								
Cefuroxime Sodium																																																																																								
Cimetidine HCl																																																																																								
Ciprofloxacin																																																																																								
Clindamycin Phosphate																																																																																								
Dexamethasone Sodium Phosphate																																																																																								
Digoxin																																																																																								
Diltiazem HCl																																																																																								
Diphenhydramine HCl																																																																																								
Dobutamine HCl																																																																																								
Dopamine HCl																																																																																								
Droperidol																																																																																								
Enalaprilat																																																																																								
Epinephrine HCl																																																																																									
Erythromycin Lactobionate																																																																																								
Esmolol HCl																																																																																								
Famotidine																																																																																								
Fentanyl Citrate																																																																																								
Filgrastim																																																																																								
Fluconazole																																																																																								
Foscarnet Sodium																																																																																								
Furosemide																																																																																								
Gentamicin Sulfate																																																																																								
Heparin Sodium																																																																																								
Hydrocortisone Sodium Succinate																																																																																								
Hydromorphone HCl																																																																																								
Imipenem-Cilastatin Sodium																																																																																								
Isoproterenol HCl																																																																																								
Labetalol HCl																																																																																								
Lidocaine HCl																																																																																								
Magnesium Sulfate																																																																																								
Meperidine HCl																																																																																								

A GUIDE TO DRUG COMPATIBILITY (continued)

	Acyclovir Sodium	Amiodarone HCl	Amikacin Sulfate	Aminophylline	Amphotericin B	Ampicillin Sodium	Ampicillin Sodium-Sulbactam Sodium	Amrinone Lactate	Atracurium Besylate	Atropine Sulfate	Aztreonam	Bretylium Tosylate	Calcium Chloride	Calcium Gluconate	Cefazolin Sodium	Cefoperazone Sodium	Cefotaxime Sodium	Cefotetan Disodium	Cefoxitin Sodium	Ceftazidime	Ceftizoxime Sodium	Ceftriaxone Sodium
Methylprednisolone Sodium Succinate	C							C			C			I								
Metoclopramide HCl	C			C		I				C	C			I								
Metronidazole	C	C	C								I				C		C			C	C	C
Mezlocillin Sodium		I									C							C				
Midazolam HCl		C	C			I			C	C				C	C					I		
Milrinone Lactate										C			C									
Morphine Sulfate		C	C			C	C		C	C	C		C		C	C	C	C	C	C	C	C
Nafcillin Sodium	C									C	I											
Nitroglycerin		C		C				C	C													
Nitroprusside Sodium								C														
Norepinephrine Bitartrate		C	C	I				C					C	C								
Ondansetron HCl	I		C	I	I	I	I				C				C	I	C		C	C	C	
Oxacillin Sodium	C																					
Pancuronium Bromide				C											C							
Penicillin G Potassium	C	C		I	I								C	C				C				
Phenylephrine HCl		C						C														
Phenytoin Sodium			I									I										
Piperacillin Sodium	C										C							C				
Piperacillin Sodium-Tazobactam Sodium	I			C	I						C			C								
Potassium Chloride	C	C		C	I	C		C	C	C	C	C		C						C		
Procainamide HCl		C							C													
Ranitidine HCl	C		C	C	I					C	C	C								C		
Sargramostim	I		C	C		I	I				C			C	C	I	C	C			C	C
Sodium Bicarbonate	C	I	C	C	C			I		C	C	C					I		C			C
Tacrolimus	C			C	C	C	C							C	C			C		C		C
Theophylline	C					C	C				C				C			C		C		
Ticarcillin Disodium	C										C							C				
Ticarcillin Disodium-Clavulanate Potassium											C											
Tobramycin Sulfate	C	C									C			C		I						
Trimethoprim-Sulfamethoxazole	C								C		C											
Vancomycin HCl	C	C	C						C					C								I
Vecuronium Bromide				C											C							
Verapamil HCl		C	C		I			C		C		C	C	C	C		C		C			
Zidovudine	C		C		C						C									C		C

	Cefuroxime Sodium	Cimetidine HCl	Ciprofloxacin	Clindamycin Phosphate	Dexamethasone Sodium Phosphate	Digoxin	Diltiazem HCl	Diphenhydramine HCl	Dobutamine HCl	Dopamine HCl	Droperidol	Enalaprilat	Epinephrine HCl	Erythromycin Lactobionate	Esmolol HCl	Famotidine	Fentanyl Citrate	Filgrastim	Fluconazole	Foscarnet Sodium	Furosemide	Gentamicin Sulfate
Methylprednisolone Sodium Succinate		C	I	C						C		C				C		I				
Metoclopramide HCl			C	C	C		C	C			C			I		C	C	C	C	C	I	
Metronidazole	C		C	C			C					C			C		C	I	C	C		C
Mezlocillin Sodium			I													C		I				
Midazolam HCl	I	C	C	C	I	C		C	I	C	C			C		C	C		C	I	I	C
Milrinone Lactate						C							C								I	
Morphine Sulfate	C	C		C	C	C	C	C	C	C	C	C		C	C	C	C	C	C	C	I	C
Nafcillin Sodium		C			C		I	C			I	C			C	C	C		C	C		I
Nitroglycerin							C		C	C		C				C	C		C		C	
Nitroprusside Sodium		C					C		C	C		C				C						
Norepinephrine Bitartrate		C					C		C							C						
Ondansetron HCl	C	C		C	C			C			C					C		C	C		I	C
Oxacillin Sodium							C			C						C			C	C		
Pancuronium Bromide	C	C							C	C			C		C		C		C			C
Penicillin G Potassium		C		C			C	C		I		C		C	C				C	C	C	
Phenylephrine HCl									C							C						
Phenytoin Sodium			I	I			I	I	I			I			C	C			C	C		
Piperacillin Sodium			C	C			C					C			C	C		I	C	C		
Piperacillin Sodium-Tazobactam Sodium		C		C	C			C	I	C	I	C				I			C		C	
Potassium Chloride	C	C	C	C	C	C	C	C		C	C	C	C	C	C	C	C	C	C		C	
Procainamide HCl									C						I	C						
Ranitidine HCl			C		C	C	C	C	C	C		C	C	C	C		C	C	C	C	C	C
Sargramostim	C	C		C	C			C		C	C					C	C		C		C	C
Sodium Bicarbonate		C		C	C				I	I			I	C	C	C	C	C			C	
Tacrolimus	C	C	C	C	C	C		C	C	C				C	C				C		C	C
Theophylline		C		C	C		C		C	C				C		C	C		C			C
Ticarcillin Disodium							C									C		C	I			I
Ticarcillin Disodium-Clavulanate Potassium							C									C		C	C	C		
Tobramycin Sulfate			C				C					C			C		C	C	C	C	C	
Trimethoprim-Sulfamethoxazole							C					C			C			C	I			
Vancomycin HCl		C			I		C					C			C		C	C	C			
Vecuronium Bromide	C	C							C	C			C		C		C		C			C
Verapamil HCl		C	C	C	C	C				C			C	C		C						C
Zidovudine		C		C	C				C	C				C				C	C			C

	Heparin Sodium	Hydrocortisone Sodium Succinate	Hydromorphone HCl	Imipenem-Cilastatin Sodium	Isoproterenol HCl	Labetalol HCl	Lidocaine HCl	Magnesium Sulfate	Meperidine HCl	Methylprednisolone Sodium Succinate	Metoclopramide HCl	Metronidazole	Mezlocillin Sodium	Midazolam HCl	Milrinone Lactate	Morphine Sulfate	Nafcillin Sodium	Nitroglycerin	Nitroprusside Sodium	Norepinephrine Bitartrate	Ondansetron HCl	Oxacillin Sodium
Methylprednisolone Sodium Succinate	C								C		C					C	I			C	I	
Metoclopramide HCl	C	C					C	C	C	C				C		C					C	
Metronidazole	C		C			C		C	C					C		C						
Mezlocillin Sodium	C		C						I							C					I	
Midazolam HCl	C	I	C	I					C		C	C				C	I	C				
Milrinone Lactate							C									C						
Morphine Sulfate		C				C	C	C	I	C	C	C	C	C	C		C				C	C
Nafcillin Sodium	C	I	C			I	C	C		I				I		C						
Nitroglycerin	C					C	C							C					C			
Nitroprusside Sodium	C						C											C				
Norepinephrine Bitartrate	C	C						C		C												
Ondansetron HCl	C	C	C	C				C	C	I	C		I			C						
Oxacillin Sodium	C	C	C			C		C	C							C						
Pancuronium Bromide	C	C			C									C		C		C	C			
Penicillin G Potassium		C	C			C	C	C	C	C	I					C						
Phenylephrine HCl							C															
Phenytoin Sodium	I		I				I		I							I		I		I		
Piperacillin Sodium	C	C	C			C		C	C					C		C					I	
Piperacillin Sodium-Tazobactam Sodium	C	C	C					C	C	C	C	C				C					C	
Potassium Chloride	C	C			C	C	C	C	C		C			C		C	C			C	C	C
Procainamide HCl	C	C					C								I							
Ranitidine HCl	C		C		C	C	C		C	C	C					C		C	C		C	
Sargramostim	C	I	I	I				C	C	I	C	C	C			I						
Sodium Bicarbonate	C	C		I	I	I		I		C	I			I	C		C			I	I	
Tacrolimus	C	C		C	C					C	C	C	C					C	C			C
Theophylline	C	C					C			C		C		C			C	C	C			
Ticarcillin Disodium	C		C					C	C							C					C	
Ticarcillin Disodium-Clavulanate Potassium	C								C							C					C	
Tobramycin Sulfate	I		C			C		C	C			C		C		C						
Trimethoprim-Sulfamethoxazole	C		C			C		C	C					I		C						
Vancomycin HCl		C	C			C		C	C					C		C					C	
Vecuronium Bromide	C	C			C									C		C		C	C			
Verapamil HCl	C	C	C		C		C	C	C	C	C				C	C		C	C	C		
Zidovudine	C			C							C					C	C				C	C

	Pancuronium Bromide	Penicillin G Potassium	Phenylephrine HCl	Phenytoin Sodium	Piperacillin Sodium	Piperacillin Sodium-Tazobactam Sodium	Potassium Chloride	Procainamide HCl	Ranitidine HCl	Sargramostim	Sodium Bicarbonate	Tacrolimus	Theophylline	Ticarcillin Disodium	Ticarcillin Disodium-Clavulanate Potassium	Tobramycin Sulfate	Trimethoprim-Sulfamethoxazole	Vancomycin HCl	Vecuronium Bromide	Verapamil HCl	Zidovudine
Methylprednisolone Sodium Succinate		C				C			C	I	C	C	C							C	
Metoclopramide HCl		I				C	C		C	C	I	C								C	C
Metronidazole						C				C		C	C			C					
Mezlocillin Sodium										C		C								I	
Midazolam HCl	C				C		C				I		C			C	I	C	C		
Milrinone Lactate								I			C									C	
Morphine Sulfate	C	C		I	C	C	C		C	I				C	C	C	C	C	C	C	C
Nafcillin Sodium							C				C		C								C
Nitroglycerin	C			I					C			C	C						C	C	
Nitroprusside Sodium	C								C			C	C						C	C	
Norepinephrine Bitartrate				I			C				I									C	
Ondansetron HCl					I	C	C		C	I	I			C	C			C			C
Oxacillin Sodium							C					C								I	C
Pancuronium Bromide									C								C	C		C	
Penicillin G Potassium							C		C			C	C							C	
Phenylephrine HCl							C				C										C
Phenytoin Sodium							I				C	C	I							C	
Piperacillin Sodium							C		C	I		C	C							C	C
Piperacillin Sodium-Tazobactam Sodium							C		C	C	C						C	I			C
Potassium Chloride		C	C	I	C	C		C	C	C	C	C	C					C		C	C
Procainamide HCl							C		C											C	
Ranitidine HCl	C	C			C	C	C	C		C		C	C	C		C		C	C		C
Sargramostim					I	C	C		C		I			C	C	I	C				C
Sodium Bicarbonate			C	C		C	C			I		C			I						
Tacrolimus		C		C	C		C		C		C					C	C	C			
Theophylline		C		I	C		C		C					C	C	C		C		C	
Ticarcillin Disodium									C	C			C							C	
Ticarcillin Disodium-Clavulanate Potassium										C	I		C								
Tobramycin Sulfate									C	I		C	C							C	C
Trimethoprim-Sulfamethoxazole	C					C				C		C							C	I	C
Vancomycin HCl	C					I	C		C			C	C						C	C	C
Vecuronium Bromide									C								C	C			
Verapamil HCl	C	C		C	C		C	C					C	C		C	I	C			
Zidovudine			C		C	C	C		C	C						C	C	C			

LEGEND

I **Incompatible**
C **Compatible**
blank **No information available or conflicting information. The primary literature should be consulted.** ***Compatibility should not be assumed.***

REFERENCES

1. Trissel, LA: Handbook on Injectable Drugs, ninth edition, American Society of Health-System Pharmacists, Bethesda, MD, 1996.
2. King, JC: Guide to Parenteral Admixtures, Pacemarq, Inc., St. Louis, 1996.

REVIEWERS

1. David DiPersio, Pharm D., Critical Care Pharmacist, Vanderbilt University Medical Center, Nashville, TN.
2. Jim Pierce, Pharm D., Clinical Specialist, Trauma Critical Care, University of Tennessee, Knoxville, TN.

Compatibility may be affected by numerous factors including temperature, drug concentration, other medications present, diluent and contact time.
This chart is not intended to be an exhaustive review. The clinician is encouraged to compare conditions in their institutions with conditions tested in the literature.
All clinicians involved in the prescribing, compounding and administration of medications have the responsibility of ensuring that medications delivered are compatible.
Abbott Laboratories cannot be responsible for events arising from use of this chart.

Abbott Laboratories
Hospital Products Division
Abbott Park, IL 60064

1-800-ABBOTT 3
1-800-222-6883
Abbott HPD Internet Address: http://www.abbotthosp.com

96-4457-20-Feb.,97

"Recommendations for Prevention of HIV Transmission in Health-Care Settings" and "Revision of the CDC Surveillance Case Definition for AIDS."

Acquired immune deficiency syndrome (AIDS) is an illness that impairs the body's ability to fight infection, making the body extremely susceptible to life-threatening disease. Researchers have isolated and identified the *human immunodeficiency virus* (HIV) as the virus that causes AIDS. This virus is transmitted through sexual contact and exposure to infected blood or blood components, and perinatally from mother to neonate. HIV has been isolated from blood, semen, vaginal secretions, saliva, tears, breast milk, cerebrospinal fluid, amniotic fluid, and urine, and is likely to be isolated from other body fluids, secretions, and excretions.

The increasing prevalence of HIV increases the risk that health-care workers will be exposed to blood from patients infected with HIV, especially when blood and body-fluid precautions are not followed for all patients. Thus, the Centers for Disease Control and Prevention recommends the need for health-care workers to consider *all* patients as potentially infected with HIV and/or other blood-borne pathogens, and to adhere rigorously to infection-control precautions for minimizing the risk of exposure to blood and body fluids of all patients. See Chapter 14 for these recommended precautions.

About 98 percent of all AIDS cases reported to date have occurred in the following groups of people:

- Sexually active homosexual and bisexual men (or men who have had sex with another man since 1977).
- Present or past abusers of illicit intravenous (IV) drugs.
- Homosexual and bisexual men who are also IV drug abusers.
- Persons who have had transfusions of blood or blood products. These cases occurred prior to the development of a laboratory test that is now used to test all units of blood for HIV-1.
- Persons with hemophilia or other blood-clotting disorders who have received blood-clotting factors.
- Heterosexual men and women (these include sex partners of persons with AIDS or at risk for AIDS, and people born in countries where heterosexual transmission is thought to be more common than in the United States).
- Infants born to mothers infected with the AIDS virus.
- About 2 percent of AIDS patients do not fall into any of these groups, but scientists believe that transmission occurred in similar ways.

During the incubation period, which may range from a few months to several years, there may be no telltale signs that suggest a person is suffering from AIDS. At this time the test for the antibodies to the HIV virus will show the individual has been exposed to the virus. This virus changes the structure of the cell it attacks. Infection with the virus can lead to AIDS. Some of those persons infected with the virus will develop symptoms of AIDS. Other people who carry the virus may remain in apparent good health. These carriers can transmit the virus during sexual contact, or an infected mother can transmit the virus to her infant before, during, or after birth.

As acquired immune deficiency syndrome progresses, symptoms become apparent. Some of these symptoms are:

- fever, including "night sweats."
- rapid weight loss for no apparent reason.
- swollen lymph glands in the neck, underarm, or groin area.
- constant fatigue.
- unexplained diarrhea.
- white spots or unusual blemishes in the mouth.

As the disease takes its toll upon the body's immune system, the patient becomes severely weakened and potentially fatal infections can occur. *Pneumocystis carinii* pneumonia and Kaposi's sarcoma account for many of the deaths of AIDS patients.

In 1993 the Centers for Disease Control and Prevention revised the classification systems for HIV infection and expanded surveillance case definition for AIDS among adolescents and adults. The following is a list of conditions included in this expanded surveillance case definition.

CDC's 1993 Revised Classification of HIV Infection and AIDS

- Candidiasis of bronchi, trachea, or lungs
- Candidiasis, esophageal
- Cervical cancer, invasive
- Coccidioidomycosis, disseminated or extrapulmonary
- Cryptococcosis, extrapulmonary
- Cryptosporidiosis, chronic intestinal
- Cytomegalovirus disease (other than liver, spleen, or nodes)
- Cytomegalovirus retinities (with loss of vision)
- Encephalopathy, HIV-related
- Herpes simplex: chronic ulcers; or bronchitis, pneumonitis, or esophagitis
- Histoplasmosis, disseminated or extrapulmonary
- Isosporiasis, chronic intestinal
- Kaposi's sarcoma
- Lymphoma, Burkitt's
- Lymphoma, immunoblastic
- Lymphoma, primary, of brain
- *Mycobacterium avium* complex or *M. Kansaii*, disseminated or extrapulmonary
- *Mycobacterium tuberculosis*, any site, (pulmonary or extrapulmonary)
- *Mycobacterium*, other species or unidentified species, disseminated or extrapulmonary
- *Pneumocystis carinii* pneumonia
- Pneumonia, recurrent
- Progressive multifocal leukoencephalopathy
- Salmonella septicemia, recurrent
- Toxoplasmosis of brain
- Wasting syndrome due to HIV

Through education and proper protection, the possibility of acquiring and/or transmitting the HIV virus can be reduced to a minimum. One must be aware of the latest information, and use all safety precautions to protect self, patients, fellow workers, and the community as a whole.

Besides the recommended precautions stated in Chapter 14, the U.S. Department of Health and Human Services, Public Health Service, recommends the following steps to protect one's self from AIDS:

- Do not have sexual contact with AIDS patients, with members of the risk groups, or with people who test positive for the HIV virus. If you do, use a *condom* and avoid practices such as anal intercourse that may injure tissue.
- Do not use IV drugs. If you do, do not share needles. Do not have sex with people who use IV drugs.
- Women who are sex partners of risk-group members or who use IV drugs should consider the risk to their babies before pregnancy. These women should have an HIV antibody test before they become pregnant and during their pregnancy.
- Do not have sex with multiple partners, including prostitutes (who may also be IV drug abusers). The more partners you have, the greater your chances of contracting AIDS.

SPOTLIGHT

HIV in Babies and Children

Much has been written about HIV and the adult, but what about the babies and children who have HIV? The following information is taken from *HIV and Your Child*, a booklet published by the U.S. Department of Health and Human Services. For more information on this subject please call the National AIDS Hotline at 1-800-342-AIDS and ask for the Agency for Health Care Policy and Research (AHCPR) HIV Guideline.

Facts about HIV in Babies and Children

- HIV can be passed to a baby during pregnancy or delivery.
- An HIV-infected woman's chances of having a baby with HIV are one in four (25 percent) for each pregnancy.
- HIV can be passed to a baby through breast milk from an HIV-infected mother.
- Like adults, children and adolescents can get HIV from contact with blood or body fluids or through sex.
- Bathing, kissing, feeding, and playing with a child are not risky and do not cause the spread of HIV.

(continued)

- In the past, some babies and children became infected through blood transfusions. Today the blood from all donors is screened for the virus, and HIV infection from this source is unlikely.
- Special blood tests can show whether an infant is infected with HIV.
- The child with HIV needs to see a health-care provider who has experience treating HIV-infected babies and children.
- **Early immunizations can help protect the baby and/or child from other HIV-related diseases.**

Immunize against Infection

With HIV infection, the baby and/or child is more likely to get common childhood illnesses, and these may be more serious. "Baby Shots" such as diphtheria, pertussis (whooping cough), and tetanus (DPT), polio (OPV or IPV) and mumps, measles, and rubella (MMR) should be given on time and at the prescribed interval.

Other immunizations may be recommended depending on the advice of the physician and after medical tests are performed. These immunizations may include: *Haemophilus influenzae* type b, hepatitis B, pneumococcal (after 2 years of age), and influenza (yearly).

Avoid Common Illnesses

Some infections cannot be prevented by immunization. A baby and/or child with HIV should be kept away from people who are sick. If the baby and/or child has been near someone with tuberculosis (TB) or other infections, the health care provider should be notified immediately.

Note: The following information is taken from the Georgia Epidemiology Report Volume 11, Number 5.

Use of Zidovudine (ZDV/AZT) for Reduction of Perinatal Transmission of HIV

The National Institutes of Health (NIH) conducted a multicenter trial of zidovudine or ZDV (also known as AZT) in HIV-infected pregnant women and their newborns and it showed a two-thirds reduction in HIV transmission from mother to infant. The trial which was randomized, double-blinded, and placebo-controlled, enrolled HIV-infected women who were at least 14-weeks pregnant, had not received any antiretroviral therapy during the current pregnancy, had no clinical indications for antenatal antiretroviral therapy, and whose CD4 count was greater than 200 cells/mm. Half the women received zidovudine 100 mg five times a day throughout the remainder of their pregnancy and intravenous zidovudine during labor, and their newborns received oral zidovudine during the first six weeks of life. The other half received placebo. By December, 1993, 415 infants had been born to women enrolled in the study. Of the 53 HIV-infected infants, 13 were on zidovudine and 40 received placebo. HIV transmission was 25.5 percent in the placebo group compared to 8.3 percent in in the zidovudine treated group, a reduction of 67 percent in in those taking zidovudine. Although the short-term side effects in the infants appear to be minimal, long-term follow-up of HIV-infected and uninfected infants born to mothers receiving zidovudine during pregnancy is necessary to determine the long term effects.

To benefit from this preventive regime, HIV-infected pregnant women must be identified early in pregnancy. Therefore, HIV screening should be incorporated into routine prenatal care. Whenever a pregnant woman who is also HIV-infected is identified, the benefits and potential risks of this therapy should be presented to her by her health-care provider. For more information you may call 1-404-657-3123, Department of Human Resources, Division of Public Health.

Special Considerations: The Child

According to a report by the Harvard-based Global AIDS Policy Coalition, HIV could infect 110 million adults and 10 million children by the end of the decade. About 12.9 million people—7.1 million men, 4.7 million women, and 1.1 million children—have been infected with the virus since AIDS was discovered in 1981. About 2.6 million have developed AIDS and 2.5 million of those with AIDS have died.

HIV infection and AIDS can be contracted by anyone and this includes children.

- HIV can be passed to a baby during pregnancy or delivery.
- HIV can be passed to a baby through breast milk from an HIV-infected mother.
- Babies and children can get HIV from contact with blood or body fluids or through sex.
- Children may have contracted HIV from a blood transfusion or from a blood product.

Hemophilia and AIDS

Hemophiliacs have a lifelong need for replacement of the clotting factors in blood. From about 1977 until 1985, many of the blood clotting factors that were prepared from human blood donors were infected with HIV.

Now about half of the nation's 20,000 hemophiliacs are HIV positive. More than 2,000 have developed AIDS and 65 percent of those have died. Of the 2,000 known to have AIDS, 179 are children under the age of 13. Of the 65 percent of those who died, 97 were children.

Today the clotting factor that hemophiliacs take is heat treated and should not carry HIV. The cost of taking the clotting factor can be as much as $100,000 a year.

Special Considerations: The Older Adult

One in 10 persons with AIDS is 50 years of age or older. Approximately 4 percent of all AIDS cases are among those age 65 or older. AIDS has been reported in more people who are 50 and older than in those 24 years old and younger. Incidence of AIDS among older adults appears to be rising faster than in younger age groups. Immune function diminishes with age and AIDS infection usually progresses more quickly in older adults.

HIV may be acquired at any age, and older adults become infected in the same ways that younger people do.

- Older adults are sexually active and usually don't use condoms, because they are no longer concerned about pregnancy and/or contracting a sexually transmitted disease.
- Homosexuality and bisexuality may also be a part of an older adult's sexual preference.
- Intravenous drug use is a high risk factor in the older adult.
- Older adults may have contracted AIDS from a blood transfusion. Screening of donated blood began in 1985 and has reduced the risk of contracting AIDS from a blood transfusion.

Possible Signs and Symptoms of AIDS in the Older Adult

- HIV/AIDS dementia (usually has a rapid onset)
- Extrapyramidal symptoms resembling parkinsonism without resting tremors
- Ataxia, leg tremors
- Peripheral neuropathy progressing to weakness and abnormal reflexes, such as a positive Babinski
- Confusion
- Opportunistic infections
- Tuberculosis
- Esophageal or recurrent genital candidiasis, toxoplasmosis
- Non-Hodgkin's lymphoma
- Kaposi's sarcoma
- *Pneumocystis carinii* pneumonia (PCP)
- Human papilloma virus infection

Differential Diagnosis

In addition to a general medical history, a social history should be taken and include questions relating to a person's sexual activities. Also, a medication history should be taken and one should ask about use of any drugs, especially those not prescribed by his/her physician. Laboratory and diagnostic tests should be used to detect or rule out possible causes of any abnormal condition presented by the patient.

Diagnosis

ELISA (enzyme-linked immunosorbent assay) test result-positive

Western blot test-positive

CD4 lymphocyte count of 700 cells/mm3 (normal is 1,000 to 1,3000 cells/mm3)

High viral load levels

The diagnosis of AIDS can be devastating to any individual, especially an older adult who has to tell his/her family about the diagnosis. Professional assistance may be necessary to help the older adult with this task. A list of agencies with addresses and phone numbers should be made available to the older adult who wishes them. Information on services available for the older adult with HIV infection and AIDS may be obtained by calling the CDC's AIDS Hotline at 1-800 342 AIDS and/or the Georgia Department of Human Resources at 1-706-724-8802.

Treatment

The treatment regimen includes treating any associated condition with proper medical intervention, and starting the patient on an antiretroviral drug or a combination of antiretroviral drugs. Drug therapy should be carefully evaluated for older adults as to pre-existing conditions, such as cardiac disease and/or renal insufficiency, that can make them less tolerant of drugs. Also, they are generally more prone to adverse drug effects than younger individuals, therefore they will need clinical evaluation and laboratory monitoring every 3–6 months and more frequently if indicated.

Teaching the Older Adult about AIDS

It would be very helpful to provide brochures and any other written materials that you could on any or all of the following subjects, so that the older adult could better understand his/her condition.

- Explain how HIV infection can and cannot be transmitted.
- Explain universal precautions and when they should be used.
- Explain the general effects of HIV infection and how AIDS is diagnosed.
- Explain the general effects of AIDS on the body.
- Instruct the patient on how to prevent the spread of AIDS and what precautions should be used during sexual acts.
- Go over the patient's medical regimen, making sure that he/she understands all aspects of drug therapy and any adverse effects that should be reported to the physician.
- Inform the patient about available home health agencies and/or visiting nurse associations.
- Inform the patient about other community resources such as "meals on wheels" and hospice care.
- Instruct the patient on how to prevent infections and ways to improve his/her immune system.

(continued)

—Explain the importance of good nutrition and the Food Guide Pyramid.

—Advise the patient not to smoke.

—Inform the patient on how to reduce stress.

—Explain the importance of regular exercise.

—Explain the importance of getting the proper amount of sleep. This is usually 6–8 hours in a given 24 hour time period.

—Advise the patient to drink at least 8 glasses of water daily.

—Talk about how to develop and keep a positive attitude.

—Teach the patient how to practice good personal hygiene. Instruct patient on how to wash his/her hands and when.

—Advise the patient to stay away from individuals who have contagious diseases.

Critical Thinking Questions/Activities

Your patient is a 62-year-old female who has been diagnosed with AIDS. As you are talking with her she says, "I didn't know that "old" people could get AIDS. I know so little about the disease and I am sure that my friends don't know very much either. We need to be educated. I often go to the local senior citizen's center where they have guest speakers who present programs on all sorts of topics. Would you be willing to present a program on AIDS for our group? It would help me to explain my disease to my friends and maybe make someone else aware that he/she could get AIDS."

With the assistance of your patient, make arrangements to present a program on AIDS to a local group of senior citizens. To assist you in formulating a program, use the information in Special Considerations: The Older Adult.

Ask yourself:

- How do older adults become infected with HIV? How can I go about explaining this to a group of senior citizens?
- What could I teach the older adult about possible signs and symptoms of AIDS?
- How can I explain the diagnosis of AIDS?
- What information could I provide the group about services available to the older adult and on HIV infection and AIDS?
- How could I explain the treatment regimen for AIDS?
- In teaching the older adult about AIDS:
  —What materials could I leave with the group, so that they could better understand AIDS?
  —What are some points and facts that I would like to emphasize about preventing the spread of AIDS?

zidovudine (Retrovir)

Zidovudine (ZDV), also called azidothymidine (AZT), is an antiretroviral drug active against human immunodeficiency virus (HIV).

Uses. Indicated for the management of certain adult patients with symptomatic HIV infection (AIDS) who have a history of cytologically confirmed *Pneumocystis carinii* pneumonia (PCP) or an absolute CD4 (T_4 helper/inducer) lymphocyte count of less than 500/mm^3 in the peripheral blood before therapy is begun.

Contraindications. Contraindicated for patients who have potentially life-threatening allergic reactions to any of the formulation.

Warnings. The full safety and efficacy profile of zidovudine has not been completely defined, particularly in regard to prolonged use, and especially in HIV-infected individuals who have less advanced disease. Use with extreme caution in patients who have bone marrow compromise evidenced by granulocyte count below 1000/mm^3 or hemoglobin less than 9.5 g/dl.

Adverse Reactions. Reported in the placebo-controlled clinical trial study of 281 patients, the most frequent adverse reactions were granulocytopenia and anemia. Other adverse reactions reported in at least 5 percent of the patients were severe headache, nausea, insomnia and myalgia. Clinical adverse events which occurred in less than 5 percent were:

- *Body as a Whole:* body odor, chills, edema of the lip, flu syndrome, hyperalgesia, back pain, chest pain, lymphadenopathy
- *Cardiovascular:* vasodilation
- *Gastrointestinal:* constipation, dysphagia, edema of the tongue, eructation, flatulence, bleeding gums, rectal hemorrhage, mouth ulcer
- *Musculoskeletal:* arthralgia, muscle spasm, tremor, twitch
- *Nervous:* anxiety, confusion, depression, emotional liability, nervousness, syncope, loss of mental acuity, vertigo
- *Respiratory:* cough, epistaxis, pharyngitis, rhinitis, sinusitis, hoarseness
- *Skin:* acne, pruritus, urticaria
- *Special senses:* amblyopia, hearing loss, photophobia
- *Urogenital:* dysuria, polyuria, urinary frequency, urinary hesitancy.

Dosage and Route

Oral: Recommended starting dose is 100 mg administered orally every four hours around the clock. Dosage adjustment is made for patients who have significant anemia and/or significant granulocytopenia.

Drug Interactions. The interaction of other drugs with zidovudine has not been studied in a systematic manner. Coadministration of zidovudine with drugs that are nephrotoxic, cytotoxic, or that interfere with RBC/WBC number or function (e.g., dapsone, pentamidine, amphotericin B, flucytosine, vincristine, vinblastine, adriamycin, or interferon) may increase the risk of toxicity. Limited data suggest that probenecid may inhibit glucuronidation and/or reduce renal excretion of zidovudine. In addition, other drugs (e.g., acetaminophen, aspirin, or indomethacin) may competitively inhibit glucuronidation.

Pregnancy. It is not known whether zidovudine can cause fetal harm when administered to a pregnant woman or affect reproductive capacity. Zidovudine should be given to a pregnant woman only if clearly needed.

Nursing Mothers. It is not known whether zidovudine is excreted in human milk. Because many drugs are excreted in human milk and because of the potential for serious adverse reactions from zidovudine in nursing infants, mothers should be instructed to discontinue nursing if they are receiving zidovudine.

Implications for Patient Care. It is most important to teach the patient that zidovudine is not a cure for HIV infections, and patients may continue to acquire illnesses associated with AIDS, including opportunistic infections. Therefore, patients should be advised to seek medical care for any significant change in health status.

Patients should be informed that the major toxicities of zidovudine are granulocytopenia and/or anemia. They should be told that they may require transfusions or dose modifications including possible discontinuation if toxicity develops. They should be told of the extreme importance of having their blood counts followed closely while on therapy. They should be cautioned about the use of other medications such as acetaminophen that may exacerbate the toxicity of zidovudine.

Patients should be instructed that Retrovir capsules are for oral ingestion only, and that they should take the medication exactly as prescribed. This means every four hours including dosing around the clock, even though it may interrupt their normal sleep.

Advise patients not to share the medication and not to exceed the recommended dose. They should be told that long-term effects of zidovudine are unknown at this time, and that zidovudine therapy has not been shown to reduce the risk of transmission of HIV to others through sexual contact or blood contamination.

didanosine (Videx)

Didanosine is an antiretroviral drug that has been approved by the Food and Drug Administration for use in adults and pediatric AIDS patients who cannot tolerate zidovudine (AZT). Clinical trials have demonstrated Videx's ability to replenish CD4 helper cells, white blood cells that bolster the immune system against infection.

Videx's use mandates careful monitoring, as serious adverse reactions such as pancreatitis and peripheral neuropathy may occur. Teach the patient to be alert for signs of pancreatitis—abdominal pain, nausea, and vomiting; and signs of neuropathy—tingling, weakness, numbness, and possible pain in extremities. If these signs occur, the drug should be stopped immediately.

zalcitabine (Hivid)

Zalcitabine is an antiretroviral drug that is used in combination with zidovudine in the treatment of advanced HIV infection. The dosage is 0.75 mg every 8 hours.

Hivid's use mandates careful monitoring, as serious adverse reactions such as pancreatitis and peripheral neuropathy may occur. Teach the patient to be alert for signs of pancreatitis—abdominal pain, nausea, and vomiting; and signs of neuropathy—tingling, weakness, numbness, and possible pain in extremities. If these signs occur, the drug should be stopped immediately.

stavudine (Zerit)

Stavudine is an antiretroviral drug that is used for the treatment of adults with advanced HIV infection who do not tolerate or respond to other forms of therapy. As with zalcitabine the major adverse reactions are pancreatitis and peripheral neuropathy. Teach the patient to be alert for signs of pacreatitis—abdominal pain, nausea, and vomiting; and signs of neuropathy—tingling, weakness, numbness, and possible pain in the extremities. If these signs occur, the drug should be stopped immediately.

Actions. Stavudine is a nucleoside analogy. It inhibits HIV replication two ways: by interfering with the enzyme, reverse transcriptase, that enables the virus's RNA genetic material to be duplicated as DNA for incorporation in the host cell's genome, and by terminating assembly of viral DNA chains.

Dosage. *Oral:* patients weighing 60 kg (132 lb) receive 40 mg twice a day; those weighing less, 30 mg twice a day. Available as capsules: 15 mg (light yellow/dark red), 20 mg (light brown), 30 mg (light orange and dark orange), and 40 mg (dark orange).

lamivudine (3TC-Epivir)

3TC-Epivir is also known as lamivudine and is approved for use in combination with AZT to treat patients with HIV infection. It appears to boost the patient's immune system and lowers the amount of the HIV virus in the blood for at least six months. The drug incapacitates a protein important in the virus' reproduction.

saquinavir (Invirase)

Saquinavir is the first of a powerful new generation of AIDS drugs called protease inhibitors. It appears to cause a decline of the virus in the body. It is recommended that it be used in combination with other AIDS drugs.

Protease inhibitors work by crippling an enzyme vital to the late stages of HIV's reproduction, while other AIDS drugs are active in the virus' early reproductive cycle. Saquinavir, in combination with other AIDS drugs, provides for treatment of HIV infection in two separate places.

Immunization

Immunity is the state of being protected from or resistant to a particular disease due to the development of antibodies. The mechanisms of immunity involve an *antigen-antibody* response. When an *antigen* enters the body, complex activities are set into motion. These activities involve chemical and mechanical forces that defend and protect the body's cells and tissues. *Antibodies* are formed and released from plasma cells, after which they enter the body fluids where they react with the invading antigen.

The mechanisms of immunity are basic on the body's ability to:

- protect itself against specific infectious microorganisms.
- defend body cells and tissues that are invaded by foreign substances.
- accept or reject another's blood or organ (blood transfusion or organ transplant).
- protect itself against cancer and immunodeficiency disease.

Note: The following portion of this unit is adapted from materials printed by the U.S. Department of Health and Human Services, Public Health Service, Centers for Disease Control and Prevention, Atlanta, GA 30333.

Immunization is a term denoting the process of inducing or providing immunity artificially by administering an immunobiologic (immunizing agent). Immunization can be active or passive.

- *Active immunization* denotes the production of antibody or antitoxin in response to the administration of a vaccine or toxoid.
- *Passive immunization* denotes the provision of temporary immunity by the administration of preformed antitoxins or antibodies. Three types of immunobiologics are used for passive immunization:
  1. pooled human IG (immune globulin)
  2. specific IG preparations
  3. antitoxin

General Recommendation for Immunization

Recommendations for immunization of infants, children, and adults are based on facts about immunobiologics and scientific knowledge about the principles of active and passive immunization, and on judgments by public health officials and specialists in clinical and preventive medicine. Benefits and risks are associated with the use of all products—no vaccine is completely safe or completely effective. The benefits range from partial to complete protection from the consequences of disease, and the risks range from common, trivial, and inconvenient side effects to rare, severe, and life-threatening conditions.

Thus, recommendations on immunization practices balance scientific evidence of benefits, costs, and risks to achieve optimal levels of protection against infectious or communicable diseases. These recommendations may apply only in the United States, as epidemiological circumstances and vaccines may differ in other countries.

Immunobiologics

The specific nature and content of immunobiologics may differ. When immunobiologics against the same infectious agents are produced by different manufacturers, active and inert ingredients among the various products may differ. Practitioners are urged to become familiar with the constituents of the products they use. The constituents of immunobiologics include:

Suspending Fluid. This frequently is as simple as sterile water or saline, but it may be a complex fluid containing small amounts of proteins or other constituents derived from the medium, or biologic system in which the vaccine is produced (serum proteins, egg antigens, cell-culture-derived antigens).

Preservatives, Stabilizers, Antibiotics. These components of vaccines are used to inhibit or prevent bacterial growth in viral culture or the final product, or to stabilize the antigen. They include such material as mercurials and specific antibiotics. Allergic reactions may occur if the recipient is sensitive to one of these additives.

Adjuvants. An aluminum compound is used in some vaccines to enhance the immune response to vaccines containing inactivated microorganisms or their products; for example, toxoids and hepatitis B virus vaccine. Vaccines with such adjuvants must be injected deeply in muscle masses, since subcutaneous or intracutaneous administration may cause local irritation, inflammation, granuloma formation, or necrosis.

Immunizing Agents

Immunobiologics include vaccines, toxoids, and antibody-containing-preparations from human or animal donors, including globulins and antitoxins.

Vaccine. A suspension of attenuated live or killed microorganisms (bacteria, viruses, or *rickettsiae*), or fractions thereof, administered to induce immunity and thereby prevent infectious disease.

Toxoid. A modified bacterial toxin that has been rendered nontoxic but that retains the ability to stimulate the formation of antitoxin.

Immune globulin (IG). A sterile solution containing antibody from human blood. It is a 15–18 percent protein obtained by cold ethanol fractionation of large pools of blood plasma. It is primarily indicated for routine maintenance of certain immunodeficient persons, and for passive immunization against measles and hepatitis A.

Specific immune globulin. Special preparations obtained from donor pools preselected for a high antibody content against a specific disease. For example: Hepatitis B Immune Globulin (HBIG), Varicella Zoster Immune Globulin (VZIG), Rabies Immune Globulin (RIG), and Tetanus Immune Globulin (TIG).

Antitoxin. A solution of antibodies derived from the serum of animals immunized with specific antigens (diphtheria, tetanus) used to achieve passive immunity or to effect a treatment.

Route and Site Selection

Route. There is a recommended route of administration for each immunobiologic. To avoid unnecessary local or systemic effects and/or to ensure optimal efficacy, the practitioner should not deviate from the recommended route of administration.

Site. Injectable immunobiologics should be administered in an area where there is minimal opportunity for local, neural, vascular, or tissue injury. Subcutaneous injections are usually administered into the thigh of infants and in the deltoid area of older children and adults. Intradermal injections are generally given on the *volar* surface of the forearms, except for human diploid cell rabies vaccine, with which reactions are less severe when given in the deltoid area.

Intramuscular Injections. Preferred sites for intramuscular injections are the anterolateral aspect of the upper thigh and the deltoid muscle of the upper arm. In most infants, the anterolateral aspect of the thigh provides the largest muscle mass and, therefore, is the preferred site. In older children, the deltoid mass is of sufficient size for intramuscular injection. An individual decision must be made for each child, based on the volume of the injected material and the size of the muscle into which it is to be injected. In adults, the deltoid is generally used for routine intramuscular vaccine administration.

The upper, outer quadrant of the gluteal region should be used only for the largest volumes of injection or when multiple doses need to be given, such as when large doses of IG must be administered. The site selected should be well into the upper, outer mass of the gluteus maximus and away from the central region of the buttocks.

Hypersensitivity to Vaccine Components

Vaccine antigens produced in systems or with substrates containing allergenic substances (for example, antigens derived from growing microorganisms in embryonated chicken eggs) may cause hypersensitivity reactions. These reactions may include anaphylaxis when the final vaccine contains a substantial amount of the allergen. Yellow fever vaccine is such an antigen. Vaccines with such characteristics should *not* be given to persons with known hypersensitivity to components of the substrates.

Screening persons by history of ability or inability to eat eggs without adverse effects is a reasonable way to identify those possibly at risk from receiving measles, mumps and influenza vaccine. Individuals with anaphylactic hypersensitivity to eggs (hives, swelling of the mouth and throat, difficulty breathing, hypotension, or shock) should *not* be given these vaccines.

Those administering vaccines should carefully review the information provided with the package insert and ascertain whether the patient is hypersensitive to any of its components. The physician must carefully evaluate each patient with known hypersensitivity before administering the vaccine.

Emergency Supplies and Medications

It is recommended that certain emergency supplies and medications be readily available when administering any drug to a patient. The recommended emergency supplies and medications are:

- epinephrine
- aminophylline
- diphenhydramine
- vasopressor (dopamine hydrochloride)
- steroids
- IV infusion materials (tourniquet, syringes, needles, alcohol swabs)
- blood pressure monitoring equipment (stethoscope and sphygmomanometer)
- oral airways
- oxygen
- cardiac support system

Altered Immunocompetence

Virus replication after administration of live, attenuated-virus vaccines may be enhanced in persons with immunodeficiency diseases, and in those with suppressed capability for immune response, as occurs with leukemia, lymphoma, generalized malignancy, or therapy with corticosteroids, alkylating agents, antimetabolites, or radiation. Patients with such conditions should *not* be given live, attenuated-virus vaccines. Also, because of the possibility of familial immunodeficiency, live, attenuated-virus vaccines should *not* be given to a member of a household in which there is family history of congenital or hereditary immunodeficiency, until the immune competence of the potential recipient is known.

Severe Febrile Illnesses

Minor illnesses, such as mild upper-respiratory infections, should not cause postponement of vaccine administration. However, immunization of persons with severe febrile illnesses should generally be deferred until they have recovered.

Immunization during Pregnancy

On the grounds of a theoretical risk to the developing fetus, live, attenuated-virus vaccines are not generally given to pregnant women or to those likely to become pregnant within 3 months after receiving vaccine(s). With some of these vaccines, particularly rubella, measles, and mumps, pregnancy is a contraindication.

There is no convincing evidence of risk to the fetus from immunization of pregnant women using inactivated virus vaccines, bacterial vaccines, or toxoids. Tetanus and diphtheria toxoid (Td) should be given to inadequately immunized pregnant women because it affords protection against neonatal tetanus.

Adverse Events Following Immunization

Modern vaccines are extremely safe and effective, but not completely so. Adverse events following immunization have been reported with all vaccines. To improve knowledge about adverse reactions, all temporarily associated events severe enough to require the recipient to seek medical attention should be evaluated and reported in detail to local or state health officials and to the vaccine manufacturer.

Sources of Vaccine Information

Official Package Circular. Manufacturers provide product-specific information along with each vaccine; some of these are reproduced in their entirety in the *Physicians' Desk Reference* (PDR) and dated.

Health Information for International Travel. Published annually by the Centers for Disease Control (CDC) as a guide to requirements and recommendations for specific immunizations and health practices for travel to various countries. It can be obtained for $5 from the Superintendent of Documents, U.S. Government Printing Office, Washington, DC 20402.

Additional Information. Division of Immunization, Centers for Disease Control and Prevention, Atlanta, Georgia 30333, telephone, (404) 657-3158 or GIST 294-3158.

Antigen(s)

Antigens are substances inducing the formation of antibodies. In some vaccines, the antigen is highly defined; for example, pneumococcal polysaccharide, hepatitis B surface antigen, tetanus or diphtheria toxoids. In other vaccines, it is complex or incompletely defined; for example, killed pertussis bacteria, live, attenuated viruses.

Immunization Schedules

In general, immunization policies have been directed toward vaccinating infants, children, and adolescents. While immunization is a routine measure in pediatric practice, it is not usually routine in the practice of physicians who treat adults.

The widespread and successful implementation of childhood immunization programs has greatly reduced the occurrence of many vaccine-preventable diseases. However, successful childhood immunization alone will not necessarily eliminate specific disease problems. A substantial proportion of the remaining morbidity and mortality from vaccine-preventable disease now occurs in older adolescents and adults. Persons who escaped natural infection or were not immunized with vaccines and toxoids against diphtheria, tetanus, measles, mumps, rubella, and poliomyelitis may be at risk of these diseases and their complications.

To reduce further the unnecessary occurrence of these vaccine-preventable diseases, all those who provide health care to older adolescents and adults should provide immunizations as a routine part of their practice. In addition, the *epidemiology* of other vaccine-preventable diseases (for example, hepatitis B, rabies, influenza, and pneumococcal disease) indicates that individuals who have special health problems are at increased risk of these illnesses and should be immunized. Travelers to some countries may be at increased risk of these illnesses and should be immunized. Travelers to some countries may be at increased risk of exposure to vaccine-preventable diseases. Several factors need to be considered before any patient is vaccinated. These include:

- the susceptibility of the patient.
- the risk of exposure to the disease.
- the risk from the disease.
- the benefits and risks from the immunizing agent.

Physicians should maintain detailed information about previous vaccinations received by each individual, including type of vaccination, date of receipt, and adverse events, if any, following vaccination. Information should also include the person's history of vaccine-preventable illnesses, occupation, and lifestyle. After the administration of any immunobiologic, the patient should be given written documentation of its receipt and information on which vaccines or toxoids will be needed in the future.

The immunization schedule in Table 19–2 applies generally to individuals in the indicated groups. For more detailed information on immunobiologics, and before administering any immunizing agent, refer to an appropriate source of information regarding indications, side effects, adverse reactions, precautions, contraindications, dosages, and route of administration.

National Health Objective: To Immunize Preschoolers

One of the most important national health objectives identified by the United States Public Health Service for the year 2000 is to immunize 90 percent of preschool children by their second birthday against diphtheria, tetanus, pertussis, poliomyelitis, measles, mumps, rubella, *Haemophilus influenzae* type b and Hepatitis B. Available data suggest that less than 60 percent of children are up-to-date for the recommended primary immunization series by their second birthday.

Table 19–2 Immunization for Children and Adults

Vaccine	Schedule
Diphtheria, Tetanus, and Pertussis (DTP)	Primary: 2, 4, 6, and (12, 15, or 18 months). Boosters: 4 to 6 years.
Haemophilus influenzae type b (Hib)	Primary: 2 and 4 months, and 6 months. (depending on type). Boosters 12–15 months.
DTP and Hib combination	Primary: 2, 4, 6, and (12, 15, or 18 months).
Polio	Primary: 2, 4, 6, and (12, 15, or 18 months). Boosters: 4 to 6 years.
Mumps	Primary: 12–15 months. Booster: 4 to 6 years or 11 to 12 years.
Rubeola	Primary: 12–15 months. Booster: 4 to 6 years or 11 to 12 years.
Rubella	Primary: 12–15 months. Booster: 4 to 6 years or 11 to 12 years.
MMR (Mumps, Rubeola, Rubella)	Primary: 12–15 months. Booster: 4 to 6 years or 11 to 12 years.
Hepatitis B	Regimen consists of 3 doses: initial, 1 month, and 6 months from initial dose. Recommended: persons of all ages at risk of contracting the virus.
Pneumococcus	Single dose given to high-risk children over 2 years, all high-risk adults, and adults at age 50 and again at age 65.
Influenza Type A and Type B	Given during the fall of the year, usually in early October. Single dose given to adults and children (6 months or older) with chronic heart or lung disorders; patients in nursing homes, or chronic care facilities; individuals with diabetes, kidney disease, and other metabolic diseases. May be given as a preventive measure to those who wish to receive the vaccine.
Bacille Calmette-Guétin (BCG)	Given in high incidence of tuberculosis.
Menomune (meningococcus serogroup C)	Given during outbreaks and for specific populations at high risk of infection.
Varivax (Varicella Virus Vaccine Live)	For Subcutaneous Injection. Children 12 months to 12 years a single dose of 0.5 mL. Adolescents and adults 13 years of age and older 0.5 mL and a second 0.5 mL dose 4 to 8 weeks later.

Table 19–2 *(Continued)*

Vaccine	Schedule
HAVRIX	For Intramuscular Injection. Protects against infection with hepatitis A virus. Primary: Adults over 18 years of age: one 1 mL/1440 ELISA units. Booster: 6–12 months after primary dose. Primary: Children and adolescents 2–18 years of age: two doses of 0.5 mL/360 ELISA units. Second dose is given 1 month after the primary dose. Booster: 6–12 months after the primary dose.

Standards for Pediatric Immunization Practices

The United States Department of Health and Human Services recommends the following standards for pediatric immunization practices.

1. Immunization services are readily available and responsive to the needs of patient.
2. There are no barriers or unnecessary prerequisites to the receipt of vaccines. Immunization services should be available on a walk-in basis at all times for both routine and new enrollee visits. Waiting time should be minimized and generally not exceed 30 minutes.
3. Immunization services are available free or for a minimal fee. In the public sector, immunizations should be free of charge. If fees must be collected, they should be kept to a minimum. In the private sector, charges should include the cost of the vaccine, and a reasonable administration fee.
4. Providers utilize all clinical encounters to screen for needed vaccines and, when indicated, immunize children.
5. Providers educate parents and guardians about the importance of immunizations, the diseases they prevent, the recommended immunization schedules, the need to receive immunizations at recommend ages, and to bring their child's immunization record to each visit.
6. Providers question parents or guardians about contraindications and, before immunizing a child, inform them in specific terms about the risks and benefits of the immunizations their child is to receive.
7. Providers follow only true contraindications. True contraindications recommended by the Advisory Committee on Immunization Practices (ACIP) and the Committee on Infectious Diseases (Red Book Committee) of the American Academy of Pediatrics (AAP) are:

General for all vaccines—anaphylactic reaction to a vaccine contraindicates further doses of that vaccine; anaphylactic reaction to a vaccine constituent contraindicates the use of vaccines containing that substance; and moderate or severe illnesses with or without fever.

DTP—encephalopathy within 7 days of administration of previous dose of DTP.

OPV—infection with HIV or a household contact with HIV; known altered immunodeficiency and immunodeficient household contact.

MMR—anaphylactic reactions to egg ingestion and to neomycin; pregnancy and known altered immunodeficiency.

8. Providers administer simultaneously all vaccine doses for which a child is eligible at the time of the visit.
9. Providers use accurate and complete recording procedures. Providers are required by statute to record, what vaccine was given, the date the vaccine was given (month, day, year), the name of the manufacturer of the vaccine, the lot number, the signature and title of the person who gave the vaccine, and the address where the vaccine was given. In addition, providers should record on the child's personal immunization record card what vaccine was given, the date the vaccine was given and the name of the provider.
10. Providers co-schedule immunization appointments in conjunction with appointments for other child health services.
11. Providers report adverse events following immunization promptly, accurately, and completely. Providers should report all such clinically significant events, including those requited by law, to the Vaccine Adverse Event Reporting System (VAERS), regardless of whether or not they believe the events are caused by the vaccine. Report forms and assistance are available by calling 1-800-822-7967.
12. Providers operate a tracking system. A tracking system should produce reminders of upcoming immunizations as well as recalls for children who are overdue.
13. Providers adhere to appropriate procedures for vaccine management. Vaccines should be handled and stored as recommended in the manufacturer's package inserts. The temperatures at which vaccines are stored and transported should be monitored daily and the expiration date for each vaccine should be noted.
14. Providers conduct semi-annual audits to assess immunization coverage levels and to review immunization records in the patient populations they serve.
15. Providers maintain up-to-date, easily retrievable medical protocols at all locations where vaccines are administered.
16. Providers practice patient-oriented and community-based approaches.
17. Vaccines are administered by properly trained individuals. Only properly trained individuals should administer vaccines.
18. Providers receive ongoing education and training on current immunization recommendations.

Why Immunize?

A Gallup survey (April, 1993) of 1,000 parents of children under 5, showed that 47 percent did not know that polio is contagious, 36 percent did not know that measles could be fatal, and 44 percent did not know that *Haemophilus influenzae* type b is the leading cause of potentially fatal childhood meningitis.

Immunizations prevent illnesses that cause pain, fever, rashes, coughs, sore throats, hearing loss, blindness, crippling, brain damage, and even death. In the United States only 56 percent of children under 2 years of age get the immunizations recommended by public health officials and the American Academy of Pediatrics. The United States ranks 70th worldwide in preschool immunization rates. To overcome this statistic and insure that all children are properly vaccinated, immunization should become a top priority for all healthcare providers.

Hepatitis B Vaccination

Hepatitis B is caused by hepatitis B virus (HBV) and usually enters the body by the parenteral route. About 300,000 people contract the hepatitis B virus each year, and the incidence is increasing. This infectious disease can destroy the liver, and each year approximately 4,000 people die from the disease.

The Centers for Disease Control and Prevention's Immunization Practices Advisory Committee recommends that all teenagers and newborns be vaccinated against hepatitis B. Vaccination is recommended in persons of all ages, especially those who are or will be at increased risk of infection with hepatitis B virus. Those who should be vaccinated include:

- Health-care personnel
- Selected patients and patient contacts
- Infants born to hepatitis B positive mothers
- Population with high incidence of the disease
- Military personnel identified as being at increased risk
- Morticians and embalmers
- Blood bank and plasma fractionation workers
- Persons at increased risk due to sexual practices
- Prisoners
- Users of illicit injectable drugs

Heptavax-B

Uses. Indicated for immunization against infection caused by all known subtypes of hepatitis B virus.

Contraindications. Hypersensitivity.

Adverse Reactions

Injection site: Soreness, erythema, swelling, warmth, and induration.

Systemic: Fatigue, asthenia, malaise, fever, chills, irritability, diaphoresis, anorexia, nausea, vomiting, abdominal pain, diarrhea, adenitis, myalgia, arthralgia, headache, dizziness, disturbed sleep, paresthesia, upper respiratory illness, and rash.

Dosage and Route. The immunization regimen consists of 3 doses of vaccine. The vaccine is given by intramuscular injection. **Do not inject intravenously or intradermally**.

	Initial	1 month	6 months
Birth to 10 years of age	0.5 ml	0.5 ml	0.5 ml
Older children and adults	1.0 ml	1.0 ml	1.0 ml
Dialysis patients and immunocompromised patients	2.0 ml	2.0 ml	2.0 ml

Recombivax-HB®

Recombivax-HB® is a genetically engineered hepatitis B vaccine. It is made by genetically programming common yeast cells to produce the antigen portion of the virus contained in its outer coat.

Uses. Indicated for immunization against infection caused by all known subtypes of hepatitis B virus.

Contraindications. Hypersensitivity to yeast or any component of the vaccine.

Adverse Reactions

Injection site: Soreness, pain, tenderness, pruritus, erythema, ecchymosis, swelling, warmth, and nodule formation.

Systemic: Fatigue/weakness, headache, fever, malaise, nausea, diarrhea, pharyngitis, and upper respiratory infection.

Dosage and Route. The immunization regimen consists of 3 doses of vaccine. The vaccine is to be given by intramuscular injection. **Do not inject intravenously or intradermally**.

	Initial	1 month	6 months
Birth to 10 years of age	0.5 ml	0.5 ml	0.5 ml
Older children and adults	1.0 ml	1.0 ml	1.0 ml

Spot Check

For childhood immunizations there are routinely recommended ages and a range of acceptable ages. For each of the vaccines listed, give the appropriate information that relates to age/ages.

Vaccine	Schedule
Hepatitis B Hep B-1 Hep B-2 Hep B-3	
Diphtheria, Tetatus, Pertussis	
H. influenzae type B (Hib)	
Polio (OPV)	
Measles, Mumps, Rubella (MMR)	

◆ Review Questions

Directions: Select the best answer to each multiple choice question. Circle the letter of your choice.

1. The ingestion and digestion of bacteria and particles by cells of the reticuloendothelial system and white blood cells is known as __________.

   a. histoplasmosis b. phagocytosis c. cryptococcosis d. lymphokines

2. Some diseases for which a physician may prescribe an antifungal agent are __________.

   a. pneumonia, genital herpes, influenza
   b. coryza, acquired immune deficiency syndrome, herpes zoster
   c. histoplasmosis, *Candida* infections, tinea
   d. hepatitis, yellow fever, diphtheria

3. Patients with *Candida* infections should be given instructions about __________.

   a. correct handwashing procedure
   b. proper personal hygiene
   c. the wearing of cotton underclothes
   d. all of these

4. The usual oral adult dose of nystatin (Mycostatin) is __________.

   a. 250,000–500,000 units tid
   b. 400,000–500,000 units tid
   c. 500,000–1,000,000 units tid
   d. 600,000–800,000 units tid

5. Genital herpes is __________.

   a. a sexually transmitted disease
   b. spread by casual contact
   c. not an infectious disease
   d. a disease that is easily cured

6. An antiviral agent that has in vitro inhibitory activity against herpes simplex types 1 and 2, varicella-zoster, Epstein-Barr and cytomegalovirus is __________.

   a. amantadine hydrochloride (Symmetrel)
   b. acyclovir (Zovirax)
   c. azidothymidine (AZT)
   d. ribavirin (Virazole)

7. __________ is the medical term for the common cold.

   a. Pertussis b. Candida c. Coryza d. Cozrya

8. __________ is the state of being protected from or resistant to a particular disease due to the development of antibodies.
   a. Immunization
   b. Vaccination
   c. Immunity
   d. Immunobiologic
9. Injectable immunobiologics should be administered in __________.
   a. the recommended route for administration for each immunizing agent
   b. an area free of nerves and vessels
   c. the lower quadrant of the gluteal muscle
   d. a and b
10. Patients who should not receive live, attenuated-virus vaccines include persons with __________.
   a. normal immune response
   b. immunodeficiency disease
   c. leukemia
   d. b and c
11. __________ are parasites, minute organisms that may invade normal cells, and cause disease.
   a. Bacteria b. Fungi c. Viruses d. Protozoa
12. __________ include molds and yeasts.
   a. Bacteria b. Fungi c. Viruses d. Protozoa
13. __________ is one of the most common causes of vaginitis in woman during the reproductive years.
   a. Crytococcosis c. Candida
   b. Cytomegalovirus d. Varicella
14. __________ agents act by exerting fungistatic or fungicidal action on both resting and growing cells.
   a. Antifungal b. Antiviral c. Antibiotic d. Immunizing
15. Monistat is an example of an __________.
   a. antifungal agent
   b. antiviral agent
   c. antibiotic
   d. immunizing agent
16. Herpes simplex virus type 2 (HSV-2) causes __________.
   a. AIDS b. cold sores c. fever blisters d. genital herpes

Case Study: Zachary Noble, 2 months old, is brought to the well-baby clinic and is given DTP and OPV-1. The parents are asked to make a return appointment with the receptionist.

17. The nurse should know that DPT is the abbreviation for __________.
    a. diphtheria, tetanus, and pertussis
    b. diphtheria, tetanus, and pertussi
    c. disseminated tetanus protein
    d. diphtheria toxoid protein
18. The nurse should know that OPV-1 is the abbreviation for oral __________.
    a. pertussis vaccine-1
    b. poliovirus vaccine-1
    c. protein vaccine-1
    d. pertussia vaccine-1
19. In scheduling a return appointment it is important to know that the infant needs to return in __________.
    a. 3 months
    b. 4 months
    c. 2 months
    d. 1 month

Matching: Place the correct letter from Column II on the appropriate line of Column I.

Column I

20. __________ Adenovirus
21. __________ Antigen
22. __________ Cytomegalovirus
23. __________ Antibody
24. __________ Antigenic
25. __________ Herpes simplex virus type 1
26. __________ Varicella
27. __________ Volar
28. __________ Human immunodeficiency virus (HIV)

Column II

A. A protein substance that is developed in response to an antigen.
B. One of a group of species-specific herpes viruses.
C. Causes cold sores or fever blisters.
D. A substance that induces the formation of antibodies.
E. One of a group of closely related viruses that can cause infections of the upper respiratory tract.
F. Capable of causing the production of an antibody.
G. Refers to the palm of the hand.
H. Chickenpox.
I. Causative agent of genital herpes.
J. Causative agent of AIDS.

CHAPTER 20

Antineoplastic Agents

OBJECTIVES

Upon completion of this chapter, you should be able to:

- Define the terms listed in the vocabulary.
- State when chemotherapy is the treatment of choice for cancer.
- List the normal cells that have the greatest sensitivity to destruction from antineoplastic agents.
- State the aim of chemotherapy.
- State who should prepare and administer antineoplastic agents.
- Describe examples of adverse reactions associated with antineoplastic agents.
- List and give the normal ranges of certain laboratory tests that are performed to establish a patient's baseline data before initiation of chemotherapy.
- Note that the dosage of antineoplastic agents is individualized for each patient.
- Describe the guidelines for handling antineoplastic agents.
- Explain the care of chemotherapy patients.
- List the signs and symptoms of breast cancer.
- Explain what one should know about the breast and one's risk factors.
- Define benign prostatic hypertrophy (BPH).
- List the symptoms of benign prostatic hypertrophy (BPH).
- Explain the treatment for benign prostatic hypertrophy (BPH).
- Describe prostate cancer.
- List the possible symptoms of prostate cancer.
- Describe the treatment for prostate cancer.
- List the guidelines for care of the older adult with cancer.
- List the cancer screening test or procedure that an individual 50 or older should have.

- Give the suggested ways that one may communicate with a child about a parent's serious illness.
- Complete the critical thinking questions/activities presented in this chapter.
- Describe the classifications of antineoplastic agents.
- Complete the Spot Check on the classification of antineoplastic agents.
- Give examples of combination chemotherapy agents.
- Describe other forms of treatment for cancer.
- Answer the review questions correctly.

Vocabulary

alopecia (al″o-pe′shi-a). Pertaining to hair loss.

anorexia (an″o-rek′si-a). A loss of appetite.

carcinogenic (kar″si-no-jen′ik). Pertaining to producing cancer.

cytotoxic (si″to-toks′ik). Destructive to cells.

dedifferentiation (de-dif″er-en″she-a′shun). The process whereby normal cells lose their specialization and become malignant.

deoxyribonucleic acid (DNA) (de-ok″si-ri″bo-nu-kle′ik as′id). A complex protein found in the nucleus of every cell.

differentiation (dif″er-en″she-a′ shun). The process whereby normal cells have a distinct appearance and specialized function.

exacerbation (eks-as″er-ba′shun). The time when the symptoms of a disease process are most severe.

extravasation (eks-trav″a-sa′shun). The process whereby fluids (especially, IV) escape into surrounding tissues.

glycoprotein (gli″ko-pro′te-in). A compound consisting of a carbohydrate and protein.

laminar airflow. Filtered air flowing along separate planes or layers. This method of airflow helps to prevent bacterial contamination and collection of hazardous chemical fumes in areas where pollution of the work environment could be detrimental to one's health. The use of a laminar airflow hood in the preparation of antineoplastic agents is recommended.

lymphokines (lim′fo-kinz). Substances released by sensitized lymphocytes when they contact specific antigens. They help to produce cellular immunity by stimulating macrophages and monocytes.

macrophage (mak′ro-fag). Cells scattered throughout the body (reticuloendothelial system) that have the power to ingest certain matter, such as bacteria.

malignant (ma-lig′nant). Literally means a "bad wandering." A cancerous tumor.

metastasis (me-tas′ta-sis). The spreading process of cancer cells from one part of the body to another.

oncologist (ong-kol′o-jist). One who specializes in tumors, especially neoplasms (new growths).

proliferation (pro-lif″er-a′shun). The process of rapid reproduction.

remission (re-mish′un). The time when the symptoms of a disease process are lessened.

ribonucleic acid (RNA) (ri″bo-nu-kle′ik as′id). A nucleic acid, found in all living cells, that is responsible for protein synthesis.

stomatitis (sto″ma-ti′tis). Inflammation of the mouth.

teratogenic (ter″a-to-jen′ik). Pertaining to producing or forming a severely malformed fetus.

Introduction

The incidence of cancer is five times greater now than it was 100 years ago. Cancer will strike one out of every four Americans, according to recent statistics from the American Cancer Society. With early detection, followed by immediate treatment, the cure rate for cancer is now one in every two.

In cancer, there is an abnormal process wherein a cell or group of cells undergoes change and no longer carries on normal cell functions. This failure of immature cells to develop specialized functions is called *dedifferentiation.* It is believed that this process involves a disturbance in the deoxyribonucleic acid (DNA) of the affected cells. Malignant cells usually multiply rapidly, forming a mass of abnormal cells that enlarges, ulcerates, and sheds malignant cells to surrounding tissues. This process destroys the normal cells, with the malignant cells taking their places. Microscopic analysis of a malignant cell reveals a loss of differentiation, anaplasia, nuclei of various sizes which are hyperchromatic, and cells in the process of rapid and disorderly division.

Oncologists have identified numerous factors that play a role in the development of cancer. These factors are environmental, hereditary, and biological. Over 200 forms of cancer have been identified.

The treatment of cancer may be any one or a combination of surgery, chemotherapy, radiation therapy, or immunotherapy. The treatment of choice depends upon the type of cancer, its location, its invasive process, and the patient's state of health. In this chapter emphasis is given to chemotherapy.

Chemotherapy with Antineoplastic Agents

Chemotherapy may be the treatment of choice when the cancer is disseminated and cannot be removed surgically. It is also used when a tumor fails to respond to radiation therapy, and is used in combination with other forms of therapy.

Antineoplastic, anticancer agents do injury to individual cells, interfere with their vital functions, and kill or destroy malignant cells. In rendering cancerous cells harmless, certain normal cells may also be destroyed. The normal cells with the greatest sensitivity to destruction are the hematopoietic cells, epithelial cells, and the hair follicles.

The plan of treatment for patients undergoing chemotherapy is individualized. The aim of chemotherapy is to put the patient in *remission* so that life may continue without *exacerbation* of symptoms.

Antineoplastic agents are potentially hazardous and fatal complications can occur. Most are *cytotoxic, mutagenic*, and *carcinogenic.*

- Only physicians or those qualified with special certification or education should prepare and administer antineoplastic agents.
- Antineoplastic drugs are curative agents in choriocarcinoma, acute lymphocytic leukemia, some cases of Hodgkin's disease, Burkitt's lymphoma, diffuse histiocytic lymphoma, certain testicular tumors, and perhaps osteogenic sarcoma.
- They accomplish tumor regression and enhance survival in acute myelocytic leukemia, non-Hodgkin's lymphoma, multiple myeloma, chronic leukemias, and adenocarcinomas of the breast and ovary.
- They are used in conjunction with surgery and radiation, and are effective in Wilm's tumor, embryonal rhabdomyosarcoma, and Ewing's sarcoma.
- They are used as an adjuvant therapy in breast cancer and other cancerous tumors.

Toxicities and Adverse Reactions

Toxicities and adverse reactions may vary with the antineoplastic agent and with each individual patient. Some examples of adverse reactions are:

Gastrointestinal. *Anorexia*, nausea, vomiting, mucositis, *stomatitis*, colitis, and liver dysfunction.

Hematopoietic. Bone marrow depression/suppression, anemia, leukopenia, thrombocytopenia, and pancytopenia.

Secondary Neoplasia. May increase incidence of a second malignant tumor.

Genitourinary. Sterile hemorrhagic cystitis, hyperuricemia, and renal failure.

Gonadal Suppression. Amenorrhea, azoospermia.

Integument. *Alopecia*, skin and fingernails may become darker, rash, maculopapular skin eruption.

Pulmonary. Interstitial pulmonary fibrosis.

Cardiac. Acute left ventricular failure, arrhythmias, cardiomyopathy.

Respiratory. Dyspnea.

Immunosuppressive Activity. May predispose patient to bacterial, viral (herpes zoster), or fungal infection.

Chromosomal Abnormalities. Mutagenic.

Teratogenic Effects. May cause fetal harm in pregnancy. Women of childbearing potential should be advised to avoid becoming pregnant.

Extravasation. Into subcutaneous tissues results in a painful inflammation. The area usually becomes indurated and sloughing of tissue may occur.

Patient Evaluation

The physician carefully evaluates each patient and determines an exact diagnosis. A plan of treatment is prescribed. When chemotherapy is the treatment regimen or part of the treatment regimen, certain laboratory tests are performed to determine the patient's baseline data before the initiation of therapy.

Tests:	*Normal Ranges:*
• Platelet Count	There are approximately 150,000–450,000 thrombocytes per cubic millimeter of blood.
• White Blood Cell Count (WBC)	There are approximately 5,000–10,000 leukocytes per cubic millimeter of blood.
• Hemoglobin	Adult female: 12–16 Gm/100 milliliter of blood Adult male: 14–18 Gm/100 milliliter of blood Children: will vary with age
• Hematocrit	Adult female: 37–47% Adult male: 40–54% Children: varies with age from 35–49% Newborn: 49–54%
• Differential	Neutrophils 40–60% Eosinophils 1–3% Basophils 0.5–1% Lymphocytes 20–40% Monocytes 4–8%

- Liver function and kidney function tests should be performed to determine these vital organs' functioning abilities.

During chemotherapy, these laboratory tests must be evaluated very carefully. When there is a deviation from normal, the physician is notified. At this time, the physician will evaluate the results of the test and determine the course of action to take.

Note: Those who prepare and/or administer antineoplastic agents should have the same laboratory tests performed before and during contact with these agents. Any deviation from normal should be carefully assessed by a physician.

Dosage

The dosage of antineoplastic agents is individualized for each patient. The dosage is based upon body surface area or kilogram of body weight. The physician will order the chemotherapy regimen, giving the patient's name, the agent or agents to use, the dose, route, rate, and time for administration. Those preparing and administering these agents should have a second qualified person check and verify the order and their preparation of the drug or drugs.

Protecting Yourself

Remember, only those qualified with special certification or education should prepare and administer antineoplastic agents. Ideally, the pharmacy department of a hospital should prepare antineoplastic agents under a vertical *laminar airflow* hood.

The National Institutes of Health (NIH) and the National Study Commission on Cytotoxic Exposure have prepared recommended guidelines for safely handling chemotherapeutic agents. The American Society of Hospital Pharmacists (ASHP) has also developed guidelines and procedures for handling cytotoxic agents. The following guidelines are based upon the aforementioned sources.

Guidelines for Handling Antineoplastic Agents

Preparations for the Procedure

- Ideally, a vertical laminar airflow hood should be available for the safe preparation of an antineoplastic agent. When such a hood is not available, a designated, secluded work area should be used. This area should be away from heating and cooling vents. Use a disposable, plastic-backed paper liner, or absorbent pad to cover the work space. Replace the liner or pad after each preparation. Correctly dispose of the liner or pad in a designated container.
- Perform medical asepsis handwash before you start the procedure.
- Wear a disposable, nonpermeable surgical gown that has a closed front and knit cuffs that completely cover your wrist.
- Wear *latex* surgical gloves. Polyvinyl gloves are permeable to some antineoplastic agents.
- Wear eyeglasses or safety glasses.
- Wear a nonpermeable surgical mask.

Preparing the Agent for Administration

- Use disposable, Luer-Lok syringe and needle units.
- Air-vent the vial to lower the internal pressure, thereby reducing the risk of spraying and spillage when the needle is removed from the vial's diaphragm.
- Make sure you have the correct amount of the agent in the syringe before removing the needle from the vial. If you have to remove air bubbles after withdrawing the needle from the vial, do not expel excess air from the syringe and needle unit at eye level. Wrap a sterile alcohol swab around the end of the needle tip while expelling the air.
- Keep a sterile alcohol swab around the needle and vial top during the withdrawal of the agent from the vial septum.
- When the agent comes in an ampule, make sure none of the agent is in the ampule tip. Wrap a sterile alcohol swab around the designated break point (neck). Hold the ampule away from your face and body. Break the neck of the ampule away from yourself.
- After preparing the agent, follow the correct protocol for removing the gown, mask, and gloves. Dispose of used garments in a designated container.
- Perform medical asepsis handwash.

Accidental Spill

- Wear two pairs of *latex* surgical gloves, a surgical gown and mask. Clean the area with 70 percent isopropyl alcohol, then rinse with water.
- If the agent comes into contact with your skin, wash the skin thoroughly with soap and water. Document the incident. Report the incident to the proper authority. Get medical attention. You should have a physical exam, plus essential laboratory tests performed.

Disposal of Used Equipment

- Dispose of used needles and syringes in a leakproof, puncture-proof container that is designated for *BIOHAZARD* equipment.
- *Do not* recap the needle or break it off from its hub.

Disposal of Patient's Waste

- *Always* wear *latex* surgical gloves to dispose of urine, feces, or vomitus from a patient receiving antineoplastic agents. Keep exposure time to a minimum.

Care of Chemotherapy Patients

Assess the patient's understanding of the disease process and the prescribed treatment regimen. Encourage the patient to express his or her emotional feelings about the disease and the treatment. Encourage the patient to ask questions and provide appropriate answers. Follow the proper protocol for preparing and/or administering antineoplastic agents.

Assess and monitor:

- Laboratory test results
- Intravenous infusion site/sites for extravasation, thrombosis or phlebitis
- Signs of adverse reactions
- Patient's response to treatment

During chemotherapy, force fluids (1, $1\frac{1}{2}$, to 2 liters) per day, unless otherwise ordered or contraindicated. Administer antiemetics and analgesics as ordered. If the patient's nausea, vomiting, and pain are not controlled by the prescribed dose, notify the physician. A more satisfactory regimen should be initiated.

Protect the patient from infection:

- Perform medical asepsis handwash.
- Maintain a clean environment.
- Administer antibiotics as ordered.
- Educate the patient, family, and visitors about the spread of infectious diseases.

Provide for nutritional needs:

- Encourage the patient to eat and take sufficient liquids.
- Assist the patient in selecting foods of choice from the menu.
- Assist the patient with eating as necessary.
- Cater to the patient's dietary needs. Provide small frequent feedings.
- Administer diet supplements, appetite stimulants, blood, blood components as ordered.

Additional measures:

- Monitor fluid and electrolyte balance.
- Record intake and output.
- Provide good mouth care. Keep the patient's mucous membranes moist. Apply lip balm as ordered. Should stomatitis occur, check with the physician for a plan of treatment.

Note: Over-the-counter mouthwashes usually contain alcohol that may be irritating to the mucosa, Lemon-glycerine swabs can irritate the mucous membranes. One teaspoon of baking soda dissolved in one cup (8 ounces) of water or a mixture of one cup of hydrogen peroxide and two cups of water are soothing mixtures. Apply with special oral-care sponges (Toothettes) or a soft-bristled toothbrush. For severe mucositis, a saline solution rinse may be used at least six times a day. Other rinses that are helpful are a 1:4 mixture of dyclonine (local anesthetic agent) and sterile water; triple mixture of equal parts 2 percent viscous lidocaine, diphenhydramine HCl elixir and Mylanta-II.

- Encourage the patient to eat moist foods.
- Encourage the patient to drink plenty of fluids. Sucking on ice chips and sugarless hard candy helps to moisten the mouth.
- Advise the patient to avoid spicy, hot, and acidic foods and beverages.
- Advise the patient not to smoke.
- Provide emotional support.

Patient Teaching

Patient teaching encompasses a wide scope of factors. The patient needs to understand the disease process and the treatment regimen. With regard to chemotherapy, the patient needs to know about possible adverse reactions and what he or she can do to lessen the side effects. It is your responsibility to inform and teach each patient about the medication being given. To do this, you must be knowledgeable about the drug. You must use appropriate reference books, such as *The Physicians' Desk Reference* (PDR), and learn about all aspects and effects of the drug.

Most antineoplastic agents cause nausea and vomiting. To lessen the severity of nausea and vomiting, you may want to advise the patient to:

- avoid hot, spicy, greasy, and acidic foods and beverages.
- avoid unpleasant odors.
- eat small frequent meals.
- take a prescribed antiemetic before chemotherapy.
- suck on ice chips and/or sugarless hard candy.
- refrain from smoking.

Teach the patient to be alert for the following signs of infection, and to report such signs to the attending physician.

- An elevated body temperature
- Sneezing, coughing, and malaise, usual indications of a viral upper respiratory infection
- Signs of inflammation, such as pain, heat, redness, swelling, and impaired function

Teach the patient to be consciously alert for the following signs of bleeding and to report such signs to the attending physician.

- Excessive bruising
- Nosebleed (epistaxis), rectal bleeding, abnormal vaginal bleeding, and bleeding gums
- Small, purplish, hemorrhagic spots on the skin (petechiae), possible indications of abnormality in blood-clotting

One of the most dreaded adverse reactions to chemotherapy is *alopecia*, the loss of hair. You may want to suggest that the patient temporarily wear a wig or some other form of scalp cover. Usually, the hair will begin to grow back after the effects of chemotherapy are eliminated from the patient's body. The new hair may be even darker than the hair that was lost.

SPOTLIGHT

Breast Cancer

This year approximately 182,000 women and approximately 1000 men will be diagnosed with breast cancer. It kills about 46,000 women a year and is the leading cause of death in women between the ages of 32 and 52. Two genes have been linked to familial breast and ovarian cancer and these are BRCA-1 and BRCA-2. These genes may encourage breast cancer to develop. The genes tell cells how to produce a protein called cyclin D, one of several proteins that tell cells to produce an extra set of genetic material to be passed along when the cell divides. If further research supports the theory, scientists may be able to develop a test that could distinguish microscopic noncancerous breast abnormalities from cancerous ones. They may also be able to develop drugs for women at high risk to slow the overactive genes.

In cancer, there is an abnormal process wherein a cell or group of cells undergoes changes and no longer carries on normal cell functions. This failure of immature cells to develop specialized functions is called dedifferentiation. It is believed that this process involves a disturbance in the DNA of the affected cells. Malignant cells usually multiply rapidly, forming a mass of abnormal cells that enlarges, ulcerates, and sheds malignant cells to surrounding tissues. This process destroys the normal cells, with malignant cells taking their places, and often results in the formation of a tumor.

If cancer is not detected and treated early, it will continue to grow, invade, and destroy adjacent tissue and spread into surrounding lymph nodes. It can be carried by the lymph and/or blood to other areas of the body and once this process, known as metastasis has occurred, the cancer is usually advanced and/or disseminated and the five-year survival rate is low. Early detection of breast cancer is extremely important. Until recently, surgical biopsy offered the only means for accurate diagnosis of breast cancer. Now, a new technique called stereotactic breast biopsy is helping reduce the need for surgical biopsy. The procedure is designed to sample millimeter-size breast lumps for malignancy with little intrusion into the body. With stereotactic breast biopsy the physician works from a computer image of the breast showing the lump's exact location. A small sampling needle is then placed inside the breast to draw out a sample of tissue to be tested.

The stereotactic breast biopsy is usually done in less than an hour and leaves the woman with little more than a temporary mark resembling a pinprick. Researchers state that this procedure is not for all women as there are circumstances where one would still do the traditional surgical biopsy. For example, if a woman had a large area or she could feel the lump, she would not be a candidate for stereotactic biopsy. The five-year survival rate for women with localized and properly treated breast cancer is 92 percent.

Approximately 50 percent of malignant tumors of the breast appear in the upper, outer quadrant and extend into the armpit. Eighteen percent of breast cancers occur in the nipple area, 11 percent in the lower outer quadrant, and 6 percent in the inner quadrant.

Signs and symptoms of breast cancer are generally insidious and may include:

- unusual secretions from the nipple.
- changes in the nipple's appearance.
- non-tender, movable lump.
- well-localized discomfort that may be described as a burning, stinging, or aching sensation.
- dimpling or peau d'orange (orange-peel appearance) may be present over the area of cancer of the breast.
- asymmetry and an elevation of the affected breast.
- nipple retraction.
- pain in the later stages.

Know Your Breast and Your Risk Factors

More than 90 percent of all breast lumps are discovered by women themselves. The majority of these lumps are benign (noncancerous) but of those that are not, early detection and treatment are essential.

Your Breast:

Being Informed Could Save Your Life
Risk Factors in Order of Importance:

1. Family history—Increased risk when breast cancer occurs before menopause in mother, sister or daughter especially if cancer occurs in both breasts.
2. Over age 50 and nullipara.
3. Having a first baby after age 30.
4. History of chronic breast disease, especially epithelial hyperplasia.
5. Exposure to ionizing radiation of more than 50 rad during adolescence.
6. Obesity.
7. Early menarche, late menopause.

Examine Your Breast Every Month
Appearance
Size, Shape, Symmetry
Tenderness, Thickening, Texture Changes

SPOTLIGHT

Abnormal Conditions of the Prostate Gland

The prostate gland is about 4 centimeters wide and weighs about 20 grams. It is composed of glandular, connective, and muscular tissue and lies behind the urinary bladder. It surrounds the first 2.5 centimeters of the urethra and secretes an alkaline fluid that aids in maintaining the viability of spermatozoa. The prostate gland produces semen, the thick fluid that carries sperm from the testicles. Normal functioning of the prostate gland depends on the male hormone testosterone, made by the testicles. Male hormones, such as testosterone, are believed to stimulate prostate cancer growth.

Benign Prostatic Hypertrophy (BPH)

Enlargement of the prostate gland may occur in men who are 50 years of age and older. As the prostate enlarges, it compresses the urethra, thereby restricting the normal flow of urine. This restriction generally causes a number of symptoms and can be referred to as prostatism. Prostatism is any condition of the prostate gland that interferes with the flow of urine from the bladder.

Symptoms usually include:

- a weak or hard-to-start urine stream.
- a feeling that the bladder is not empty.
- a need to urinate often, especially at night.
- a feeling of urgency (a sudden need to urinate).
- abdominal straining, a decrease in size and force of the urinary stream.
- interruption of the stream.
- acute urinary retention.
- recurrent urinary infections.

Treatment for Benign Prostatic Hypertrophy

Surgery—Transurethral resection of the prostate (TURP or TUR) is the most common form of surgery used for benign prostatic hypertrophy. During this procedure an endoscopic instrument that has ocular and surgical capabilities is introduced directly through the urethra to the prostate and small pieces of the prostate gland are removed by using an electrical cutting loop.

Medication—Proscar (finasteride) an oral medication, may be prescribed by a physician to help relieve the symptoms of BPH. It lowers the levels of dihydrotestosterone (DHT) which is a major factor in enlargement of the prostate. Lowering of DHT leads to shrinkage of the enlarged prostate gland in most men. Although this can lead to gradual improvement in urine flow and symptoms, it does not work for all cases. Sometimes the prostate may shrink without improvement in symptoms and it may take 6 months or more to determine if it is working for an individual. Side effects may include impotence and less desire for sex. Proscar can alter the Prostate-Specific Antigen test (PSA) that is used to screen for prostate cancer.

Balloon Dilation—During this procedure a balloon catheter is placed in the distal urethra and inflated by injecting a dilute contrast media at high pressure. The balloon is left in place for approximately 10 minutes and then the pressure is released and the catheter is removed.

Prostate Cancer

By age 60, four out of five men may have enlarged prostate and suffer urinary difficulties. By age 75, one in ten men may develop prostate cancer. Approximately 200,000 new cases of prostate cancer occur each year with a death toll of 38,000 lives.

A malignant neoplasm that affects the prostate tissue is known as prostatic cancer. It tends to spread to other parts of the body, often spreading to the bones of the spine or pelvis. The majority of these neoplasms are classified as adenocarcinomas. This disease is rare before the age of 50, however it is the second leading cause of cancer deaths in men.

The exact cause of prostate cancer is not known. It has been reported that researchers have found a genetic defect they think might trigger prostate cancer by robbing cells of an enzyme that fights the disease. The enzyme glutathione S-transferase is part of a group of chemicals produced in the body that fights cancer. A genetic change, which apparently alters the body's natural cancer-fighting mechanisms, appeared in 91 prostate victims that were studied, and was not found in the tissues of healthy men. If continued research confirms this hypothesis, tests might be developed that could identify future prostate cancer patients before the disease progresses.

It is recommended that men ages 40 and up, should have a digital rectal exam each year and that men ages 50 and over, should have a Prostate-Specific Antigen (PSA) blood test each year. Those men who are at high-risk should have the exam and blood test at an earlier age.

A rectal examination will help in diagnosing a tumor, but a biopsy is essential for a positive diagnosis. To localize and gauge the extent of the tumor, a computed tomography scan or ultrasonography may be used. The Prostate-Specific Antigen (PSA) blood test can detect prostate cancer by measuring the concentration in the blood of a protein made in the prostate.

Although prostate cancer frequently develops with no noticeable signs, possible symptoms may include:

- inability to urinate.
- frequent urination especially at night:

(continued)

- pain or burning sensation when urinating or ejaculating.
- blood or pus in the urine or semen.
- persistent pain in the back, hips, and pelvis.
- fatigue and anemia.

These symptoms may also be caused by benign prostate conditions. Benign conditions, including infections, prostate stones and BPH are common as men age.

Treatment for Prostate Cancer

Doctors have varying opinions on which treatment, if any, is best for the patient with prostate cancer. The *New England Journal of Medicine* published a study concluding that, for many men, observation may be just as effective as surgery or radiation. Surgery can have serious side effects, such as impotency and incontinence. And men in their 70s and 80s are likely to die from other causes before their prostate cancer becomes deadly, some doctors argue. But it is not easy for men to live with a potentially fatal disease. It is recommended that the best thing that a man who has been diagnosed with prostate cancer can do is to become educated about the options that are available. The most common treatments are:

Radical Prostatectomy—The total removal of the prostate gland that involves general anesthesia and a several-day hospital stay. This is the most common treatment, but some doctors are now saying that older men shouldn't have surgery. Surgery leaves 1 to 2 percent of men incontinent, and 15 to 20 percent sexually impotent.

Radiation—Regular doses of high-energy x-rays are targeted to the prostate area. The risk of incontinency and impotency are the same as with surgery.

Interstitial Implantation Therapy—Using needles, radioactive seeds are implanted in the prostate to kill cancerous tissue. Impotency rate is about 10 percent and incontinence is rare.

Hormones—Often used in conjunction with radiation or surgery, they reduce the levels of testosterone, the male hormone that promotes the growth of prostate cancer. Causes impotence in a small number of men.

Cryosurgery—An experimental outpatient procedure that freezes cancerous tissues. Carries the risk of impotence and incontinence.

About one in 10 American men will develop prostate cancer by the age of 85. Age is a risk factor of developing prostate cancer. More than 80 percent of all prostate cancers are diagnosed in men older than 65. It is unclear whether family history, environment or diet play a role in developing prostate cancer. Blacks contract the disease almost twice as often as whites.

Almost 60 percent of all prostate cancers are discovered while still confined to the prostate. The five-year survival rate for patients at this stage is 92 percent. The survival rate for all stages of prostate cancer is 78 percent. For more information about cancer one may call the National Cancer Institute's toll-free number: 1-800-422-6237.

Special Considerations: The Older Adult

Guidelines for Care of the Older Adult with Cancer

Explain the probable course of the disease including the diagnosis, hospital stay, treatment regimen, and follow-up care. Provide information about support groups and hospice care. Also:

- Modification of chemotherapy should be employed.
- Anxiety and depression should be anticipated and treated.
- Fatigue that can be debilitating should be recognized.
- Bone marrow function should be evaluated.
- Skin changes should be noted:
  —xerosis (dry skin) is common
  —loss of skin moisture
  —the aging skin is more prone to developing skin cancers
  —carcinomas appear on the nose, eyelid, or check from sun exposure
- Realize that modifications in life-style will be hard to accomplish and provide assistance when applicable.
- Anorexia, nausea, vomiting, and alopecia may be intensified.
- Recognize that fear of death may be present and provide needed understanding.

Early Diagnosis and Prompt Treatment

Early diagnosis and prompt treatment of cancer could save more than 50 percent of all cancer patients. The five-year survival rate for women with localized and properly treated breast cancer is 92 percent. Almost 60 percent of all prostate cancers are discovered while still confined to the prostate. The five-year survival rate for patients at this stage is 92 percent. The American Cancer Society recommends that individuals who are 50 and older should have the following cancer screening test or procedure performed on a regular basis.

Test or Procedure	Gender	Frequency
Digital rectal exam	Men and Women	Every year
Prostate-Specific Antigen (PSA)	Men	Every year
Stool Guaiac Slide Test	Men and Women	Every year
Sigmoidoscopy	Men and Women	Every 3 to 5 years
Pap test	Women	Every year
Breast self-exam	Women	Every month
Breast physical exam	Women	Every year
Mammogram	Women	Every year

Special Considerations: The Child

A diagnosis of cancer has a great impact on the patient, his or her family, and especially the patient's child or children. Researchers at the University of Washington who have studied the responses of children to their mothers' breast cancer found that an almost universal reaction among children is that they do not want to add to their mother's burden, so they try to hide their fears.

The following are suggested ways that may help encourage communication about a parent's serious illness. Each should be based upon the age of the child and his/her level of understanding.

- Create a comfortable environment. Sitting around a kitchen table or on a sofa, ask open-ended questions. Share information about the disease process, treatment, and possible outcome. Spread the sharing of this information over a given time period. Do not overload the child with too much information at one time.
- Draw pictures to illustrate the disease. Encourage the child to ask questions. Answer the questions openly and honestly.
- Plan ahead how to answer the question, "Are you going to die?" One may explain that all living things die sooner or later and then talk about death.
- Many times a child is going to feel guilty because he/she cannot understand what is happening and may think that he/she caused the illness. When this occurs the parent should reassure the child and provide any additional information about the condition that would help alleviate feelings of guilt.
- Involve the child in daily living activities. Let the child help out around the house. Simple tasks such as picking up toys, clothes, etc. may foster a sense of security for the child.
- The parent should provide extra time for "hugs and kisses."
- The parent should plan for time spent away from the family, such as hospitalization. Tape-recorded bedtime stories and songs can be a big help to a child when a parent is away. Hearing a mother's or father's voice can often quiet distressing feelings.
- The other parent or another adult should be involved in all phases of communicating with the child or children regarding a serious illness. By being present and involved, this individual may provide additional support to all concerned.
- Household routines should be kept as close to normal as possible, as this provides stability to the family.
- One should be informed about support groups and seek professional assistance when applicable. For information on cancer one may call 1-800-4 CANCER or 1-800-422-6237 or 1-800-ACS-2345.

Critical Thinking Questions/Activities

Your patient is a 32-year-old mother of two who has been diagnosed with advanced breast cancer. She is very upset, nervous, and says, "How am I going to tell my children about this?" Formulate your response by using the information provided in Special Considerations: The Child. Ask yourself:

- What are the ages of the children, and why is this so important for me to know?
- What information on cancer can I provide for my patient, so that she can explain this disease to her children?
- What suggestion can I give, that will help her illustrate this disease process to her children?
- How can I find out more information on death, so that I can help my patient talk about this?
- How can I help my patient plan for the time she is going to have to spend away from her family? What can I recommend that she do?
- How can I help her learn about support groups?
- What professional assistance is available for this patient?

Classifications of Antineoplastic Agents

Antineoplastic agents prevent the development, growth, or proliferation of malignant cells. The following are the primary classifications of antineoplastic agents.

Alkylating Agents

Alkylating agents are chemical compounds that cause chromosome breakage and prevent the formation of new DNA, thereby interfering with cell division. They affect all rapidly proliferating cells, and often cause toxicity to the hematopoietic system. Bone marrow depression/suppression, anemia, leukopenia, thrombocytopenia, and pancytopenia may occur. Most alkylating agents disrupt cells within the gastrointestinal tract, thereby producing nausea and vomiting.

Examples:

busulfan (Myleran)
carmustine (BiCNU)
chlorambucil (Leukeran)
cisplatin (Platinol)
cyclophosphamide (Cytoxan)
lomustine (CCNU or CeeNU)
mechlorethamine HCl (Mustargen)
melphalan (Alkeran)
streptozocin (Zanosar)
triethylenethiophosphoramide (Thiotepa)

Antimetabolites

Antimetabolites are substances that interfere with the metabolic process of the cell, thus preventing cell reproduction. They act only on dividing cells, and are most effective in treating rapidly proliferating malignant cells. These agents often cause toxicity to the hematopoietic system. Bone marrow depression/suppression, anemia, leukopenia, thrombocytopenia, and pancytopenia may occur. They also cause nausea and vomiting.

Examples:

cytarabine (Cytosar)
floxuridine (FUDR)
fluorouracil (5-FU)
mercaptopurine (Purinethol)
methotrexate
thioguanine (Tabloid)

Antibiotics

Certain *antibiotics* have an antineoplastic effect. These antibodies are derived from species of microorganisms and are not to be confused with antibiotics that are used in the treatment of infections. Their action is not known, but it appears they act by interfering with one or more stages of RNA and/or DNA synthesis. They interfere with the malignant cell's ability to grow and reproduce. These antibiotics do cause toxicity.

Examples:

bleomycin sulfate (Blenoxane)
dactinomycin (Cosmegen)
daunorubicin HCl (Cerubidine)
doxorubicin HCl (Adriamycin)
mitomycin (Mutamycin)
plicamycin (Mithracin)

Vinca Alkaloids

Vinca alkaloids are compounds that interfere with cell division by interacting with the cell's miotic process.

Examples:

vinblastine sulfate (Velban)
vincristine sulfate (Oncovin)

Hormones

Hormones are used to treat endocrine-related tumors (carcinoma of the breast, prostate, endometrium, ovary, kidney, and thyroid) and nonendocrine malignant neoplasms (leukemia, lymphomas). They have been used in antineoplastic therapy because they are capable of suppressing the growth of certain tissues of the body without exerting cytotoxic action.

Corticosteroids (prednisone and prednisolone) are used in conjunction with antineoplastic agents in the treatment of acute lymphoblastic leukemia and malignant lymphomas. Corticosteroids do produce a wide variety of adverse reactions after extended use, such as Cushingoid features, edema, hypertension, heart failure, potassium loss, "paper thin" skin, euphoria, and poor wound healing.

The following are examples of the different types of hormones used in antineoplastic therapy and some of the more common adverse reactions.

	Adverse Reactions
Estrogens	
chlorotrianisene (Tace) conjugated estrogens (Premarin) diethylstilbestrol (Stilbestrol, DES) diethylstilbestrol diphosphate (Honvol) ethinyl estradiol (Estinyl)	edema, nausea, anorexia, changes in libido, breast tenderness, abdominal cramps, dizziness, irritability, and urinary frequency when used for prostatic carcinoma-gynecomastia and impotence
Androgens	
dromostanolone propionate (Drolban) fluoxymesterone (Android-F) methyltestosterone (Android) testolactone (Teslac)	fluid retention, masculinization with clitoral enlargement, hirsutism, deepening of the voice, increased libido, acne, alopecia, and erythrocythemia
Progestins	
hydroxyprogesterone caproate (Delalutin) medroxyprogesterone acetate (Depo-Provera) megestrol acetate (Megace)	anorexia, fluid retention, and pain at site of injection
Antiestrogen	
tamoxifen citrate (Nolvadex)	nausea, vomiting, hot flashes, vaginal bleeding or discharge
Androgen-suppressing	
ketoconazole (Nizoral)	hepatic toxicity, hypersensitivity
Hypothalamic-like	
leuprolide (Lupron)	potential exacerbations of symptoms
Adrenal corticosteroids	
prednisone prednisolone	Cushingoid features, edema, hypertension, heart failure, potassium loss, "paper thin" skin, euphoria, and poor wound healing

Spot Check

For each of the classifications of antineoplastic agents given, list several examples of drugs and their action. Give the major toxicity of each classification.

Classification	Action	Major Toxicity
Alkylating Agents		
Antimetabolites		
Antibiotics		
Vinca Alkaloids		
Hormones		

Combination Chemotherapy

The combination of certain antineoplastic agents has proven to be effective in treating acute leukemia; Hodgkin's disease; non-Hodgkin's lymphoma; carcinoma of the breast, testis, and ovary; childhood neuroblastoma; Wilm's tumor; and osteogenic sarcoma. The physician who prescribes combination chemotherapy weighs the anticipated benefits against the possible additive toxic effects of the drugs. The following are some examples of combination chemotherapy.

MOPP	mechlorethamine (Mustargen) vincristine (Oncovin) procarbazine (Matulane) prednisone
ABVD	doxorubicin (Adriamycin) bleomycin (Blenoxane) vinblastine (Velban) dacarbazine (DTIC-Dome)
CMF	cyclophosphamide (Cytoxan) methotrexate (Mexate) fluorouracil (5-FU)
CAMP	cyclophosphamide (Cytoxan) doxorubicin (Adriamycin) methotrexate (Mexate) procarbazine (Matulane)
CMFP	cyclophosphamide (Cytoxan) methotrexate (Mexate) fluorouracil (5-FU) prednisone

Miscellaneous Agents

Certain antineoplastic agents are not easily classified. These are called *miscellaneous*. The following are examples of miscellaneous antineoplastic agents.

asparaginase (Elspar)
dacarbazine (DTIC)
hydroxyurea (Hydrea)
mitotane (Lysodren)
procarbazine HCl (Matulane)

Other Forms of Treatment for Cancer

Due to scientific investigation and the advent of genetic engineering, new forms of treatment for cancer have emerged. A new anticancer drug, N-methylformamide, is being tested on humans. It has demonstrated good activity against colon cancer. N-methylformamide is one of a class of drugs called *differentiation* agents or *maturation* agents. These drugs invade cancer cells and somehow cause them to mature into cells that are almost normal. It is not known how the drugs work.

Interleukin-2 (IL-2), a genetically engineered immune-boosting drug, has been approved by the Food and Drug Administration for use in the treatment of certain types of cancer. It stimulates the patient's immune system to produce more lymphocytes. Side effects of the drug are fever, fluid retention, severe weight gain, irregularities in kidney and cardiovascular function, dyspnea, and even death.

Human interleukin-3 (IL-3) is a naturally occurring substance that stimulates blood-cell growth. It may open up a new way to treat infections and even cancer by getting extremely high levels of blood cells normally involved in fighting infections.

Interleukin-4a is a natural, hormone-like substance that stimulates human immune-system cells to fight cancer and infectious diseases. It is genetically engineered and requires several more years of study before it will be ready for use.

Intraoperative Radiation Therapy

This is the delivery of tumoricidal doses of radiation directly onto a tumor bed while the surgical wound is still open. The surgeon and radiotherapist decide on the target area, and then the radiotherapist positions the sterile treatment cone in the incision. The treatment is usually for 15 to 30 min, and the incision is closed after the treatment is completed.

Photodynamic Therapy

This is the use of a red laser to kill cancerous cells. Hematoporphyrin derivative (Hpd), a light-sensitizing agent, is intravenously injected, and 3 days after the injection the physician uses the red laser. Normal cells eliminate Hpd and are not harmed during the treatment. Cancerous cells retain Hpd, and the red light kills them.

Recombinant Interferon Therapy

This is a genetically engineered immune system activator. It strengthens the body's immune system and helps it fight cancer cells. It is indicated for use in the treatment of hairy cell leukemia in people 18 years of age or older.

Tumor Necrosis Factor (TNF)

This is a lymphokine produced by macrophages (white blood cells). It triggers the macrophages to destroy malignant tumors. It is being tested in the treatment of low-grade lymphoma.

Whole Body Hyperthermia

This is the process of elevating the patient's body temperature to 108°F (42.2°C) to enhance the effect of radiation or chemotherapy. Cancer cells are sensitive to heat, so after radiation therapy, hyperthermia is employed to inhibit the cancer cells from repairing themselves. It is used before chemotherapy to increase the vulnerability of the cancer cells to the drug being used in the treatment process.

ondansetron (Zofran)

An antiemetic for preventing the nausea and vomiting that occurs in up to 90 percent of patients receiving cancer chemotherapy. It inhibits the vomiting reflex that occurs when chemotherapeutic agents damage the intestinal mucosa and cause release of the neurotransmitter serotonin. It is a selective serotonin antagonist, preventing vomiting by blocking serotonin receptors on sensory nerve endings and in the portion of the brain that controls vomiting. Dosage is 0.15 mg/kg infused IV thirty minutes before chemotherapy and four and eight hours after chemotherapy. Side effects during clinical trials were diarrhea and headache.

filgrastin (Neupogen)

A human granulocyte colony stimulating factor (G-CSF) produced by recombinant DNA technology and approved to fight infection in patients receiving chemotherapeutic agents that commonly cause severe neutropenia with fever. The recommended starting dose is 5 mcg/kg/day subcutaneously or IV. It is given 24 hours or more after the last dose of chemotherapy and at least 24 hours before the next dose. It should be given daily for up to two weeks and the dosage may be increased in increments of 5 mcg/kg/day if necessary.

Adverse reactions are bone pain and subclinical splenomegaly detectable by scanning.

sargramostim (Leukine, Prokine)

A recombinant granulocyte-macrophage colony stimulating factor (GM-CSF) used to treat patients with Hodgkin's disease, non-Hodgkin's lymphoma, and acute lymphoblastic leukemia who undergo autologous bone marrow transplantation. Treatment is begun not less than 24 hours after the last chemotherapeutic dose and 12 hours after the last dose of radiotherapy. Recommended dose is 250 mcg/m/day for 21 days as a two-hour IV beginning two to four hours after autologous bone marrow infusion. Side effects include malaise, weakness, fever, rash, and fluid retention.

paclitaxel (Taxol)

Promising anti-cancer drug processed from the bark of the Pacific yew tree. It is strictly controlled by the National Cancer Institute because so little of it is harvested each year. It has shown to be effective in treating ovarian cancer. It appears to shrink the tumor. Researchers are testing taxol as a possible treatment for several other types of cancer.

tamoxifen citrate (Nolvadex)

A hormonal drug that may prevent recurring breast tumors. It blocks estrogen receptors on tumor cells, preventing cancer cells from getting the estrogen they need to grow.

Bone Marrow Transplants for Recurring Breast Cancer

High-dose chemotherapy and marrow transplantation involves the removal of bone marrow from the patient's hip bone with a syringe and freezing. Large doses of antineoplastic drugs are used to kill cancer cells left in the body and in the remaining bone marrow. The bone marrow is thawed and infused into the patient's vein. The marrow should begin replenishing itself and churning out new white blood cells. The treatment takes place in several stages and over several months.

ifosfamide (Ifex)

An alkylating agent that attaches to proteins in the cancer cell, preventing them from carrying on metabolic activities. It lengthens the lives of some of the 25 percent of patients with testicular cancer who don't respond to other antineoplastic drugs. It is used in combination with Platinol (cisplatin), VePesid (etoposide), and Velban (vinblastine).

Interferon

Interferon is a natural *glycoprotein* released by cells that are invaded by viruses. It acts as a regulator of cell growth and has a variety of effects on the immune system. Interferon belongs to the group known as immune system activators, *lymphokines.* When assaulted by a foreign substance, usually a protein, white blood cells produce lymphokines in small amounts. The lymphokines move from cell to cell, telling the immune system how to cope with the invading foreign substance.

The breakthrough for the production of interferon was made possible through biotechnology and genetic engineering. Roferon®-A (Interferon alfa-2a, recombinant) by Roche Laboratories is a sterile protein product for use by subcutaneous or intramuscular injection. It is indicated for use in the treatment of hairy cell leukemia in people 18 years of age or older. Intron®-A (Interferon alfa-2b, recombinant) by Schering Corporation is a purified sterile lyophilized recombinant interferon for use by subcutaneous or intramuscular injection. It is also indicated for use in the treatment of hairy cell leukemia in people 18 years of age or older.

cladribine (Leustatin)

Leustatin is a potent antineoplastic agent that has been approved for use in selected patients with hairy cell leukemia. The drug should be administered under the supervision of a qualified physician experienced in the use of antineoplastic therapy. Suppression of bone marrow function should be anticipated. This is usually reversible and appears to be dose dependent. Patients should be monitored closely for hematologic and non-hematologic toxicity. Leustatin is for intravenous infusion only. The treatment regimen is for 7 consecutive days and the dose is 0.09 mg/kg/day. Patients may experience complete or partial remission for 8 to 25 months.

With continued scientific investigation, and the advent of genetic engineering, it is anticipated that many new drugs will be available to treat viral diseases and certain types of cancer. It is most important that you become knowledgeable about the advances that are being made in the medical field, and keep up with current trends and practices. New drugs are being approved all the time, and it is impossible for a textbook on pharmacology to contain a complete drug listing.

♦ Review Questions

Directions: Select the best answer to each multiple choice question. Circle the letter of your choice.

1. The process whereby normal cells have a distinct appearance and specialized function is known as __________.
   a. dedifferentiation
   b. differentiation
   c. remission
   d. exacerbation
2. The medical term for loss of appetite is __________.
   a. anorexia
   b. alopecia
   c. stomatitis
   d. cytotoxic
3. Chemotherapy is the treatment of choice when the cancer is __________.
   a. disseminated
   b. surgically inoperable
   c. localized
   d. a and b
4. The normal cells that are most sensitive to chemotherapy are __________.
   a. hematopoietic cells
   b. epithelial cells
   c. hair follicles
   d. all of these

5. Antineoplastic agents may be prepared and administered by __________.
   a. any nurse or health professional
   b. physicians only, who are qualified to do so
   c. those qualified with special certification or education
   d. b and c
6. Adverse reactions to antineoplastic agents include __________.
   a. nausea and vomiting
   b. bone marrow depression
   c. alopecia
   d. all of these
7. The normal range of thrombocytes per cubic millimeter of blood is __________.
   a. 100,000–300,000
   b. 150,000–450,000
   c. 200,000–400,000
   d. 150,000–600,000
8. Patients who are receiving chemotherapy need:
   a. special consideration
   b. physical and emotional support
   c. education about their disease, support groups, and ways to lessen the severity of the disease
   d. all of these
9. When the patient's nausea, vomiting, and pain are not controlled by the prescribed medication, you should __________.
   a. notify the physician
   b. seek a more satisfactory regimen
   c. a and b
   d. none of these
10. To lessen the severity of nausea and vomiting, the patient should __________.
    a. avoid unpleasant odors
    b. avoid hot, spicy, greasy foods
    c. eat small frequent meals
    d. all of these
11. You should teach your patient to be alert for signs of bleeding and to report such signs to the physician. Signs of bleeding include __________.
    a. epistaxis
    b. petechiae
    c. excessive bruising
    d. all of these
12. Antineoplastic agents may be classified as __________.
    a. alkylating agents
    b. antimetabolites
    c. antibiotics
    d. all of these
13. __________ is the time when the symptoms of a disease process are most severe.
    a. Extravasation
    b. Exacerbation
    c. Malignant
    d. Remission

14. __________ is the time when the symptoms of a disease process are lessened.
    a. Extravasation
    b. Exacerbation
    c. Malignant
    d. Remission
15. __________ is a genetically engineered immune-boosting drug that stimulates the patient's immune system to produce more lymphocytes.
    a. Zofran
    b. Interleukin-2
    c. Interferon
    d. Leukine
16. The treatment of cancer may be one or a combination of __________.
    a. surgery
    b. chemotherapy
    c. radiation therapy and/or immunotherapy
    d. all of these
17. There are approximately __________ to __________ leukocytes per cubic millimeter of blood.
    a. 150,000, 450,000
    b. 12,000, 15,000
    c. 5,000, 10,000
    d. 1, 2 million
18. Recommended guidelines for safely handling chemotherapeutic agents have been prepared by the __________.
    a. National Institutes of Health (NIH)
    b. National Study Commission on Cytotoxic Exposure
    c. American Society of Hospital Pharmacists (ASHP)
    d. all of these

Case Study: A 56-year-old female is admitted with the diagnosis of possible ovarian carcinoma. She has ascites, edema of the legs, and pain in the abdomen and back of the legs. She is scheduled for surgical exploration with the possibility of a total abdominal hysterectomy and bilateral salpingo-oophorectomy with biopsies of the liver and the diaphragm.

During surgery a positive diagnosis was made. Biopsy of the liver and diaphragm showed no evidence of metastasis. A total abdominal hysterectomy and bilateral salpingo-oophorectomy were performed. The patient was placed on cisplatin and cyclophosphamide.

19. The nurse should know that cisplatin and cyclophosphamide are __________.
    a. antimetabolites
    b. alkylating agents
    c. antibiotics
    d. hormones

20. These antineoplastic agents are chemical compounds that __________.
    a. interfere with the metabolic process of the cell
    b. interfere with RNA and/or DNA synthesis
    c. cause chromosome breakage and prevent formation of new DNA, thereby interfering with cell division
    d. suppress the growth of certain tissues of the body
21. These antineoplastic agents often cause toxicity to the __________.
    a. hematopoietic system
    b. nervous system
    c. endocrine system
    d. skeletal system
22. In caring for this patient it is important to __________.
    a. encourage and/or force fluids
    b. provide good mouth care
    c. be alert for adverse reactions
    d. all of these
23. The Patient expresses her concern about possible hair loss. Which of the following responses would be best for you to give?
    a. "Usually, hair will begin to grow back after the effects of chemotherapy are eliminated from the body."
    b. "Alopecia is one of the adverse reactions to chemotherapy."
    c. "You may want to buy a wig and wear it when you go out."
    d. "You don't need to worry about hair loss with this type of medication."

Matching: Place the correct letter from Column II on the appropriate line of Column I.

Column I	Column II
24. __________ Alopecia	A. Loss of appetite.
25. __________ Cytotoxic	B. Producing cancer.
26. __________ Teratogenic	C. Loss of hair.
27. __________ Carcinogenic	D. Inflammation of the mouth.
28. __________ Proliferation	E. Producing or forming a severely malformed fetus.
29. __________ Stomatitis	F. The process of rapid reproduction.
30. __________ Malignant	G. Destructive to cells.
	H. A "bad wandering."

CHAPTER 21

Vitamins and Minerals

OBJECTIVES

Upon completion of this chapter, you should be able to:

- Define the terms listed in the vocabulary.
- State the importance of vitamins and minerals to the human body.
- Explain what "5 A Day for Better Health" means.
- List the foods that one should include in his/her diet at least once a week.
- Describe antioxidants.
- List the six food groups that make up the "Food Guide Pyramid".
- Describe the factors that may affect an older adult's dietary regimen.
- State the importance of folic acid for the child.
- Complete the critical thinking questions/activities presented in this chapter.
- Differentiate between fat-soluble and water-soluble vitamins.
- Give the functions, food sources, USRDA, and indications of deficiency of selected vitamins and minerals.
- State the symptoms of hypervitaminosis for vitamins A, D, and E.
- Describe the importance of cations and anions in electrolyte balance.
- Complete the Spot Check on selected vitamins and minerals.
- Answer the review questions correctly.

Vocabulary

avitaminosis (a-vi″ta-mi-no′sis). A deficiency disease that is due to a lack of vitamins in the diet.

hypervitaminosis (hi″po-vi″ta-min-o′sis). A condition caused by an excessive amount of vitamins, especially from the taking of too many vitamin pills.

hypovitaminosis (hi″po-vi″ta-min-o′sis). A condition due to a lack of vitamins, especially from an inadequate diet. The signs of hypovitaminosis may include fatigue, pain and aches throughout the body. It can be corrected by a well-balanced diet.

International Unit (I.U.). An internationally accepted amount of a substance.

megadose (meg'a-dose). An extremely large dose. It is more than five times the RDA of a fat-soluble vitamin or ten times the RDA of a water-soluble vitamin.

RDA. The Recommended Daily Allowance. The nutrient level of intake that is considered by the National Research Council (NRC) and Nutrition Board to be adequate for most healthy individuals.

USRDA. The United States Recommended Daily Allowance.

Introduction

Carbohydrates, fats, proteins, water, electrolytes, vitamins, and minerals are nutrients that are essential for life. Carbohydrates and fats furnish heat and energy. Proteins provide energy and build and repair body tissues. Water and electrolytes are essential for maintaining the body's acid-base balance. Vitamins, minerals, and water help regulate such body processes as circulation, respiration, digestion, and elimination.

The Food Guide Pyramid

Through proper selection of foods from the Food Guide Pyramid, Figure 21–1, most healthy adults can receive the nutrients essential for life. During infancy, childhood, ado-

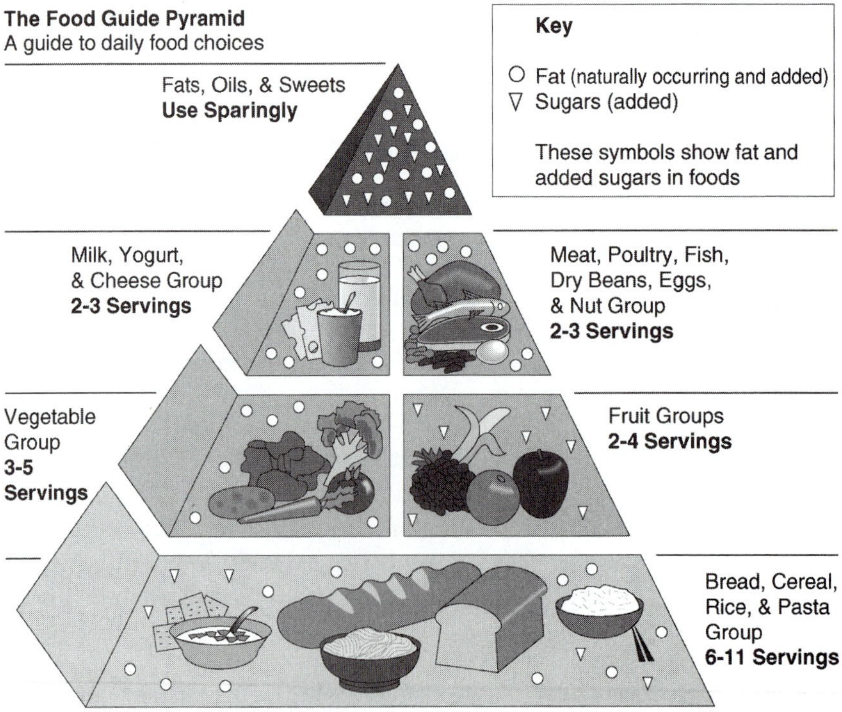

Figure 21–1 The Food Guide Pyramid *(Courtesy of U.S. Department of Agriculture)*

lescence, the aspects of aging, pregnancy, lactation, surgery, and disease, one's body may require additional nutrients. The physician carefully evaluates each patient to determine his or her nutritional needs. When supplemental vitamins and minerals are prescribed, the patient needs to understand that these are drugs and should be taken as ordered.

The role of nutrition in health and disease is being recognized as one of the forces that makes a person who he or she is. The McGovern Commission recommends reducing fat intake and increasing intake of fiber-rich foods, and makes specific dietary recommendations for preventing heart disease and cancer. Health-conscious individuals are very aware of foods that are good for them. At the same time, a substantial proportion of the diet consumed by many Americans consists of processed and "fast" food. It has been estimated that the "average" American consumes 120 pounds of sugar and 125 pounds of fat each year. Obesity, diabetes, diseases of the heart, blood vessels, and some forms of cancer are being linked to diet.

As a person engaged in the delivery of health care, it is essential that you have an understanding of nutrients and their roles in health. In this chapter, emphasis is placed on vitamins and minerals.

SPOTLIGHT

Proper Nutrition—A Plan to Improve Health

You have heard the saying, "you are what you eat." The correlation between dietary habits and health has become a much researched topic. Much has been learned about fat intake and heart disease; calcium intake and osteoporosis; sodium and hypertension; and fiber-containing grain products, fruits, and vegetables and cancer.

According to the National Institutes of Health, over one-third of cancer deaths in 1992 could have been related to diet. This Institute has launched a program called "5 A Day for Better Health." It recommended eating at least five servings of fruits and vegetables daily as a way of reducing the risk of cancer.

Some dietary substances showing anticarcinogenic activity in animal studies include vitamins A, C, E, and beta-carotene, the minerals calcium and selenium, and some forms of fiber.

Some foods are better than others, and the following are foods that you should include in your diet, at least once a week.

1. Broccoli contains a nutrient that is believed to help protect against cancer. If you don't like broccoli try cauliflower, cabbage, and/or turnips.
2. Dry beans provide protein, without fat or cholesterol.
3. Nonfat yogurt is a good source of calcium.

(continued)

4. Fish (most) provides protein without excess fat. Some fish, such as tuna, salmon, mackerel, herring, and sardines, contain small amounts of omega-3 oils, that help fight heart disease.
5. Whole wheat bread, pasta, and cereals are high in fiber that aids in digestion and helps prevent constipation and possible colorectal cancer.
6. Oatmeal is high in soluble fiber and it is believed to help lower cholesterol. Other sources of soluble fiber are apples, peas, dried beans, prunes, and lentils.

Antioxidants

Antioxidants are chemical substances that neutralize free radicals, the highly-reactive and unstable molecules that can cause significant cellular damage. The body makes antioxidants and antioxidants are found in various foods, herbs, and nutritional supplements. Vitamins C, E and beta carotene are known as antioxidant vitamins.

Vitamin C is found in many fruits and vegetables, including oranges, grapefruit, strawberries, broccoli, kale and tomatoes. Vitamin E is found in nuts, certain vegetable oils, and leafy greens. Beta carotene is found in dark green leafy vegetables such as spinach, and in yellow-orange fruits and vegetables such as cantaloupes, peaches, carrots and sweet potatoes. Tea leaves also contain antioxidants called polyphenols, which can prevent damage to DNA.

Antioxidants help to protect the body's cells. The billions of cells in the body are continually exposed to free radicals that are produced through normal bodily processes, as well as external sources such as air pollution and tobacco smoke. It is believed that this cellular damage, along with other factors may lead to aging, and the development of chronic diseases such as cancer, cataracts, and heart disease.

The positive benefits of proper nutrition are many. It is believed that if one eats a variety of foods, maintains desirable weight, avoids too much fat, sugar, and sodium, eats high-fiber foods, and consumes beverages and foods containing antioxidants, the quality of life will be improved, and certain diseases may be prevented.

In 1992, the United States Department of Agriculture unveiled the new "Food Guide Pyramid" made up of six food groups. This pyramid provides a guide to choosing the proper foods one should eat on a daily basis.

The Six Food Groups

- Bread, Cereal, Rice, and Pasta (6–11 servings/day)
- Fruit (2–4 servings/day)
- Vegetable (3–5 servings/day)
- Milk, Yogurt, and Cheese (2–3 servings/day)
- Meat, Poultry, Fish, Dry Beans, Eggs, and Nuts (2–3 servings/day)
- Fats, Oils and Sweets (use sparingly)

Special Considerations: The Older Adult

Carbohydrates, fats, proteins, vitamins, minerals, and water are essential ingredients needed for the proper functioning of the human body. Because of reduced physical activity and a decline in metabolic processes, an older adult generally needs fewer calories than when they were younger. It is suggested that calories should be reduced by 7 percent to 8 percent every 10 years after a person has reached age 25. Although the older adult needs to reduce calories, the intake of salt, cholesterol, and saturated fats, a balanced diet still needs to include the six basic food groups.

- Bread, Cereal, Rice, and Pasta (6–11 servings/day)
- Fruit (2–4 servings/day)
- Vegetables (3–5 servings/day)
- Milk, Yogurt, and Cheese (2–3 servings/day)
- Meat, Poultry, Fish, Dry Beans, Eggs, and Nuts (2–3 servings/day)
- Fats, Oils and Sweets (use sparingly)

It is estimated that 25 percent of U.S. households do not have nutritionally balanced diets. There are many reasons for this and some of these are: lack of knowledge about nutrients and the proper amount of nutrients to make up a balanced diet and food sources rich in these nutrients; too little time to prepare balanced meals; loss of vitamin content during food preparation; taste preference for less nutritious foods; and lack of knowledge about their individual nutrient needs. In addition to these, older adults may have other factors affecting their dietary regimen such as:

- reduced income that limits their purchase of nutritional foods.
- lack of adequate cooking facilities.
- loneliness and having to eat alone.
- physically unable to prepare meals.
- loss of teeth of poorly fitting dentures.
- lack of means to go grocery shopping.
- loss of interest in food.
- depression.
- many older adults take multiple medications that may affect the taste of food and their desire to eat.
- disease or multiple disease processes that affect their desire to eat.

The older adult who is able, needs to continue to participate in food selection and preparation. Likes and dislikes need to be discussed and a meal plan should be formulated that covers all the essential nutrients that the body needs. For those individuals who need assistance with meals, "Meals on Wheels" is a good program. For those individuals who can attend a community senior citizens center, daily lunches can be enjoyed at a minimal cost. In addition to a good meal, the older adult may enjoy the socialization and recreational activities provided at these centers.

Special Considerations: The Child

The U.S. Food and Drug Administration has ordered that most breads, flour, pasta and other food from grains be fortified with folic acid. Folic acid is a trace B vitamin found in citrus fruits and dark, leafy vegetables such as spinach and lettuce. It is also available in multiple vitamin supplements. The U.S. Recommended Daily Allowance for children under 4 years of age is 0.2 mg and for the child over 4 years of age and older, 0.4 mg. Women of childbearing age should consume 0.4 mg of folic acid daily, but it is estimated that most women consume about half that amount. Folic acid is required to make DNA, the genetic building blocks of life. When pregnant women consume too little folic acid, infants may have malformations of the spinal cord such as spina bifida and/or anencephaly. In addition to improving the lives of children, folic acid may reduce the possibility of heart attacks and strokes. A study in the *Journal of the American Medical Association* presented strong evidence that folic acid reduces a chemical, homocysteine, that is associated with high risk of heart attacks and strokes.

Critical Thinking Questions/Activities

Analyze your own eating habits by charting what you actually eat and drink for 5 days. You may use the following chart to assist you.

Bread, cereal, rice, and pasta	Fruit	Vegetables	Milk, yogurt, cheese	Meat, poultry, fish, dry beans, eggs, nuts
Day 1				
Day 2				
Day 3				
Day 4				
Day 5				

Ask yourself:

- How many servings of bread, cereal, rice, and pasta did I have each day?
- How many servings of fruit did I have each day?
- How many servings of vegetables did I have each day?
- How many servings of milk, yogurt, and cheese did I have each day?
- How many servings of meat, poultry, fish, dry beans, eggs, and nuts did I have each day?
- How well did I choose the proper foods that I should eat on a daily basis?
- How can I improve my eating habits?

Vitamins

Vitamins are organic substances that are essential for normal metabolism, growth, and development of the human body. They are complex chemical substances that may be obtained naturally from plants, animals, and sunshine, or they may be made commercially.

Vitamins may be classified as fat-soluble and water-soluble (see Table 21–1). The fat-soluble vitamins are: A, D, E, and K. The water-soluble vitamins are: Thiamine (B_1), Riboflavin (B_2), Niacin (nicotinic acid), Pyridoxin (B_6), Folic acid, Cyanocobalamin (B_{12}), Biotin, and C (ascorbic acid).

The fat-soluble vitamins are stored in adipose tissue and the liver. The water-soluble vitamins are not stored in the body. They are essential to health and need to be replaced on a daily basis. The United States Recommended Daily Allowance (USRDA) for each vitamin is given in Table 21–1. When an individual follows these recommended allowances, conditions such as *avitaminosis, hypovitaminosis,* and *hypervitaminosis* can be prevented.

Some of the commonly prescribed vitamin products are Theragran, Centrum, Citracal, B–C–Bid, Therabid, Vicon–C, Vicon Forte, Vita-plus H, Nico–400, Os-Cal Forte, cyanocobalamin—vitamin B_{12} (Redisol, Rubramin), folic acid (Folvite), folinic acid (Leucovorin), and vitamin K (Aqua MEPHYTON).

Minerals

Minerals are nonorganic substances that are essential constituents of all body cells. Minerals play an important role in maintaining the water balance of the body (see Table 21–2).

Table 21–1 Vitamins

Vitamin and Function	Food Sources	USRDA	Indications of Deficiency	Hypervitaminosis
A Important for healthy mucous membranes, skin, epithelial cells, development of bones and teeth, and for vision in dim light.	Dairy products, fish liver oils, animal liver, green and yellow vegetables.	5,000 I.U.	Retarded growth, susceptibility to disease, skin lesions, and night blindness.	Anorexia, loss of hair, pain in long bones, fragility of bones, dry skin, pruritus, enlarged liver and spleen.
D Aids in the proper use of calcium and phosphorus in the body.	Ultraviolet rays, dairy products and commercial foods that contains supplemental vitamin D (milk and cereals) and fish liver oils.	400 I.U.	*Childhood:* Rickets. *Adults:* Osteomalacia, muscle spasms, and spontaneous fractures.	Demineralization (softening) of bone, hypercalcemia, calcium deposits in soft tissue, hypertension, diarrhea, and deafness.
E May promote normal reproduction, and helps in the formation of muscles and red blood cells.	Leafy green vegetables, wheat germ, margarine.	30 I.U.	Edema, ataxia, absence of reflexes.	Not definitely known. Large doses may destroy vitamin K in the intestine.
K Essential in the formation of prothrombin in the liver that is necessary for normal blood clotting.	Dairy products, leafy green vegetables, cauliflower, soybeans, liver, peas, potatoes, and tomatoes.		Poor blood clotting, even hemorrhage.	
C Important for maintenance of bones, teeth, and small blood vessels. Prevents scurvy and promotes healing of wounds and formation of protein collagen. Aids in the absorption of calcium. *May* help in preventing the common cold.	Citrus fruits, tomatoes, melons, fresh berries, raw vegetables, and sweet potatoes.	60 mg	Fatigue, irritability, fleeting joint pain, tendency to bruise, and small petechiae under the tongue.	
B_1 Essential for the release of energy from carbohydrates and nerve conduction.	Yeast, wheat germ, lean meats, pork, dried beans and peas, dairy products, poultry, eggs, dark green vegetables, and whole-grain enriched foods.	1.5 mg	Beriberi, malaise, polyneuritis, numbness and tingling in the extremities.	

B_2 Essential for cellular oxidation and the storage of energy. Helps maintain the skin and mucous membranes.	Organ meats, lean meats, milk, green vegetables, eggs, poultry, and yeast.	1.7 mg	Skin and lip lesions, seborrheic dermatitis, inflamed tongue, lack of vigor, and ocular changes.	
Niacin Important for cellular respiration, glycolysis, and lipid synthesis.	Liver, lean meats, fish, poultry, whole grain, and enriched flour and cereals.	20 mg	Pellagra, dermatitis, irritability, dizziness, skin and mucous membrane lesions.	
B_5 Aids in the metabolism of foods. Also helps the work of certain hormones and chemicals in the nervous system.	Whole and enriched grain products, dried beans and peas, legumes, dairy products, eggs, organ meats, lean meats, poultry, dark green vegetables, and fish.	10 mg	Not known.	
B_6 Necessary for the metabolism of amino acids and fatty acids. Also aids in the production of red blood cells.	Muscle meats, liver, yeast, molasses, and whole grain cereals.	2 mg	Skin lesions, anemia, hypochromic anemia, insomnia, numbness in extremities.	
B_{12} Vital for the production of red blood cells and genetic material. Helps the nervous system function properly.	Liver, kidney, milk, fish, and muscle meats.	6 mcg.		
Folic Acid Necessary for the synthesis of amino acids, DNA, and formation of red blood cells.	Liver, yeast, green leafy vegetables, and most food groups.	0.4 mg	Fatigue, sore tongue, low RBC count, and macrocytic anemia.	
Biotin Regulates amino acid and fatty acid metabolism.	Liver, kidney, egg yolk, yeast, nuts, legumes, and cauliflower.	0.3 mg	Dermatitis, glossitis, anorexia, and muscle pain.	

Table 21–2 Minerals

Minerals and Function	Food Sources	RDA	Indications of Deficiency	Toxicity
Sodium (Na) Chief *cation* in the extracellular fluid. Important for maintaining acid-base balance, regulating osmotic pressure in cells and body fluids, controlling fluid volume in the body. Helps in maintaining normal heart action, regulating muscle and nerve irritability.	Meats, sardines, cheese, green olives, table salt, baking soda, baking powder, milk, eggs, beets, spinach, and is added to many foods such as nuts, potato chips, soups, butter, breads, cakes, sauces, salad dressings, and cereals.	1100–3300 mg/daily	Hyponatremia, loss of weight, weakness, cramps, "salt hunger," and nervous disorders.	Hypernatremia, confusion, and coma
Potassium (K) Chief *cation* in the intracellular fluid. Helps maintain the acid-base balance. Important in nerve impulse conduction and muscle tissue excitability.	Cereals, dried peas and beans, fresh vegetables, fresh or dried fruits (especially bananas, prunes, and raisins), sunflower seeds, nuts, meats, molasses, oranges, and orange juice.	50–150 mEq/daily	Hypokalemia, muscle weakness, thirst, dizziness, mental confusion, arrhythmias.	Hyperkalemia, confusion, and coma.
Calcium (Ca) Plays a key role in blood clotting and lactation. Helps in maintaining acid-base balance. Activates enzymes. Needed for proper functioning of the nerves and muscles. Maintains cell membrane permeability. In combination with phosphorus helps form strong bones and teeth.	Dairy products, beans, cauliflower, egg yolk, molasses, leafy green vegetables, tofu, sardines, clams, and oysters.	800–1200 mg/daily	Hypocalcemia, brittle bones, poor development of bones and teeth, rickets, tetany, excessive bleeding, and irritability.	Hypercalcemia, gastrointestinal atony, renal stones or failure, psychosis, drowsiness, and lethargy.
Magnesium (Mg) Important in maintaining muscle and nerve irritability. Helps regulate body temperature, aids in bone and tooth development. Activates certain enzymes.	Widely distributed in foods, especially whole grains, fruits, milk, nuts, vegetables, seafoods, and meats.	400 mg daily	Hypomagnesemia, tetany, muscle tremor and weakness, mental confusion, depression, and ataxia.	Hypermagnesemia, respiratory failure, cardiac disturbances.

Phosphorus (P) Needed for metabolism of fats, carbohydrates, and proteins. Helps the body extract energy from foods. Important for healthy bones, teeth, and tissues. Helps maintain acid-base balance.	Dairy products, eggs, fish, poultry, meats, dried peas and beans, whole grain cereals and nuts.	800–1200 mg/daily	Hypophosphatemia, irritability, weakness, retarded growth, poor tooth and bone development, rickets, anorexia, malaise, and pain in bones.	Hyperphosphatemia.
Iron (Fe) Essential to hemoglobin formation. Component of proteins in the blood and muscle.	Liver, soybean flour, muscle meats, dried fruits, egg yolk, enriched breads and cereals, potatoes, dark green leafy vegetables.	18 mg/daily	Anemia, dizziness, weakness, fatigue, loss of weight, pallor, spoon-shaped nails, poor resistance to infection, and anorexia.	Hemochromatosis.
Iodine (I) Important in the development and functioning of the thyroid gland, formation of thyroxine (T_4) and triiodothyronine (T_3). Aids in the prevention of goiter.	Seafood, iodized salt.	150 mg/daily	Simple goiter, cretinism.	Occasional hyxedema.
Copper (Cu) Helps iron form blood cells and aids to enzyme activity. Helps the central nervous system function properly.	Liver, nuts, shellfish, kidney, fruits, and dried peas and beans.	2 mg/daily	Anemia	Hepatolenticular degeneration.
Zinc (Zn) Aids in enzyme activity, wound healing, and growth.	Meats, liver, eggs, and seafood.	15 mg/daily	Retarded growth, hypogonadism, anorexia, impaired wound healing, night blindness, and white spots on nails.	

Electrolytes

The body's weight is 60–70 percent water. All cells are bathed by an aqueous solution that brings nourishment to the cells and removes wastes. Electrolytes (acids, bases, and salts) are suspended in this solution. *Electrolytes* are particles that result from disintegration of compounds. They are found dissolved in body fluids as *ions* that carry electrical charges. *Cation* is an ion with a positive charge of electricity. *Anion* is an ion with a negative charge of electricity. Cations and anions are involved in metabolic activities, and are essential to the normal function of all cells. The normal fluid state in which positive and negative ions are in balance is called *homeostasis.*

The chief cations and anions are:

Cations		Anions	
Na^+	Sodium	Cl^-	Chloride
K^+	Potassium	HCO_3^-	Carbonate
Ca^{++}	Calcium	HCO_4^-	Phosphate
Mg^{++}	Magnesium	SO_4^-	Sulfate

Selected minerals and their functions, food sources, RDA, indications of deficiency and toxicity are described in Table 21–2 in this unit. Minerals are excreted daily from the body; therefore, it is most important to replace them through a well-balanced diet.

Minerals may be grouped as macrominerals and microminerals. *Macrominerals* are magnesium, sodium, potassium, chlorine and sulfur. *Microminerals* are minerals that are required in small amounts. They are also known as trace elements. This group includes iron, copper, iodine, manganese, zinc, fluorine, cobalt, chromium, tin, selenium, vanadium, silicon, nickel and molybdenum.

Spot Check

Vitamins and minerals are very important nutrients that are needed for proper functioning of the human body. For each selected vitamin and mineral, provide the function and USRDA.

Vitamin/Mineral	Function	USRDA
Vitamin A		
Vitamin D		

Vitamin E		
Vitamin C		
Folic Acid		
Sodium		
Potassium		

◆ Review Questions

Directions: Select the best answer to each multiple choice question. Circle the answer of your choice.

1. A deficiency disease that is due to a lack of vitamins in the diet is known as __________.
   a. hypervitaminosis
   b. megadose
   c. avitaminosis
   d. none of these
2. Nutrients that help regulate body processes such as circulation, respiration, digestion, and elimination are __________.
   a. carbohydrates, fats, and proteins
   b. vitamins, minerals, and water
   c. sugars, starch, and fats
   d. proteins, vegetables, and fruit

3. Most healthy adults can receive the nutrients essential for life by __________ .
   a. selecting foods from the "food guide pyramid"
   b. eating processed and "fat" food
   c. taking large amounts of commercially prepared vitamins
   d. selecting foods deficient in vitamins and minerals
4. Daily servings from the "food guide pyramid" for a healthy adult include:
   a. 6–11 servings of grains; 3–8 servings of vegetables; 2–6 servings of fruit; 2–3 servings of milk and meat
   b. 5–10 servings of grains; 3–5 servings of vegetables; 2–8 servings of fruit; 2–4 servings of milk and meat
   c. 6–11 servings of grains; 3–5 servings of vegetables; 2–4 servings of fruit; 2–3 servings of milk and meat
   d. 6–11 servings of grains; 3–7 servings of vegetables; 3–5 servings of fruit; 2–3 servings of milk and meat
5. Vitamin __________ is important for healthy mucous membranes, skin, epithelial cells, development of bones and teeth, and for vision in dim light.
   a. C b. A c. D d. K
6. An indication of deficiency of vitamin D is __________ .
   a. poor blood clotting
   b. beriberi
   c. rickets
   d. pellagra
7. Vitamin __________ is important for maintenance of bones, teeth, and small blood vessels. It prevents scurvy and promotes healing of wounds.
   a. B_1 b. E c. D d. C
8. Vitamin __________ is vital for the production of red blood cells and genetic material.
   a. biotin b. niacin c. B_5 d. B_{12}
9. The chief *cations* are sodium, __________.
   a. chloride, calcium, sulfate
   b. carbonate, magnesium, chloride
   c. potassium, phosphate, sulfate
   d. potassium, calcium, magnesium
10. Cereals, dried peas and beans, fresh vegetables, fresh or dried fruits, sunflower seeds, nuts, meats, molasses, oranges, and orange juice are food sources of __________.
   a. sodium b. potassium c. calcium d. iodine

11. Indications of iron deficiency are __________.
    a. simple goiter
    b. anemiac
    c. hyponatremia
    d. hypokalemia
12. It has been estimated that the "average" American consumes __________ pounds of sugar and __________ pounds of fat each year.
    a. 10, 20 b. 75, 90 c. 20, 25 d. 120, 125
13. Obesity, diabetes, diseases of the heart, blood vessels, and some forms of cancer are linked to __________ .
    a. exercise b. rest c. diet d. sleep
14. __________ are organic substances that are essential for normal metabolism, growth, and development of the human body.
    a. Minerals
    b. Vitamins
    c. Electrolytes
    d. Cations
15. __________ are particles (acids, bases, and salts) that result from disintegration of compounds.
    a. Minerals
    b. Vitamins
    c. Electrolytes
    d. Cations
16. The fat-soluble vitamins are __________.
    a. niacin and folic acid
    b. biotin and ascorbic acid
    c. B_1, B_2, B_6, and B_{12}
    d. A, D, E, and K

Case Study: The physician wants the patient to increase the intake of vitamin A in the diet. Which of the following foods should the nurse encourage the patient to eat?

17. a. Citrus fruits, tomatoes
    b. Organ meats, eggs
    c. Dairy products, green and yellow vegetables
    d. Grains and cereals
18. a. Orange juice
    b. Liver and fried eggs
    c. Carrots and sweet potatoes
    d. Bread and oatmeal

Case Study: The patient has been advised to increase his/her intake of iron. Which of the following would indicate to the nurse that the patient understands the dietary source of iron.

19. a. Selecting a peanut butter sandwich
    b. Selecting an egg salad sandwich
    c. Selecting a lettuce and tomato sandwich
    d. Selecting a jelly sandwich
20. a. Selecting liver smothered with onions
    b. Selecting a chef salad
    c. Selecting a fruit salad
    d. Selecting sardines and crackers

Matching: Place the correct letter from Column II on the appropriate line of Column I.

Column I	Column II
21. ________ USRDA	A. Minerals required in large amounts.
22. ________ RDA	B. A good source of calcium, sodium magnesium, and phosphorus.
23. ________ Minerals	C. United States Recommended Daily Allowance.
24. ________ Milk	D. An ion with a positive charge of electricity.
25. ________ Meats	E. A good source of carbohydrates.
26. ________ Bread and cereals	F. A good source of fats and protein.
27. ________ Cation	G. Nonorganic substances that are essential constituents of all body cells.
28. ________ Macrominerals	H. Minerals required in small amounts.
29. ________ Microminerals	I. The Recommended Daily Allowance.
	J. Minerals required in excessive amounts.

CHAPTER 22

Psychotropic Agents

OBJECTIVES

Upon completion of this chapter, you should be able to:

- Define the terms listed in the vocabulary.
- Define stress.
- State five diseases/conditions that may be implicated in stress.
- Describe symptoms of anxiety.
- List possible stressors for the older adult.
- List the symptoms of stress overload.
- Give several general guidelines for reducing stress.
- Explain how stress, anxiety, and/or depression could affect a child.
- Complete the critical thinking questions/activities presented in this chapter.
- Describe the four classifications of psychotropic drugs.
- State the actions, uses, contraindications, adverse reactions, dosages, routes, and implications for patient care of selected antianxiety, antidepressive, antipsychotic, and antimanic agents.
- List the symptoms of marked elevation of blood pressure.
- List the foods and beverages a person should avoid when taking Monoamine Oxidase inhibitors.
- List the early symptoms of lithium intoxication.
- Complete the Spot Check on psychotropic agents.
- Answer the review questions correctly.

Vocabulary

limbic system. A group of brain structures that is activated by motivated behavior and arousal. The endocrine and autonomic motor nervous systems are influenced by the limbic system.

serotonin (ser″ro-ton′in). A chemical present in gastrointestinal mucosa, platelets, mast cells, and in carcinoid tumors. It is a vasoconstrictor and affects sleep and sensory perception.

mast cells. Connective tissue cells that contain heparin and histamine.

endogenous (en-doj′e-nus). Pertaining to being produced or arising from within a cell or organism.

anticholinergic (an″ti-ko″lin-er′jik). An agent that blocks parasympathetic nerve impulses.

adrenergic (ad-ren-er′jik). Pertaining to nerve fibers that, when stimulated, release epinephrine at their endings.

orthostatic hypotension (or′tho-stat′ik). A condition in which there is a decrease of systolic and diastolic blood pressure below normal. It is due to a sudden change in body position, especially when arising from a lying position to a standing position.

affective (a-fek′tiv). Pertaining to an emotion or mental state; feeling, mood, emotional response.

tyramine (ti′ra-men). Intermediate product in the conversion of tyrosine to epinephrine. Tyramine is found in most cheeses, beer, and protein foods that are aged.

tyrosine (ti′ro-sin). An amino acid that is present in many proteins.

dopamine (do′pa-men). A catecholamine synthesized by the adrenal gland that acts to increase blood pressure, especially the systolic phase. It also increases urinary output.

catecholamine (kat″e-kol′a-men). Biochemical substances, epinephrine, norepinephrine, and dopamine that have a marked effect on the nervous system, cardiovascular system, metabolic rate, temperature, and smooth muscle.

extrapyramidal (eks″tra-pi-ram′i-dal). Descending tracts of the spinal cord (lateral, ventral, and ventrolateral).

bioavailability (bi″o-a-val″a-bil′i-te). The rate and extent to which an active agent/drug or metabolite enters the general circulation. Bioavailability of such a substance is determined either by measuring the concentration of the drug in body fluids (blood) or by the magnitude of the pharmacologic response.

metabolite (me-tab′o-lit). Pertaining to any product of metabolism.

Introduction

Health is defined by the World Health Organization as a state of complete physical, mental, and social well-being. When a deviation from normal occurs in any of these states a process known as disease, illness, or disorder generally appears.

Mental health may be defined as a state of well-being of the mind. When there is a disturbance in the functioning of the mind, a state of emotional and/or mental disorder may appear. The exact cause of mental illness is not known. Contributing factors may include genetics, environment, biochemical changes occurring in the brain, and certain drugs.

The treatment of emotional and/or mental disorders encompasses a wide scope of factors. In this chapter, emphasis is given to the four classifications of drugs that are prescribed to reduce and control symptoms of emotional disturbances.

The physician determines a diagnosis and then prescribes a plan of treatment. This plan has to be carefully monitored on a continuous basis to determine the effectiveness of the program. Psychotropic drugs are usually only a part of the prescribed treatment plan. The dosage is individualized for each patient and is carefully evaluated for maximum effectiveness.

Drugs that affect psychic function, behavior, or experience are called *psychotropic*. These drugs may be classified as:

- *Antianxiety agents.* Drugs that counteract or diminish anxiety are called *anxiolytic.*
- *Antidepressant agents.* Drugs that elevate a person's mood.
- *Antimanic agents.* Drugs used to treat the manic episode of bipolar disorder.
- *Antipsychotic agents.* Drugs that modify psychotic behavior are called *neuroleptics.*

Psychotropic drugs are among the most frequently prescribed medications in the United States. It should be noted that these drugs when misused can cause physical and/or psychological dependence.

SPOTLIGHT

Stress and Anxiety

There seems to be a lump in your throat. Your stomach feels as though it is tied in knots and your heart is beating rapidly. Your fingers are cold as ice, but your palms are sweaty. You know these signs of stress and anxiety because you have had them before. Stress may be defined as the physical and/or psychological forces that are experienced by an individual. According to the *Occupational Health and Safety News*, U.S. Chamber of Commerce, U.S. Department of Human Services, and the National Institute of Drug Abuse an estimated 14 percent of all occupational disease claims were stress related with a cost of approximately $34 billion dollars.

Stress is implicated in immune system dysfunction, cancer, hypertension, heart disease, and ulcers. An agent or condition that is capable of causing stress is called a stressor. There are many conditions that can be stressors and these will vary with each individual. Finances, health problems, birth, death of a loved one, school, peer pressure, relationships, crime, and things beyond one's control are only a few conditions that may be stressors. It is believed that a certain amount of stress helps the body maintain homeostasis, a state

(continued)

of balance. When stress becomes more powerful than an individual can handle, certain physical symptoms appear.

The body responds to stressful situations the same way it responds to physical danger. It automatically prepares one for combat or retreat. This is known as the "fight-or-flight" response produced when the hypothalamus flashes signals through the nervous and endocrine systems. The anterior pituitary gland secretes the hormone adrenocorticotropic (ACTH) into the bloodstream, thereby stimulating the adrenal glands. During this alarm reaction, the adrenal medulla releases epinephrine (adrenaline; Adrenalin) and norepinephrine directly into the bloodstream.

Epinephrine elevates the systolic blood pressure; increases the heart rate and cardiac output; increases glycogenolysis, thereby hastening the release of glucose from the liver. It is through this action that the blood sugar level is elevated and the body is supplied with a "spurt-of-energy"; it also dilates the bronchial tubes and the pupils. Norepinephrine acts as a vasoconstrictor and elevates the systolic blood pressure.

As stress continues, perspiration increases and the palms become moist. Blood flow is slowed to the extremities and the fingers and toes feel "cold." The digestive process is slowed down, and under prolonged stress, hydrochloric acid within the stomach begins to eat away at the stomach lining. Muscles tense up and breathing may become rapid and then shallow.

Anxiety may be defined as a feeling of uneasiness, apprehension, worry, or dread. It is an involuntary or reflex reaction of the body to stress. When its negative effects cause a change in one's behavior or performance and it continues for a long period of time, persistent underlying anxiety may be diagnosed.

It is important to recognize the symptoms of stress and anxiety, and to find out what is causing the symptoms. Once this is done, the stressor may be eliminated or the individual must learn to cope with the situation. Developing coping skills is a technique that one can learn. Find out what works for you, such as taking a warm bath/shower, talking to a friend, taking a walk, reading a book, and so on.

You have heard the saying "laughter is the best medicine" and to relieve stress and anxiety, it certainly can work wonders. Try it. Just laugh out loud and see how you feel.

Symptoms of Anxiety

Physical:

fast heart rate
palpitations
shortness of breath
hot flashes
chills
dry mouth
dizziness
light-headedness
nausea
dyspepsia
diarrhea
cold, sweaty, tremulous hands
smothering sensation
frequent urination
lump in throat
band-like pressure about the head

Tension:

restlessness	trembling, twitching or feeling shaky
fatigue	

Emotional:

irritability	extreme feeling of worry
keyed-up feeling	inability to concentrate
problems with sleeping	

Special Considerations: The Older Adult

For the older adult, many times stress is just a part of daily life. With the increase in health care cost and the cost of just about everything, the "worries" of how one is going to pay the bills on a fixed income can be a major stressor of daily living. Other stressors that may affect the older adult are related to health problems, loss of physical and mental abilities, death of a spouse, and loneliness. How the older adult adjusts to stress is an individual process and depends upon many factors. When one cannot control stress and/or adapt to it, overload can occur and certain symptoms signal that it is time for one to say, "I must do something about this."

The symptoms of stress overload may include:

- headache
- stomachache
- sleeplessness
- backache
- irritability (snapping at others)
- forgetfulness

What can the older adult do about reducing stress? Naturally, this is going to depend on the cause of the stress and the individual.

General Guidelines for Reducing Stress:

- Analyze your financial situation. Make a budget that works for you. Plan for unexpected expenses.
- Take control. When one has control over situations in his/her life, stress is reduced and the harmful effects of stress can be lessened.
- Reach out to others. Sharing feelings and concerns often lessens the burden and stress is reduced. Try to do something nice for someone else each day.
- Develop healthy habits. A good diet, rest, and exercise help to control stress. Avoid heavy use of alcohol, tobacco, caffeine, and self-medication.

(continued)

- Strive for balance. Include time for yourself each day. Work hard, but also learn to play hard. Do work that you are capable of doing, that you really enjoy.
- Avoid negative thoughts. Learn to think positively.
- Be realistic—don't expect too much of yourself. Take one thing at a time.
- Keep fit emotionally. Know your own strengths and weaknesses. Get involved in things that you are comfortable doing. Avoid things that are unpleasant for you.
- Find out where to go for help if and when you need assistance. The local mental health center or hospital(s) may offer services for reducing stress. In addition to your physician there are many professionals who deal with stress such as psychiatrists, psychologists, clergy, social workers, nurses, mental health counselors, or state or local health associations. Do not be afraid to get help when help is needed.
- It has been shown that having a pet reduces stress. There are programs that have adapted this theory by placing pets in nursing homes and other long-term care facilities. Pets give love and seek very little in return. They can provide comfort and companionship. It has been shown that they may lower blood pressure, reduce feelings of loneliness, and provide the older adult with a purpose in life.

The older adult should have a complete physical examination regularly. There is more evidence that mental health plays a role in physical health. A study found that skin wounds heal more slowly in people suffering chronic stress. The findings suggest that stress reduction might speed healing in people who are recovering from accidents or surgery, according to researchers at Ohio State University in Columbus. The study involved 13 women ages 47 to 81 who were caring for relatives with dementia and who scored high on tests of psychological stress, and 13 women who were not caregivers and who scored low on stress tests. Researchers removed a tiny piece of skin from their forearms. The women in the no-stress group healed after 39 days and the stressed group took ten days longer. It is unclear how stress may slow healing, but researchers noted that the women under stress had lower levels of an immune system compound called interleukin-1 beta, which is known to play a role in wound repair.

Special Considerations: The Child

At some time in life, almost every individual experiences stress and/or depression. Experts have known that adolescents are as prone to depression as adults. Recently they have begun to realize that children as young as three and four can experience the blues. Clinical depression affects roughly 2.5 percent of school-age children. When a child generally behaves well and then suddenly becomes irritable or disrespectful, one should suspect a medical or psychological problem. Children who are depressed will typically "act up" and undergo a total behavior change. The usual calm child may turn demonstrably angry; the happy-go-lucky child may become sullen and hide in a corner, closet, basement, or some other part of the house.

Symptoms of Depression in the Child:

- **Toddlers:** sadness; inactivity; stomachaches; and in rare cases, self-destructive behavior.
- **Elementary-School-Age Children:** unhappiness; poor school performance; irritability; refusal to take part in activities one used to enjoy; occasional thoughts of suicide.
- **Adolescents:** sadness; withdrawal; feelings of hopelessness or guilt; changes in sleeping or eating habits; frequent thoughts of suicide.

A child does not understand feelings of stress, anxiety, and/or depression. He/she does not know how to ask for help, so when a child exhibits dramatic mood or behavior shifts, a physician should be consulted immediately. A physician may recommend psychotherapy or prescribe an antidepressant for children who are at least five years of age or older.

Critical Thinking Questions/Activities

Your patient is a 66-year-old female who has been admitted with pneumonia. You recognize her as being one of your former instructors from college. She seems to be irritable and complains of a headache and stomachache. She states, "I just can't get a good night's sleep anymore. I wake up around 3 o'clock in the morning, and I just can't go back to sleep. This is wearing me out." You recall that it had been about three months since the death of her husband.

Ask yourself:

- What do the symptoms: headache, stomachache, irritability, and sleeplessness signal?
- What are some of the factors that cause this condition in the older adult?
- Which of the guidelines for reducing stress would benefit my patient?
- How am I going to discuss these guidelines with my patient? What approach should I use?
- What are some available community resources that deal with stress? Should I provide the addresses and telephone numbers for such resources?

Antianxiety Agents

Antianxiety agents are chemical substances that relieve anxiety and muscle tension. They are indicated when anxiety interferes with a person's ability to function properly. The signs and symptoms of anxiety vary with the cause and an individual's response to the distressing situation. The physiologic signs may include palpitation, heart pain, nausea, anorexia, dyspepsia, constriction of the throat, muscle tension, pressure about the head, and cold, sweaty, tremulous hands. The psychological symptoms may include feelings of nervousness, apprehension, tension, inadequacy, indecisiveness, and insomnia.

Benzodiazepines

Benzodiazepines are a group of drugs with similar chemical structure and pharmaceutical activity. They are the most widely prescribed drugs for the treatment of anxiety.

Actions. The precise mechanism of action of the benzodiazepines is not known. They appear to exert their primary action on the *limbic system* of the brain. The benzodiazepines suppress the response to conflict or aggression in animals; they produce muscle relaxation and control induced seizures in experimental test models.

Uses. Benzodiazepines are used for the management of anxiety disorders, for the short-term relief of symptoms of anxiety, withdrawal symptoms of acute alcoholism, and preoperative apprehension and anxiety.

Contraindications. Hypersensitivity to benzodiazepines.

Adverse Reactions. Drowsiness, daytime sedation, ataxia, dizziness, fatigue, muscle weakness, dryness of the mouth, nausea, vomiting, increased irritability, insomnia, hyperactivity, blood dyscrasias.

Dosage and Route. The dosage and route of administration is determined by the physician. The dosage is individualized for each patient and regulated according to the effectiveness of the medication. See Table 22–1 for selected benzodiazepines.

Implications for Patient Care. Observe the patient for any signs of hypersensitivity. Note the effectiveness of the drug. Are the signs and symptoms improved? Observe for adverse reactions. Be especially aware of possible signs of blood dyscrasias such as a sore throat, fever, purpura, jaundice, excessive and progressive weakness. Report any adverse reactions to the proper authority or to the physician.

During hospitalization, provide for safety measures, monitor vital signs, and record intake and output when indicated. In geriatrics and/or debilitated patients, be especially aware of signs of confusion, drowsiness, and ataxia. Provide adequate protection.

Patient Teaching. Inform the patient that benzodiazepines may impair mental and/or physical abilities; therefore, one should not operate machinery or drive a motor vehicle while on these medications. Teach the patient that alcohol and/or other central nervous system depressants have an additive effect, and should not be used while on these medications. Teach the patient that smoking may enhance the metabolism of benzodiazepines and larger doses may be needed to maintain a sedative effect. Advise the patient who smokes to discuss this matter with his/her physician.

Table 22–1 Selected Benzodiazepines

Generic Name	Trade Name	Route	Usual Dosage
alprazolam	Xanax	Oral:	*Adults:* 0.25–2 mg tid *Geriatrics* or *Debilitated Patients:* 0.25 mg bid or tid
chlordiazepoxide HCl	Librium	Oral:	*Adults:* Mild and moderate anxiety: 5–10 mg tid or qid Severe anxiety: 20–25 mg tid or qid *Geriatrics* or *Debilitated Patients:* 5 mg 2–4 times daily *Children:* 6–12 years old 5 mg 2–4 times daily may be increased in some children to 10 mg 2–3 times daily
diazepam	Valium	Oral:	*Adults:* 2–10 mg 2–4 times daily *Geriatrics* or *Debilitated Patients:* 2–2.5 mg 1–2 times daily *Children:* 6 months and older 1–2.5 mg 3–4 times daily
lorazepam	Ativan	Oral:	*Adults:* 2–6 mg daily in 2–3 divided doses *Geriatrics* or *Debilitated Patients:* 1–2 mg/day in divided doses
oxazepam	Serax	Oral:	*Adults:* Mild and moderate anxiety: 10–15 mg tid or qid Severe anxiety: 15–30 mg tid *Geriatrics* or *Debilitated Patients:* 10 mg tid
clorazepate	Tranxene	Oral:	*Adults:* 15–60 mg daily in divided doses For elderly or debilitated: 7.5–15 mg daily in divided doses

Inform the patient that physical dependence may occur. Withdrawal symptoms will be similar to those produced by dependence on alcohol or barbiturates. Insomnia, anxiety, irritability, headache, muscle tremor, weakness, anorexia, nausea, and vomiting are symptoms of withdrawal from an addictive substance. Instruct the patient to take the medication as ordered. If the prescribed dosage does not produce the desired results, the patient should notify his or her physician. One should not stop taking the drug abruptly.

Benzodiazepines should be kept out of the reach of children, or those who may have a tendency to abuse drugs.

> **CAUTION:** Benzodiazepines have been used in suicide attempts. When taken in large amounts and mixed with alcohol or other central nervous system depressants, the effects may be fatal.

The patient should be advised to inform his or her physician about:

- all over-the-counter drugs being taken.
- any plans to become pregnant.
- being pregnant.
- presently breast feeding.
- all other prescription medication being taken.
- consumption of alcohol.

Antidepressant Agents

Antidepressant agents are chemical substances that relieve the symptoms of depression. They are indicated when depression interferes with a person's ability to function properly. The signs and symptoms of depression vary with the cause and each individual. Most individuals experience some form of depression during their lifetimes. When the feelings of depression occur every day and persist for weeks, a severe depressive illness may be present. This form of depression is called an affective disorder.

An *affective disorder* is characterized by a disturbance of mood, accompanied by a manic or depressive syndrome. This syndrome is not caused by any other physical or mental disorder. *Mood* is a pervasive and sustained emotion that may play a key role in an individual's perception of the world. With depression there is generally a loss of interest in food, sex, work, family, friends, and hobbies, among others. Feelings of helplessness, worthlessness, and guilt prevail in a person with this form of depression. Suicide is often contemplated or attempted.

There are various forms of depression. Depression is one of the most common illnesses in America today. It is estimated that 18 million Americans are affected by clinical depression every year. Twenty-five percent of all women and 13 percent of men suffer at least one episode of serious depression during their lifetimes. It is estimated that 20 percent to 40 percent of older adults experience depressive symptoms, with the highest rates of depression found among those who are medically ill or in long-term care. Depression is not something that occurs normally as a result of the aging or illness. In three out of ten depressed older adults, the depression is related to treatable physical illness, or adverse effects of medications. For others, it is a recurring and disabling illness that is unrelated to any other health problem or medications.

When depression lasts more than a few weeks and gets in the way of living, it is more than a mood. It is an illness that needs to be treated by a professional. The symptoms of clinical depression include a deep sense of sadness, a noticeable change in appetite or sleep patterns, a loss of interest in pleasurable activities, fatigue or loss of energy, a feeling of worthlessness, recurrent thoughts of death or suicide, plus other possible symptoms.

Clinical Depression Test

If one answers yes to five or more of the following questions and if the symptoms described have been present nearly every day for 2 weeks or more, one should seek professional assistance.

- Are there persistent feelings of sadness, emptiness, pessimism, or anxiety?
- Are there feelings of helplessness, hopelessness, guilt, or worthlessness?
- Is it difficult to make decisions, concentrate, or remember?
- Is there loss of interest or pleasure in everyday activities?
- Is there loss of drive or energy?
- Is there a significant change in sleep patterns (insomnia, early-morning waking, oversleeping)?
- Is there a significant change in appetite or weight change when not dieting?
- Are there symptoms such as headache, stomachache, backache, or chronic aches and pains of the joints and muscles? Sometimes depressive disorders masquerade as chronic physical symptoms that do not respond to treatment.
- Are there feelings of restlessness or irritability?
- Is there a significant change in smoking and drinking habits?
- Are there thoughts about death or suicide?

For more information on depression, you can call The National Institutes of Mental Health's hotline at 1-800-421-4211.

The physician who diagnoses and prescribes treatment for depression carefully evaluates each individual. After an accurate diagnosis is made, the physician may prescribe antidepressant agents as part of the patient's treatment regimen.

fluoxetine HCl (Prozac)

Prozac is an antidepressant agent that is unrelated to tricyclic or other antidepressant agents.

Actions. It is believed that fluoxetine blocks the uptake of serotonin, but not of norepinephrine, into human platelets. It seems to elevate mood, producing a feeling of sufficient well-being so that one can continue functioning without despair and futility.

Uses. Prozac is used for the relief of symptoms of depression.

Contraindications. Hypersensitivity to fluoxetine.

Adverse Reactions. Anxiety, nervousness, insomnia, drowsiness, fatigue, asthenia, tremor, sweating, anorexia, nausea, diarrhea, dizziness, lightheadedness.

Dosage and Route. Prozac is an oral antidepressant drug and the dosage is prescribed by the physician. Adults: Initially 20 mg daily in morning. May be increased if needed after several weeks. Doses greater than 20 mg/day are given in two divided doses (morning and noon). Maximum dose is 80 mg/day.

Implications for Patient Care. Observe the patient for any signs of hypersensitivity. Note the effectiveness of the drug. Are the symptoms improved? Observe for adverse reactions. Report any adverse reactions to the proper authority or to the physician. Evaluate the patient for history of drug abuse and be aware of the possibility of misuse or abuse. Be aware and ever alert to the possibility of suicide.

Patient Teaching. Inform the patient that Prozac may impair mental and/or physical abilities; therefore, one should not operate machinery or drive a motor vehicle. Advise the patient to inform the physician if he/she is taking or plan to take any prescription or over-the-counter medication or alcohol. The patient should advise the physician if she becomes pregnant or intends to become pregnant or if breast-feeding an infant.

Instruct the patient to take the medication as ordered. Inform the patient to keep the medication out of the reach of children.

Inform the patient to report any adverse reactions to this medication, especially a rash or hives.

Encourage the patient to seek medical attention if symptoms do not improve.

> **CAUTION:** With the combined administration of MAO inhibitors and tricyclics, at least 14 days should elapse between discontinuation of an MAO inhibitor and initiation of treatment with fluoxetine.

venlafaxine HCl (Effexor)

Effexor is a structurally novel antidepressant for oral administration. It is chemically unrelated to tricyclic, tetracyclic, or other available antidepressant agents.

Actions. It is believed that venlafaxine potentiates neurotransmitter activity of the central nervous system. Preclinical studies have shown that it inhibits serotonin and norepinephrine reuptake and is a weak inhibitor of dopamine reuptake.

Uses. Indicated for the treatment of depression.

Contraindications. Hypersensitivity to venlafaxine.

Adverse Reactions. General weakness, sweating, nausea, constipation, anorexia, vomiting, sleepiness, dry mouth, dizziness, nervousness, anxiety, tremor, blurred vision, abnormal ejaculation or orgasm in men, and impotence.

Dosage and Route. Effexor is an oral antidepressant drug and the dosage is prescribed by the physician. The recommended dosage is 75 mg/day. Depending on tolerability and the need for further clinical effect, the dose may be increased to 150 mg/day. When discontinuing Effexor after more than 1 week of therapy, it is generally recommended that the dose be tapered to minimize the risk of discontinuation symptoms. Patients who have received Effexor for 6 weeks or more should have their dose tapered gradually over a 2-week-period.

Implications for Patient Care. Observe the patient for signs of hypersensitivity. Note the effectiveness of the drug. Are the symptoms improved? Observe for adverse reactions. Report any adverse reactions to the proper authority. Evaluate the patient for history of drug abuse and be aware of the possibility of misuse or abuse. Be aware and ever alert to the possibility of suicide.

Patient Teaching. Inform the patient that Effexor may impair mental and/or physical abilities; therefore, one should not operate machinery or drive a motor vehicle. Advise the patient to inform the physician if he/she is taking or plans to take any prescription or over-the-counter medication or alcohol. The patient should advise the physician if she becomes pregnant or intends to become pregnant or if breast-feeding an infant. If the patient has high blood pressure he/she should inform the physician, as Effexor can cause sustained increases in blood pressure. If the patient has liver or kidney disease, and/or a history of seizures, the physician should be informed before initiation of drug therapy.

Instruct the patient to take the medication as ordered. Inform the patient to keep the medication out of reach of children.

Inform the patient to report any adverse reactions to this medication, especially a rash or hives.

Encourage the patient to seek medical attention if symptoms do not improve.

> **CAUTION:** Taking Effexor in combination with a monoamine oxidase inhibitor (MAO) or within 14 days of stopping MAOI therapy can cause serious side effects and/or fatalities. At least 14 days should elapse between discontinuation of an MAOI and initiation of therapy with Effexor. In addition, at least 7 days should be allowed after stopping Effexor before starting an MAOI. Some common prescribed MAOIs include Nardil (pheneizine sulfate) and Parnate (tranylcypromine sulfate).

Tricyclic Antidepressants

Tricyclic antidepressants share a chemical configuration that is characterized by a three-ring or *tricyclic* structure. They are used in the treatment of depression.

Actions. The precise mechanism of action in humans is not known. These agents are believed to block norepinephrine and serotonin uptake shortly after administration. They seem to elevate mood, increase physical activity and mental alertness, and improve appetite and sleep. In 60 to 70 percent of patients with endogenous depression, morbid preoccupation was reduced. Anticholinergic and alpha-adrenergic blocking activities are adverse actions to note.

Uses. Tricyclic antidepressants are used for the relief of symptoms of depression. Endogenous depression is more likely to be alleviated than other depressive states.

Contraindications. Hypersensitivity to tricyclic antidepressants.

Adverse Reactions. The most common adverse reactions of these agents are due to their *blocking parasympathetic nerve impulses (anticholinergic)* and *alpha-adrenergic blocking activities:* flushing, diaphoresis, blurred vision, disturbance of accommodation, increased intraocular pressure, constipation, paralytic ileus, urinary retention, and dilatation of urinary tract.

Other adverse reactions that may occur are: hypotension—particularly orthostatic hypotension; hypertension; tachycardia; palpitation; confusion; excitement; anxiety; insomnia; numbness, tingling, and paresthesias of the extremities; ataxia; tremors; seizures; skin rash; nausea; vomiting; anorexia; diarrhea; dizziness; fatigue; headache; weight gain or loss; and drowsiness.

> ***Note:*** Cimetidine (Tagamet) may increase the bioavailability of certain tricyclic antidepressants. This drug interaction may produce severe anticholinergic adverse reactions, such as dizziness, and orthostatic hypotension.

Dosage and Route. The dosage and route is prescribed by the physician and individualized for each patient. See Table 22–2 for selected tricyclic antidepressants.

Implications for Patient Care. Observe the patient for any signs of hypersensitivity. Note the effectiveness of the drug. Are the symptoms improved? Observe for adverse reactions. Report any adverse reactions to the proper authority or to the physician.

During hospitalization, provide for safety measures, monitor vital signs, especially the blood pressure (orthostatic hypotension may occur). Be aware and ever alert to the possibility of suicide.

Patient Teaching. Inform the patient that tricyclic antidepressants may impair mental and/or physical abilities; therefore, one should not operate machinery or drive a motor vehicle. Advise the patient not to arise suddenly. Teach the patient that alcohol and/or other central nervous system depressants have an additive effect and should not be used while on these medications.

Instruct the patient to take the medications as ordered. Inform the patient to keep these medications out of the reach of children.

Table 22–2 Selected Tricyclic Antidepressants

Generic Name	Trade Name	Route	Usual Dosage
amitriptyline HCl	Elavil	Oral:	*Adults:* Outpatients: 75 mg–150 mg daily in divided doses Hospitalized patients: 100–200 mg daily in divided doses *Adolescent and Geriatrics:* 10 mg tid with 20 mg at bedtime
amoxapine	Asendin	Oral:	*Adults:* 200–300 mg daily *Geriatrics:* 25 mg bid or tid
desipramine HCl	Norpramin	Oral:	*Adults:* 100–200 mg daily *Adolescent and Geriatrics:* 25–100 mg daily
doxepin HCl	Adapin	Oral:	*Adults:* 75–100 mg daily
imipramine HCl	Tofranil	Oral:	*Adults:* Outpatients: 75–150 mg daily Hospitalized patients: 100–300 mg daily *Adolescent and Geriatrics:* 30–40 mg daily; not to exceed 100 mg/day
protriptyline HCl	Vivactil	Oral:	*Adults:* 15–40 mg a day divided into 3 or 4 doses *Adolescent and Geriatrics:* 5 mg tid
trimipramine maleate	Surmontil	Oral:	*Adults:* Outpatients: 75–150 mg daily in divided doses Hospitalized patients: 100–200 mg daily in divided doses *Adolescents and Geriatrics:* 50–100 mg/day
trazodone HCl	Desyrel	Oral:	*Adults:* Outpatients: Initial dose of 150 mg/day in divided doses. The dose may be increased by 50 mg/day every 3–4 days. The maximum dose should not exceed 400 mg/day in divided doses. Inpatients may be given up to, but not in excess of, 600 mg/day in divided doses.

Inform the patient to report any adverse reactions to his or her physician. Encourage the patient to seek medical attention if symptoms do not improve.

CAUTION: Tricyclic antidepressants should not be given with monoamine oxidase inhibitors. When it is desired to replace a monoamine oxidase inhibitor with one of these agents, a minimum of 14 days should be allowed to elapse after the former is discontinued.

Note: The possibility of suicide in depressed patients remains until significant remission occurs. Potentially suicidal persons should not have access to a large quantity of these agents.

Monoamine Oxidase (MAO) Inhibitors

Monoamine oxidase inhibitors are antidepressants that inhibit the oxidase enzyme that breaks down monoamine transmitters in the body. They may be considered as the drugs of choice in such nonendogenous types of depression as agoraphobia and hysteroid dysphoria. They appear to be less effective than the tricyclic antidepressants in patients with endogenous depression and their use generally requires strict dietary control. See Table 22–3.

Actions. MAOIs inhibit the monoamine oxidase enzyme that catalyzes the inactivation of serotonin, norepinephrine, and dopamine, thereby increasing the brain concentrations of these substances. In theory, this increased concentration of monoamines in the brain-stem is the basis for the antidepressant activity of MAO inhibitors. *In vivo* and *in vitro* studies demonstrated inhibition of amine-oxidase in the brain, heart, and liver.

Uses. MAOIs may be used in agoraphobia, hysteroid dysphoria, and in patients who have not responded to treatment with tricyclic antidepressants.

Table 22–3 Monoamine Oxidase (MAO) Inhibitors

Generic Name	Trade Name	Route	Usual Dosage
isocarboxazid	Marplan	Oral:	*Adults:* Starting dose 30 mg daily, given in single or divided dose. Maintenance dose 10–20 mg (or less) daily.
phenelzine sulfate	Nardil	Oral:	*Adults:* Initial dose 15 mg (one tablet) tid. Early phase treatment 60 mg/day or up to 90 mg/day. Maintenance dose 15 mg/day or every other day.
tranylcypromine sulfate	Parnate	Oral:	*Adults:* Starting dose 20 mg/day. 10 mg in A.M. and 10 mg in the afternoon. Maintenance dose 20 mg/day or 10 mg/day.

Contraindications

- In patients with known hypersensitivity to the drug.
- In patients with cerebrovascular defects or cardiovascular disorders.
- In the presence of pheochromocytoma.
- In combination with MAO inhibitors or with dibenzazepine-related entities.
- In combination with sympathomimetics.
- In combination with meperidine.
- In combination with cheese or other foods with a high tyramine content.
- In patients undergoing elective surgery.
- In patients with impaired renal and/or liver function.
- In combination with narcotics, alcohol, and hypotensive agents.
- Cautious use with anti-parkinsonism drugs.

Adverse Reactions. Orthostatic hypotension, drowsiness, dryness of the mouth, blurred vision, dysuria, constipation, restlessness, insomnia, weakness, nausea, diarrhea, abdominal pain, tachycardia, anorexia, edema, palpitation, chills, impotence, headache, dizziness, vertigo, tremors, muscle twitching, and photosensitivity are some of the adverse reactions.

Dosage and Route. The dosage and route is determined by the physician. The dosage is individualized for each patient and regulated according to the effectiveness of the medication. The patient has to be carefully monitored by the prescribing physician.

Implications for Patient Care. Observe the patient for any signs of hypersensitivity. Note the effectiveness of the drug. Observe for adverse reactions.

During hospitalization, provide for safety and carefully monitor the patient's blood pressure.

> **CAUTION:** Hypertension crises may occur with the use of MAO inhibitors. These crises may be fatal.

Know the symptoms of marked elevation of blood pressure: occipital headache which may radiate frontally, palpitation, neck stiffness or soreness, nausea or vomiting, sweating (sometimes with fever and sometimes with cold), and photophobia. Either tachycardia or bradycardia, chest pain and dilated pupils may occur. Notify the physician immediately if these symptoms appear. The medication should be discontinued and measures to lower the blood pressure should be initiated. Be observant for signs of orthostatic hypotension.

Patient Teaching. Instruct the patient to notify the physician immediately if headache, stiff neck, pounding heartbeat, feelings of nausea, or vomiting occur. Instruct the patient not to suddenly arise from a lying position. If the patient feels dizzy upon arising, instruct him or her to lie back down until the dizziness disappears.

Inform the patient not to drink alcoholic or caffeine beverages or take over-the-counter medications while using MAO inhibitors. Inform the patient to be sure to tell the physician about all other medications that he or she may be taking. If the patient is seeing more than one physician, each physician should be informed of the patient's medication regimen. Advise the patient who is taking insulin and/or oral sulfonylureas to monitor blood glucose levels very carefully, as MAO inhibitors may have an additive hypoglycemic effect when taken with these drugs. The diabetic patient should discuss this information with his/her physician.

Be sure that the patient understands that large amounts of tyramine can lead to a hypertensive crisis. Provide the patient with a list of foods and beverages to *avoid*. You may use the following list.

When taking MAO inhibitors, the following foods and beverages should be *avoided*:

Cheese	Avocados	Chianti winc
Sour cream	Chocolate	Sherry
Pickled herring	Soy sauce	Beer
Liver	Fava beans	Protein foods that are aged
Canned figs	Yeast extracts	Chicken livers
Raisins	Meats prepared with tenderizers	Pickles
Bananas		Yogurt

Antimanic Agent(s)

Lithium is considered the drug of choice for the treatment of the manic episode of bipolar disorder. *Bipolar disorder* is a major affective disorder that is characterized by episodes of mania and depression. It was previously called manic-depressive psychosis. Bipolar disorder is subdivided into three types: manic, depressed, and mixed. In the manic phase, there are excessive emotional displays such as excitement, euphoria, hyperactivity, boisterousness, impaired ability to concentrate, decreased need for sleep, exalted feelings, delusions of grandeur, and overproduction of ideas. In the depressive phase, there is marked apathy, underactivity, and feeling of profound sadness, loneliness, and guilt. In the mixed phase elements of both mania and depression may be present.

Lithium

Actions. The specific biochemical mechanism of lithium action in mania is unknown. It counteracts mood changes without producing sedation. Studies have shown that lithium alters sodium transport in nerve and muscle cells and effects a shift toward intraneuronal metabolism of catecholamines.

Uses. Specific antimanic drug for prophylaxis and treatment of bipolar disorder (manic-depressive).

Warnings. Generally not given to patients with significant renal or cardiovascular disease, severe debilitation or dehydration, or sodium depletion, since the risk of lithium toxicity is high in such patients. Lithium may cause fetal harm when administered during pregnancy.

Adverse Reactions. Fine hand tremor, polyuria, and mild thirst may occur during initial therapy and may persist throughout the treatment. During the first few days of lithium administration, there may be transient and mild nausea and general discomfort.

Early signs of lithium intoxication are: diarrhea, vomiting, drowsiness, muscular weakness, and lack of coordination. These signs may appear at serum lithium levels below 2.0 mEq/L. At higher levels, ataxia, giddiness, tinnitus, blurred vision, and polyuria may occur. Serum lithium levels above 3.0 mEq/L may cause a complex of signs and symptoms involving various organs and systems of the body. Refer to the *Physicians' Desk Reference* for further information.

Dosage and Route. The dosage is individualized according to the serum lithium level and the patient's clinical response. A threshold level of lithium in body tissues must be reached before it is effective. This may take three to five days of therapy. Lithium is available as:

- Eskalith—300 mg tablets and capsules; 450 mg controlled-release tablets
- Lithobid—300 mg slow-release tablets
- Cibalith-S Syrup—300 mg of lithium carbonate in each 5 ml
- Lithium carbonate—300 mg tablets and capsules
- Lithium Citrate Syrup—8 mEq/5 ml (300 mg of lithium carbonate)

Implications for Patient Care. The patient should have a complete physical examination before the initiation of lithium therapy.

Close clinical observation and frequent monitoring of serum lithium levels is essential. Serum lithium levels should be determined two to three times weekly during the acute manic phase, then on a monthly basis during maintenance therapy. During the initial stage of therapy, the blood level should be maintained between 1 and 1.5 mEq/L of serum. During maintenance therapy, the blood level should be between 0.6–1.2 mEq/L of serum. Observe for adverse reactions. Report to the proper authority or to the physician.

During hospitalization, provide for safety measures and support to the patient and his or her family. Establish rapport with the patient. Assess the patient's mental status: *cognitive function; alertness; level of orientation; attention span; memory; language function*; and *spatial ability*.

Patient Teaching. The patient and his or her family should be informed of the early symptoms of lithium intoxication or toxicity and instructed to discontinue the medication and contact the physician immediately.

Early Symptoms of Lithium Intoxication:

drowsiness, vomiting, muscle weakness, ataxia, dryness of the mouth, lethargy, abdominal pain, dizziness, slurred speech, diarrhea, tremor, and nystagmus

Inform the patient that the metallic taste in the mouth may be temporary and will usually decrease with a lower dose of lithium. Teach the patient how to perform good oral hygiene. Advise the patient to take the medication as prescribed and not to discontinue the medication unless symptoms of lithium intoxication occur.

To diminish nausea, lithium may be given with meals. Stress the importance of good nutrition and emphasize that the patient should maintain a normal intake of sodium and fluids. Lithium may enhance sodium depletion which could enhance lithium toxicity. Instruct the patient to drink 10–12 eight ounce glasses of water daily to prevent possible toxicity. The patient should be advised to refrain from drinking caffeine liquids and alcoholic beverages. Instruct the patient not to change the brand of the prescribed medication.

Advise female patients against becoming pregnant during the time they are taking lithium.

Advise the patient to inform other health-care providers of his or her lithium therapy.

Stress to the patient the importance of returning to his or her attending physician, as scheduled, for lithium blood analysis.

Antipsychotic Agents

Antipsychotic agents modify psychotic behavior and are called *neuroleptics.* Antipsychotic drugs are classified as phenothiazines and nonphenothiazines. *Phenothiazine* is an organic compound used in the manufacture of certain tranquilizers. *Thorazine,* the first antipsychotic agent to be introduced in the early 1950s, is a phenothiazine derivative.

Neuroleptics

Actions. The precise mechanism of action is not known. They are believed to control the symptomatology of psychosis by reducing excessive dopamine activity, by blocking post-synaptic dopamine receptors in the cerebral cortex, basal ganglia, limbic system, brain stem, and hypothalamus.

Antipsychotic agents have varying degrees of antihistaminic, anticholinergic, and alpha-antiadrenergic activities. These activities account for a number of the adverse reactions associated with antipsychotic agents.

Uses. Antipsychotic agents are used in the treatment of acute and chronic schizophrenia, organic psychoses, the manic phase of bipolar affective disorder, and psychotic disorders.

Contraindications. Hypersensitivity to the specific antipsychotic agent. Most antipsychotic agents are contraindicated in comatose patients; patients receiving large doses of CNS depressants; and in patients with bone marrow depression, blood dyscrasias, or liver damage.

Adverse Reactions. Antipsychotic agents may cause a wide gamut of adverse reactions. Some that may occur are: drowsiness, sedation, convulsive seizure, dryness of mouth, constipation, urinary retention, blurred vision, orthostatic hypotension, tachycardia, fainting, dizziness, dystonia, motor restlessness, nasal congestion, toxic psychosis, photosensitivity, jaundice, skin pigmentation, and ocular changes.

Other adverse reactions include: *extrapyramidal symptoms* (EPS)—these symptoms appear to be dose related and are the most frightening to the patient. *Dystonia*—difficult or bad muscle tone may appear as spasm of the neck muscles, torticollis, rigidity of back muscles, carpopedal spasm, trismus, swallowing difficulty, oculogyric crisis, and protrusion of the tongue. *Akathisia* (acathisia)—an inability to sit down. The patient has a feeling of restlessness and an urgent need of movement. Pacing, fidgeting, and agitation are classic symptoms of akathisia.

Pseudo-parkinsonism—a neuroleptic-induced reaction. Symptoms may include mask-like expression (facies), drooling, tremors, rigidity, bradykinesia, shuffling gait, postural abnormalities, and hypersalivation. These symptoms may occur within a few weeks to a few months after initiating therapy, and may be controlled by an antiparkinsonism agent.

> ***Note:*** *Levodopa* has not been found to be effective in the treatment of pseudoparkinsonism.

Tardive Dyskinesias—a syndrome characterized by rhythmical involuntary movement of the tongue, face, mouth, jaw, trunk and extremities. These symptoms may appear in some patients on long-term therapy. They may also appear after drug therapy has been discontinued. Tardive (lateness) dyskinesias (difficult movement) may occur in patients of any age, but is more common in older women. There is no known effective treatment for this syndrome.

Dosage and Route. The dosage and route of administration is determined by the physician. The dosage is individualized for each patient and regulated according to the effectiveness of the medication. See Table 22–4 for selected antipsychotic agents.

Implications for Patient Care. The patient who takes antipsychotic agents needs special care. It is essential that you understand the patient's diagnosis and his or her treatment regimen. Remember that drug therapy is only a part of the treatment plan. The patient

Table 22–4 Selected Antipsychotic Agents

Generic Name	Trade Name	Route	Usual Dosage
chlorpromazine HCl	Thorazine	Oral:	*Adults:* Excessive anxiety, tension and agitation: 10 mg tid or qid or 25 mg bid or tid. More severe cases: 25 mg tid; daily dosage may be 200–800 mg. *Children:* Office patients, outpatients: $\frac{1}{4}$ mg/lb of body weight every 4–6 h, PRN.
fluphenazine HCl	Permitil	Oral:	*Adults:* 0.5–10 mg in divided doses.
mesoridazine	Serentil	Oral:	Schizophrenia: Starting dose 50 mg tid, daily dose range 100–400 mg/day.
perphenazine	Trilafon	Oral:	Moderately disturbed nonhospitalized psychotic patients: 4–8 mg tid or 1–2 REPETABS bid (initially). Hospitalized psychotic patients: 8–16 mg bid to qid or 1–4 REPETABS bid; avoid dosage in excess of 64 mg daily.
prochlorperazine	Compazine	Oral:	*Adults:* Nonpsychotic anxiety: 5 mg 3–4 times daily, psychotic disorders (mild) office patients, outpatients: 5–10 mg 3–4 times daily. Moderate-severe hospitalized or adequately supervised patients: 10 mg 3–4 times daily (initially); 50–75 mg/daily. More severe patients: optimum dosage is 100–150 mg daily.
promazine HCl	Sparine	Oral:	*Adults:* Psychotic disorders: 10–200 mg at 4–6 hour intervals; dose limit 1000 mg/day. *Children:* Over 12 years: 10–25 mg every 4–6 hours.
thioridazine HCl	Mellaril	Oral:	*Adults:* 50–100 mg tid (starting dose); maximum to 800 mg a day. Daily dosage range 200–800 mg divided into 2–4 doses. *Children:* Ages 2–12 years: 0.5–3.0 mg/kg/day.
trifluoperazine HCl	Stelazine	Oral:	*Adults:* Nonpsychotic anxiety: 1–2 mg bid. Psychotic disorders: 2–5 mg bid. *Children:* 6–12 years hospitalized or under close supervision: 1 mg once a day or bid (starting dose).
Nonphenothiazines			
haloperidol	Haldol	Oral:	*Adults:* Moderate symptomatology: 0.5–2.0 mg bid or tid. Severe symptomatology: 3.0–5.0 mg bid or tid. Geriatric or debilitated: 0.5–2.0 mg bid or tid. Chronic or resistant patients: 3.0–5.0 mg bid or tid. *Children:* 3–12 years: psychotic disorders: 0.05 mg/kg/day to 0.15 mg/kg/day.

Table 22–4 *(Continued)*

Generic Name	Trade Name	Route	Usual Dosage
loxapine	Loxitane	Oral:	Initially 10 mg bid. Severely disturbed: up to 50 mg/day. Maintenance 60–100 mg/day.
molindone HCl	Moban	Oral:	Initially 50–75 mg/day; increase to 100 mg/day in 3–4 days. An increase to 225 mg/day may be required in patients with severe symptomatology. Maintenance: Mild: 5–15 mg 3–4 times a day. Moderate: 10–25 mg 3–4 times a day. Severe: 225 mg/day.
pimozide	Orap	Oral:	Initially 1–2 mg a day in divided doses. Maintenance: 0.2 mg/kg/day.
thiothixene HCl	Navane	Oral:	Initially (mild) 2 mg tid. Severe 5 mg bid. Optimal dose 20–30 mg daily.

needs emotional, physical, and social support. It is important that the patient's family be included in the planning and implementation of patient care.

Observe the patient for signs of hypersensitivity and adverse reactions. Notify the proper authorities or physician of any adverse reactions. Note the effectiveness of the medication. Are the symptoms improved? During hospitalization, provide for safety measures, monitor vital signs, and record intake and output when indicated.

Patient Teaching. Inform the patient that antipsychotic agents may impair mental and/or physical abilities; therefore, one should not operate machinery or drive a motor vehicle while on these medications. Teach the patient that alcohol and/or other central nervous system depressants have an additive effect and should not be used while on these medications.

Instruct the patient to take the medications as ordered. If the patient is unable to manage his or her own plan of treatment, inform the proper family member or other responsible person of any and all essential information.

Assess the patient's mental status: *cognitive function; alertness; level of orientation; attention span; memory; language function; spatial ability;* the presence of *delusions* or *hallucinations; agitation;* and *withdrawal.* Assess the patient's behavioral status: *purposefulness* of activity; *sleeping* pattern; *eating* pattern; *appropriate* responses; and *speech* patterns.

Teach the patient to report adverse reactions to his or her physician. Inform the patient to avoid exposure to ultraviolet rays (sunlight or artificial). Instruct the patient not to suddenly arise from a lying position. Inform the patient to be sure to tell the physician about all other medications that he or she may be taking. If the patient is seeing more than one physician, each physician should be informed of the patient's medication regimen.

Encourage the patient to eat a balanced diet and to drink sufficient fluids. Keeping the mucous membranes moist will help relieve dryness of the mouth. If desired, the patient may suck on ice chips or sugarless hard candy to help moisten the mouth. When the patient has constipation, the physician should order an appropriate stool softener and/or laxative.

Spot Check

For each of the psychotropic agents given, list several aspects of patient teaching and implications for patient care.

Psychotropic Agent	Patient Teaching	Implications for Patient Care
Benzodiazepines		
Prozac		
Tricyclic Antidepressants		
Lithium		

◆ Review Questions

Directions: Select the best answer to each multiple choice question. Circle the letter of your choice.

1. The medical term that means pertaining to an emotion or mental state; feeling, mood, emotional response, is known as __________.
   a. endogenous
   b. entrapyramidal
   c. limbic
   d. affective
2. Biochemical substances, epinephrine, norepinephrine, and dopamine are called __________.
   a. tyrosines
   b. catecholamines
   c. metabolites
   d. adrenergies
3. Drugs that affect psychic function, behavior, or experience are called __________.
   a. psychotropic
   b. anticholinergic
   c. adrenergic
   d. antibiotic
4. __________ agents are chemical substances that relieve anxiety and muscle tension.
   a. Antidepressive
   b. Antipsychotic
   c. Antimanic
   d. Antianxiety
5. When a patient is taking benzodiazepines it is your responsibility to teach the patient that __________.
   a. impairment of mental and/or physical abilities may occur
   b. alcohol and/or other CNS depressants have an additive effect
   c. physical dependence may occur
   d. all of these
6. The usual adult dose of diazepam (Valium) is __________.
   a. 2–10 mg 2–4 times daily
   b. 0.25–5.0 mg tid
   c. 20–40 mg 3–4 times daily
   d. 15–30 mg tid
7. __________ agents are chemical substances that relieve the symptoms of depression.
   a. Antidepressive
   b. Antipsychotic
   c. Antimanic
   d. Antianxiety
8. The most common adverse reaction to tricyclic antidepressants are __________.
   a. flushing, diaphoresis, blurred vision, disturbance of accommodation
   b. increased intraocular pressure, constipation, paralytic ileus
   c. urinary retention and dilatation of urinary tract
   d. all of these

9. Orthostatic __________ is a condition in which there is a decrease of systolic and diastolic blood pressure below normal due to a sudden change in body position.
   a. hypertension
   b. pneumonia
   c. hypotension
   d. none of these
10. Tricyclic antidepressants should not be given with __________.
   a. protein foods that are aged
   b. cheese
   c. monoamine oxidase inhibitors
   d. caffeine
11. The usual adult dose of imipramine (Tofranil) for an outpatient is __________.
   a. 100–225 mg daily
   b. 75–150 mg daily
   c. 10 mg tid
   d. 15–40 mg a day in divided doses
12. Monoamine oxidase inhibitors may be used in __________.
   a. agoraphobia
   b. hysteroid dysphoria
   c. patients who have not responded to tricyclic antidepressants
   d. all of these
13. When a patient is taking MAO inhibitors, it is your responsibility to teach the patient __________.
   a. to notify the physician immediately if headache, stiff neck, pounding heartbeat, feelings of nausea, or vomiting occur
   b. not to arise suddenly from a lying position
   c. about foods and beverages he or she is to *avoid*
   d. all of these
14. The usual adult dose of isocarboxazid (Marplan) is __________.
   a. 30 mg daily, given in single or divided dose
   b. maintenance dose 10–20 mg (or less) daily
   c. 50 mg daily, given in single or divided dose
   d. a and b
15. __________ is/are considered the drug of choice for the treatment of the manic episode of bipolar disorder.
   a. Monoamine oxidase inhibitors
   b. Tricyclic antidepressants
   c. Lithium
   d. Elavil
16. The early signs of lithium intoxication are __________.
   a. diarrhea, vomiting, drowsiness, muscular weakness, and lack of coordination
   b. dryness of the mouth, lethargy, abdominal pain
   c. dizziness, slurred speech, tremor and nystagmus
   d. all of these

17. During the initial stage of lithium therapy the blood level should be maintained between __________.
    a. 2–3.0 mEq/L
    b. 1–1.5 mEq/L
    c. 0.6–1.2 mEq/L
    d. 1–3.5 mEq/L

18. When a patient is taking lithium it is your responsibility to teach the patient __________.
    a. to recognize the early signs/symptoms of lithium intoxication
    b. how to perform good oral hygiene
    c. to refrain from drinking caffeine liquids and alcoholic beverages
    d. all of these

19. __________ __________ modify psychotic behavior and are called neuroleptics.
    a. Antidepressive agents
    b. Antipsychotic agents
    c. Antimanic agents
    d. Antianxiety agents

20. Adverse reactions to pheothiazines that appear to be dose related and are most frightening to the patient are __________.
    a. dystonia, akathisia, and pseudo-parkinsonism
    b. dryness of the mouth, constipation, and tachycardia
    c. dizziness, nasal congestion, and blurred vision
    d. photosensitivity, jaundice, and skin pigmentation

21. __________ __________ is a syndrome characterized by rhythmical involuntary movement of the tongue, face, mouth, jaw, trunk and extremities.
    a. Pseudo-parkinsonism
    b. Tardive dyskinesias
    c. Toxic psychosis
    d. none of these

22. When a patient is taking an antipsychotic agent, it is your responsibility to teach the patient __________.
    a. that impairment of mental and/or physical abilities may occur
    b. that alcohol and other CNS depressants have an additive effect
    c. to avoid exposure to ultraviolet rays
    d. all of these

Case Study: Mrs. Alice Allen, age 42, is brought to the physician's office by her husband who says that he is worried about her behavior. He states that she has not dressed for three days and has no interest in food, sex, or her family.

23. Mrs. Allen experiences many of the major symptoms of depression. Which one of the following behaviors is a major symptom?
    a. Hallucinations and delusions
    b. Increase in physical activity
    c. Loss of interest
    d. Increased interest in surroundings

24. Mrs. Allen states that she feels helpless and worthless. The nurse should know that this type of statement may indicate signs of __________.
    a. hallucinations
    b. delusions
    c. suicide
    d. mood disturbance

25. After careful evaluation, Mrs. Allen is diagnosed as having depression. The physician admits the patient to the hospital and orders that she receive Elavil 75 mg stat and then again at bedtime. The nurse should know that Elavil is a tricyclic antidepressant and has anticholinergic effects. This means that __________.
    a. parasympathetic nerve impulses are blocked
    b. sympathetic nerve impulses are blocked
    c. peripheral nerves are blocked
    d. central nervous impulses are blocked

26. During hospitalization it is important to monitor the patient's blood pressure for signs of __________.
    a. hypertension
    b. hypotension
    c. orthostatic hypotension
    d. essential hypertension

27. Before Mrs. Allen is discharged from the hospital she should be taught certain basic facts about her medication. These facts include not to __________.
    a. arise suddenly from a lying position
    b. use alcohol and other CNS depressants
    c. operate machinery or drive a motor vehicle
    d. all of these

Matching: Place the correct letter from Column II on the appropriate line of Column I.

Column I

28. __________ Endogenous
29. __________ Anticholinergic
30. __________ Serotonin

Column II

A. A vasoconstrictor that affects sleep and sensory perception.
B. Produced or arising within a cell or organism.
C. Agent that blocks parasympathetic nerve impulses.
D. Agent that stimulates parasympathetic nerve impulses.

CHAPTER 23

Substance Abuse

OBJECTIVES

Upon completion of this chapter, you should be able to:

- Define the terms listed in the vocabulary.
- Describe problems that are associated with substance abuse.
- Understand how an individual becomes involved with substance abuse.
- Explain why the rate of alcoholism is expected to increase in the older population.
- Describe alcohol as a psychotropic drug.
- List the effects that alcohol has as a multisystem toxin and a central nervous system depressant.
- Be aware of some drugs that interact with alcohol.
- Describe alcohol abuse as the number-one drug problem of American children.
- Complete the critical thinking questions/activities presented in this chapter.
- State the effects that amphetamines have upon the body.
- Give some of the street names for amphetamines.
- Describe cocaine as a central nervous system stimulant, and explain how it is used as an abused substance.
- List the adverse effects of cocaine.
- State how barbiturates are abused, and explain their effects upon the body.
- Describe how narcotic analgesics are abused, and explain their effects upon the body.
- State the physical dangers associated with opiate abuse.
- Describe marijuana as an abused substance.
- Describe how phencyclidine (PCP) is an abused substance, and its illegal use.

- Give some of the names that PCP is known by.
- State that lysergic acid diethylamide (LSD) is a hallucinogenic agent and describe its effects upon the body.
- Describe inhalants as psychoactive vapors, and explain their effects upon the body.
- State the nurse's role in recognizing substance abuse and the action to take when substance abuse is suspected.
- Describe substance abuse in the workplace.
- List the warning signs of substance abuse in the workplace.
- Complete the Spot Check on interactions of selected drugs and alcohol.
- Answer the review questions correctly.

Vocabulary

Attention deficit disorder. A disease characterized by inappropriate inattention, impulsivity, and hyperactivity. It occurs in infancy and/or childhood, and may be known as hyperkinetic syndrome, hyperactivity, minimal brain damage, minimal brain dysfunction, and minimal cerebral dysfunction.

dependency (de-pend′en-cy). The psychic craving for a drug or a substance. It may or may not be accompanied by physiological dependency.

euphoria (u-for′e-a). A feeling of good health. It is a term that also means an exaggerated feeling of well-being; elation.

narcolepsy (nar′ko-lep″se). A chronic condition whereby the patient is unable to control recurrent attacks of drowsiness and sleep.

obesity (o-be′si-te). Excessive amount of fat on the body. *Exogenous* obesity is due to excessive intake of food.

withdrawal (with-draw′al). The removal of a substance to which the individual has become addicted. Sudden withdrawal of certain substances can be very dangerous. This also refers to a set of physiological symptoms that occur when an individual is no longer taking a substance he or she has become addicted to.

Introduction

The abuse of alcohol, nicotine, certain drugs, and other chemical substances is a health and social problem that affects everyone. The cost of substance abuse runs into the billions of dollars; most of which goes to combat crime by drug users, to pay for property and personal injury resulting from accidents involving substance abuse, and for social and psychiatric services to victims of drug abuse. Increased taxation and higher insurance are pocketbook expenses that can be calculated in measurable terms. Not so easily measured is the absenteeism from school or work, the defective products produced by affected workers, and the waste of human potential epitomized by the addict.

So widespread is the practice of substance abuse that no community is without the problem. The abuse of alcohol and tobacco is well known because these substances have been marketed to the public for hundreds of years. All but the smallest child can recognize when a person is under the influence of alcohol because the physiologic changes caused by the use of this drug are well known. Less well known are the serious organ damage and sociological problems that can result when social drinking degenerates into the disease of alcoholism.

Smoking was an accepted part of adult behavior until it was linked by medical evidence to cancer, heart disease, and other serious health problems. These health risks, emphasis on fitness, and the efforts of antismoking advocates have succeeded in reducing the number of nicotine addicts.

Other legal and illegal drugs are less well understood by the public and, when abused, can be more dangerous than alcohol and nicotine because their potency may vary widely and the user may have little or no experience with the adverse effects of an overdose. The use of psychoactive (mind altering) substances by large numbers of people of both sexes and from all socioeconomic strata is a relatively recent occurrence that has spread to all parts of the United States since the 1960s. The proliferation of drug use by the general population in all age groups has awakened national concern over the illegal use of certain drugs, and the abuse of other common chemical agents.

Getting Started on Drugs

Today's typical American is better informed and more health conscious than ever before, but most will succumb to peer pressure or their own curiosity and try beer, wine, liquor, and tobacco before they reach the minimum age for purchasing such products. Consumption of alcohol in moderate amounts is a socially accepted practice throughout the world. As such, there are numerous role models for the young people who want to continue drinking into adulthood.

The same social pressures that influence young people to try alcohol are responsible for introducing people of all ages to marijuana, cocaine, PCP, LSD, heroin, amphetamines, and other chemical substances. Because it is easier to prevent drug abuse than it is to break an established habit, most antidrug campaigns focus on the young, often giving the impression that older people are not drug abusers. Nothing could be further from the truth.

Special Considerations: The Older Adult

According to an article in the Journal of the American Medical Association (JAMA), doctors should prepare for an increase in the number of elderly alcoholics. If the alcoholism rate remains constant, it is expected to have jumped by 50 percent between 1970 and the turn of the century. This information is based upon the aging of the population. A U.S. Census Bureau projection indicates that by the year 2030 there will be more people over 65 years of age than people under 18 years of age. Alcohol is a psychotropic drug that affects mood, judgment, behavior, concentration, and consciousness. It is a direct multisystem toxin and central nervous system depressant. Alcohol can cause drowsiness, incoordination, slurring of speech, sudden mood changes, aggression, belligerency, grandiosity, and uninhibited behavior. It can also cause stupor, coma, and death if taken excessively. Because of the increased susceptibility of older adults to the toxic effects of alcohol, a person can develop alcohol problems just by becoming older, and this may occur without necessarily increasing the amount of alcohol consumed. Manifestations of alcohol abuse in older adults are generally more subtle, atypical, and nonspecific than in younger people.

Some Drugs That Interact with Alcohol

- **Antibiotics:** chloramphenicol, furazolidone, griseofulvin, metronidazole, some cephalosporins may interact with acute alcohol consumption and produce a disulfiram-like (Antabuse-like) reaction which is a severe hypersensitivity to alcohol. Symptoms that may occur are: flushing, chest pain, palpitations, tachycardia, hypotension, syncope (fainting), and arrhythmias.
- **Salicylates and aspirin:** alcohol increases the tendency of salicylates to cause gastrointestinal bleeding. Aspirin increases alcohol absorption and results in elevated blood alcohol levels.
- **Acetaminophen:** may increase susceptibility to acetaminophen-induced liver toxicity.
- **Tricyclic antidepressants:** alcohol may accelerate the clearance of these antidepressants and depressed patients who mix alcohol and these drugs may not achieve the appropriate blood levels of the antidepressant.
- **Sedatives and anxiolytics:** alcohol enhances the sedative action and causes psychomotor impairment.
- **Monoamine oxidase inhibitors (MAOIs):** may produce disulfiram-like (Antabuse-like) effects. Dark beers and red wines contain tyramine and may produce hypertensive episodes.
- **Opioids:** respiratory depressant effects of both alcohol and opioids may be potentiated.
- **Anticoagulants:** long-term drinkers metabolize warfarin more rapidly and careful monitoring of anticoagulant therapy/blood studies is essential.
- **Cimetidine, ranitidine, and rizatidine:** may increase blood alcohol levels by reducing alcohol metabolism in the stomach.
- **Oral hypoglycemic agents:** when ingested with alcohol, significant decreases in blood sugar levels may be produced.
- **Lithium:** may reduce alcohol-induced intoxication as information processing in the brain is reduced.
- **Certain antihistamines:** alcohol enhances sedative effect.
- **Certain cardiovascular drugs:** may markedly increase alcohol's effects.

Special Considerations: The Child

Alcohol abuse is the number-one drug problem of American children. Although most states have legal drinking ages of between 18 and 21 years of age, these laws have not prevented younger individuals from drinking. It is estimated that there are 3.3 million problem drinkers among 14- to 17-year-olds—19 percent of the population.

The first drinking experience generally occurs at about 12 years of age and the amount and frequency of drinking increases with age. Alcohol is a mind-altering drug that works as a depressant. The abusive effects of alcohol on a child's body systems can cause vomiting, diarrhea, ulcers, cirrhosis of the liver, pancreatitis, and brain damage.

Alcohol is also the drug most commonly abused by females of childbearing age. No "safe" level of alcohol intake during pregnancy is known. Three cans of beer per day, three glasses of wine or three mixed drinks per day, and/or repetitive binge drinking is known to increase the risk of alcohol-related infant defects. Maternal use of alcohol can cause spontaneous abortion and Fetal Alcohol Syndrome (FAS), which includes growth retardation before and after birth, facial and cranial abnormalities, and mental retardation and developmental delay.

The U.S. Department of Education has designed a quiz for parents to help them learn about drug abuse and how it impacts families. To assist you in your learning about substance abuse, the following are the questions and answers to this quiz.

1. What is the most commonly used drug in the United States?
   a. heroin
   b. cocaine
   c. *alcohol*
   d. marijuana
2. Name the three drugs most commonly used by children. *Alcohol, tobacco, and marijuana.*
3. Which drug is associated with the most teenage deaths? *Alcohol.*
4. Which of the following contains the most alcohol?
   a. a 12-ounce can of beer
   b. a cocktail
   c. a 12-ounce wine cooler
   d. a 5-ounce glass of wine
   e. *all contain equal amounts of alcohol (1.5 ounces)*
5. Crack is a particularly dangerous drug because it is:
   a. cheap
   b. readily available
   c. highly addictive
   d. *all of the above*

6. Fumes from which of the following can be inhaled to produce a high?
   a. spray paint
   b. model glue
   c. nail polish remover
   d. whipped cream canisters
   e. *all of the above*

7. People who have used alcohol and other drugs before their 20th birthday:*
   a. have no risk of becoming chemically dependent
   b. are less likely to develop a drinking problem or use illicit drugs
   c. *have an increased risk of becoming chemically dependent*

   *children who use alcohol before age 15 are very likely to have drug-related problems later in life

8. A speedball is a combination of which two drugs? *Cocaine and heroin.*

9. Anabolic steroids are dangerous because they result in:
   a. development of female characteristics in males
   b. development of male characteristics in females
   c. stunted growth
   d. damage to liver and cardiovascular system
   e. overly aggressive behavior
   f. *all of the above*

10. How much alcohol can a pregnant woman safely consume?*
    a. a 6-ounce glass of wine with dinner
    b. two 12-ounce cans of beer
    c. five 4-ounce shots of whiskey a month
    d. *none*

    *there have been no "safe" limits established

Critical Thinking Questions/Activities

Prepare a presentation on alcohol abuse among American children. Using the information in Special Considerations: The Child and any other reference that you need: Ask yourself:

- What is the legal drinking age in the state where I live?
- How many problem drinkers exist among the 12- to 17-year-old age group?
- At what age do most children first try drinking?
- What are some of the abusive effects of alcohol on a child's body?
- What amount of beer, wine, or mixed drinks per day can increase the risk of alcohol-related infant defects?
- What quiz could I use to help others understand about drug abuse?

Getting Hooked on Drugs

Not everyone who drinks becomes an alcoholic, but millions are habitual users of this drug because they are seeking the effects that alcohol has on the central nervous system. Habitual use of other psychoactive drugs may or may not lead to psychological and/or physical dependency; however, many of these substances are much more likely to cause dependency than is alcohol. Just as no one begins drinking with the objective of becoming an alcoholic, neither does the drug abuser plan to become drug dependent. Unfortunately, the body develops a tolerance for most abused substances. Increases in both dosage and frequency of use are needed in order to achieve the same degree of effect that was once possible with smaller or less frequent doses. Abuse with high doses of psychoactive substances leads to dependency. Physical dependency occurs when one or more of the body's physiologic functions becomes dependent on the presence of the abused drug. Psychological dependency does not involve the body's physiologic functions; rather, it is a psychic craving for the effects produced by the abused substance.

Groups of Drugs

Amphetamines

Drugs of the amphetamine group are prescription medications designed for oral use in the treatment of exogenous obesity, narcolepsy, and attention deficit disorder. *Amphetamine sulfate, dextroamphetamine sulfate* (Dexedrine), *methamphetamine sulfate* (Desoxyn), *methylphenidate HCl* (Ritalin), and *phenmetrazine HCl* (Preludin) have a high potential for abuse and are classed as Schedule II drugs under the Federal Controlled Substances Act. These drugs stimulate the central nervous system and cause increased alertness, elevation of mood, reduction of appetite, and a diminished sense of fatigue.

The misuse and abuse of amphetamines relates to the effects these drugs have upon the central nervous system. They have been taken to avoid sleep while studying or driving, and they have also been taken by athletes in an attempt to improve performance. Primarily, these drugs are abused by those seeking euphoric excitement, or by those who want to counter the effects of depressant drugs. Street names for amphetamines are *speed, crystal, bennies, wake-ups*, and *pep pills.*

Euphoria, excitement, anorexia, and insomnia are but a few of the possible effects of amphetamines. Those abusing these drugs may also experience dilated pupils, talkativeness, nervousness, agitation, dizziness, increased or decreased blood pressure, palpitations, tachycardia or bradycardia, pallor or flushing, dry mouth, abdominal pain, chills, fever, and fatigue.

If amphetamine use is abruptly stopped, the heavy user exhibits withdrawal symptoms. These symptoms usually include fatigue, long but disturbed sleep, irritability, strong hunger, and deep depression that may lead to attempted suicide.

Cocaine

Like the amphetamines, cocaine is a central nervous system stimulant. This drug is extracted from the leaves of *Erythroxylon coca*, a plant that can be found in a number of South American countries. Cocaine hydrochloride (HCl), a fine, white, crystal-like powder, is the most available form of the drug and is used medically for surface anesthesia of the ear, nose, throat, rectum, and vagina. Cocaine has a high potential for abuse and is classified as a Schedule II drug under the Federal Controlled Substances Act.

As an abused substance, cocaine is usually sniffed or snorted into the nose, although some users inject it or smoke a form of the drug called *crack* or *freebase*. Cocaine is readily absorbed through mucous membranes; thus the reason for snorting it into the nasal passageway. Its effects begin within a few minutes, reach a peak within 15 to 20 minutes, and subside within an hour. These effects include dilated pupils, increases in blood pressure, heart rate, breathing rate, and body temperature. The drug's high potential for abuse relates to its ability to cause feelings of euphoria, excitement, and a sense of well-being. In addition, other desirable effects are feeling more energetic or alert, and a reduction of appetite.

Crack or freebase cocaine is made by chemically converting cocaine HCl to a purified, altered form of the drug that is more suitable for smoking. This altered form of the drug resembles beige or brownish clumps of sugar which, when smoked, produces an intense feeling of euphoria in less than 10 seconds. This instant "high" lasts only 5 to 25 minutes and is followed, almost immediately, by an equally intense depression. To avoid the depression, there is a strong need to smoke more of the drug. Crack can cause serious psychological dependency in as little as two weeks and, of those addicted to crack, experts predict 9 out of 10 will continue to abuse the drug despite efforts at rehabilitation.

Cocaine hydrochloride, while not as powerful as crack, is a very dangerous, dependency-producing drug. The feeling of well-being produced by cocaine can cause some of its users to center their lives around seeking and using this drug. Street names for cocaine are *blow, coke, flake, gold dust, nose candy, rock, snow*, and *white girl*. The street name for the combination of cocaine and heroin is *speedball*.

The adverse effects of cocaine use include perforated nasal septum, chills, fever, runny nose, ventricular fibrillation, cocaine psychosis, and death from respiratory and circulatory failure.

Barbiturates

The barbiturates are a group of drugs derived from barbituric acid. Although they may vary in onset of action, potency, and duration of effect, all are central nervous system depressants. Barbiturates are used medically as sedatives, to relieve anxiety, to treat insomnia, and in the control of epilepsy. Misuse of barbiturate drugs may grow out of poorly supervised prescription use of these agents. Patients may arbitrarily increase the dosage and frequency of use in response to self-perceived needs. Misuse of barbiturates can lead to their abuse because prolonged use results in tolerance and dependency.

Because of their potential for abuse, barbiturates are classified as Schedule II, III, and IV drugs under the Federal Controlled Substances Act. Those classified as Schedule II are *amobarbital* (Amytal), *pentobarbital* (Nembutal), and *secobarbital* (Seconal). Street names for barbiturates are *barbs, blues, downers, goof balls, yellow jacket (pentobarbital) red devil (secobarbital),* and *blue devil (amobarbital).* These drugs are generally taken orally in tablet or capsule form, but may be prepared as a solution for intravenous injection.

Relief from anxiety and sedation occurs when dosages of barbiturates are taken as prescribed. Higher doses may produce slurred speech, confusion, poor motor coordination, impaired judgment, and drowsiness. Very high doses can produce coma, respiratory arrest, circulatory collapse, and death.

Abrupt discontinuance of barbiturates can induce withdrawal symptoms that can be fatal. Such symptoms include apprehension, weakness, dizziness, tremors, nausea, vomiting, sweating, disturbed vision, insomnia, hypotension, headache, delirium, and convulsion.

Narcotic Analgesics (Opiates)

Opiates, sometimes referred to as narcotics, are a group of drugs derived from *opium*, some of which are used medically to relieve pain. Opiates have a high potential for abuse and can cause dependency if abused or when occasional use extends over a long period of time. Opium is a dark brown substance obtained by air-drying the juice of unripe seed pods of Asian poppy plants. A number of other drugs, including *morphine, codeine*, and *heroin*, have been derived from opium. Other opiates, such as *meperidine* (Demerol) and *hydromorphone hydrochloride* (Dilaudid) are synthetic or semisynthetic drugs with morphine-like qualities.

The use of opium is prohibited in the United States. Heroin is a Schedule I drug under the Federal Controlled Substances Act because of its high abuse potential and the lack of any acceptable medical use. Other natural and synthetic opiates are listed as Schedule II drugs which have medical applications.

Heroin, sometimes called *junk* or *smack*, accounts for 90 percent of the opiate abuse in the United States in spite of the fact that its sale or possession is illegal. Most street preparations are "cut" with other substances such as sugar or quinine and appear as a white or brownish powder. Because the effects of heroin (or morphine) are significantly diminished when taken orally, intravenous injection is the route of administration preferred by drug abusers.

Patients beginning treatment with an opiate, and those misusing these drugs for the first time, often experience nausea, vomiting, itching, and restlessness. This initial unpleasantness precedes a feeling of relaxation, drowsiness, and/or euphoria. With continued use, the unpleasant side effects of these drugs are diminished. Users develop a drug tolerance and larger dosages are required to produce the same effects. Drug dependence is easily established with opiate use. Finding and using the drug often becomes the primary focus in the lives of users. Since heroin use is very expensive, those addicted to this opiate often resort to criminal acts to pay for their habit.

The physical dangers associated with opiate abuse depend on the specific drug used, its source, the dose, and the route of administration. Most of the danger can be attributed to using too much of the drug, use of unsterile hypodermic needles, contamination of the drug itself, or combining the drug with other substances. Infections from contaminated solutions, syringes, and needles can cause liver disease, tetanus, serum hepatitis, and acquired immune deficiency syndrome (AIDS).

When the opiate-dependent person stops taking the drug, withdrawal symptoms become evident within 4 to 6 hours of the last dose. Symptoms include uneasiness, diarrhea, abdominal cramps, chills, sweating, nausea, runny nose, and tearing of the eyes. The intensity of withdrawal symptoms correlates with the dosage taken, the frequency of use, and the length of time that the user has been dependent on the drug. Withdrawal symptoms for most opiates grow stronger approximately 24 to 72 hours after they begin and subside within 7 to 10 days; however, symptoms such as sleeplessness and drug craving can last for months.

Marijuana

Two widely abused substances, marijuana and hashish, are obtained from the hemp plant *Cannabis sativa.* Both drugs owe their popularity to the same psychoactive component, *tetrahydrocannabinol,* better known as THC. The major differences in these two drugs are their appearance and the amount of THC each contains.

Marijuana is composed of the flowering tops and leaves of the plant. The seeds and stems of the plant may also be included when preparing marijuana for use by drug abusers. It may range in color from greyish-green to greenish brown, and vary in texture from fine to coarse. The fine textured marijuana resembles the spice oregano whereas the coarse textured drug looks like tea. The street names for marijuana are *Acapulo gold, grass, joint, Mary Jane, pot, reefer, roach, tea,* and *weed.*

Hashish is the dried resin extracted from the flowers, tops, and leaves of the female plant. This gummy extract, when dried, may range in color from light brown to black and in texture from soft to hard. Hashish also differs from marijuana in that an equal amount of hashish can contain five to ten times as much THC, thereby making it a much more potent drug.

Although it is possible to chew or swallow these substances, the most common method of use is by smoking. Marijuana is usually prepared for use as hand-rolled cigarettes, although it may be smoked in special pipes. Hashish is usually smoked in small pipes. Smoking these substances produces the euphoric effect of THC quicker than other methods of administration. The use of marijuana or hashish has been shown to produce moderate tolerance to the effects of THC; thereby requiring increased usage to produce similar effects.

The effects produced by marijuana and hashish are dose related and can be influenced by such factors as the user's level of tolerance for the drug, the method of use, the concurrent use of other drugs such as alcohol, and the user's psychological state of mind. The use of moderate amounts of marijuana or hashish produces feelings of euphoria, relaxation, and drowsiness. The user may become less inhibited, talking and laughing more than usual. Coordination and judgement may be affected in much the same way as they are by alcohol. With larger doses, there is the tendency to misjudge the passage of time, and the user's perceptions of sound, color, and taste may be sharpened or distorted. In very large doses, the effects of cannabis may cause hallucinations. The effects of marijuana and hashish generally last for several hours. About 5 percent of regular users of these drugs will develop some degree of psychological dependence. Physical dependence and withdrawal symptoms are not usually associated with these drugs.

Aside from the euphoric effect that gives these drugs their high potential for abuse, they tend to increase the heart rate, decrease pulmonary function, and increase appetite. To this end, their use may aggravate an existing medical condition such as heart disease or hypertension. Although marijuana has been reported as beneficial in reducing nausea suffered by patients undergoing cancer chemotherapy, it remains classified as a Schedule I drug under the Federal Controlled Substances Act.

Phencyclidine (PCP)

Phencyclidine (PCP) was originally developed for use as a surgical anesthetic; however, its unwanted and undesirable side effects caused its experimental use with humans to be discontinued. Today, the only legal use for phencyclidine is with animals through licensed veterinary clinics. Unfortunately, limiting this drug's use to veterinary medicine has not prevented its abuse by those acquainted with its psychoactive properties. PCP is readily available from illegal suppliers because it is easily made. The chemicals needed to manufacture this drug are readily available to illegal labs across the country that are interested in making a profit.

The street names for PCP are *angel dust, cosmos, jet, mist, peace pill, rocket fuel, superjoint, tranq*, and *whack*. Since it is cheaply manufactured, PCP is frequently used to "cut" more expensive drugs; thereby increasing the drug dealer's profits. It may be found as a powder, in tablet form, or as a capsule. In that PCP is usually produced illegally, the size, shape, and color of the tablet may vary, making it possible to masquerade it as other popular street drugs.

For the same reasons that researchers discontinued medical use of PCP, many drug abusers have also labeled it as a bad drug. Its effects are often unpredictable and, since it is produced illegally, one cannot tell how much PCP is in a powder, tablet, or capsule. The most popular method for taking the drug is by sprinkling the powder on a marijuana cigarette and smoking the combination of drugs. Other methods include taking it orally in any of its available forms, or injecting a solution containing the drug.

Users of PCP often have difficulty describing its effects; however, most agree that it gives them a feeling that is different from other drugs. The psychoactive effects are described as hallucinogenic, sometimes pleasant, sometimes not, but usually associated with a world of fantasy. As the effects of the drug wear off, users report feeling depressed, irritated, and somewhat alienated from their surroundings. While under the influence of PCP, users may appear confused, expressionless, or intoxicated. Speech is often confused, vision distorted, and the user has difficulty thinking and remembering. Some users become violent and aggressive, while others withdraw and resist communicating with others. High doses of PCP can induce prolonged stupor or even coma for periods of a few days to several weeks. Long-term users of PCP are subject to recurring episodes of anxiety or depression, and regularly experience disturbances in memory, judgment, concentration, and perception, even after they have stopped taking the drug. Accidental death in which the victim fails to perceive danger is more likely to occur while under the influence of PCP than is death by chemical overdose. Users have been known to drown in shallow water, fall from buildings, and die of burns in circumstances that would have been avoided by less disoriented people.

SPOTLIGHT

Inhalant Abuse and the Return of LSD

Inhalant use is on the rise, particularly among middle-age school children. One in five eighth-graders, 20 percent, has done some sniffing during their lifetime, making inhalants the drug of choice for that age group, according to Patrick O'Malley, a University of Michigan researcher who surveyed teenagers on inhalant use.

The American Council for Drug Education says sniffing products, even just one time can lead to brain damage, kidney failure, loss of concentration, and death. In Georgia in 1993, two teenagers died of intentional inhalant exposure. A 14-year old boy inhaled butane fuel, and a 16-year old inhaled VCR tape-head cleaner. Both died immediately. There are probably more deaths that don't get reported as such because doctors classify them as heart failure or drug abuse.

Nationally, estimates on inhalant deaths per year range from 100 to 1,000. Researchers rely on surveys because it is difficult to determine how many kids use inhalants. One sniff can kill, yet teenagers are huffing household products at a numbing rate. Most household products, such as fabric protectors and paint thinners, have warning labels that specify the dangers of inhaling.

"Once I figured it out, I started looking for things that said 'Do Not Inhale'," said a 14-year old eighth-grader who is now in a recovery program. Another 14-year old, also now in a treatment program, said that she could get a "strange floating sensation" by sniffing a fabric protector that she found at home. "I would spray it on my sweater and put my mouth up to it to inhale. I would put it in my backpack and when the teacher wasn't looking I'd spray it on my sweater all day. Everybody was kind of into it, but after awhile, they said to me, 'Maybe you should cool it with that stuff.'"

She didn't cool it. She had easy access to it because it was always around her house. But after three months, her mother caught on to her strange behavior. The girl's mother said she noticed that her daughter, an honor student who excelled at gymnastics and dance, became a very angry child during that time. She detected a faint smell, but figured the teenager was just spraying her shoes with a lot of Scotchguard.®

(continued)

Instant death is always a possibility when using inhalants. The impact of inhalants is unpredictable and could be affected by the user's size, general health, amount inhaled, and type of product.

What happens to the body when one uses inhalants?

- Brain: euphoric, floating sensation. Can cause brain damage, headache, dizziness, disorientation, memory loss, blurry vision, fainting, impaired speech, learning disabilities, death.
- Lungs: irritation of airway passage, chest tightness, coughing, difficulty in breathing, suffocation, death.
- Heart: adrenaline rushes to the heart. The heart reacts with fast, irregular beats, heart failure, sudden death.
- Body: damage to kidneys and liver, vomiting, bone marrow disorders, leukemia, coma, death.

The popularity of inhalants tends to decrease slightly as the students get older and move on to hard drugs, such as marijuana and LSD according to the study conducted by Patrick O'Malley at the University of Michigan. According to Joe Sullivan, a special agent with the U.S. Drug Enforcement Administration in Atlanta, the use of lysergic acid diethylamide (LSD) has surged nationwide, especially among suburban, middle- and upper-class white teens and young adults.

School officials in suburban Atlanta say they are seeing increasing problems with LSD. A student collapsed in choir class after ingesting LSD, and a high school student was charged with selling LSD to another student. Sullivan says young people are enticed into trying LSD in the belief it will give them an intellectual experience.

To be sure, LSD is not the drug of choice for most teenagers who abuse alcohol, marijuana, and inhalants far more frequently than hallucinogens. Scientists at the University of Michigan Institute for Social Research, have documented dramatic increases in reported use of marijuana and LSD among secondary school students in the 1990's, as well as other hallucinogens, inhalants, stimulants, barbiturates, and cocaine and crack.

Warning Signs of Inhalant Abuse

- Chemical smell
- Drunken appearance
- Flu-like symptoms (headache, nausea, runny nose)
- Lack of attention (difficulty in staying awake)
- Paraphernalia (soda cans, plastic bags, rags and old socks that smell of chemicals)
- Rash or sores around the mouth or nose
- Weight loss

Lysergic Acid Diethylamide (LSD)

Lysergic acid diethylamide (LSD) or "acid" as it is sometimes called, is a hallucinogenic agent that has no accepted medical use. As such, LSD is classified as a Schedule I drug under the Federal Controlled Substances Act. The psychoactive effects of the drug are influenced by such factors as the environment in which it is being used, the user's personality, and the user's state of mind at the time the drug was taken. When LSD is taken in pleasant surroundings by a stable, unthreatened personality, the effect on the user can be pleasant and has been described as a "good trip." Alter any of these circumstances and this mood-related drug can provoke unpleasant hallucinations, and a "bad trip."

LSD is usually taken orally, often by absorbing the drug in a sugar cube or other substance. Because it is an extremely potent drug, a dose as small as 25 mcg is capable of producing psychoactive effects in some users. Higher doses of LSD have been associated with effects such as alteration of perception wherein the user can "hear" colors, "taste" sounds, and see structural changes as they occur in objects. Those who use LSD may also experience mood changes that range from euphoria to deep depression.

Whether or not LSD produces lasting physical changes in those who take the drug is a subject that is under examination. There is some evidence that long-term use can cause chromosome damage and lead to subsequent birth defects. Incidences of serious adverse reactions to LSD have rarely been reported when the dosage taken was not excessive. There have been incidences where users suffered prolonged adverse psychological effects from LSD; however, the greatest danger presented by the drug appears to be from accidents and suicide attempts by those under its influence.

Inhalants

Inhalants are breathable chemicals that produce psychoactive vapors. These substances are most often abused by those under the age of 17 and include such common products as gasoline, nail polish remover, lighter fluid, cleaning fluids, airplane glue, and aerosol sprays. Other less easily obtained inhalants that have been abused include *amyl nitrite, butyl nitrite*, and the anesthetics *nitrous oxide* (laughing gas) and *halothane*.

Amyl nitrite is used with heart patients and for diagnostic purposes because it dilates blood vessels and increases the rate of heartbeat. Available by prescription only, amyl nitrite is a clear, yellowish liquid. Because it is contained in sealed bulb-like containers that cause a snapping sound when broken, amyl nitrite has also been referred to as "poppers" or "snappers."

Since 1979, when amyl nitrite was restricted to prescription use only, there has been an increase in the abuse of butyl nitrite. This substance is packaged in small bottles and sold under such street names as "locker room" and "rush." When inhaled, it produces a "high" that lasts from a few seconds to several minutes. More specifically, butyl nitrite causes a decrease in blood pressure, an increase in heart rate, flushing of the face and neck, dizziness, and headache.

Other inhalants are abused because they also cause similar effects. At low doses, the user may feel somewhat stimulated. Somewhat higher doses of an inhalant can result in a reduction of inhibition or loss of consciousness. Inhalant abuse may result in negative effects on the body that range from nausea and vomiting to heart failure and death. Breathing concentrated vapors from paper bags increases the risk of central nervous system depression and suffocation. Continued abuse of inhalant substances can cause damage to the liver, kidneys, blood, and bone marrow.

Recognizing Substance Abuse

As a member of a health-care team, the nurse is likely to encounter patients who are substance abusers. Aside from the usual disease conditions that might cause an individual to seek medical attention, those who abuse drugs are at greater risk of sustaining accidental injury or infection as a result of drug use. Additionally, there are patients who will attempt to simulate a disease condition that could result in a prescription for a dependency-producing drug.

Obvious signs of drug abuse are needle tracks on the arms or other parts of the patient's body. They may be observed when taking vital signs or doing other medical procedures. Less obvious indicators of possible drug abuse are jaundice, nasal ulceration, dilated or constricted pupils, slurred speech, confusion, impaired reflex action, neglected appearance, poor hygiene, and early withdrawal symptoms. When substance abuse is suspected, the nurse should reflect a nonjudgmental attitude toward the patient and inform the physician at the earliest opportunity. All information obtained from patients, including evidence of drug abuse, is confidential. Those who provide health care are not allowed to disclose such information unless it becomes necessary to do so during a medical emergency.

Substance Abuse in the Workplace

According to the National Institute on Drug Abuse (NIDA), ten to 23 percent of Americans abuse drugs and alcohol at work. Chemical dependency has an overwhelming impact on industry with the annual cost expressed in absenteeism, waste, theft, lost productivity, and property damage at a cost of $140 billion.

Marijuana and cocaine are the most used illegal drugs, but alcohol and nicotine pose a far wider problem. It is estimated that 6 percent of all workers always have alcohol in their bloodstream. It is believed that one in three Americans use or have recently used drugs at work.

Warning Signs of Substance Abuse in the Workplace

- Performance Deteriorates: Inconsistent work quality and low productivity; increased mistakes, poor concentration, carelessness.
- Poor Attendance and Absenteeism: Absenteeism and tardiness, particularly around weekends; increased physical complaints, vaguely defined illnesses; leaves early for lunch, long breaks, unexplained absences.
- Attitude/Physical Appearance Change: Loss of pride in work, blames others for mis-

takes; avoids contact with co-workers and superiors; drastic change in appearance and hygiene; complaints from co-workers about covering up for him/her.

- Health/Safety Hazards: Increase in on-the-job accidents, carelessness in handling equipment, disregard for co-workers' safety.
- Domestic Problems Emerge: Complaints about family problems, talk of separation divorce; recurring financial problems.

Services Available

There are many services available for individuals who are substance abusers. These services provide information and pamphlets and offer assistance to anyone who is a substance abuser. The following is a list of some of the local, state, and national addresses and/or telephone numbers that offer help.

1. National Clearinghouse for Drug Abuse Information
   P.O. Box 1706
   Rockville, MD 20850
2. National Institute on Drug Abuse (NIDA)
   Prevention Branch
   Room 11 A-33
   5600 Fishers Lane
   Rockville, MD 20857
3. Action Drug Prevention Program
   806 Connecticut Avenue, N.W.
   Washington, DC 20525
4. American Council for Drug Education
   6193 Executive Boulevard
   Rockville, MD 20852
5. National Federation of Parents for Drug Free Youth (NFP)
   P.O. Box 722
   Silver Springs, MD 20901
6. Parent Resources Institute on Drug Education (PRIDE)
   Robert W. Woodroff Building
   100 Edgewood Avenue
   Atlanta, GA 30303
7. American Cancer Society
8. Division of Mental Health, Mental Retardation and Substance Abuse
   Informtion Center
   878 Peachtree St. N.E., Room 321
   Atlanta, GA 30309
   (404) 894-4204

9. Department of Health and Human Services
Public Health Service
Alcohol, Drug Abuse, and Mental Health Administration
Washington, DC 20402

10. Telephone Directory (Yellow Pages)
Drug Abuse and Addiction (Information and Treatment)
Alcoholism Information and Treatment Centers

11. Toll-free telephone numbers
1-800-Cocaine 1-800-USA-2525
1-800-241-7946 OR 1-800-658-2548

Spot Check

It is known that some drugs interact with alcohol. Give the interaction(s) of the following selected drug(s) when taken with alcohol.

Drug(s)	Interaction
Antibiotics	
Salicylates and Aspirin	
Acetaminophen	
Anticoagulants	

Cimetidine	
Lithium	
Certain Antihistamines	

◆ Review Questions

Directions: Select the best answer to each multiple choice question. Circle the letter of your choice.

1. __________ is the psychic craving for a drug, a substance.
   a. Euphoria
   b. Narcolepsy
   c. Dependency
   d. Withdrawal
2. Amphetamines stimulate the central nervous system and cause __________.
   a. increased alertness, elevation of mood, and reduction of appetite
   b. decreased alertness, depression of mood, and stimulation of appetite
   c. increased sense of fatigue
   d. all of these
3. Street names for amphetamines are speed, __________.
   a. downers, and uppers
   b. bennies, wake-ups, and pep pills
   c. amphies, and pep pills
   d. poppers, and pep pills

4. Sudden stoppage of amphetamines in a heavy user may cause the following withdrawal symptoms.
   a. Elation, loss of appetite, and restful sleep
   b. Disturbed sleep, irritability, strong hunger, and deep depression
   c. Disturbed sleep, elation, and anorexia
   d. all of these
5. Cocaine's high potential for abuse relates to its ability to cause __________.
   a. depression, excitement, and stimulation
   b. elation, stimulation, and irritability
   c. euphoria, excitement, and a sense of well-being
   d. none of these
6. __________ or __________ cocaine is made by chemically converting cocaine HCl to a purified, altered form of the drug that is more suitable for smoking.
   a. Crack, freebase
   b. Coke, freebase
   c. Smack, freebase
   d. all of these
7. The adverse effects of cocaine are __________.
   a. perforated nasal septum, chills, fever
   b. runny nose, ventricular fibrillation
   c. cocaine psychosis, and death from respiratory and circulatory failure
   d. all of these
8. Misuse of barbiturates can lead to their abuse because prolonged use results in __________.
   a. sedation and addiction
   b. tolerance and dependency
   c. elation and addiction
   d. none of these
9. Very high doses of barbiturates can produce __________.
   a. coma, respiratory arrest
   b. circulatory collapse
   c. death
   d. all of these
10. The following are all true statements about heroin except it __________.
   a. accounts for 90 percent of the opiate abuse in the United States
   b. is a legal drug
   c. is sometimes called junk or smack
   d. is usually injected
11. The physical dangers associated with opiate abuse may include __________.
   a. the use of unsterile hypodermic needles which could cause AIDS
   b. using too much of the drug
   c. contamination of the drug itself
   d. all of these

12. All of the following are true statements about marijuana except __________.
    a. it is usually smoked
    b. it causes feelings of euphoria, relaxation, and drowsiness
    c. its effects can be felt for several days
    d. regular users will develop some degree of psychological dependency
13. All of the following are true statements about PCP except __________.
    a. it is readily available from legal suppliers
    b. it is known as angel dust, killer weed, and crystal cyclone
    c. its psychoactive effects are described as hallucinogenic
    d. some users become violent and aggressive
14. Lysergic acid diethylamide (LSD) is classified as a Schedule __________ drug.
    a. I b. II c. III d. IV
15. Higher doses of LSD can cause the user to __________.
    a. "hear" colors
    b. "taste" sounds
    c. see structural changes as they occur in objects
    d. all of these
16. __________ are breathable chemicals that produce psychoactive vapors.
    a. Amphetamines
    b. Barbiturates
    c. Opiates
    d. Inhalants
17. All of the following are true statements about the abuse of butyl nitrite except it __________.
    a. is packaged in small bottles
    b. is called "locker room" and "rush"
    c. produces a "low" that lasts from a few seconds to several minutes
    d. causes a decrease in blood pressure
18. The nurse should be aware of signs of possible substance abuse. These signs may include __________.
    a. needle tracks on the arms or other parts of the body
    b. jaundice, nasal ulceration, slurred speech
    c. dilated or constricted pupils, neglected appearance
    d. all of these

Case Study: At 12:35 A.M. a young male is brought into the emergency room by two police officers. The youth has multiple injuries to his head and appears to be in respiratory distress. One of the police officers states that they found the youth face down in front of a local store.

The patient is taken to trauma room 1. An airway is established and 4 liters of oxygen per minute is administered via a Venturi mask. Upon assessing vital signs you notice needle track marks on the antecubital area of the left arm. His vital signs are: BP 160/102, P 120, R 32, T 101.

The patient's nostrils are red and swollen and his pupils are dilated. Crack overdose is suspected.

Based on the clinical data described and your knowledge of substance abuse, select the best answer to each of the following questions.

19. The nurse should know that crack is a form of __________.
    a. morphine
    b. opium
    c. cocaine
    d. heroin
20. Crack produces an intense feeling of euphoria in less than __________.
    a. 30 seconds
    b. 10 seconds
    c. 30 minutes
    d. 10 minutes
21. The most dangerous adverse effects of crack include __________.
    a. respiratory and circulatory failure
    b. perforated nasal septum and chills
    c. fever and runny nose
    d. psychosis and fever
22. Needle marks in the antecubital space indicate __________.
    a. IV drug use
    b. IM drug use
    c. Intradermal drug use
    d. Subcutaneous drug use
23. Crack is a __________.
    a. central nervous system stimulant
    b. central nervous system depressant
    c. peripheral nervous system stimulant
    d. autonomic nervous system stimulant

Matching: Place the correct letter from Column II on the appropriate line of Column I.

Column I	Column II
24. ________ Euphoria	A. Removal of a substance.
25. ________ Narcolepsy	B. Excessive amount of fat on the body.
26. ________ Dependency	C. A feeling of good health.
27. ________ Obesity	D. A chronic condition whereby the patient is unable to control recurrent attacks of drowsiness and sleep.
28. ________ Amphetamines (street names)	E. Angel dust, cosmos, and peace pill.
29. ________ Phencyclidine (PCP) (street names)	F. Speed, crystal, bennies, and pep pills.
30. ________ Withdrawal	G. The psychic craving for a drug.
	H. The physical craving for a drug.

SECTION 5

Effects of Medications on Body Systems

CHAPTER 24

Medications Used for Circulatory System Disorders

OBJECTIVES

Upon completion of this chapter, you should be able to:

- Define the terms listed in the vocabulary.
- State the function of the circulatory system.
- Describe heart disease as the number one cause of death in the United States.
- List the warning signs of a heart attack.
- Describe two primary causes of chest pain.
- List the established risk factors for heart disease.
- Explain why age complicates the treatment regimen for the older adult.
- Describe some factors that can affect the actions, absorption, metabolism, and excretion of cardiovascular drugs.
- Complete the critical thinking questions/activities presented in this chapter.
- Describe three ways that drugs may affect heart action.
- Explain the action of digitalis products.
- State the usual initial or digitalizing dose, the usual maintenance dose, and adverse reactions of selected digitalis products.
- State the actions, uses, contraindications, warnings, adverse reactions, dosage and route, implications for patient care, patient teaching, and special considerations for digitalis preparations, antiarrhythmic agents, vasopressors, nitrate preparations, antihypertensive agents, anticoagulants, antiplatelet drug (aspirin), thrombolytic agents, hematinic agents, agents used in treating megaloblastic anemia, and antilipemic agents.
- Describe the step-care approach to treating hypertension.
- Describe hemostatic agents and their uses.

- Complete the Spot Check on selected drugs that are used to treat circulatory system disorders.
- Answer the review questions correctly.

Vocabulary

adrenergic (ad-ren-er′jik). Pertaining to nerve fibers that, when stimulated, release norepinephrine at their endings.

angiotensin (an″je-o-ten′sin). A vasopressor substance that is formed in the body by interaction of renin and angiotensinogen.

angiotensinogen (an″je-o-ten-sin′o-jen). A serum globulin fraction formed in the liver.

glycoside (gli″ko′sid). A substance that is derived from plants and upon hydrolysis yields a sugar plus additional products.

mast cells. Connective tissue cells that contain heparin and histamine.

megaloblastic anemia (meg″a-lo-blast′ik a-ne′me-a). An anemia in which megaloblasts (large-size nucleated abnormal red blood cells) are found in the blood. Also known as pernicious anemia.

plasminogen (plaz-min′o-jen). A protein that is found in many body tissues and fluids, important in the prevention of fibrin clot formation.

Synopsis: The Circulatory System

The heart and a complex network of arteries, veins, and capillaries make up the circulatory system. The arteries take blood away from the heart to the various organs of the body. Blood, leaving the left side of the heart, enters the aorta and is carried by even smaller arteries to all parts of the body. Within the tissues, tiny arteries empty into microscopic vessels known as *capillaries.* The thin, porous walls of these vessels are easily penetrated by molecules of sugars, salts, gases, and other substances needed by surrounding cells. It is in this network of capillaries that the primary function of the circulatory system is carried out. That function is to bring oxygen and needed nutrients to the cells adjacent to the capillary, and to pick up carbon dioxide and metabolic wastes that need to be removed from the body.

As blood passes through the capillaries, it enters into tiny veins. These veins link up with larger and larger veins and ultimately carry the blood back to the heart. Venous blood enters the right side of the heart and is pumped out again into the pulmonary artery that takes it to the lungs. Once in the lungs, the waste carbon dioxide in the venous blood is removed and a new supply of oxygen is absorbed. The blood is now ready to circulate back through the left side of the heart and the arteries to supply the needs of the body once again. See Figure 24–1 for a drawing of the circulatory system.

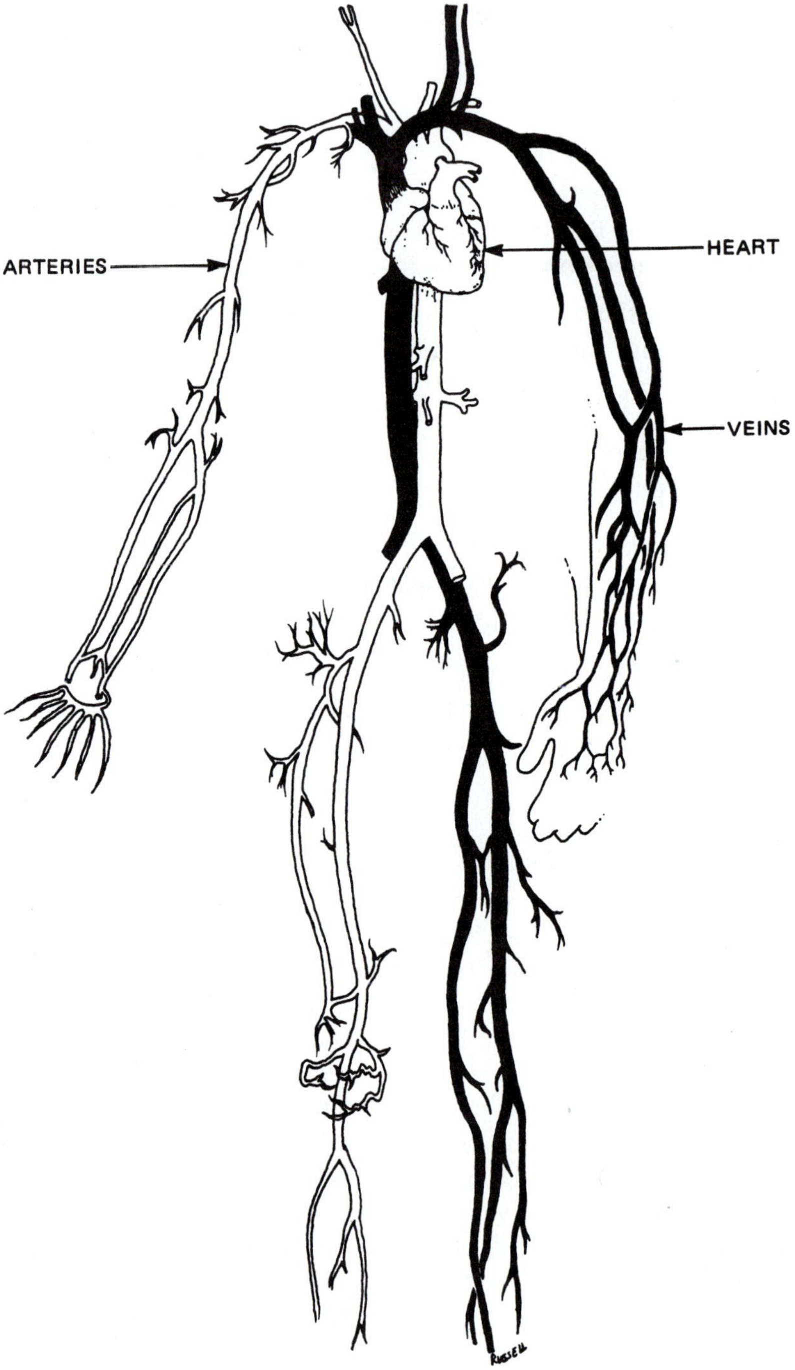

Figure 24–1 The circulatory system *(Courtesy of James Russell, Jr.)*

SPOTLIGHT

Heart Disease

In the United States, one out of four adults is at risk for heart disease. Coronary heart disease is the number one cause of death in the United States, outnumbering the deaths from cancer and accidents combined. It is said that every minute an American suffers a heart attack. Of the Americans alive today, 4.8 million have a history of heart attack, angina, or both. This year, 1.5 million Americans will have a heart attack. About 600,000 will die and of this number 350,000 die before they reach medical help. It is said that the average heart attack victim waits three hours after symptoms occur to seek help. Many times they try to ignore the symptoms or say "it's just indigestion."

The American Heart Association lists the following as warning signs of heart attack:

- Pressure, fullness, squeezing pain in the center of the chest that lasts two minutes or longer.
- Pain that spreads to the shoulders, neck or arms.
- Dizziness, fainting, sweating, nausea, or shortness of breath.

Chest pain can be caused by a variety of conditions, including angina, myocardial infarction, stress, anxiety, and gastrointestinal disorders. It is essential that the physician determine the cause of the pain and treat it appropriately.

The two primary causes of chest pain.

	Angina Pectoris	Myocardial Infarction
Cause(s):	Decreased blood flow through the coronary arteries that causes less oxygen to reach the myocardium.	Occlusion of a coronary artery. Area becomes necrotic (infarct). May be caused by an embolus, vasoconstriction of the arteries, or sudden atherosclerotic changes in the vessels.
Predisposing Factors:	• atherosclerosis • hypertension • diabetes mellitus • syphilis • rheumatic heart disease	• atherosclerosis • hypertension • diabetes mellitus • obesity • family history • smoking • blood cholesterol level: 200–239 borderline high 240 high LDL 130–159 borderline/ 160 high-risk

(continued)

Symptoms:	Sudden, agonizing pain in the substernal region, may radiate to left shoulder and arm, up to jaw; skin cold and clammy; pulse normal; B/P little or no change; anxious, apprehensive.	Severe, crushing pain in the substernal region and upper abdomen, radiates to shoulders, arms, jaw; skin cold and clammy; pulse rapid, weak, irregular; nausea and possible vomiting; B/P drops; extremely apprehensive.

Established Risk Factors

- Male sex
- Family history (heredity)
- Smoking
- Hypertension
- Diabetes mellitus
- Obesity
- Elevated blood cholesterol level
- History of cerebrovascular or occlusive vascular disease

Special Considerations: The Older Adult

More than 2.7 million persons over 60 years of age live with heart disease. Four out of five people who die of heart attacks are 65 years of age or older. With maturity the body begins the inevitable process of aging and the body's ability to restore and repair itself decreases. The heart must work harder to pump against the hardening of the arteries and the increasing systolic blood pressure that is common as one ages. Reduced blood flow, elevated blood lipids (fats), and defective endothelial repair common in aging accelerates the course of cardiovascular disease.

Age is directly related to the development of heart disease, and age complicates the treatment regimen for the older adult because of the normal physiologic changes that occur with aging —the presence of chronic diseases such as arthritis, diabetes, COPD and others, in addition to heart disease, the taking of multiple drugs (polypharmacy), and the possibility of nutritional deficiencies and/or substance abuse. The functional, cognitive, and sensory capacities of the older adult should be carefully evaluated before and during drug therapy. Some other factors that can affect the actions, absorption, metabolism, and excretion of cardiovascular drugs are:

- Slowed intestinal motility. With aging, blood flow to the entire digestive system decreases thereby slowing drug entry into the general circulation. This delay in absorption may weaken the drugs' potency and extend the duration of action.

- Decrease in learn body mass and total body water makes it necessary for smaller dosages of some medications to maintain therapeutic levels without causing toxicity.
- Low serum albumin levels in older adults may allow too much free circulation of drugs that bind with albumin, such as digoxin. The increased risk of adverse effects and toxicity may occur because the drug's plasma concentration is too high.
- Age or disease related cardiovascular changes can slow drug distribution to tissues and prolong the time until onset and duration of action.
- The efficiency of the kidneys and liver can decline with age, decreasing their ability to excrete drugs, which may necessitate drug dosage reductions.

Special Considerations: The Child

Pulse, respiration, blood pressure, and hematologic values vary with the age of the child. In the newborn, the pulse may vary from 110–160 beats per minute, respirations 40–50 per minute, and blood pressure 50–52/25–30. The newborn's circulation begins to function shortly after birth and if proper adaptations do not take place, congenital heart disease may occur. Annually, approximately 25,000 babies in the United States are born with congenital heart defects.

The development of the fetal heart is usually completed during the first 2 months of intrauterine life. It is completely formed and functioning by 10 weeks, and most congenital heart defects develop before the tenth week of pregnancy. Pediatric cardiologists have recognized more than 50 congenital heart defects. If the left side of the heart is not completely separated from the right side, various septal defects develop. If the four chambers of the heart do not occur normally, complex anomalies form such as tetralogy of Fallot, a congenital heart defect involving pulmonary stenosis, ventricular septal defect, dextro position of the aorta, and hypertrophy of the right ventricle.

The causes of congenital heart disease may be classified as exogenous congenital heart disease, and chromosomal abnormalities are among the most important endogenous causes.

- Viruses—during the first 3 months of pregnancy, the rubella (German measles) virus is associated with a high incidence of congenital heart disease in the infant. It is believed that the virus enters the fetal circulation and damages the developing heart.
  Prevention: rubella can be prevented by immunization.
- Alcohol—affects the fetal heart directly and interferes with its development. Fetal alcohol syndrome is often associated with heart defects.
  Prevention: there is no "safe" level of alcohol consumption for the pregnant female. All alcohol should be avoided during pregnancy.

Critical Thinking: Questions/Activities

Your patient is a 72-year-old male who has been admitted with angina pectoris and hypertension. He complains of having experienced a sudden, agonizing pain in his chest, that radiated to his left shoulder, and his skin is cold and clammy and he appears anxious. His physician has ordered blood studies, a chest x-ray, and an electrocardiogram stat. He has asked that the patient continue his sublingual nitroglycerin PRN and atenolol (Tenormin) 50 mg once daily. Ask yourself:

- What are some of the factors that cause angina pectoris and hypertension in the older adult?
- What are some factors that may complicate the treatment regimen for an older adult?
- What are some other factors that can affect the actions, absorption, metabolism, and excretion of cardiovascular drugs?
- What type of cardiovascular drug is nitroglycerin?
- What should I teach the patient about this medication?
- What type of cardiovascular drug is atenolol (Tenormin)?
- What should I teach the patient about this medication?

Drugs That Affect the Heart

The agents discussed in this chapter may affect heart action in one or more of the following ways:

1. Exert a positive or negative inotropic effect by increasing or decreasing the force of myocardial contraction.
2. Exert a positive or negative chronotropic effect by increasing or decreasing heart rate.
3. Exert a positive or negative dromotropic effect by increasing or decreasing the conduction of electrical impulses through the heart muscle.

Digitalis

In the treatment of congestive heart failure, therapy usually includes the use of a digitalis drug together with a diuretic, a low-sodium diet, and a reduction of physical activities. This combination of drugs, diet, and change in lifestyle is designed to increase cardiac output while reducing pulmonary congestion and the lower-body edema that is characteristic of this disorder.

Digitalis is obtained by crushing into a powder the dried leaves of the plant *Digitalis purpurea* or purple foxglove. A similar drug, digoxin, is obtained from the leaves of *Digitalis lanatas.* The primary use for these and other digitalis compounds is the treatment of various types of heart failures and, together, they belong to a chemical classification known as *cardiac glycosides* , Table 24–1. These drugs exert a positive inotropic effect on the heart. They strengthen the heart muscle (myocardium), increase the force of systolic contraction, slow the heart, and improve the muscle tone of the myocardium. As a result of these effects on the heart, there is a decrease in venous pressure as the heart takes in larger amounts of venous blood. Improving the effectiveness of the heart's pumping action reduces the size of the heart and increases the flow of blood to the kidneys; thereby causing a diuretic effect and the removal of some excess fluid from the body. Additional fluids are removed through the use of diuretic drugs.

The pharmacologic actions of all digitalis compounds are similar, but these products differ in their potency, onset of action, and the rate at which they are absorbed. Digitalis drugs may be given parenterally, although the oral route is generally preferred.

When first started, an *initial* or *digitalizing* dose is often given to bring the serum level of the drug up to the desired level. The effect of the initial dose is then sustained by smaller daily *maintenance doses.* When a digitalizing dose is not given, the administration of maintenance doses over a period of about seven days will usually result in sufficient accumulation of the drug to produce the desired serum level. The amount of the initial and maintenance doses may vary, depending upon the size of the patient and whether or not there is normal renal or hepatic function. Frequently, maintenance doses of digitalis drugs must be taken throughout the remainder of a patient's lifetime.

Digitalis intoxication can occur when there is excess accumulation of the drug in the body. This can occur when the initial or digitalizing dose is administered too rapidly, or from maintenance doses that are larger than necessary. The difference between therapeutic and toxic doses of digitalis is generally not great. Signs of digitalis intoxication have been reported in up to 20 percent of hospitalized patients receiving the drug; therefore, those who administer this medication should observe the patient for possible toxic reactions.

Table 24–1 Digitalis Drugs (Cardiac Glycosides)

Medication	Usual Initial or Digitalizing Dose	Usual Maintenance Dose
deslanoside (Cedilanid-D)	1.6 mgh IM or IV.	Not used for maintenance.
digitoxin (Crystodigin) (Digitaline)	Oral, IV: 06 mg initially followed by 0.4 mg and then 0.2 mg at 4–6 hour intervals; or 0.2 mg twice daily for 4 days.	0.05–0.3 mg daily.
digoxin (Lanoxin)	Oral: 0.5–0.75 mg initially, then 0.25–0.5 mg every 6–8 hours until therapeutic levels are obtained. IV: 0.4–0.6 mg initially, then 0.25 mg every 4–6 hours until therapeutic levels are reached.	0.125–0.5 mg daily.

Digitalis Preparations

Actions. Digitalis drugs strengthen the heart muscle, increase the force and velocity of myocardial systolic contraction (positive inotropic effect), slow the heart rate (negative chronotropic effect), and decrease conduction velocity through the atrioventricular (AV) node.

Uses. Congestive heart failure, atrial fabrillation, atrial flutter, paroxysmal atrial tachycardia.

Contraindications. Contraindicated in patients with known hypersensitivity to any of its ingredients and in ventricular fibrillation.

Warnings:

1. The use of digitalis drugs for the treatment of obesity is unwarranted and dangerous. They can cause potentially fatal arrhythmias or other adverse reactions.
2. Anorexia, nausea, vomiting and arrhythmias may be indications of digitalis intoxication.
3. Use caution in patients with renal disease, severe respiratory disease, acute myocardial infarction, AV block, and/or hypothyroidism, also in the geriatric patient and during pregnancy/lactation.

Adverse Reactions. Unifocal or multiform ventricular premature contractions, ventricular tachycardia, atrioventricular dissociation, atrial tachycardia, excessive slowing of the pulse (clinical sign of digitalis overdose), complete heart block, anorexia, nausea, vomiting, diarrhea, blurred or yellow vision, headache, weakness, dizziness, apathy, psychosis, gynecomastia, maculopapular rash, drowsiness, confusion, depression.

Dosage and Route. The dosage and route of administration is determined by the physician and individualized for each patient. See Table 24–1.

Implications for Patient Care. Assess the apical pulse for one minute before administering digitalis drugs. Withhold the medication if the pulse is below 60 or the minimum specified by the prescribing physician. Monitor intake and output ratio, daily weight, liver function studies, serum electrolytes, creatinine, and drug levels. Be alert for signs of digitalis toxicity and hypokalemia. Evaluate therapeutic response of medication (decreased edema, weight loss, increased urine output, improved heart rate, and rhythm).

Signs and Symptoms of Digitalis Toxicity

The most common early symptoms of digitalis toxicity are anorexia, nausea, vomiting, and arrhythmias. Other signs and symptoms according to body system are:

Gastrointestinal: anorexia, nausea, vomiting, diarrhea, abdominal pain.

Nervous System: headache, restlessness, irritability, drowsiness, depression, confusion, disorientation, insomnia, psychosis, convulsions, coma, blurred or yellow vision.

Cardiovascular: bradycardia, tachycardia, atrial tachycardia with varying AV block, ventricular bigeminy, ventricular tachycardia, second-degree AV block, complete AV block.

Musculoskeletal: severe weakness.

Patient Teaching

Educate the patient:

- about possible adverse reactions and the signs and symptoms of digitalis toxicity.
- to notify his/her physician without delay if toxic symptoms appear.
- about the importance of taking the medication as prescribed.
- to not stop taking the drug unless the physician so orders.
- to avoid over-the-counter medications unless ordered by the physician.
- to include foods high in potassium (Unless the patient is taking a potassium-sparing diuretic), and low in sodium in his/her diet.
- and his/her family about how to take a pulse and how to recognize changes in rate, volume and rhythm.
- to weight him/herself weekly and report a weight gain of 5 pounds or more to the physician.
- to wear or carry a Medic Alert ID stating that he/she is on digitalis.

Special Considerations

- Potassium-depleting corticosteroids and diuretics may be major contributing factors to digitalis toxicity.
- Rapid intravenous administration of calcium may produce serious arrhythmias in patients receiving digitalis.
- Quinidine, verapamil, and amiodarone cause a rise in serum digoxin concentration, with the implication that digitalis intoxication may result.
- Antacids, kaolin-pectin, sulfasalazine, neomycin, cholestyramine and certain anti-cancer drugs may interfere with intestinal digoxin absorption, resulting in expectedly low serum concentration.

- The additive effects of beta adrenergic blockers or calcium channel blockers and digitalis can result in complete heart block.
- There are numerous precautions and drug interactions associated with digitalis drugs. Please refer to a current edition of the *Physicians' Desk Reference* for more information.

Antiarrhythmic Agents

The heartbeat is controlled by neuromuscular tissue within the heart. The sinoatrial node (SA), located in the upper wall of the right atrium, is considered to be the source of the heartbeat. This specialized network of Purkinje fibers has the property of automaticity and is sometimes referred to as the *pacemaker* of the heart.

Normally, impulses from the sinoatrial node cause contraction of both left and right atria. The impulse also stimulates the atrioventricular node below the endocardium of the right atrium which, in turn, transmits the impulse to the atrioventricular bundle (Bundle of His) and causes contraction of the left and right ventricles.

Disorders of the SA node that interfere with impulsive formation, or disorders of the conduction system (AV node, Bundle of His) result in a variety of cardiac arrhythmias. The term *arrhythmia* means irregularity or loss of rhythm and is commonly used to describe an irregular heartbeat. Some cardiac arrhythmias do not require treatment while others may result in death if not treated by drug therapy or the use of an artificial pacemaker.

Antiarrhythmic drugs are used to control many cardiac arrhythmias. Some of the drugs used to threat this condition are found in Table 24–2.

Actions. Antiarrhythmic agents are classified as Class IA, Class IB, Class IC, Class II, Class III, and Class IV. The action of the drug varies with the classification and the drug's chemical properties.

- **Class IA:** quinidine sulfate (Quinidex Extentabs) depresses excitability of cardiac muscle, slows the rate of spontaneous rhythm, decreases vagal tone, and prolongs conduction and effective refractory period.

  Procainamide hydrochloride (Pronestyl) increases the effective refractory period, reduces impulse conduction velocity, and reduces myocardial excitability.

  Disopyramide (Norpace) decreases rate of diastolic depolarization (phase 4) in cells with augmented automaticity, decreases the upstroke velocity (phase 0), increases the action potential duration of normal cardiac cells, and decreases the disparity in refractories between infarcted and adjacent normally perfused myocardium.
- **Class IB:** tocainide (Tonocard) decreases sodium and potassium conductance, thereby decreasing the excitability of myocardial cells.

  Lidocaine (Xylocaine) attenuates (phase 4) diastolic depolarization and decreases automaticity and causes a decrease or no change in excitability and membrane responsiveness.

Table 24–2 Antiarrhythmic Drugs

Medication	Usual Dosage
flecainide acetate (Tambocor)	Oral: 100 mg every 12 hours with increases of 50 mg bid every 4 days until efficacy is achieved.
lidocaine HCl (Xylocaine HCl)	IM: 2 mg/lb (4.3 mg/kg) of 10% solution as needed.
propranolol HCl (Inderal)	Oral: 10–30 mg 3–4 times daily before meals and at bedtime. IV: 1–3 mg under careful monitoring.
procainamide HCl (Pronestyl)	Oral: 50 mg/kg per day in divided doses every 3 hours. IM: 0.5–1 Gm every 4–8 hours.
(Procan SR)	Oral: (maintenance): 50 mg/kg per day in divided doses every 6 hours starting 2–3 hours after the last dose of standard oral procainamide.
quinidine sulfate (Quinidex Extentabs)	Oral: 200–300 mg 3–4 times daily.
tocainide HCl (Tonocard)	Oral: Initial dosage: 400 mg every 8 hours; then 1200–1800 mg/day in a 3 dose daily divided regimen.
bretylium (Bretylol)	Severe ventricular fibrillation: Adult: IV bolus 5 mg/kg, increase to 10 mg/kg repeated every 15 min. Not to exceed 30 mg/kg/day. IV infusion: 1–2 mg/min or 5–10 mg/kg over 10 min every 6 hours (maintenance). Ventricular dysrhythmias: Adult: IV infusion 500 mg diluted in 50 ml D5W or NS, infuse over 10–30 min, may repeat in 1 hour, maintain with 1–2 mg/min or 5–10 mg/kg over 10–30 min every 6 hours. IM: 5–10 mg/kg undiluted; repeat in 1–2 hours if needed; may repeat with 3rd dose every 6–8 hours.
verapamil (Calan)	Oral: 240–480 mg/day in divided (3–4 times) doses.
disopyramide (Norpace)	Oral: 600 mg/day in divided doses (150 mg every 6 hours).
(Norpace CR)	Oral: 600 mg/day in divided doses (300 mg every 12 hours). For patients less than 110 pounds (50 kg) the recommended dosage is 400 mg/day in dividend doses (Norpace—100 mg every 6 hours; Norpace CR—200 mg every 12 hours).

- **Class IC:** flecainide acetate (Tambocor) produces a dose-related decrease in intracardiac conduction in all parts of the heart with the greatest effect on the His-Purkinje system. It also causes a dose-related and plasma-level related decrease in single and multiple PVCs and can suppress recurrence of ventricular tachycardia.
- **Class II:** propranolol hydrochloride (Inderal) is a nonselective beta-adrenergic receptor blocking agent that blocks receptor sites in the conduction system of the heart, thereby slowing SA node automaticity and the conduction of the AV node and other cells.

- **Class III:** bretylium tosylate (Bretylol) inhibits norepinephrine release by depressing adrenergic nerve terminal excitability. It also suppresses ventricular fibrillation and ventricular arrhythmias.
- **Class IV:** verapamil hydrochloride (Calan) is a calcium ion antagonist that exerts its pharmacologic effects by modulating the influx of ionic calcium across the cell membrane of the arterial smooth muscle as well as in conductible and contractile myocardial cells. By decreasing the influx of calcium, Calan prolongs the effective refractory period within the AV node and slows AV conduction in a rate-related manner, thereby slowing the ventricular rate in patients with chronic atrial flutter or fibrillation.

Uses

- quinidine sulfate (Quinidex Extentabs): premature atrial and ventricular contractions, paroxysmal atrial tachycardia, paroxsymal A-V junctional rhythm, atrial flutter, paroxysmal atrial fibrillation, paroxysmal ventricular tachycardia when not associated with complete heartblock, maintenance therapy after electrical conversion of atrial fibrillation and/or flutter.
- procainamide hydrochloride (Pronestyl): life-threatening ventricular arrhythmias. Treatment of some patients with less severe, symptomatic ventricular arrhythmias.
- disopyramide (Norpace): suppression and prevention of recurrence of unifocal and multifocal premature (ectopic) ventricular contractions, paired premature ventricular contractions, and episodes of ventricular tachycardia.
- tocainide (Tonocard): life-threatening ventricular arrhythmias.
- lidocaine (Xylocaine): acute management of ventricular arrhythmias such as those occurring in relation to acute myocardial infarction, or during cardiac manipulation, such as cardiac surgery.
- flecainide acetate (Tambocor): treatment of documented ventricular arrhythmias, such as sustained ventricular tachycardia, that in the judgment of the physician, are life-threatening.
- propranolol hydrochloride (Inderal): treatment of supraventricular arrhythmias, ventricular tachycardias, tachyarrhythmias of digitalis intoxication, resistant tachyarrythmias due to excessive catecholamine action during anesthesia.
- bretylium tosylate (Bretylol): indicated in the prophylaxis and therapy of ventricular fibrillation, and in the treatment of life-threatening ventricular arrhythmias, such as ventricular tachycardia, that have failed to respond to adequate doses of a first-line antiarrhythmic agent, such as lidocaine.
- verapamil hydrochloride (Calan): used in association with digitalis for the control of ventricular rate at rest and during stress in patients with chronic atrial flutter and/or fibrillation. Also used as prophylaxis of repetitive paroxysmal sypraventricular tachycardia.

Dosage and Route. The dosage and route of administration is determined by the physician and individualized for each patient. See Table 24–2.

Implications for Patient Care

- **Class IA:** quinidine sulfate (Quinidex Extentabs): Assess ECG for increase in PR or QRS segments. Reduce the dose or discontinue the medication if these increases occur. Notify the physician. Assess the blood pressure for fluctuations, hypotension and/or hypertension. Monitor pulse, respirations, intake and output ratio, blood level of the drug, electrolytes (K, Na, Cl), and for signs of cinchonism (quininism).

  procainamide HCl (Pronestyl): Assess ECG for increase in PR or QRS segments. Discontinue the medication if these increases occur. Notify the physician. Monitor pulse, respirations, intake and output ratio, blood level of the drug, electrolytes (K, Na, Cl).

  disopyramide (Norpace): Assess apical pulse for one minute, if less than 60, check again in one hour. Notify the physician if the pulse is less than 60. Assess ECG for increase in QT and widening QRS segments. Discontinue the medication if these increases occur. Notify the physician. Monitor weight daily and report any rapid weight gain. Check for dehydration and/or hypovolemia. Monitor intake and output ratio, electrolytes (K, Na, Cl), liver and kidney function studies, blood pressure for hypotension and/or hypertension. Assess diabetic patient for signs of hypoglycemia.
- **Class IB:** tocainide (Tonocard): Assess chest x-ray, pulmonary function tests, and liver enzymes during treatment. Monitor CBC, intake and output ratio, blood level of the drug, blood pressure, pulse, respirations, and lung fields for rales. Be aware of possible adverse reactions: increased respirations and pulse (discontinue drug and notify the physician); toxicity: fine tremors, dizziness; blood dyscrasias: fatigue, sore throat, fever, bruising.

  lidocaine (Xylocaine): Assess ECG for increase in PR or QRS segments. Reduce the dose or discontinue if these increases occur. Notify the physician. Assess blood pressure for fluctuations, pulse, respirations, and blood level of the drug. Monitor intake and output ratio, electrolytes (K, Na, Cl). Be aware of possible adverse reactions: increased respirations and pulse (discontinue drug and notify the physician); malignant hyperthermia: tachycardia, tachypnea, changes in B/P, elevated temperature; CNS effects: dizziness, confusion, psychosis, paresthesia, convulsions (discontinue drug and notify the physician).
- **Class IC:** flecainide acetate (Tambocor): Before administration assess for hypokalemia and/or hyperkalemia. If present these should be corrected before administration. Monitor blood pressure for fluctuations, pulse, respirations, and blood level of the drug. Be aware of possible adverse reactions: increased respirations and pulse (discontinue drug and notify the physician); malignant hyperthermia: tachycardia, tachypnea, changes in B/P, elevated temperature; CNS effects: dizziness, confusion, psychosis, paresthesia, convulsions (discontinue drug and notify the physician).

- **Class II:** propranolol HCl (Inderal): Assess ECG, blood pressure, pulse, respirations, and weight daily. Monitor intake and output ratio and hepatic enzymes. Evaluate therapeutic response.
- **Class III:** bretylium tosylate (Bretylol): Assess ECG, blood pressure, pulse and respirations. Monitor intake and output ratio, and for signs of dehydration and/or hypovolemia. Place patient in the supine position and have suction equipment available. Monitor blood pressure for rebound hypertension after 1–2 hours. Evaluate cardiac status.
- **Class IV:** verapamil (Calan). Assess ECG (PR, QRS, and QT segments), blood pressure, pulse and respirations. Evaluate therapeutic response.

Table 24–3 Contraindications and Adverse Reactions of Selected Antiarrhythmic Drugs

Medication	Contraindications	Adverse Reactions
quinidine (Quinidex)	Complete A-V block, intraventricular conduction defects, hypersensitivity to quinidine, myasthenia gravis.	Cinchonism (Loss of hearing, ringing in the ear, nausea, dizziness, headache, lightheadedness, disturbed vision) nausea, vomiting, abdominal pain, diarrhea, anorexia, headache, vertigo
tocainide (Tonocard)	Hypersensitivity, second or third degree atrioventricular block in the absence of an artificial pacemaker.	tiredness, drowsiness, hypotension, bradycardia, palpitations, chest pain, nausea, vomiting, anorexia, diarrhea, dizziness, vertigo, headache, rash
lidocaine (Xylocaine)	Hypersensitivity, Stokes-Adams syndrome, Wolff-Parkinson-White syndrome, severe degrees of sinoatrial, atrioventricular, or intraventricular block in the absence of an artificial pacemaker.	nervousness, lightheadedness, euphoria, dizziness, drowsiness, vomiting, double vision, respiratory depression, bradycardia, hypotension, cardiovascular collapse
flecainide (Tambocor)	Preexisting second- or third degree AV block, or with rigid right bundle branch block, cardiogenic shock, hypersensitivity.	cardiac arrest, new or worsened arrhythmias, dizziness, dyspnea, headache, nausea, chest pain, asthenia, edema
propranolol (Inderal)	Cardiogenic shock, sinus bradycardia and greater than first degree block, bronchial asthma, congestive heart failure.	bradycardia, CHF, hypotension, intensification of AV block, mental depression, nausea, vomiting, diarrhea, bronchospasm, agranulocytosis
bretylium (Bretylol)	No contraindications in the treatment of ventricular fibrillation or life-threatening refractory ventricular arrhythmias.	hypotension, postural hypotension, nausea, vomiting, vertigo, syncope, dizziness, bradycardia, substernal pain, initial increase in arrhythmias
verapamil (Calan)	Severe left ventricular dysfunction, hypotension (systolic less than 90 mm Hg), cardiogenic shock, sick sinus syndrome and second- or third-degree AV block (except in patients with a functioning artificial ventricular pacemaker), atrial flutter/fibrillation, Wolff-Parkinson-White, Lown-Ganong-Levine syndromes, hypersensitivity.	heart failure, hypotension, elevated liver enzymes, AV block, constiption, dizziness, nausea, edema, headache, pulmonary edema, fatigue

Patient Teaching

Educate the patient:

- about possible adverse reactions and the signs and symptoms of toxicity.
- to notify his/her physician without delay if toxic symptoms appear.
- about the importance of taking the medication as prescribed.
- to not stop taking the drug unless directed by the physician to do so.
- to avoid alcohol and over-the-counter medications.
- to make body position changes slowly (during early treatment).
- to avoid hazardous activities if dizziness or blurred vision occurs.
- and his/her family about how to take a pulse and how to recognize changes in rate, volume, and rhythm.
- to weigh him/herself weekly and report a weight gain of 5 pounds or more to the physician.
- to wear or carry a Medic Alert ID stating what drug he/she is taking.

Special Considerations

- There are numerous precautions and drug interactions associated with antiarrhythmic drugs. Please refer to a current edition of a *Physicians' Desk Reference* for information on precautions and drug interactions. See Table 24-3.
- Antiarrhythmic drugs may cause serious adverse reactions. Emergency equipment, supplies and medications should be readily available for use.
- Treatment of overdose: oxygen, artificial ventilation, dopamine for circulatory depression, diazepam or thiopental for convulsions. Monitor ECG.

Vasopressors and Vasodilators

There are many uses for drugs that act to either constrict (narrow) or dilate (widen) the walls of blood vessels. Based simply upon their primary action, these medications can be classified as vasopressors and vasodilators.

Vasopressors are drugs that cause contraction of the muscles associated with capillaries and arteries; thereby narrowing the space through which the blood circulates. This narrowing increases the resistance to blood flow and results in an elevation of blood pressure. Drugs classified as vasopressors are useful in the treatment of patients suffering from shock. See Table 24–4.

Vasopressors

Actions. Dopamine HCl (Intropin; Dopastat) exerts an inotropic effect on the myocardium resulting in an increased cardiac output. Metaraminol bitartrate (Aramine) has a positive inotropic effect and a peripheral vasoconstriction action. Norepinephrine (Levophed Bitartrate) acts as a peripheral vasoconstrictor (alpha-adrenergic); as an inotropic

Table 24–4 Selected Vasopressors

Medication	Usual Dosage	Adverse Reactions
dopamine HCl (Intropin) (Dopastat)	IV: 2–50 mcg/kg/min as needed after dilution with appropriate sterile solution recommended by manufacturer.	ectopic beats, nausea, vomiting, tachycardia, anginal pain, dyspnea, headache, hypotension, and vasoconstriction
metraraminol bitartrate (Aramine)	IM, SC: 2–10 mg IV infusion: 15–100 mg in 500 ml of Sodium Chloride Injection at rate adequate to maintain blood pressure at desired level.	sinus or ventricular tachycardia, or other arrhythmias, especially in patients with myocardial infarction
norepinephrine (Levophed Bitartrate)	IV infusion: 4 ml per 1000 ml of 5% dextrose solution. Give at rate of 8–12 mcg of base per minute.	occasional bradycardia, headache may indicate overdosage and extreme hypertension
phenylephrine HCl (Neo-Synephrine 1% Injection)	IM, SC: 2–5 mg. IV: 0.2 mg.	headache, reflex bradycardia, excitability, restlessness

stimulator of the heart and dilator of coronary arteries (beta-adrenergic). Phenylephrine HCl (Neo-Synephrine) is a powerful postsynaptic alpha-receptor stimulant with little effect on the beta receptors of the heart.

Uses. Shock, hypotension.

Contraindications. Contraindicated in patients with known hypersensitivity to any of its ingredients. Other contraindications depend upon the drug. For example: Dopamine is contraindicated in ventricular fibrillation, tachydysrhythmias, and pheochromocytoma.

> **CAUTIOUS USE:** During pregnancy, lactation, arterial embolism, and peripheral vascular disease. Please use a current reference book for contraindications of other vasopressor drugs.

Adverse Reactions. Adverse reactions depend upon the drug. For example: Dopamine may have the following adverse reactions: headache, palpitations, tachycardia, hypertension, ectopic heart beats, angina, nausea, vomiting, diarrhea, necrosis, tissue sloughing with extravasation, gangrene.

Dosage and Route. The dosage and route of administration is determined by the physician and individualized for each patient. See Table 24–4.

Implications for Patient Care. Assess intake and output ratio, and ECG during administration. Monitor blood pressure. Take blood pressure and pulse every 5 minutes after parenteral route. Dosage adjustment according to blood pressure. Administer IV slowly, after reconstituting. Reconstituted solution (refrigerated) may not be stored more than 24 hours. Do not use discolored solution. Check paresthesia and coldness of extremities; peripheral blood flow may decrease. Check injection site for tissue sloughing (administer phentolamine mixed with normal saline if this occurs). Evaluate therapeutic response increased blood pressure with stabilization.

Patient Teaching

Educate the patient about:

- the therapeutic response.
- the reason for the medication.

Special Considerations for Dopamine HCl

- Should not be used within 2 weeks of MAO inhibitors, since hypertensive crisis may occur.
- Dysrhythmia may occur when used with general anesthetics.
- Beta-blockers may decrease the action of dopamine.
- Drug is incompatible with alkaline solutions.

Vasodilators are medications that cause the relaxation of blood vessels. This action dilates the vessels; thereby increasing their ability to carry blood. This eases resistance to blood flow and lowers blood pressure.

Coronary vasodilators are used primarily for the treatment of *angina pectoris*, a condition caused by an insufficient supply of blood to the heart. The treatment of this condition usually involves the nitrate group of drugs. Nitrate tablets are rapidly absorbed through the mucous membrane of the mouth or stomach. See Table 24–5.

Nitrate Preparations

Nitrates include erythrityl tetranitrate, isosorbide dinitrate, nitroglycerin, and pentaerythritol tetranitrate. These drugs are available in various doses and forms. See Table 24–5.

Actions. Nitrates relax vascular smooth muscle. This action dilates the vessels; thereby increasing their ability to carry blood. This eases resistance to blood flow and lowers blood pressure. Myocardial oxygen demand is increased by both the arterial and venous effects of nitrates, and a more favorable supply-demand ratio can be achieved.

Uses. Angina pectoris, prophylaxis of angina pain, congestive heart failure associated with acute myocardial infarction, control of blood pressure in perioperative hypertension, and in the production of controlled hypotension during surgical procedures.

Contraindications. Contraindicated in patients with known hypersensitivity to any of its ingredients and in severe anemia, increased intracranial pressure, cerebral hemorrhage.

Table 24–5 Coronary Vasodilators

Medication	Usual Dosage	Adverse Reactions
amyl nitrate	0.18 to 0.3 ml by inhalation.	cutaneous vasodilation, marked lowering of systemic pressure, occasional headache, nausea
isosorbide dinitrate (Isordil) Sorbitrate)	Sublingual: 2.5–5 mg every 3 hours. Chewable: 5 mg initially every 2–3 hours. Oral: 5–20 mg 4 times daily. Oral (sustained-release): 40 mg every 6–12 hours.	headache, hypotension, cutaneous vasodilation with flushing, transient episodes of dizziness
nitroglycerin (Nitro-Bid) (Nitroglyn) (Nitrospan) (Nitrostat) (Transderm Nitro) (Nitrolingual Spray) (Nitrogard)	Topical: Spread in a thin layer over a 2–6 inch area every 3–4 hours when needed. Sublingual: 0.15–0.6 mg under tongue as needed for acute angina. Oral (sustained-release): 2.5 mg 3–4 times daily. Transdermal: 2.5–20 mg released over a 24-hour period. Lingual aerosol: 1–2 metered doses onto or under the tongue. Transmucosal: 1 mg placed on the oral mucosa between cheek and gum.	headache, hypotension, cutaneous vasodilation with flushing, and occasional drug rash or exfoliative dermatitis; refer to nitrate preparation for other adverse reactions
pentaerythritol tetranitrate (Peritrate)	Oral (sustained-release): 10–40 mg 4 times a day.	rash, headache, mild gastrointestinal distress, cutaneous vasodilation with flushing, transient episodes of dizziness

CAUTIOUS USE: During pregnancy, lactation, postural hypotension, and in patients who have severe hepatic or renal disease.

Adverse Reactions. Headache, tachycardia, nausea, vomiting, apprehension, restlessness, muscle twitching, retrosternal discomfort, palpitations, dizziness, abdominal pain, cutaneous flushing, weakness, drug rash or exfoliative dermatitis.

Dosage and Route. The dosage and route of administration is determined by the physician and individualized for each patient. See Table 24–5.

Implications for Patient Care. Assess blood pressure, pulse and respirations during initial therapy. Evaluate pain: time started, activity being performed, duration, severity, and length. Monitor patient for adverse reactions. Headache, lightheadedness, and decreased blood pressure are signs that may indicate a need to reduce the dosage. Evaluate therapeutic response.

Patient Teaching

Educate the patient:

- about possible adverse reactions.
- to avoid hazardous activities if dizziness occurs.
- about the importance of taking the medication as prescribed.
- that when pain is not relieved by the medication, he/she should go to an emergency room without delay.
- to avoid alcohol.
- to make position changes slowly to prevent possible fainting.

Special Considerations

- Most drug interactions with nitrates adversely affect the cardiovascular system. Alcohol may cause severe hypotension; anticholinergics delay sublingual absorption due to dryness of the mouth; antihypertensives and phenothiazines may cause hypotension produced by additive effects of the drugs.

Peripheral vasodilators are used in the treatment of peripheral vascular disease (VD), although many are classified by the Food and Drug Administration as only "possibly effective." They are used for the relief of symptoms of cerebral and peripheral vascular insufficiency. See Table 24–6.

Table 24–6 Peripheral Vasodilators

Medication	Usual Dosage	Adverse Reactions
cyclandelate (Cyclospasmol)	Oral: Initial dose, 1200–1600 mg per day in divided doses before meals and at bedtime; with clinical response, reduce dose by 200 mg decrements until maintenance dose (400–800 mg/day) is reached.	gastrointestinal distress, mild flush, headache, feeling of weakness, or tachycardia
ethaverine HCl (Ethaquin) (Ethatab)	Oral: 100–200 mg 3 times a day. Oral (sustained-release): 150 mg every 12 hours.	nausea, anorexia, abdominal distress, flushing, sweating, cardiac arrhythmia, headache, hypotension, drowsiness
isoxsuprine HCl (Vasodilan)	Oral: 10–20 mg 3–4 times daily. IM: 5–10 mg 2–3 times daily.	occasional hypotension, tachycardia, nausea, dizziness, chest pain, rash
nylidrin HCl (Arlidin)	Oral: 3–12 mg 3–4 times daily.	trembling, nervousness, weakness, dizziness, nausea and vomiting
papaverine HCl (Cerespan) (Pavabid)	Oral (sustained-release): 150 mg every 8–12 hours.	nausea, abdominal distress, anorexia, constipation, headache, drowsiness, sweating

Antihypertensive Agents

Hypertension can be defined as a condition wherein the patient has a higher arterial blood pressure than that judged to be normal. The primary factor in hypertension is increased resistance to blood flow resulting from the narrowing of peripheral blood vessels. The specific cause for hypertension can be determined for only a small percentage of patients with the condition. When no physical cause can be determined, the patient is said to have *essential* or *primary* hypertension.

When left untreated, those with elevated blood pressure are at risk for stroke and/or progressive deterioration of cardiac and renal function.

Drugs used in the treatment of hypertension may be categorized as *diuretics*, adrenergic blocking agents, or sympatholytics, calcium channel blockers, direct vasodilators, and angiotensin antagonists. Diuretics act by reducing extracellular fluid volume.

Adrenergic blocking agents disrupt sympathetic nervous system function. They are classified according to their site of action.

1. Alpha-blockers interrupt the actions of sympathomimetic agents at alpha-adrenergic receptor sites, relaxing vascular smooth muscle, increasing peripheral vasodilation and decreasing blood pressure.
2. Beta-adrenergic blockers prevent sympathetic nervous system stimulation by inhibiting the action of catecholamines and other sympathomimetic agents at beta-adrenergic receptor sites. Used as an antianginal agent.
3. Autonomic ganglionic blockers inhibit the action of acetylcholine, reduce or prevent the transmission of impulses in the autonomic nervous system. Limited chemical use as it has a potent hypotensive effect.
4. Mixed alpha- and beta-adrenergic blocking agents and norepinephrine depletors.

Calcium channel blockers block the flow of calcium ions into myocardial muscle cells and myocardial pacemaker cells. They produce antianginal effects and act on vascular smooth muscle cells.

Direct vasodilators act on arteries, veins, or both to reduce blood pressure. They relax smooth muscle, thereby reducing blood pressure.

Angiotensin antagonist agents reduce blood pressure by inhibiting the enzyme that converts angiotensin I to angiotensin II, a potent vasoconstrictor. They also decrease aldosterone release, thereby preventing sodium and water retention. See Table 24–7 for selected antihypertensive agents.

The Step-Care Approach to Treating Hypertension

The step-care approach to treating hypertension provides the physician with a means of tailoring therapy to individual patient variables. In this approach, the physician initially prescribes a diuretic and/or a mild antihypertensive drug, followed by an increase in the dose(s) to control the patient's blood pressure. When the patient's blood

Table 24–7 Selected Antihypertensive Agents

Medication	Drug Action	Usual Dosage	Adverse Reactions
bendroflumethiazide (Naturetin)	thiazide diuretic	Oral: 5–20 mg as an initial dose, then 5 mg/day.	anorexia, nausea, dizziness, photosensitivity, rash
furosemide (Lasix)	loop diuretic	Oral (Adult): 20–80 mg/day. Oral (Child): initial, 2 mg/kg.	anorexia, oral and gastric irritation, nausea, dizziness, anemia, purpura
spironolactone (Aldactone)	potassium-sparing diuretic	Oral: 50–100 mg/day.	gynecomastia, drowsiness, cramping and diarrhea, headache, lethargy
clonidine HCl (Catapres)	centrally acting *adrenergic* agent	Oral: 0.2–0.8 mg daily in divided doses.	dry mouth, drowsiness, sedation, anorexia, nausea, constipation, headache
methyldopa (Aldomet)	central and peripherally acting adrenergic agent	Oral: 0.5–2.0 Gm daily divided into 2–4 doses.	drowsiness, dry mouth, nasal congestion, nausea, vomiting, diarrhea
guanethidine sulfate (Ismelin)	peripherally acting adrenergic agent	Oral: 10–50 mg/day.	fatigue, nausea, nasal congestion, abdominal distress, weight gain
metoprolol tartrate (Lopressor)	beta-adrenergic blocking agent	Oral: 50–100 mg twice daily.	tiredness, dizziness, depression, mental confusion, headache
hydralazine HCl (Apresoline)	direct-acting vasodilator	Oral: 10–50 mg 4 times daily.	headache, anorexia, nausea, vomiting, diarrhea, palpitations, tachycardia
captopril (Capoten)	angiotensin-converting enzyme (ACE) inhibitor	Oral: 12.5–50 mg 3 times daily.	proteinuria, rash, hypotension, loss of taste perception
methyldopa-hydrochlorothiazide (Aldoril)	combination of two antihypertensive agents	Oral: 1 tablet 2 or 3 times/day.	sedation, headache, bradycardia, nausea, rash
guanfacine HCl (Tenex)	alpha–2 adrenergic receptor agonist	Oral: 1–2 mg daily, given at bedtime.	sedation, weakness, dizziness, dry mouth, constipation, and impotence
verapamil HCl (Isoptin SR)	calcium channel blocker	Oral: 240 mg once daily in the morning.	constipation, dizziness, nausea, hypotension, edema, headache
prazosin HCl (Minipress)	alpha-1 adrenergic receptor agonist	Oral: adjusted according to patient's blood pressure. Initial dose: 1 mg 2–3 times a day. Maintenance dose: Slowly increased to a total daily dose of 20 mg given in divided doses.	dizziness, headache, drowsiness, palpitations and nausea

(continued)

Table 24–7 Selected Antihypertensive Agents *(Continued)*

Medication	Drug Action	Usual Dosage	Adverse Reactions
terazosin HCl (Hytrin)	alpha-1 selective adrenoceptor blocking agent	Oral: adjusted according to patient's blood pressure. Initial dose: 1 mg at bedtime. Subsequent dose: Slowly increased. Range 1 mg to 10 mg once a day.	asthenia, back pain, headache, palpitations, postural hypotension, tension, tachycardia, nausea
atenolol (Tenormin)	beta-1 selective adrenoreceptor blocking agent	Oral: 50 mg given as one tablet a day.	bradycardia, leg pain, cold extremities, vertigo, postural hypotension, dizziness, fatigue, depression, diarrhea, nausea, dyspnea
losartan (Cozaar)	angiotensin II receptor antagonist	Oral: 50 mg once daily.	diarrhea, dyspepsia, headache, muscle cramps, myalgia, dizziness, cough, insomnia, fatigue, nasal congestion, sinusitis

pressure is not controlled by this approach, the physician adds or substitutes one drug after another in varying doses as needed, until the blood pressure is controlled. During the step-care approach the patient's blood pressure is carefully monitored. The goals of this approach is to provide the patient with the best drug therapy that will maintain a diastolic pressure below 80 mm Hg.

- **STEP 1 DRUGS:**
  Diuretics
  Beta-adrenergic blockers
- **STEP 2 DRUGS:**
  Angiotensin antagonists
  Calcium channel blockers
  Beta-adrenergic blocker
  Diuretics
- **STEP 3 DRUGS:**
  Direct vasodilators
  Angiotensin antagonists
  Calcium channel blockers
  Beta-adrenergic blockers
  Diuretics
- **STEP 4 DRUGS:**
  Direct vasodilators
  Angiotensin antagonists
  Calcium channel blockers
  Beta-adrenergic blockers
  Diuretics

Implications for Patient Care. Assess blood pressure for therapeutic response to the prescribed medication. Monitor blood studies (neutrophils, decreased platelets, potassium and sodium levels), and renal studies (protein, BUN, creatinine-increased levels may indicate nephrotic syndrome). Be aware of possible adverse reactions to the prescribed medication.

Patient Teaching

Educate the patient:

- to take the medication as prescribed.
- that he/she may have to take high blood pressure medicine for the rest of his/her life.
- that the medication does not cure hypertension, but helps to control it, and one must continue to take the medication even if he/she feels better.
- about possible adverse reactions.
- to avoid alcohol, over-the-counter drugs (especially cough, cold, and allergy medicines).
- not to operate hazardous machinery or drive a motor vehicle if dizziness occurs.
- about the factors that tend to increase blood pressure: obesity, smoking, consumption of alcohol, stress, lack of exercise, and excessive intake of sodium.
- in ways to reduce the factors that may be contributing to hypertension.
- who is taking diuretics that may deplete potassium to eat foods rich in potassium. (See Chapter 27 for more information on diuretics.)

Drugs That Affect the Blood

A number of medications have been developed that affect the clotting of blood. Simply put, these drugs either assist in the clotting process or work to inhibit the formation of a clot. The formation of a blood clot within a blood vessel is a life-threatening event; therefore, agents that interfere with the clotting process are important. These drugs are the anticoagulants and the thrombolytic agents.

Anticoagulants are used therapeutically after a *thrombus* or blood clot has formed. They do not alter the size of an existing thrombus; however, they do act to prevent further growth and reduce the possibility of embolization. If a thrombus is detached from the point at which it formed, it becomes an *embolus* moving within the vascular system. An embolus that occludes (blocks) the flow of blood can cause serious damage to an organ, as in the case of a coronary embolism.

Thrombolytic agents will dissolve existing fresh thrombi and emboli. These drugs diffuse into the clot and activate plasminogen that is trapped therein. *Plasminogen* is a protein that is important in the prevention of fibrin clot formation. After a thrombolytic agent has been employed, anticoagulants are used to prevent recurrence of a blood clot.

Heparin

Heparin is a potent anticoagulant that has been used for that purpose for many years. It is produced by *mast cells* found in the liver, lungs, and other parts of the body. Clinically, heparin is used during open heart surgery, during renal hemodialysis, and in the treatment of deep venous thrombosis or pulmonary infarction. Subcutaneous administration of low doses of heparin has been shown to diminish post-operative pulmonary embolism in older adults. The administration of heparin is by either *subcutaneous* or *intravenous* injection.

Actions. Prevents conversion of fibrinogen to fibrin.

Uses. Anticoagulant therapy in prophylaxis and treatment of venous thrombosis and its extension. Used for prevention of postoperative deep venous thrombosis and pulmonary embolism, prevention of clotting in arterial and heart surgery, prophylaxis and treatment of peripheral arterial embolism, atrial fibrillation with embolization, disseminated intravascular clotting syndrome, as an anticoagulant in blood transfusions, extracorporeal circulation, and dialysis procedures and in blood samples for laboratory purposes.

Contraindications. Contraindicated in patients with known hypersensitivity to any of its ingredients and in patients with severe thrombocytopenia and uncontrollable active bleeding.

Warnings:

1. Used with extreme caution in hemophilia, leukemia with bleeding, peptic ulcer disease, hepatic disease (severe), renal disease (severe), blood dyscrasias, pregnancy, severe hypotension, subacute bacterial endocarditis, acute nephritis.
2. Heparin is not intended for intramuscular use.
3. Hemorrhage can occur at almost any site in patients receiving heparin.

Adverse Reactions. Hemorrhage. Local irritation, erythema, mild pain, hematoma or ulceration may follow deep subcutaneous injection. Hypersensitivity reactions with chills, fever, and urticaria. Other adverse reactions are asthma, rhinitis, lacrimation, headache, nausea, vomiting, anaphylactoid reactions, including shock.

Dosage and Route. The dosage and route of administration (IV or subcutaneous) is determined by the physician and individualized for each patient. See Table 24–8.

Implications for Patient Care. Parenteral drug products should be inspected visually for particulate matter and discoloration prior to administration. Slight discoloration does not alter potency. **Never administer by intramuscular injection.** Before adding to an infusion solution for continuous intravenous administration, the container should be inverted at least six times to insure adequate mixing and prevent pooling of the heparin in the solution. The dosage of heparin should be adjusted according to the patient's coagulation test results; these should be monitored very carefully. Be aware of signs of bleeding: petechiae, ecchymosis, black tarry stools, bleeding gums, hematuria. Be alert for signs of adverse reactions.

Table 24–8 Anticoagulants

Medication	Usual Dosage	Adverse Reactions
heparin sodium	(Adult): 5,000 U by IV injection, followed by 10,000–2,000 U of a concentrated solution. Maintenance: 8,000–10,000 U every 8 hours or 15,000–20,000 U every 12 hours. IV intermittent (Adult): 10,000 units followed by 5,000–10,000 units every 4–6 hours. IV infusion, (Adult): 5,000 units by IV injection followed by 20,000–40,000 units daily.	hemorrhage, hematoma, hypersensitivity reaction include chills, fever, and urticaria
dicumarol	Oral, (Adult): 200–300 mg on the first day, followed by 25–200 mg daily.	hemorrhage, flatulence, and diarrhea
warfarin sodium (Coumadin)	Oral, (Adult): 40–60 mg the first day, followed by 2–10 mg daily.	hemorrhage, alopecia, dermatitis, urticaria

Patient Teaching

Educate the patient:

- about the purpose of the medication.
- about adverse reactions.

Special Considerations

- Heparin sodium is not effective by oral administration and should be given by intermittent intravenous injection, intravenous infusion, or deep subcutaneous injection.

Oral Anticoagulants

Anticoagulants that are administered *orally* do not produce an immediate effect. Their action is usually evident within 12 to 24 hours of administration. As with other anticoagulants, the use of these drugs may produce a cumulative effect; therefore, dosages must be individualized and based upon the patient's clotting time, using a blood coagulation test. See Table 24–8.

warfarin sodium (Coumadin)

Actions. Coumadin and other coumarin anticoagulants act by inhibiting the synthesis of vitamin K dependent coagulation factors.

Uses. Indicated for the prophylaxis and/or treatment of venous thrombosis and its extension, pulmonary embolism, atrial fibrillation with embolization, and as an adjunct in the prophylaxis of systemic embolism after myocardial infarction.

Contraindications. Contraindicated in patients with known hypersensitivity to any of its ingredients and in patients where the hazard of hemorrhage might be greater than the potential clinical benefits of anticoagulation such as pregnancy, hemorrhagic tendencies or blood dyscrasias, recent or contemplated surgery, bleeding tendencies associated with active ulceration or overt bleeding, threatened abortion, and in unsupervised senility, alcoholism, and/or psychosis.

Warnings:

1. Hemorrhage can occur at almost any site in patients on anticoagulant therapy.
2. Anticoagulant therapy with Coumadin may enhance the release of atheromatous plaque emboli.
3. Cautious use during lactation, severe to moderate hepatic or renal insufficiency, trauma which may result in internal bleeding, surgery or trauma resulting in large exposed raw surfaces, and in patients with indwelling catheters, severe to moderate hypertension, known or suspected deficiency in protein C, polycythemia vera, vasculitis, severe diabetes, severe allergic and anaphylactic disorders.

Precautions:

1. A patient receiving Coumadin must have periodic and carefully monitored prothrombin time or other suitable coagulation tests.
2. There are numerous factors that can affect anticoagulant response. Please refer to a current *Physicians' Desk Reference.*

Adverse Reactions. Hemorrhage. Necrosis of skin and other tissues. Other adverse reactions are alopecia, urticaria, dermatitis, fever, nausea, diarrhea, abdominal cramping, systemic cholesterol microembolization, a syndrome called "purple toe," cholestatic hepatic injury, and hyperensitivity reactions.

Dosage and Route. The dosage and route of administration is determined by the physician and individualized for each patient. See Table 24–8.

Implications for Patient Care. Assess prothrombin time and therapeutic response to medication. Monitor blood pressure, blood studies (hematocrit, platelet count), stools and urine for blood. Be aware of signs of bleeding. Be alert for signs of adverse reactions.

Patient Teaching

Educate the patient:

- about the purpose of the medication.
- about adverse reactions.

- to take the medication as prescribed and to have periodic (monitored) prothrombin time evaluations.
- to avoid alcohol, salicylates (aspirin), large amounts of green vegetables and/or drastic changes in dietary habits, which may affect Coumadin therapy.
- that Coumadin may cause a red-orange discoloration of alkaline urine.

Special Considerations

- The patient should notify the physician if any illness, such as diarrhea, infection or fever develops or if any unusual symptoms, such as pain, swelling, prolonged bleeding from cuts, increased menstrual bleeding, nosebleeds, bleeding of gums from brushing of teeth, unusual bleeding or bruising, red or dark brown urine and/or red or tarry stools.

Antiplatelet Drug: Aspirin (Used as an Antiplatelet Drug)

Aspirin may be recommended by physicians to reduce the risk of a second heart attach and/or to reduce the risk of having a heart attack and/or a stroke. Aspirin has been shown to inhibit an essential enzyme cells use to manufacture prostaglandin production, a hormone-like substance that takes an active role in many cellular activities. By inhibiting prostaglandin production it also inhibits platelet clumping, the first stage of the blood clotting process.

Aspirin helps keep platelets from sticking together to form clots. With this clotting activity reduced, the blood flows more freely and oxygen is more easily supplied to the heart, brain, and other organs. Clots are less likely to form, thus reducing the possibility of a clot forming and breaking away and lodging in the heart and/or brain.

It is generally recommended that an individual take aspirin (80, 160, or 325 mg) per day to prevent thromboembolic disorders.

Contraindications. Hypersensitivity, gastrointestinal bleeding, bleeding disorders, children under 3 years of age, children with flu-like symptoms, pregnancy, lactation, vitamin K deficiency, peptic ulcer.

Precautions. Anemias, hepatic and/or renal disease, Hodgkin's disease.

Adverse Reactions. Thrombocytopenia, agranulocytosis, leukopenia, neutropenia, hemolytic anemia, increased pro-time, drowsiness, dizziness, confusion, convulsions, headache, flushing, hallucinations, coma, nausea, vomiting, GI bleeding, heartburn, anorexia, rash, urticaria, bruising, ototoxicity, tinnitus, hearing loss, rapid pulse, hyperpnea, hypoglycemia, hypokalemia, hepatotoxicity, renal dysfunction, visual changes.

Implications for Patient Care. Assess liver, renal, and blood studies. Monitor prothrombin time and intake and output ratio. Decreased output may indicate renal failure (long-term therapy). Be aware of adverse reactions, especially hepatotoxicity (dark urine, clay-colored stool, jaundice, itching, abdominal pain, fever, diarrhea), allergic reactions (rash, urticaria), renal dysfunction (decreased urine output), ototoxicity (tinnitus, ringing in ears, loss of hearing), visual changes (blurring, halos, corneal, retinal damage), edema in feet, ankles, legs.

Patient Teaching

Educate the patient:

- to take the medication as prescribed.
- about adverse reactions.
- to visit his/her physician on a regular basis.
- to have liver, renal, and blood studies performed.
- not to take over-the-counter medications unless prescribed by his/her physician.
- to avoid alcohol, caffeine, and nicotine

Special Considerations

- Patient taking anticoagulant drugs should not take aspirin unless prescribed by his/her physician. Prothrombin time should be performed on a regular basis and monitored carefully.
- Antacids, steroids, urinary alkalizers may decrease the effectiveness of the drug.
- Anticoagulants, insulin, and methotrexate may increase the effectiveness of the drug.

Thrombolytic Agents

Approximately 80 percent of all acute myocardial infarctions are caused by a thrombus that occludes a coronary artery. Unless contraindicated, thrombolytic therapy is the treatment of choice for an MI patient who reaches the hospital within six hours of the onset of chest pain. In some hospitals the time period for administering thrombolytic agents has been extended to 12 and 24 hours.

Thrombolytic agents act to dissolve an existing thrombus when administered soon after its occurrence. These agents dissolve the clot, reopen the artery, restore blood flow to the heart, and prevent further damage to the myocardium.

Thrombolytic agents that have been approved for treating acute myocardial infarction are: streptokinase (Kabikinase, Streptase), anistreplase—which is also called APSAC (Eminase), alteplase (Activase), urokinase (Abbokinase) that is used to dissolve obstructive thrombi in the peripheral circulation and acute pulmonary emboli, and a single-chain urokinase plasminogen activator that converts to urokinase at the site of the clot. See Table 24-9.

Table 24–9 Thrombolytic Agents

Medication	Usual Dosage	Implications for Patient Care
alteplase (Activase)	Bolus dose of 6–10 mg IV over 1–2 minutes, then a lytic dose of 50–54 mg over 60 minutes, followed by a maintenance dose of 40 mg over 2 hours. Total dose: 100 mg IV over 3 hours.	Assess vital signs every 30 minutes. Monitor activated partial thromboplastin time every 4 hours for 48 hours. Check cardiac isoenzymes every 3 hours for 12 hours, then every 6 hours for 12 hours. Perform neurological assessment every 30 minutes to detect early signs of intracranial bleeding. Monitor ECG. Be alert for signs of bleeding and/or hypersensitivity.
anistreplase (Eminase)	30 units IV push over 2–5 minutes.	Same as above.
streptokinase (Kabikinase, Streptase)	1.5 million units IV over 60 minutes by controlled drip.	Same as above.

Contraindications. Hypersensitivity, active internal bleeding, recent (within 2 months) cerebrovascular accident, intracranial or intraspinal surgery, intracranial neoplasm, severe uncontrolled hypertension.

Warnings:

1. Bleeding is the most common complication encountered during thrombolytic therapy. Internal bleeding may involve the gastrointestinal tract, genitourinary tract, retroperitoneal or intracranial sites. Superficial or surface bleeding may occur at invaded or disturbed site (venous cutdown, arterial puncture, sites of recent surgical intervention). Intramuscular injections and nonessential handling of the patient should be avoided during treatment.
2. Should serious bleeding (not controlled by local pressure) occur, treatment with a thrombolytic agent should be stopped immediately.
3. Each patient being considered for therapy must be carefully evaluated and anticipated benefits weighed against potential risks associated with thrombolytic therapy.

Adverse Reactions. Bleeding, allergic reactions, anaphylactic and anaphylactoid reactions, fever.

Hemostatic Agents

Hemostatic agents may be administered systemically to overcome specific coagulation defects, or applied topically to control surface bleeding. Certain of these drugs are used in the treatment of hemophilia (Humafac, Proplex) and for hypofibrinogenemia

(Amicar, Vitamin K). Other products, known as *locally absorbable* hemostatics, are applied topically to control capillary oozing and surface bleeding. Examples of these are gelatin sponge (Gelfoam), oxidized cellulose (Surgicel), microfibrillar collagen (Avitene) and thrombin.

Hematinic Agents: Irons

Oral hematinic agents that are used to treat iron deficiency anemia are: ferrous fumarate, ferrous gluconate, and ferrous sulfate. These iron preparations are available in various trade name products such as ferrous fumarate (Eldofe, Farbegen, Fecot, Femiron, Feostat, Hemocyte, Ircon, Maniron, Neofer, Palmiron); ferrous gluconate (Fergon, Ferralet, Simiron); ferrous sulfate (Feosol, Fer-in-Sol, Ferolix, Irospan, Mol-Iron, Slow-Fe, Telefon).

Actions. Provides the body with iron that is needed for red blood cell development, energy and oxygen.

Uses. Iron deficiency and iron-deficiency anemia.

Contraindications. Contraindicated in patients with known hypersensitivity and in patients with ulcerative colitis, regional enteritis, hemosiderosis, hemochromatosis, peptic ulcer disease, hemolytic anemia, cirrhosis.

Warnings:

1. Oral iron preparations interfere with the absorption of oral tetracycline antibiotics. These products should not be taken within two hours of each other.
2. Cautious use in pregnancy and/or lactation.

Adverse Reactions. Nausea, constipation, epigastric pain, vomiting, diarrhea, tarry stools.

Dosage and Route. The dosage and route of administration is determined by the physician and individualized for each patient. See Table 24–10.

Implications for Patient Care. Assess hematocrit, hemoglobin, reticulocyte, and bilirubin determinations before initiation of therapy and monthly during treatment. Liquid preparation should be diluted and given through a plastic straw to avoid discoloration of tooth enamel. Store medication in a tight, light-resistant container. Monitor patient for signs of toxicity: nausea, vomiting, diarrhea (green then tarry stools), hematemesis, pallor, cyanosis, shock, coma. Assess patient's nutritional needs. Evaluate therapeutic response.

Patient Teaching

Educate the patient:

- about the purpose of the medication.
- about adverse reactions.

Table 24–10 Hematinic Agents: Iron Preparations

Medication	Usual Dosage
ferrous fumarate	Oral, (Adult): 200 mg tid-qid.
ferrous gluconate	Oral, (Adult): 200–600 mg tid.
ferrous sulfate	Oral, (Adult): 0.750–1.5 gm/day in divided doses, tid.
iron dextran	IM, (Adult): Test dose 0.5 ml. Less than 50 kg: 100 mg/day. More than 50 kg: 250 mg/day.

- to take the medication as prescribed.
- to have monthly blood studies evaluated by his/her physician.
- to take the medication between meals for best absorption and not to take with milk or antacids.
- to take liquid iron preparations through a plastic straw.
- that iron may cause dark green or black stools.
- about the proper method of storage for the medication.
- to include iron-rich foods in his/her diet. (Foods rich in iron are: liver, beef, veal, lamb, pork, turkey, chicken, oysters, eggs, peanut butter, soybeans, dried apricots, peaches, prunes, dates, figs, raisins, molasses, dried beans, enriched breads and cereals, dark green leafy vegetables.)

Special Considerations

- Tablets should not be crushed.
- In case of accidental overdose, contact physician and/or poison control center immediately.
- Do not substitute one iron preparation for another.

iron dextran (Imferon)

Iron dextran (Imferon) is a parenteral preparation that is available for IM/IV administration. It is administered only after test dose of 0.5 ml by preferred route and if well tolerated the remaining portion of the dose is administered after a one hour wait. The Z-track method of intramuscular injection is used and a 19–20 gauge, 2–3 inch needle is used for the average adult patient. For patients who are more than average, a longer needle is used to ensure that the drug is deep in muscle tissue, as the drug may be irritating to subcutaneous tissue and cause discoloration. IV injection is administered only by physicians.

Contraindications. Hypersensitivity, all anemias excluding iron deficiency anemia, hepatic disease.

Adverse Reactions. Headache, paresthesia, dizziness, shivering, weakness, seizures, nausea, vomiting, abdominal pain, rash, pruritus, urticaria, fever, sweating, chills, brown skin discoloration at injection site, necrosis, sterile abscess, phlebitis, chest pain, shock, hypoension, tachycardia, dyspnea, leukocytosis, anaphylaxis.

Implications for Patient Care. Assess patient for signs of adverse reactions. Monitor cardiac status: chest pain, hypotension, tachycardia. Monitor for hypersensitivity reaction: rash, pruritus, fever, chills, anaphylaxis. Store medication at room temperature in cool environment. Patient should remain in the recumbent position for 30 minutes after an injection of Imferon.

Agents Used in Treating Megaloblastic Anemias

Megaloblastic anemias result from decreased erythrocyte formation and the immaturity, fragility, and early destruction of these cells. There is a defective DNA synthesis, usually from vitamin B_{12}.

folic acid (Vitamin B_9)

Actions. Increases red blood cell, white blood cell and platelet formation in megaloblastic anemias.

Uses. Megaloblastic or macrocytic anemia caused by folic acid deficiency; liver disease, alcoholism, hemolysis, intestinal obstruction. Cautious use during pregnancy.

Contraindications. Hypersensitivity, anemias other than megaloblastic/macrocytic anemia, vitamin B_{12} deficiency.

Adverse Reactions. Bronchospasm.

Dosage and Route. Megaloblastic/macrocytic anemia: Oral, IM, SC: (Adult and child over 4 years of age) 1 mg every day times 4–5 days.

Implications for Patient Care. Assess folate blood levels. Store medication in light-resistant container. Evaluate therapeutic response and nutritional status of patient.

Patient Teaching

Educate the patient.

- about sources of folic acid (meat, eggs, green leafy vegetables).
- about the therapeutic response.
- on how to properly store the medication.

cyanocobalamin (Vitamin B_{12})

Actions. Replaces vitamin B_{12} that the body would normally absorb from the diet.

Uses. Vitamin B_{12} deficiency, pernicious anemia, vitamin B_{12} malabsorption syndrome.

Contraindications. Hypersensitivity, optic nerve atrophy. Cautious use during pregnancy and lactation.

Adverse Reactions. Flushing, optic nerve atrophy, diarrhea, congestive heart failure, peripheral vascular thrombosis, pulmonary edema, itching, rash, hypokalemia.

Dosage and Route. Pernicious anemia: (Adult) IM 100–1000 micrograms every day times 2 weeks, then 100–1000 micrograms every month.

Implications for Patient Care. Assess gastrointestinal function, potassium blood level, and complete blood count. Be aware of signs of adverse reactions. Evaluate therapeutic response and nutritional status of patient.

Patient Teaching

Educate the patient:

- about the importance of taking the medication exactly as prescribed by his/her physician.
- that treatment is for life when one has pernicious anemia.
- about foods rich in vitamin B_{12}.

epoetin alfa (Epogen, Amgen)

Epoetin alfa (Epogen, Amgen) is a genetically engineered hemopoietin that stimulates the production of red blood cells. It is a recombinant version of erythropoietin and is indicated for treating anemia in patients with chronic renal failure and in AIDS patients taking zidovudine (AZT).

Contraindications. In patients with uncontrolled hypertension, known hypersensitivity to mammalian cell-derived products and known hypersensitivity to albumin (human).

Warnings:

1. Blood pressure should be properly controlled before initiation of therapy. It must be monitored carefully during therapy.
2. Seizures have occurred in patients with chronic renal failure.
3. Please refer to a current *Physicians' Desk Reference* for additional warnings and precautions.

Adverse Reactions. Hypertension, headache, arthralgia, nausea, edema, fatigue, diarrhea, vomiting, chest pain, skin reactions, asthenia, dizziness, clotted vascular access, seizure, myocardial infarction.

Dosage and Route. Starting dose: 50–100 U/kg three times weekly IV for dialysis patients; IV or SC for non-dialysis patients. Reduce dose when 1) target range is reached, or 2) hematocrit increases above 4 points in any two-week period. Increase dose if hematocrit does not increase by 5–6 points after 8 weeks of therapy, and hematrocrit is below target range.

Implications for Patient Care. Carefully monitor blood pressure for signs of hypertension. Assess hematocrit for therapeutic range. Do not shake the container as shaking may denature the glycoprotein, rendering it biologically inactive. Inspect parenteral drug product for particulate matter and discoloration. Do not use vial if either or both are apparent. Use aseptic technique. Use only one dose per vial; do not re-enter vial. Discard unused portions. Do not administer in conjunction with other drug solutions.

Antilipemic Agents

Antilipemic agents are used to lower abnormally high blood levels of fatty substances (lipids) when other treatment regimens fail. Lipids may accumulate in the walls of blood vessels as atherosclerotic plaques and this accumulation can contribute to hypertension, increase the risk of coronary artery disease, and decrease the flow of oxygenated blood to the heart and other body organs. See Table 24–11.

Lipids include sterols (cholesterol and cholesterol esters), free fatty acids (FFA), triglycerides (glycerol esters of FFA), and phospholipids (phosphoric acid esters of lipid substances). Lipids may be exogenous (derived from foods and oils that are high in saturated fat) and endogenous (produced by the liver from the end products of lipid and carbohydrate metabolism).

Saturated fats (usually solid at room temperature) raise low density lipoprotein (LDL)-cholesterol, the fatty substance that can accumulate in the walls of blood vessels. Foods high in saturated fats include butter, cheese, chocolate, coconut oil, egg yolk, lard, meats, palm oil, whole milk, shell fish, and sardines. Other types of lipoprotein include very low density lipoprotein (VLDL) and high density lipoprotein (HDL). High density lipoprotein are "H"ighly "D"esirable and are known as the "good type of cholesterol." Elevations in total cholesterol and low density lipoprotein are associated with the development of coronary heart disease.

Antilipidemic agents are not usually the first treatment of choice for lowering lipids in the blood. Diet, weight and stress management, exercise, and proper treatment of other conditions such as hypertension and diabetes are tried before the physician prescribes an antilipidemic agent. When the blood cholesterol is not lowered by these other means, then one of several medications may be ordered. Some of these medications are: niacin (Nicolar, Nicobid), lovastatin (Mevacor), probucol (Lorelco), gemfibrozil (Lopid), clofibrate (Atromid-S), colestipol (Colestid), and cholestyramine (Questran, Cholybar). See Table 24–12.

Implications for Patient Care. Assess cholesterol blood level, liver function studies and renal function studies in patients with compromised renal system. A slit lamp examination of the eye should be performed one month after treatment begins and then annually (lens opacities may occur). Evaluate therapeutic response to medication. Administer medication as prescribed.

Patient Teaching

Educate the patient:

- to take the medication as prescribed.
- about adverse reactions.

- to report any adverse reactions to his/her physician.
- to continue to see his/her physician on a regular basis for cholesterol and liver function tests.
- about diet, exercise, life-style changes, and stress management.

Table 24–11 Cholesterol Values and Associated Risk Level

Total Cholesterol	LDL	Risk Level
Below 200 mg/dL	Below 130 mg/dL	Desirable level
200–239 mg/dL	130–159 mg/dL	Borderline-High
240 mg/dL	160 mg/dL	High

Table 24–12 Selected Antilipemic Agents

Medication	Usual Dosage	Adverse Reactions
niacin (Nicolar, Nicobid)	300–600 mg daily, orally.	flushing, skin rash, pruritus, GI upset, exacerbation of peptic ulcer, hyperglycemia, hyperuricemia
lovastatin (Mevacor)	20–80 mg daily, orally.	muscle pain and inflammation, increased liver function studies, rhabdomyolysis, acute muscle deterioration, headache, skin rash, pruritus, nausea, diarrhea, constipation, gas
probucol (Lorelco	500 mg bid, orally.	nausea, diarrhea, prolonged QT interval on ECG, increased risk of ventricular tachycardia and fibrillation, insomnia, headache
gemfibrozil (Lopid)	600 mg bid, orally 30 minutes before morning and evening meal.	nausea, flatulence, diarrhea, epigastric pain, abdominal pain
clofibrate (Atromid-S)	500 mg qid, orally.	nausea, vomiting, dyspepsia, increased liver enzyme studies, stomatitis, flatulence, gastritis, weight gain, hepatomegaly, increased cholelithiasis
colestipol (Colestid)	15–30 gm/day in 2–4 divided doses.	constipation, abdominal pain, nausea, fecal impaction, vomiting, hemorrhoids, flatulence, peptic ulcer, steatorrhea
cholestyramine (Questran, Cholybar)	4 gm ac and hs, orally.	headache, dizziness, vertigo, tinnitus, muscle and joint pain, abdominal pain, constipation, nausea, fecal impaction, hemorrhoids, flatulence, vomiting, peptic ulcer, steatorrhea
simvastatin (Zocor)	5–10 mg once a day in the evening. range 5–40 mg/day single dose in the evening.	muscle cramps, myalgia, tremor, dizziness, headache, vertigo, memory loss, anorexia, vomiting, constipation, diarrhea, alopecia, pruritus, gynecomastia, loss of libido, blurred vision
atorvastatin calcium (Lipitor)	10 mg once daily.	constipation, flatulence, dyspepsia, and abdominal pain
fluvastatin sodium (Lescol)	20 mg once daily at bedtime.	rash, back pain, coughing, dyspepsia, diarrhea, abdominal pain, nausea, constipation, flatulence, dizziness, headache

Spot Check

There are many medications that may be used to treat circulatory system disorders. For each of the selected drugs and/or drug classifications list several aspects of patient teaching and several implications for patient care.

Drug(s)	Patient Teaching	Implications for Patient Care
Digitalis		
Antiarrhythmics		
Vasopressors		
Nitrates		
Antihypertensives		

Anticoagulants		
Antilipemics		

◆ Review Questions

Directions: Select the best answer to each multiple choice question. Circle the letter of your choice.

1. A protein that is found in many body tissues, fluids, and is important in the prevention of fibrin clot formation is __________.
   a. angiotensinogen
   b. angiotensin
   c. plasminogen
   d. adrenergic
2. The primary function of the circulatory system is carried out in the __________.
   a. arteries
   b. veins
   c. aorta
   d. capillaries
3. Inotropic effect means increasing or decreasing __________.
   a. heart rate
   b. the force of myocardial contraction
   c. the conclusion of electrical impulses
   d. all of these
4. Cardiac glycosides (digitalis drugs) __________.
   a. strengthen the myocardium
   b. increase the force of the systolic contraction
   c. slow the heart, and improve muscle tone
   d. all of these

5. The usual initial or digitalizing dose of digitoxin is __________.
   a. 0.5–0.75 mg, then 0.25–0.5 mg every 6–8 hours
   b. 1.2 Gm daily in divided doses every 6 hours
   c. 0.6 mg, followed by 0.4 mg and then 0.2 mg at 4–6 hour intervals
   d. 0.4–0.6 mg, then 0.25 mg every 4–6 hours
6. The most common early symptoms of digitalis toxicity are anorexia, __________.
   a. constipation, vomiting, arrhythmias
   b. nausea, vomiting, arrhythmias
   c. dizziness, vomiting, arrhythmias
   d. pruritus, vomiting, arrhythmias
7. Vasopressors are drugs that __________.
   a. cause dilation of the muscles associated with capillaries and arteries
   b. cause contraction of the muscles associated with capillaries and arteries
   c. are useful in the treatment of patients suffering from shock
   d. b and c
8. Coronary vasodilators are used primarily for the treatment of __________.
   a. congestive heart failure
   b. angina pectoris
   c. hypertension
   d. peripheral vascular disease
9. The usual dose of papaverine HCl (Cerespan or Pavabid) is __________.
   a. 3–12 mg 3–4 times daily
   b. 100–200 mg 3 times a day
   c. 150 mg every 8–12 hours
   d. 10–20 mg 3–4 times daily
10. Drugs used in the treatment of hypertension may be categorized as __________.
    a. diuretics
    b. vasodilators
    c. angiotensin antagonists
    d. all of these
11. Heparin is a potent __________.
    a. anticoagulant
    b. antiarrhythmic
    c. antihypertensive agent
    d. vasopressor
12. Agents used in the treatment of megaloblastic anemias include __________.
    a. folic acid
    b. quinidine
    c. Vitamin B_{12}
    d. a and c
13. In the treatment of congestive heart failure, therapy usually includes a ________.
    a. low-sodium diet
    b. reduction of physical activities
    c. digitalis drug
    d. all of these

14. The pharmacologic actions of all digitalis compounds are similar, but these products differ in their __________.
    a. potency
    b. onset of action
    c. the rate of absorption
    d. all of these

15. The __________ is referred to as the pacemaker of the heart.
    a. Bundle of His
    b. sinoatrial node (SA)
    c. atrioventricular node
    d. Purkinje fibers

16. The term __________ means irregularity or loss of rhythm.
    a. bradycardia
    b. tachycardia
    c. arrhythmia
    d. anrhythmia

17. The treatment of angina pectoris usually involves the __________ group of drugs.
    a. nitrate
    b. anticoagulant
    c. thrombolytic
    d. hemostatic

18. __________ can be defined as a condition wherein the patient has a higher arterial blood pressure than that judged to be normal.
    a. Hypotension
    b. Hypertension
    c. Pulse pressure
    d. Venous pressure

> **Case Study:** Mr. Barry Anderson, a 56-year-old lawyer is admitted to the coronary care unit with a diagnosis of acute myocardial infarction. His pain began 3 hours before admission to the hospital. He is placed on bedrest and his physician orders streptokinase 1.5 million units IV over 60 minutes by controlled drip. Other orders include oxygen via nasal cannula and morphine for pain. Mr. Anderson has a Transderm Nitro patch on his left upper chest and he has been taking gemfibrozil (Lopid) 600 mg bid for the past six weeks.

19. The nurse should know that streptokinase is a/an __________.
    a. anticoagulant agent
    b. antiarrhythmic agent
    c. thrombolytic agent
    d. antihypertensive agent

20. For streptokinase to be most effective it should be administered within __________ hours of the onset of pain.
    a. 4
    b. 6
    c. 26
    d. 32

21. __________ is the most common complication encountered during the administration of streptokinase.
    a. Seizure
    b. Convulsion
    c. Bleeding
    d. Urticaria

22. The action of Transderm Nitro is to relax __________.
    a. vascular smooth muscle
    b. skeletal muscle
    c. the myocardium
    d. all of the above
23. The nurse should know that gemfibrozil (Lopid) is a/an __________.
    a. anticoagulant agent
    b. antiplatelet agent
    c. antilipemic agent
    d. antiarrhythmic agent
24. For best results Lopid should be administered __________.
    a. 30 minutes before morning and evening meals
    b. 15 minutes before morning and evening meals
    c. early in the morning and at bedtime
    d. in 2–4 divided doses

Matching: Place the correct letter from Column II on the appropriate line of Column I.

Column I

25. __________ Adrenergic
26. __________ Angiotensin
27. __________ Angiotensinogen
28. __________ Glycoside
29. __________ Antilipemic agents
30. __________ Megaloblastic anemia
31. __________ Plasminogen

Column II

A. A protein that is found in many body tissues and fluids. It is important in the prevention of fibrin clot formation.
B. A serum globulin fraction formed in the liver.
C. An anemia in which megaloblasts are found in the blood.
D. Pertaining to nerve fibers that, when stimulated, release norepinephrine at their endings.
E. A vasopressor substance that is formed in the body by interaction of renin and angiotensinogen.
F. A substance that is derived from plants, and upon hydrolysis yields a sugar plus additional products.
G. Used to lower blood cholesterol.
H. An increased amount of fibrinogen in the blood.

CHAPTER 25

Medications That Affect the Respiratory System

OBJECTIVES

Upon completion of this chapter, you should be able to:

- Define the terms listed in the vocabulary.
- Describe respiration.
- Describe the causes of respiratory conditions and/or diseases.
- State the actions, uses, contraindications, warnings, adverse reactions, dosage and route, implications for patient care, patient teaching, and special considerations for antihistamines, decongestants, antitussives, expectorants and mucolytics, and bronchodilators.
- Describe inhalational corticosteroids.
- State the dosage and route of selected inhalational corticosteroids.
- Give the adverse reactions of selected inhalational corticosteroids.
- Describe cromolyn sodium and state its usage.
- Describe tuberculosis.
- List the symptoms of tuberculosis.
- Explain how tuberculosis is diagnosed.
- Describe the treatment regimen for tuberculosis.
- List the CDC guidelines for reducing the risk of tuberculosis transmission in health-care settings.
- State the usual dosage and adverse reactions of the primary drugs used to treat tuberculosis.
- State the usual dosage and adverse reactions of the secondary drugs used to treat tuberculosis.
- Explain why there may be an increased risk of developing tuberculosis in the older adult.
- Explain why a child may be at greater risk of contracting tuberculosis.
- Complete the critical thinking questions/activities presented in this chapter.
- Complete the Spot Check on recommended children's dosages for selected antituberculosis drugs.
- Answer the review questions correctly.

Vocabulary

allergen (al′er-jen). Any substance that causes allergy.

allergy (al′er-je). An individual hypersensitivity to a substance, usually an antibody-antigen reaction.

anaphylaxis (an″a-fi-lak′sis). An allergic hypersensitivity reaction of the body to a foreign substance, usually to a protein substance or a drug. Anaphylactic shock usually occurs suddenly and can be life threatening.

allergic rhinitis (a-ler′jik ri-ni′tis). Inflammation of the nasal mucosa that is due to the sensitivity of the nasal mucosa to an allergen. Also known as *hay fever.*

common cold. A general term for *coryza.* An inflammation of the respiratory mucous membranes caused by a rhinovirus.

rhinovirus (ri″no-vi′rus). One of a subgroup of viruses that cause the common cold in man.

urticaria (ur-ti-ka′re-a). A vascular reaction of the skin that is characterized by wheals and severe itching. Also known as *hives.*

pruritus (proo-ri′tus). Severe itching.

histamine (his′ta-min). A substance that is normally present in the body. When released from injured cells it causes increased mucous secretions, dilation of capillaries, constriction of bronchial smooth muscle, and increased gastric secretions.

rhinorrhea (ri″no-re′a). Flow of thin watery discharge from the nose.

Synopsis: The Respiratory System

The organs of the respiratory system are the nose, pharynx, larynx, trachea, bronchi, and lungs. These structures provide for the passage of respiratory gases to and from the lungs during the act of breathing. The lungs do not contain muscle tissue; therefore, they are dependent upon the movement of surrounding structures (the rib cage and the diaphragm) in order to function. The contraction of the intercostal (rib) muscles and the diaphragm expands the volume of the thoracic cavity and causes the intake (inspiration) of air into the lungs. The relaxation of these muscles decreases the volume of the cavity and forces air out of the lungs (expiration). The rhythmic contraction and relaxation of rib and diaphragm muscles involved in breathing is controlled by nerve impulses from the respiratory center of the brain.

The act of breathing brings oxygen-rich air into the lungs where a very important exchange of gases occurs. Air that enters the lungs travels through a multi-branched network of smaller and smaller bronchial tubes until it reaches clusters of tiny, thin-walled air sacs called *alveoli.* There are about 300 million alveoli, each in close contact with equally thin-walled capillaries filled with pulmonary blood. This close contact between air and oxygen-poor blood allows an exchange of gases to take place. Carbon dioxide,

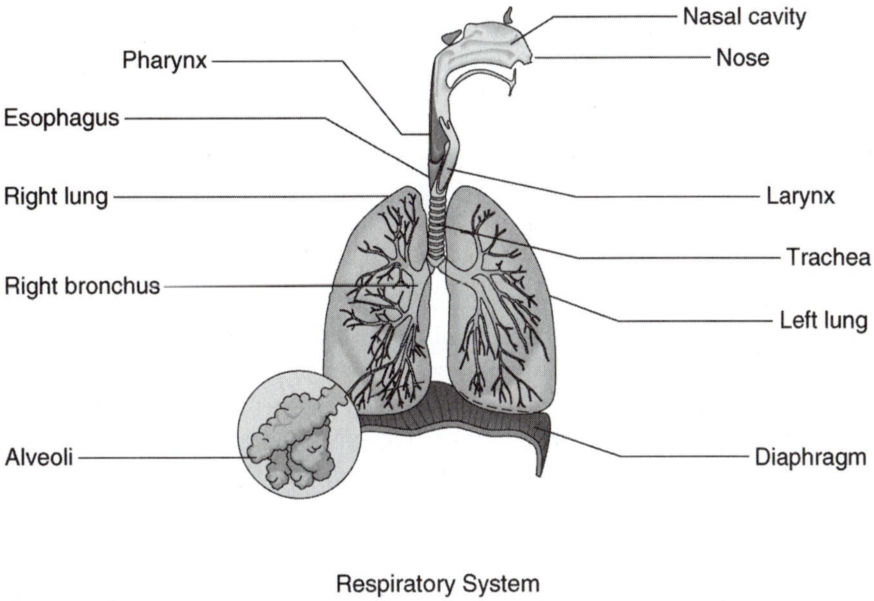

Figure 25–1 Structures of the respiratory system

carried from tissue cells by pulmonary blood, is released into the air to be exhaled. As this gas is given up, oxygen molecules diffuse from the air into the blood and are carried to body cells that use it in metabolizing foods. See Figure 25–1.

Introduction

Respiratory conditions/diseases may be caused by viruses, allergies, pathogenic organisms, fungi, environmental and/or hereditary factors. Rhinoviruses, the cause of the common cold, affect the average adult two to three times a year and children an average of twelve times a year. There is no cure for the common cold and it generally runs its course with or without treatment. It is estimated that there are 71 million colds a year.

Some researchers feel that the cold virus is spread by direct contact with an infected person or the things he has contaminated. Other researchers say the viruses float through the air, taking root in nasal mucosa of unsuspecting passers-by. Regardless of the method by which the virus is spread, the common symptoms: sniffling, sneezing, hacking cough, and malaise are experienced by many during a year. Antihistamines, decongestants, antitussives, and analgesics/antipyretics are some of the medications that may be used to treat the *symptoms* of the common cold. In children, aspirin should not be used as an analgesic/antipyretic because of the risk of Reye's syndrome.

Allergy is an individual hypersensitivity to a substance, usually an antibody-antigen reaction. The most common allergens are pollens, animal dander, house dust, house dust mites, molds, certain drugs, insect stings, and many foods. There are many other substances that act as allergens such as dyes, perfumes, tobacco, feathers, chemicals, metals, and gases. Allergies affect over 25 million Americans.

An allergic condition may manifest itself as hay fever, asthma, eczema, conjunctivitis, dermatitis, urticaria/hives, food allergy, occupational allergy, and anaphylaxis. Antihistamines, decongestants, corticosteroids, and cromolyn sodium are the major drug agents used to treat allergic disease.

Pathogenic organisms are the cause of many respiratory diseases, such as sinusitis, laryngitis, pharyngitis, pleuritis, bronchitis, pneumonia, tuberculosis, pneumocystis pneumonia, and bronchomycosis. Antimicrobials/antibiotics and antifungals are the drugs of choice for the treatment of respiratory diseases caused by pathogenic organisms.

Environmental factors like smoke, chemicals, metals, and gases may cause certain respiratory diseases such as pneumoconiosis and emphysema (chronic obstructive pulmonary disease). Bronchodilators and mucolytics are the drugs of choice for the treatment of respiratory diseases that may be caused by environmental factors.

Antihistamines, decongestants, antitussives, expectorants, mucolytics, bronchodilators, corticosteroids by inhalation, cromolyn sodium, and drugs used to treat tuberculosis are described in this chapter.

PLEASE NOTE: Many of the medications described in this chapter may be given in combination with each other. This is especially true of antihistamines, decongestants, and antitussive agents. When this occurs, one should be aware of the combined effects of the drugs, the possible adverse reactions, contraindications, warnings, and special considerations for each.

Antihistamines

Antihistamines are chemical agents that are structurally related to histamine and act to counter its effects by blocking histamine 1 (H_1) receptors. They do not interfere with the production and release of histamine.

Actions. Antihistamines appear to compete with histamine for cell receptor sites on effector cells. Histamine-related allergic reactions and tissue injury are blocked or diminished in intensity.

Uses. The primary use for antihistamine agents is the treatment of allergy symptoms that have resulted from the release of histamine. They are effective in the treatment of perennial and seasonal allergic rhinitis, contact dermatitis, urticaria, pruritus, for amelioration of allergic reactions to substances such as blood, plasma, insect stings, plant poisons, and as an adjunctive therapy during anaphylactic shock. Some antihistamines are used for the prevention and control of motion sickness and others are used in combination cold remedies to decrease mucus secretion and at bedtime for sedation.

Contraindications. Antihistamines are contraindicated in patients who are known to be hypersensitive to any of its ingredients. They should not be used in newborn or premature infants and nursing mothers.

Warnings:

Antihistamines should be used with considerable caution in patients with narrow-angle glaucoma, stenosing peptic ulcer, liver function problems, pyloroduodenal obstruction, symtomatic prostatic hypertrophy, or bladder-neck obstruction.

Seldane (terfenadine) and Hismanal (astemizole) might cause irregular heartbeats and death when combined with other medicines. Patients taking Seldane and/or Hismanal along with antibiotics such as erythromycin, TAO (troleandomycin), Biaxin (clarithromycin) and antifungal medicines like Nizoral (ketoconazole), Sporanox (itraconazole) could suffer serious cardiovascular events.

Adverse Reactions. The most frequent adverse reactions to antihistamines are sedation, sleepiness, dizziness, disturbed coordination, epigastric distress, and thickening of bronchial secretions. Other adverse reactions are dryness of mouth, nose, and throat, hypotension, headache, palpitations, nervousness, tremor, irritability, vertigo, tinnitus, anorexia, nausea, vomiting, diarrhea, constipation, wheezing, and nasal stuffiness.

Dosage and Route. The dosage and route of administration is determined by the manufacturer, but a physician should be consulted when needed. See Table 25–1 for selected antihistamines.

Implications for Patient Care. The nurse should know that many antihistamines have an atropine-like action and therefore should be used with caution in patients with a history of bronchial asthma, increased intraocular pressure, hyperthyroidism, cardiovascular disease or hypertension.

Patient Teaching

Educate the patient that antihistamines:

- may impair mental alertness; therefore, one should not operate machinery or drive a motor vehicle, until his/her response to the medication has been determined.
- taken with alcohol or other sedative drugs may enhance drowsiness.
- should not be taken if monoamine oxidase inhibitor(s) or anticoagulants are part of the patient's drug regimen.
- such as Seldane and Hismanal may cause serious cardiovascular problems when taken with erythromycin, TAO, Biaxin, Nizoral and/or Sporanox.

Special Considerations

- The action of oral anticoagulants may be diminished by antihistamines.
- Antihistamines have additive effects with alcohol and other CNS depressants (tranquilizers, sedatives, hypnotics).

Table 25–1 Antihistamines

Medication	Usual Dosage	Adverse Reactions
azatadine maleate (Optimine)	Oral, (Adult): 1–2 mg twice daily.	drowsiness, dizziness, epigastric distress, thickening of bronchial secretions
brompheniramine maleate (Dimetane)	Oral, (Adult): 16–24 mg/daily or 16–36 mg/daily (time-release form). Oral, (Child 6–12): 10–24 mg/day. (Child 2–6): 6 mg/day.	drowsiness, dryness of mouth, nose, and throat, thickening of bronchial secretions
chlorpheniramine maleate (Chlor-Trimeton)	Oral, (Adult): 6–16 mg/daily or 8–36 mg/daily (time-release form). IM, IV, SC (Adult): 5–20 mg. Oral, (Child 6–11): 3–8 mg/day.	drowsiness, excitability in children
clemastine fumarate (Tavist, Tavist-1)	Dosage should be individualized according to the needs and response of the patient. Refer to a *Physicians' Desk Reference.*	drowsiness, urticaria, drug rash, anaphylactic shock, photosensitivity, chills, dryness of the mouth, nose and throat
diphenhydramine HCl (Benadryl)	Oral, (Adult): 25–50 mg 3–4 times daily. IV, deep IM, (Adult): 10–100 mg 3–4 times daily. Oral, (Child over 20 lb): 12.5–25 mg 3–4 times daily. IV, deep IM, (Child): 5 mg/kg/day in 4 divided doses.	drowsiness, dizziness, epigastric distress, thickening of bronchial secretions
terfenadine (Seldane)	Oral, (Adult, Child 12 and over): 60 mg twice daily.	tachycardia, palpitations, headache, dizziness, nausea, restlessness, tremor, weakness, pallor, respiratory difficulty, dysuria, insomnia, arrhythmias, cardiovascular collapse with hypotension
astemizole (Hismanal)	Oral, (Adults and Children 12 years and over): maintenance dose 10 mg daily. Take on an empty stomach, 2 hours after a meal and no food for 1 hour after dose.	drowsiness, headache, fatigue, nervousness, dizziness, nausea, diarrhea, abdominal pain, dry mouth

- Antihistamines are most likely to cause dizziness, sedation, and hypotension in patients over 60 years of age.
- Antihistamines should only be taken when needed. One may develop tolerance to a certain antihistamine.
- Antihistamines may cause respiratory tract to dry and mucus to thicken; therefore, one should drink plenty of fluids while taking to thin secretions and keep tissue moist.

Decongestants

Congestion of the nasal mucosa may occur as a result of infection, allergy, inflammation, or emotional upset. Decongestants are commonly used for symptomatic relief of nasal congestion.

Actions. Decongestants act by stimulating alpha adrenergic receptors of vascular smooth muscle. As a result, dilated arterioles in the nasal mucosa are constricted. This reduces blood flow to the affected area, slows the formation of mucus, improves drainage, and opens obstructed nasal passages.

Uses. For the temporary relief of nasal congestion associated with the common cold, hay fever and/or other upper respiratory allergies, and sinusitis.

Contraindications. Decongestants are contraindicated in patients who are allergic to adrenergic agents, narrow-angle glaucoma, and patients who are taking MAO inhibitors or tricyclic antidepressants.

Warnings:

1. If recommended dosage is exceeded, nervousness, dizziness, sleeplessness, rapid pulse, or high blood pressure may occur.
2. Medication should not be taken more than 7 days. If symptoms do not improve or fever occurs, patient should see a physician.
3. Patients with heart disease, hypertension, thyroid disease, glaucoma, diabetes, or prostatic hypertrophy should not take decongestants without the permission of their physician.
4. Patients who are pregnant or nursing babies should not take decongestants without the permission of their physician.

Adverse Reactions. Rebound nasal congestion, dryness and stinging of the mucosa, sneezing, lightheadedness, headache, anxiety, palpitations, drowsiness, nausea, vomiting, and anorexia.

Dosage and Route. The dosage and route of administration is determined by the manufacturer, but a physician should be consulted when needed. See Table 25–2 for selected decongestants.

Implications for Patient Care. Since most decongestants are taken as over-the-counter medications, the implications for patient care mainly involve teaching the patient about the medication.

Patient Teaching

Educate the patient that:

- long term use of nasal sprays or solutions increase the risk of sensitization which often causes a rebound effect or an increase in symptoms.

Table 25–2 Decongestants

Medication	Usual Dosage	Adverse Reactions
oxymetazoline HCl (Afrin)	Topical, (Adults, children over 6 years): 2–3 drops or sprays of 0.5% solution in each nostril twice daily. Topical, (Children 2–5 years): 2–3 drops of 0.025% solution in each nostril twice daily.	mild adverse effects include dryness and stinging of the mucosa, sneezing, light-headedness, and headache
phenylephrine HCl (Coricidin) (Neo-Synephrine HCl) (Super Anahist Nasal Spray	Topical, (Adults and older children): several drops of a 0.25–1.0% solution in each nostril as needed. Topical, (Infants): 0.125% solution used as above.	drowsiness, excitability in children, rebound nasal congestion, anxiety
phenylpropanolamine HCl (Propagest)	Oral, (Adult): One tablet every 4 hours not to exceed 6 tablets in 24 hours. Oral, (Children, 6–12 years): One-half tablet every 4 hours not to exceed 3 tablets in 24 hours.	nervousness, dizziness, sleeplessness, rapid pulse or high blood pressure can occur at higher doses
pseudoephedrine HCl (Sudafed) (Symptom 2)	Oral, (Adult): 60 mg 3–4 times daily Oral, (Child): 4 mg/kg daily in four divided doses.	drowsiness, rebound nasal congestion, anxiety, headache, palpitation
xylometazoline HCl (Sinutab Long-Lasting Sinus Spray)	Topical, (Adult): 2–3 drops of 0.1% solution or 1–2 inhalations of the 0.1% spray in each nostril every 8–10 hours. Topical, (Child): 2–3 drops of 0.05% solution in each nostril every 8–10 hours. Topical, (Infant): 1 drop of 0.05% solution in each nostril every 6 hours if necessary.	mild adverse effects include local stinging, sneezing, dryness of the nose, headache, drowsiness, palpitations. Chronic swelling of the nasal mucosa may occur with prolonged or excessive use.

- decongestants should not be taken if antihypertensive agents, MAO inhibitors or tricyclic antidepressants are part of the medication regimen.

Special Considerations

- Topical decongestants must be administered correctly to avoid systemic absorption.
- Physician should be notified if irregular heart beat, insomnia, dizziness, or tremors occur.
- Environmental humidification may decrease drying of the mucosa.

Antitussives

Cough is a physiologic reflex. It is a protective action that clears the respiratory tract of secretions and foreign substances. Coughing helps to maintain an open airway in individuals with asthma, chronic obstructive pulmonary disease, and cystic fibrosis. In other individuals, coughing may be associated with smoking, viral upper respiratory infections, allergy, and numerous other causes. Often, cough can be alleviated by treating the underlying cause. Although antitussives have no effect on the underlying condition, they ease respiratory discomfort, facilitate sleep, and reduce irritation.

Actions. Non-narcotic antitussive agents anesthetize the stretch receptors located in the respiratory passages, lungs, and pleura by dampening their activity and thereby reducing the cough reflex at its source. Narcotic antitussive agents depress the cough center that is located in the medulla, thereby raising its threshold for incoming cough impulse.

Uses. For symptomatic relief of cough.

Contraindications. Antitussive agents are contraindicated in individuals who are hypersensitive to any of its ingredients. They should not be used by newborn or premature infants, pregnant women, and nursing mothers.

Adverse Reactions. Non-narcotic antitussive agents may produce sedation, headache, mild dizziness, pruritus, nasal congestion, constipation, nausea, and GI upset. Narcotic antitussive agents may produce nausea, vomiting, constipation, lightheadedness, and drowsiness.

Dosage and Route. The dosage and route of administration is determined by the manufacturer, but a physician should be consulted when needed. See Table 25–3 for selected antitussives.

Implications for Patient Care. Since most non-narcotic antitussives are taken as over-the-counter medications, the implications for patient care mainly involve teaching the patient about medication. For narcotic antitussives the nurse should monitor the patient for signs of improvement, adverse reactions, dependency and/or tolerance.

Patient Teaching

Educate the patient that:

- narcotic antitussive agents may be habit forming and may cause drowsiness.
- the medication may impair mental alertness; therefore, one should not operate machinery or drive a motor vehicle, until his/her response to the medication has been determined.

Special Considerations

- Medication should not be chewed or allowed to dissolve in the mouth as it could anesthetize the throat and lead to choking.
- Liquid medication should not be taken with or followed by water as this could diminish its effect.

Table 25–3 Antitussives

Medication	Usual Dosage	Adverse Reactions
benzonatate (Tessalon)	Oral, (Adults, children over 10): 100 mg 3–6 times daily. Oral, (Children under 10 years): 8 mg/kg/day in 3–6 divided doses.	mild adverse effects include constipation, rash, drowsiness, nasal congestion, headache, and hypersensitivity reactions
codeine codeine phosphate codeine sulfate	Oral, (Adult): 10–20 mg every 4–6 hours (maximum 120 mg/24 hrs). Oral, (Children 6–12): 5–10 mg every 4–6 hours (maximum of 60 mg/day). Oral, (Children 2–6): 2.5–5 mg every 4–6 hours (maximum of 30 mg/day).	respiratory and circulatory depression with overdose (particularly with children), nausea, vomiting, constipation, light-headedness, drowsiness
dextromethorphan hydrobromide	Oral, (Adults): 10–20 mg every 4 hours (maximum, 120 mg/day). Oral, (Children 6–12): 5–10 mg every 4 hours. Oral, (Children 2–6): 2.5–5 mg every 4 hours.	mild adverse effects include drowsiness, nausea, dizziness
diphenhydramine HCl (Benylin)	Oral, (Adult): 25 mg every 4 hours (maximum, 100 mg/day). Oral, (Children 6–12): one-half the adult dose above. Oral, (Children 2–5): 6.25 mg every 4 hours (maximum of 25 mg/day).	drowsiness, dry mouth, constipation, may interfere with expectoration by making secretions thicker
hydrocodone bitartrate (Codone) (Dicodid)	Oral, (Adult): 5–10 mg 3–4 times daily. Oral, (Child): 0.6 mg/kg/day in 3–4 divided doses.	nausea, dizziness, constipation

Expectorants and Mucolytics

Among the drugs used to treat a cough are expectorants and mucolytics. An expectorant is an agent that stimulates and decreases the *thickness* of respiratory tract secretions. Mucolytics are drugs that reduce the *viscosity* of respiratory tract fluids. The actions of these medications are theoretically useful in treating coughs, because such actions should facilitate removal of irritants and phlegm. Despite studies that show some agents to be effective, conclusive evidence of the effectiveness of these medications is yet to be reported.

Expectorants

Actions. Expectorants enhance the output of lower respiratory tract fluids and help make them less viscid. This promotes and facilitates the removal of mucus.

Uses. To help loosen phlegm (mucus) and to thin bronchial secretions to make cough more productive.

Contraindications. Expectorants are contraindicated in patients who are hypersensitive to any of its ingredients and in those with persistent cough.

Adverse Reactions. Drowsiness, nausea, vomiting, and anorexia.

Dosage and Route. The dosage and route of administration is determined by the physician. See Table 25–4 for selected expectorants.

Implications for Patient Care. The nurse should monitor the patient for signs of improvement and adverse reactions.

Patient Teaching

Educate the patient:

- on how to cough to facilitate the removal of phlegm and the proper disposal of the coughed-up secretions. (The patient should be in the upright position, take several slow, deep breaths, place a tissue over his/her mouth, and then cough. The color, amount, and character of the sputum should be noted. The tissue should be placed in a proper container.)
- to drink plenty of fluids to help keep mucous membranes moist and loosen secretions.

Table 25–4 Expectorants and Mucolytics

Medication	Usual Dosage	Adverse Reactions
EXPECTORANTS		
guaifenesin (Robitussin)	Oral, (Adult): 100–400 mg every 4 hours (maximum, 2400 mg/day). Oral, (Children 6–12): 100–200 mg as above (maximum, 1200 mg/day). Oral, (Children 2–6): 50–100 mg as above (maximum, 600 mg/day).	drowsiness, nausea, vomiting, and anorexia
saturated solution of potassium iodide (SSKI)	Oral, (Adults): 0.3–0.6 ml diluted in 1 glassful of water, fruit juice or milk 3–4 times daily.	skin rash, swelling or tenderness of salivary glands
terpin hydrate elixir terpin hydrate and codeine elixir	Oral (terpin hydrate elixir): 5 ml, repeated in 3–4 hours, if necessary. (terpin hydrate and codeine elixir): 5 ml 3–4 times a day.	gastrointestinal upset
MUCOLYTICS		
acetylcysteine (Mucomyst)	Nebulization-face mask, mouth piece, tracheostomy: 3–5 ml of 20% solution, or 6–10 ml of 10% solution 3–4 times/day.	stomatitis, nausea, vomiting, fever, rhinorrhea, drowsiness, clamminess, chest tightness, bronchoconstriction

Special Considerations

- The patient should notify the physician if cough does not improve or if he/she develops a fever, rash, or a persistent headache.
- Environmental humidification may decrease drying of the mucosa and help loosen secretions.
- Saturated Solution of Potassium Iodide (SSKI) should be diluted in water or fruit juice before administering.

Mucolytics

Actions. Mucolytics break chemical bonds (disulfide linkage) in mucus, thereby lowering the viscosity.

Uses. As adjuvant therapy for patients who have abnormal, viscid or thickened mucous secretions in such conditions as chronic obstructive pulmonary disease(s), cystic fibrosis, and pneumonia.

Contraindications. Contraindicated in patients who are hypersensitive to any of its ingredients.

Warnings:

1. Asthmatics using Mucomyst should be watched carefully. If bronchospasm progresses, immediately discontinue the medication.
2. After proper use, an increased amount of liquefied bronchial secretions may occur. When coughing is inadequate, an open airway must be maintained by mechanical suction.

Adverse Reactions. Most patients tolerate Mucomyst very well. Adverse reactions that may occur are stomatitis, nausea, vomiting, fever, rhinorrhea, drowsiness, clamminess, chest tightness, and bronchospasm.

Dosage and Route. The dosage and route of administration is determined by the physician. See Table 25–4 for Mucomyst.

Implications for Patient Care. The nurse should know that this medication should not be mixed with antibiotics, iron, copper, or rubber products.

Patient Teaching

Educate the patient:

- about good oral hygienic practices.
- that the unpleasant odor experienced with use of Mucomyst will decrease after repeated use, and that discoloration of solution after the bottle is opened does not impair the effectiveness of the medication.

Special Considerations

- Medication should be stored in a refrigerator and used within 96 hours of opening.
- Medication should be given $\frac{1}{2}$–1 hour before meals for better absorption and to decrease nausea.
- May be used as an antidote for acetaminophen overdose.

Bronchodilators

Bronchodilators are used to improve pulmonary airflow in patients with chronic obstructive pulmonary disease. They are important in the treatment of asthma, a condition characterized by episodic, reversible obstruction of the peripheral airways. These agents include sympathomimetic and xanthine drugs. Inhalational corticosteroids are also used in the treatment of bronchial asthma, but do not act as bronchodilators. See Tables 25–5 and 25–6 for selected bronchodilators and Table 25–7 for selected inhalational corticosteroids.

Actions. Sympathomimetics act on beta 2 adrenoreceptors to relax smooth muscle cells of the bronchi. They also produce a vasoconstriction response throughout the body by stimulating alpha receptors. This response reduces edema in the bronchial mucosa. Some sympathomimetics also stimulate beta 1 receptors and this results in an increased heart rate and its force of contraction. Xanthine bronchodilators relax smooth muscle of the bronchial airways and pulmonary blood vessels by blocking phosphodiesterase, which increases adenosine monophosphate (AMP). By preventing the breakdown of cyclic AMP, smooth muscles relax and bronchodilation occurs, thus relieving dyspnea. They may also produce cardiac stimulation, coronary vasodilation, stimulation of skeletal muscles, cerebral stimulation, and diuresis.

Uses. Bronchodilators are used in the prevention and relief of bronchospasm in patients with asthma, bronchitis, and emphysema.

Contraindications. Bronchodilators are contraindicated in patients who are hypersensitive to any of its ingredients.

Warnings:

1. The potential for paradoxical bronchospasm should be kept in mind and if it occurs, discontinue the medication immediately.
2. Metered-dose aerosol units are under pressure. Do not puncture, use or store near heat or flame.
3. Keep out of the reach of children.

Table 25–5 Sympathomimetic Bronchodilators

Medication	Usual Dosage	Adverse Reactions
albuterol (Proventil) (Ventolin)	Inhalation, (Adult, children 12 and older): 2 inhalations every 4–6 hours. Oral: 2 mg or 4 mg three or four times a day.	palpitations, tachycardia, hypertension, nausea, nervousness
bitolterol mesylate (Tornalate)	Inhalation, (Adults, children 12 and older): 2 inhalations every 8 hours to prevent bronchospasm, or the 2 inhalations 1–3 minutes apart to treat bronchospasm.	tremors, nervousness, headache, throat irritation, coughing
epinephrine epinephrine HCl (Adrenalin)	IM, SC, (Adult): 0.2–0.5 mg (0.2–0.5 ml of 1:1,000 solution) every 2 hours as necessary. IM, SC, (Child): 0.01 mg/kg every 4 hours as needed (maximum of 0.5 mg/day).	anxiety, headache, palpitations, tremor, tachycardia
isoproterenol HCl (Isuprel)	Inhalation: 1–2 deep inhalations from nebulizing unit; dose may be repeated up to 5 times daily.	tachycardia, palpitations, headache, nervousness
metaproterenol sulfate (Alupent)	Inhalation, (Adults, children 12 and older): Usual single dose is 2–3 inhalations, every 3–4 hours. Total dosage should not exceed 12 inhalations. Oral, (Adults): 20 mg 3 or 4 times a day. Oral, (Children, six to nine years or weight under 60 lb): 10 mg 3–4 times a day.	tachycardia, hypertension, palpitations, nervousness, tremor, nausea and vomiting
terbutaline sulfate (Brethine) (Bricanyl)	Oral, (Adult): 2.5–5 mg 3 times daily (maximum, 15 mg/day). Oral, (Adolescent): 2.5 mg 3 times/day (maximum, 7.5 mg/day). SC, (Adult): 0.25 mg.	tremor, nervousness, headache
ephedrine sulfate	Oral, SC, IV, (Adults): 25–50 mg every 3–4 hours as needed. (Children): 2–6 years: 0.3–0.5 mg/kg every 4–6 hours. (Children): 6–12 years: 6.25–12.5 mg every 3–4 hours as needed.	tremors, anxiety, insomnia, headache, confusion, anorexia, nausea, dyspnea

Adverse Reactions. Palpitations, increase in blood pressure, tremors, nausea, vomiting, dizziness, heartburn, nervousness, urticaria, and headache.

Dosage and Route. The dosage and route of administration is determined by the physician. See Table 25–6 for selected xanthine bronchodilators and Table 25–7 for inhalational corticosteroids.

Table 25–6 Xanthine Bronchodilators

Medication	Usual Dosage	Adverse Reactions
aminophylline	Oral, (Adults): 500 mg, then, 250–500 mg every 6–8 hours. (Children): 7.5 mg/kg, then 3–6 mg/kg every 6–8 hours. Rectal, (Adults): 250–500 mg every 6–8 hours. IM, (Adults): 500 mg as necessary.	anxiety, restlessness, insomnia, headache, palpitations, nausea, vomiting, anorexia, increase in blood pressure
theophylline (Tedral SA)	Oral, (Adults): 1 every 12 hours. Do not chew.	epigastric distress, palpitations, tremor, CNS stimulation, insomnia
theophylline (Theo-24)	Oral, (Adults): initially 400 mg as single daily dose. Maximum without serum monitoring: 13 mg/kg/day, up to 900 mg/day. (Children): 30-35 kg: initially 300 mg once daily.	cardiac arrhythmias, nausea, headaches, diuresis, rash
oxtriphylline (Choledyl)	Oral, (Adults): 200 mg 4 times daily. (Children): 2–12 years: 3.7 mg/kg 4 times daily.	cardiac arrhythmia, nausea, headache, tachypnea, irritability, diuresis, rash
dyphylline (Lufyllin)	Oral, (Adults): Up to 15 mg/kg every 6 hours. IM, (Adult): 250–500 mg (1–2 ml) every 2–6 hours (maximum of 15 mg/kg every 6 hours).	headache, nausea, palpitations
theophylline (Elixophyllin)	Oral, (Adults and children): 6 mg/kg initially, followed by 3–4 mg/kg every 4–6 hours.	nausea, vomiting, headache, dizziness, nervousness, epigastric pain

Implications for Patient Care. The nurse should be aware that many sympathomimetic bronchodilators may also stimulate beta 1 receptors located in the heart. They may be dangerous to use in patients who have heart disease. Monitor all patients for changes in cardiac function and blood pressure. With xanthine bronchodilators, monitor the patient for disruption of cardiac function, insomnia, and hyperexcitability. Be aware of increased potential for convulsive activity. The serum levels of the medication should be checked on a regular basis. Therapeutic range should be 10–20 mcg/ml.

Patient Teaching

Sympathomimetic Bronchodilators: Educate the patient:

- to take the medication as prescribed and not to exceed the dosage.
- to notify the physician immediately if symptoms do not improve, if he/she experiences bronchial irritation, dizziness, chest pain, and/or insomnia.
- not to take any other medication unless it is prescribed by the physician.

- to drink plenty of fluids, especially water, to help moisten mucous membranes and reduce the thickness of mucus.
- that the medication should be protected from light and if the color of the solution changes, it should be discarded.

Xanthine Bronchodilators: Educate the patient that:

- oral xanthine bronchodilators may be taken with food to avoid GI upset, but the medicine should not be crushed or chewed.
- cola drinks, coffee, tea, and chocolate contain xanthine and they should not be consumed while on medication.

Special Considerations

- Sympathomimetic bronchodilators should not be used with MAO inhibitors as sympathomimetic activity could be increased and hypertensive crises may occur.
- Patients using antihistamines, tricyclic antidepressants, and thyroid hormone may experience greater sympathomimetic activity with the use of a sympathomimetic bronchodilator.
- Xanthine bronchodilators may enhance CNS stimulation of ephedrine, sympathomimetics, and amphetamines.
- Certain antibiotics (erythromycin, lincomycin, and clindamycin) may increase blood levels of xanthines.
- Xanthines may interact with beta-blocking agents, digitalis, anticoagulants, lithium, and furosemide.

Inhalational Corticosteroids

Corticosteroids are anti-inflammatory agents that are chemically related to the naturally occurring hormone cortisone. There are many uses for corticosteroids, but inhalational forms are used in the treatment of bronchial asthma, and in seasonal or perennial allergic conditions when other forms of treatment are not effective. Examples of inhalation via metered-dose inhaler steroids are dexamethasone phosphate (Decadron Phosphate Turbinaire), beclomethasone dipropionate (Beclovent, and Vancenase Nasal Inhaler), flunisolide (Aerobid and Nasalide), and triamcinolone acetonide (Azmacort). See Table 25–7 for selected corticosteroids.

Cromolyn Sodium

Cromolyn sodium inhibits the degranulation of sensitized mast cells which occurs after exposure to specific antigens. It inhibits the release of histamine and SRS-A (the slow-reacting substance of anaphylaxis, i.e. leukotrienes). Cromolyn sodium is used for the prophylactic treatment of bronchial asthma and for the prevention and treatment of the symptoms of allergic rhinitis.

Table 25–7 Inhalational Corticosteroids

Medication	Usual Dosage	Adverse Reactions
dexamethasone (Decadron)	Inhalation, (Adults), Initially 2 sprays in each nostril 2–3 times a day, Maximum 12 sprays per day. (Children over 6 years), Initially 1–2 sprays in each nostril 2 times a day. Maximum 8 sprays per day.	nasal irritation and dryness, headache, nausea, epistaxis, rebound congestion, light-headedness
flunisolide (Aerobid)	Inhalation, (Adults): 2 inhalations twice daily, morning and evening. Maximum 8 inhalations/day. (Children 6–15): 2 inhalations twice daily.	diarrhea, nausea, sore throat, headache, URI, dizziness
triamcinolone acetonide (Azmacort)	Inhalation, (Adults): 2 inhalations 3–4 times daily. Maximum 16 inhalations daily. (Children 6–12): 12 inhalations 3–4 times daily. Maximum12 inhalations daily.	hoarseness, dry mouth and throat, wheezing, cough, oral fungal infections
beclomethasone (Beclovent)	Inhalation, (Adults): 2 inhalations 3–4 times daily or 4 inhalations twice daily. Maximum 20 inhalations daily. (Children 6–12): 1–2 inhalations 3–4 times daily or 4 inhalations twice daily. Maximum 10 inhalations daily.	hoarseness, dry mouth, bronchospasm, rash, oral fungal infections

SPOTLIGHT

Tuberculosis

Tuberculosis is a contagious disease caused by the bacillus *Mycobacterium tuberculosis*. It is spread from person to person by airborne transmission. An infected person releases large and small droplets through talking, coughing, sneezing, laughing, or singing. The large droplets settle, while the small droplets remain suspended in the air and are inhaled by the susceptible person.

Tuberculosis, once called "consumption" is not a new disease. At one time it was the number one killer in the United States and it is still a major cause of death worldwide. One of public health's oldest enemies is back, and with a vengeance. An estimated 10 million Americans are infected with the TB bacterium. Compounding the problem are drug-resistant strains of TB that can shrug off as many as seven of the antibiotics traditionally used to treat this disease.

(continued)

At the present time TB is occurring primarily among AIDS patients, the homeless, drug abusers, prison inmates, and immigrants. Health officials are concerned about the rapid spread of this disease and the risks for the general public. Virtually anyone who comes in contact with an infected person is at risk contracting TB. Studies show that exposure to an infected person in confined quarters such as in homes and classrooms increases an individual's risk.

Symptoms

Symptoms include a chronic cough, fatigue, low grade fever, night sweats, weakness, chills, anorexia, weight loss, hemoptysis, and in the early stages scanty, whitish, or grayish-yellow, frothy sputum.

During the early stages of TB the sputum is expectorated in small quantities, but later when consolidation takes place it becomes more copious, tenacious and yellowish-gray. In the late stages of TB, the sputum becomes mucopurulent, musty and fetid, containing fibers and tubercle bacilli, and blood-tinged or mixed with blood.

Diagnosis

To determine a diagnosis of tuberculosis, a careful history is taken and a complete physical examination is performed. After evaluation of the patient, the physician may order a tuberculin test (if the patient has not had a previous positive reaction), chest x-ray, a bronchoscopy, or a sputum analysis for a positive diagnosis.

Treatment

Treatment of TB requires long-term drug therapy (6 to 9 months), often utilizing a regimen that includes a combination of antituberculosis agents. The use of multiple drugs is indicated in all but a few active cases, because any large population of *Mycobacterium tuberculosis* will have naturally occurring mutants that are resistant to each of the drugs administered. The primary drug regimen for active tuberculosis combines the drugs isoniazid (INH), rifampin (RIF), and ethambutol (EMB). Other drugs that are also used are streptomycin (SM) and pyrazinamide (PZA). Diet and rest are also important aspects of treatment for this disease. See Table 25–10 for selected antituberculosis agents.

The effectiveness of treatment can be evaluated by monitoring patients' sputum smear results. It takes about two weeks for the drugs to kill enough bacteria so that they can't infect other people. It takes six to nine months of continuous drug therapy for a cure. Follow-up care is essential. A sputum culture is essential to confirming a diagnosis, determining an infections's susceptibility to drugs, and assessing response to treatment. If the TB bacteria become resistant to two of the drugs that are used to treat tuberculosis then MDR TB (multi-drug resistant tuberculosis) is suspected and appropriate measures must be instituted promptly to treat and prevent the spread of MDR-TB.

Some persons are at high risk for drug-resistant TB: persons who have been recently exposed to drug-resistant TB, especially if they are immunocompromised; TB patients who failed to take medications as prescribed; TB patients who were prescribed an ineffective treatment regimen; and persons previously treated for TB.

CDC Guidelines

The Centers for Disease Control and Prevention has published a booklet called *Guidelines for Preventing the Transmission of Tuberculosis in Health-Care Settings*. The following specific actions are used to reduce the risk of tuberculosis transmission:

- Screening patient for active TB and TB infection.
- Providing rapid diagnostic services.
- Prescribing appropriate curative and preventive therapy.
- Maintaining physical measures to reduce microbial contamination of the air.
- Providing isolation rooms for persons with, or suspected of having, infectious TB.
- Screening health-care-facility personnel for TB infection.
- Promptly investing and controlling out-breaks.

Transmission-Based Precautions

The Centers for Disease Control and Prevention (CDC) released transmission-based precautions in 1996 to reduce the risk of airborne, droplet, and contact transmission of pathogens. These precautions are to be used in addition to standard precautions, and are intended for patients diagnosed with or suspected of specific highly transmissible diseases, such as tuberculosis. See Tables 25–8 and 25–9.

Special Considerations: The Older Adult

With aging there may be an increased risk of developing tuberculosis. Two factors that may contribute to an increased incidence of tuberculosis among the older adult are:

1. Previous exposure to the *Mycobacterium tuberculosis* bacillus as a child.
2. Actually having had an active case of tuberculosis as a younger person and the disease process was not treated sufficiently.

(continued)

Table 25–8 Airborne Precautions, One Category of Transmission-based Precautions

AIRBORNE PRECAUTIONS
(in addition to Standard Precautions)

VISITORS: Report to nurse before entering.

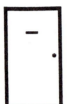

Patient Placement
Use **private room** that has:
Monitored negative air pressure,
6 to 12 air changes per hour,
Discharge of air outdoors or HEPA filtration if recirculated.
Keep room door closed and patient in room.

Respiratory Protection
Wear an **N95 respirator** when entering the room of a patient with known or suspected infectious pulmonary **tuberculosis**. **Susceptible** persons should not enter the room of patients known or suspected to have **measles** (rubeola) or **varicella** (chickenpox) if other immune caregivers are available. If susceptible persons must enter, they should wear an **N95 respirator**. (Respirator or surgical mask not required if immune to measles and varicella.)

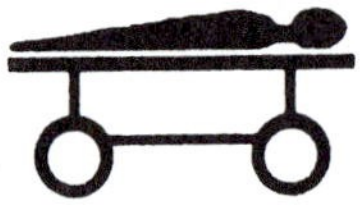

Patient Transport
Limit transport of patient from room to essential purposes only.
Use **surgical mask** on patient during transport.

(Courtesy of Brevis Corp.)

The *Mycobacterium tuberculosis* bacillus can remain dormant in a person's body for years. With the aging of the immune system, the dormant bacillus can become active and tuberculosis can emerge again. In addition to age-related immune system changes, the presence of chronic diseases often seen in the older adult can make him/her more susceptible to infection. Some age-related changes seen in the older adult's respiratory system that may make him/her more susceptible to infection are:

- Decline in the protective mechanisms of the respiratory mucosa.
- Decrease in the effectiveness of bronchial cilia.
- Changes in the connective tissues of the lungs and chest.
- Decline in elastic recoil of the lungs.

Table 25–9 Droplet Precautions, One Category of Transmission-based Precautions

DROPLET PRECAUTIONS
(in addition to Standard Precautions)

VISITORS: Report to nurse before entering.

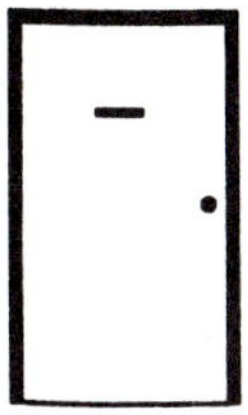

Patient Placement
Private room, if possible. Cohort or maintain spatial separation of **3 feet** from other patients or visitors if private room is not available.

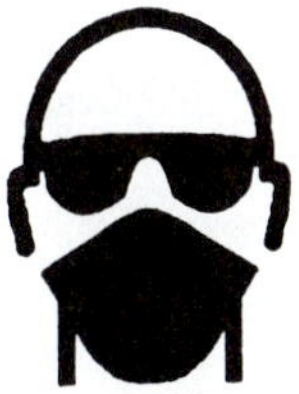

Mask
Wear mask when working within **3 feet** of patient (or upon entering room).

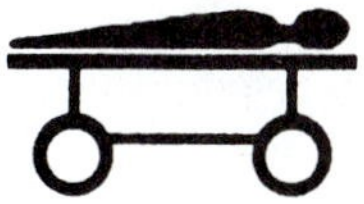

Patient Transport
Limit transport of patient from room to essential purposes only. Use **surgical mask** on patient during transport.

(Courtesy of Brevis Corp.)

- Increase in the stiffness of the chest wall decreases the lung's air moving efficiency.
- Decreased airflow delivers less oxygen to the blood and body's tissues.

Symptoms, Diagnosis, and Treatment

The classic symptoms of tuberculosis may not be obvious in the older adult. The older adult may only have weight loss and anorexia as presenting symptoms. The diagnosis and treatment are the same for the older adult as they are for anyone with tuberculosis. The exception is in the monitoring of drug therapy. Adverse reactions are more likely to occur in the older adult. One should be especially aware of possible toxic effects of streptomycin: deafness, dizziness, unsteadiness of gait, ringing in the ears, or severe headache; and for isoniazid: numbness, tingling, and weakness of the extremities. Additionally, individuals who have a previous history of drug treatment for tuberculosis may be at an increased risk of developing drug-resitant TB, and their regimen should be monitored very carefully.

Table 25–10 Antituberculosis Agents

Medication	Usual Dosage	Adverse Reactions
PRIMARY DRUGS		
ethambutol HCl (Myambutol)	Oral: 15–25 mg/kg/day in a single dose.	dose-related ocular toxicity
isoniazid (INH) (Nydrazid)	Oral, IM: 300 mg daily in a single dose, or 4–5 mg/kg of body weight per day.	hepatotoxicity, peripheral neuritis
rifampin (Rifadin) (Rimactane)	Oral, (Adult): 600 mg daily in a single dose 1 hour before or 2 hours after a meal. Oral, (Child): 10–20 mg/kg/day.	gastrointestinal disturbances, headache, flu-like symptoms, orange-tinged body fluids
SECONDARY DRUGS		
para-aminosalicylic acid (PAS)	Oral: 150 mg/kg/day in 2–3 doses after meals.	nausea, vomiting, diarrhea, hepatotoxicity
capreomycin sulfate (Capastat Sulfate)	IM, (deep): 1 Gm/day for 60–120 days followed by 1 Gm 2–3 times weekly.	nephrotoxicity, ototoxicity, hypokalemia
cycloserine (Seromycin)	Oral: 0.5–1 Gm daily in divided doses monitored by blood levels.	psychoses, convulsions, tremor, seizures
pyrazinamide	Oral: 20–35 mg/kg/day in divided doses.	hepatotoxicity, hyperuricemia, symptoms of gout
streptomycin sulfate	IM: 0.75–1 Gm daily, then reduced to 1 Gm 2–3 times weekly.	ototoxicity, nephrotoxicity
ethionamide (Trecator-SC)	Oral, (Adult): 0.5 Gm to 1 Gm daily in divided doses.	gastrointestinal intolerance, peripheral neuritis, optic neuritis, psychic disturbances

Special Considerations: The Child

When exposed to the *Mycobacterium tuberculosis* bacillus, a child may be at greater risk of contracting tuberculosis because of the following factors.

1. The airway diameter is smaller in a child and this increases the potential for obstruction.
2. The airway mucous membranes are highly vascular and susceptible to trauma, edema, infection, and spasm.
3. The accessory muscles of respiration are not as strong in a child as in an adult.
4. The child with respiratory problems is more prone to infections.

Symptoms, Diagnosis, and Treatment

The classic symptoms of tuberculosis may be more difficult to identify in a child than in an adult. The child may appear weak, have a history of weight loss, anorexia, and a low grade fever. Since there are several conditions that could cause the same symptoms, a careful analysis of the child's physical state should be evaluated and a differential diagnosis should include a tuberculin test, chest x-ray, and a positive smear or sputum culture indicating the presence of acid-fast bacteria (AFB).

When a positive diagnosis is determined the child is placed on antituberculosis agents for six to nine months. The drug regimen is determined by the attending physician and the dosage is based upon kilogram of body weight. The following dosage chart is taken from the Centers for Disease Control and Prevention: *TB/HIV The Connection, What Health Care Workers Should Know.*

Dosage Recommendations for the Treatment of TB in Children (12 years of age and younger)

Drug	Daily Dose	Twice-Weekly Dose	Thrice-Weekly Dose
Isoniazid	10–20 mg/kg Max. 300 mg	20–40 mg/kg Max. 900 mg	20–40 mg/kg Max. 900 mg
Rifampin	10–20 mg/kg Max. 600 mg	10–20 mg/kg Max. 600 mg	10–20 mg/kg Max. 600 mg
Pyrazinamide	15–30 mg/kg Max. 2 gm	50–70 mg/kg	50–70 mg/kg
Ethambutol*	15–25 mg/kg Max. 2.5 gm	50 mg/kg	25–30 mg/kg
Streptomycin	20–40 mg/kg Max. 1 gm	25–30 mg/kg	25–30 mg/kg

*Ethambutol is generally not recommended for children whose visual acuity cannot be monitored (children under 6 years of age). However, ethambutol should be considered for all children with organisms resistant to other drugs, if susceptibility to ethambutol has been demonstrated or susceptibility is likely.

Critical Thinking Questions/Activities

An estimated 10 million Americans are infected with the TB bacterium. To help protect yourself, your family, and your patients, you should know certain facts about tuberculosis. Ask yourself:

- How is tuberculosis spread?
- What are the symptoms of tuberculosis?
- How is tuberculosis diagnosed?

(continued)

- What is the treatment regimen for tuberculosis?
- How is the effectiveness of the treatment regimen evaluated?
- What is MDR TB?
- What persons are at high risk for MDR TB?
- What are the recommended CDC guidelines for preventing the transmission of tuberculosis in health-care settings?

Spot Check

There are several medications that may be used to treat tuberculosis. For each of the selected drugs listed, give the recommended children's dosage.

DrugDaily Dose	Twice-Weekly Dose	Thrice-Weekly Dose
Isoniazid		
Rifampin		
Pyrazinamide		
Ethambutol		
Streptomycin		

◆ Review Questions

Directions: Select the best answer to each multiple choice question. Circle the letter of your choice.

1. Allergic rhinitis is also known as __________.
   a. rhinovirus b. coryza c. hay fever d. hives
2. __________ is an inflammation of the respiratory mucous membrane caused by a rhinovirus.
   a. Urticaria c. Pruritus
   b. Coryza d. Rhinorrhea
3. Antihistamines are effective in the treatment of __________.
   a. allergy symptoms c. urticaria and pruritus
   b. seasonal upper respiratory disorders d. all of these
4. The most frequent adverse reactions to antihistamines are __________.
   a. sedation, sleepiness, dizziness, disturbed coordination, epigastric distress, and thickening of bronchial secretions
   b. dryness of mouth, nose, and throat
   c. hypotension, headache, palpitations
   d. nervousness, tremor, vertigo, anorexia
5. The usual adult dose of chlorpheniramine maleate (Chlor-Trimeton) is__________.
   a. 5–20 mg/day c. 6–16 mg/daily
   b. 1–2 mg twice daily d. 6 mg/day
6. The usual dose of terfenadine (Seldane) is __________.
   a. 60 mg twice daily c. 10–100 mg 3–4 times daily
   b. 25–50 mg 3–4 times daily d. 75 mg twice daily
7. Decongestants that are commonly used for symptomatic relief of nasal congestion produce the following effects. They:
   a. dilate the nasal mucosa
   b. increase blood flow to the affected area
   c. slow the formation of mucus
   d. close nasal passages
8. Adverse reactions to pseudoephedrine HCl (Sudafed) are __________.
   a. drowsiness, rebound nasal congestion, anxiety, headache, and palpitation.
   b. sneezing, dryness of the mouth, light-headedness, and headache
   c. sneezing, stinging of the mucosa, light-headedness, and headache
   d. nausea, vomiting, diarrhea, and hypotension

9. Although antitussives have no effect on the underlying coughing condition, they do __________.
   a. increase respiratory discomfort
   b. facilitate sleep
   c. reduce irritation
   d. b and c
10. Adverse reactions to diphenhydramine (Benylin) are __________.
    a. nausea, dizziness, and constipation
    b. drowsiness, dry mouth, and constipation
    c. nausea, constipation, light-headedness
    d. headache, rash, drowsiness
11. The usual children's (6–12 years) dose of guaifensin (Robitussin) is __________.
    a. 100–200 mg every 4 hours
    b. 0.3–0.6 ml 3–4 times daily
    c. 200–400 mg every 4 hours
    d. 50–100 mg every 4 hours
12. Adverse reactions to epinephrine HCl (Adrenalin) are __________.
    a. nausea, vomiting, and diarrhea
    b. anxiety, headache, palpitations, tremor, and tachycardia
    c. bradycardia, hypotension, nausea, and vomiting
    d. constipation, tremor, headache, and vomiting
13. The primary drug regimen for active tuberculosis combines the drugs __________.
    a. para-aminosalicylic acid, cycloserine, and rifampin
    b. streptomycin, capreomycin, and ethambutol
    c. isoniazid, rifampin, and ethambutol
    d. isoniazid, streptomycin, and para-aminosalicylic acid
14. The usual oral dose of isoniazid (INH) is __________ mg daily in a single dose.
    a. 300
    b. 600
    c. 500
    d. 375
15. Adverse reactions to rifampin (Rifadin) are __________.
    a. nephrotoxicity, ototoxicity, hypokalemia
    b. psychoses, convulsions, tremor, seizures
    c. peripheral neuritis and hepatotoxicity
    d. gastrointestinal disturbance, headache, flu-like symptoms
16. Respiratory conditions/diseases may be caused by __________.
    a. nonpathogenic organisms, allergens, fungi
    b. pathogenic organisms, allergies, viruses
    c. fungi, environmental and/or hereditary factors
    d. b and c
17. The thin-walled air sacs of the lungs are called:
    a. alveoli
    b. bronchi
    c. bronchus
    d. aveoli

Case Study: Mr. Cole Dawson, a 64-year-old retired engineer is admitted with a diagnosis of COPD and pneumonia. Admitting vital signs are: B/P 32/84; P 98, T 100.8, R 14, shallow and labored. Medications ordered are aminophylline 500 mg tabs stat, then 500 mg every 6 hours; amoxicillin 500 mg tabs every 8 hours; acetaminophen 650 mg tabs every 4 hours with food or milk.

18. The nurse should know that aminophylline is a/an __________ bronchodilator.
    a. xanthine
    b. sympathomimetic
    c. anticholinergic
    d. cholinergic
19. This type of bronchodilator relaxes smooth muscle cells of the bronchi by __________.
    a. acting on beta 1 receptors
    b. acting on beta 2 adrenoreceptors
    c. blocking phosphodiesterase
    d. stimulation of alpha adrenergic receptors
20. To evaluate the effectiveness of aminophylline, the nurse should monitor the __________.
    a. pulse
    b. rate and rhythm of respirations
    c. blood pressure
    d. temperature
21. When a patient is taking aminophylline, the serum level of the medication should be checked on a regular basis. Therapeutic range should be ________.
    a. 10–20 mcg/ml
    b. 15–30 mcg/ml
    c. 5–15 mcg/ml
    d. 20–30 mcg/ml
22. Adverse reactions to observe the patient for are __________.
    a. nausea, diarrhea, anorexia
    b. nausea, constipation, anorexia
    c. palpitations, increase in B/P, vomiting, headache
    d. polyuria, anorexia, nausea
23. Mr. Dawson should be taught not to consume cola drinks, coffee, tea and/or chocolate while on aminophylline because they contain __________.
    a. diuretics
    b. xanthine
    c. polypeptides
    d. proteins
24. The nurse should know that amoxicillin is a/an __________.
    a. broad-spectrum antibiotic
    b. narrow-spectrum antibiotic
    c. antifungal agent
    d. antiviral agent

25. Amoxicillin is contraindicated in patients who are __________.
    a. anemic
    b. hypertensive
    c. hypersensitive to penicillin
    d. diabetics
26. Mr. Dawson is receiving acetaminophen for __________.
    a. hypertension
    b. fever
    c. rapid pulse
    d. shallow respirations
27. After several days of hospitalization, Mr. Dawson states that his breathing is easier, but he feels very nervous, is nauseated, and has a severe itching. The nurse should know that these symptoms could be an adverse reaction to aminophylline. The best action to take is __________.
    a. reassure the patient, assess vital signs, notify the physician
    b. reassure the patient, stop the medication
    c. ignore the symptoms
    d. notify the physician

Matching: Place the correct letter from Column II on the appropriate line of Column I.

Column I	**Column II**
28. __________ Allergic rhinitis	A. One of a subgroup of viruses that causes the common cold in man.
29. __________ Coryza	B. Severe itching.
30. __________ Histamine	C. An inflammation of the nasal mucosa that is due to the sensitivity of the nasal mucosa to an allergen.
31. __________ Pruritus	D. The flow of thin watery discharge from the nose.
32. __________ Rhinorrhea	E. Hives.
33. __________ Rhinovirus	F. A substance that is normally present in the body.
34. __________ Urticaria	G. The common cold.
35. __________ Robitussin	H. Antihistamine.
	I. Expectorant.

C H A P T E R 26

Medications Used for Gastrointestinal System Disorders

OBJECTIVES

Upon completion of this chapter, you should be able to:

- Define the terms listed in the vocabulary.
- Describe the digestive process.
- State the actions, uses, contraindications, adverse reactions, dosage and route, implications for patient care, patient teaching, and special considerations for antacids, histamine H_2-receptor antagonists, and antispasmodics/anticholinergics.
- State the action, uses, contraindications, adverse reactions, dosage and route, and interactions for sucralfate (Carafate).
- Describe misoprostol (Cytotec) and state its use, contraindications, adverse reactions, and dosage and route.
- Describe an ulcer that is associated with the *Helicobacter pylori* bacteria.
- State the treatment regimen for an ulcer associated with the *Helicobacter pylori* bacteria.
- Give the reported problems associated with the drug regimen for an ulcer caused by the *Helicobacter pylori* bacteria.
- List the side effects associated with the drug regimen that is used to treat ulcers caused by the *Helicobacter pylori* bacteria.
- Describe the symptoms of a peptic ulcer.
- List the changes that occur in gastrointestinal functioning of the older adult.
- State the signs and/or symptoms of gastrointestinal disorders in the child.
- List the signs of dehydration in the child.
- Complete the critical thinking questions/activities presented in this chapter.
- State the usage, classifications, actions, usual dosage, onset of action, patient teaching, and special considerations for laxatives.
- Describe diarrhea and state eight possible causes.

- State the usual dosage, adverse reactions, and special considerations for antidiarrheal agents.
- State the usage, contraindications, and dosage of apomorphine HCl and Ipecac syrup.
- Complete the Spot Check on selected drugs used to treat ulcers.
- Answer the review questions correctly.

Vocabulary

defecation (def-e-ka'shun). The process of emptying the bowel.

histamine antagonist (his'ta-min an-tag'o-nist). An agent that inhibits the action of histamine at the histamine H_2 receptor site. The H_2 receptor site is located on the parietal cells of the stomach.

peptic ulcer (pep'tik ul'ser). An ulcer occurring in the lower end of the esophagus; along the lesser curvature of the stomach; or in the duodenum.

dyspepsia (dis-pep'si-a). Difficulty in digestion; indigestion.

constipation (kon"sti-pa'shun). Infrequent passage of hard, dry feces; difficult defecation.

Synopsis: The Gastrointestinal System

The gastrointestinal system enables the body to extract absorbable nutrients from food during the digestive process. During this process, food passes from the mouth, down the esophagus, to the stomach where it is converted to a near-liquid mass by hydrochloric acid, various enzymes, and the churning motions of the stomach walls. This partially digested mass, known as *chyme*, leaves the acidic environment of the stomach through its lower orifice (pylorus) and passes into the first part of the small intestine (duodenum). Here, the acid chyme is made alkaline as it is mixed with bile, pancreatic juice, and intestinal secretions. As this near-liquid mass passes through the small intestine, the products of digestion are absorbed, passed into the blood and lymph, and are eventually carried throughout the body. The residue of digestion is passed into the ascending colon where reabsorption of water begins. The now semi-solid waste passes from the ascending colon, through the transverse and descending colons, to the rectum. Here, it is stored until there is an opportunity for defecation, Figure 26–1.

The digestive process involves a combination of mechanical and chemical processes coordinated by the autonomic nervous system. Typical complaints and disorders of the gastrointestinal system include dyspepsia (indigestion), pyrosis (heartburn), ulcers, nausea, vomiting, diarrhea, constipation, and infection. Many of these complaints may be symptomatic of conditions other than disorders of the gastrointestinal system.

Antacids

Many gastrointestinal complaints are simply the result of poor eating habits, stress, over indulgence, alcohol, smoking, and can be said to be the result of the patient's

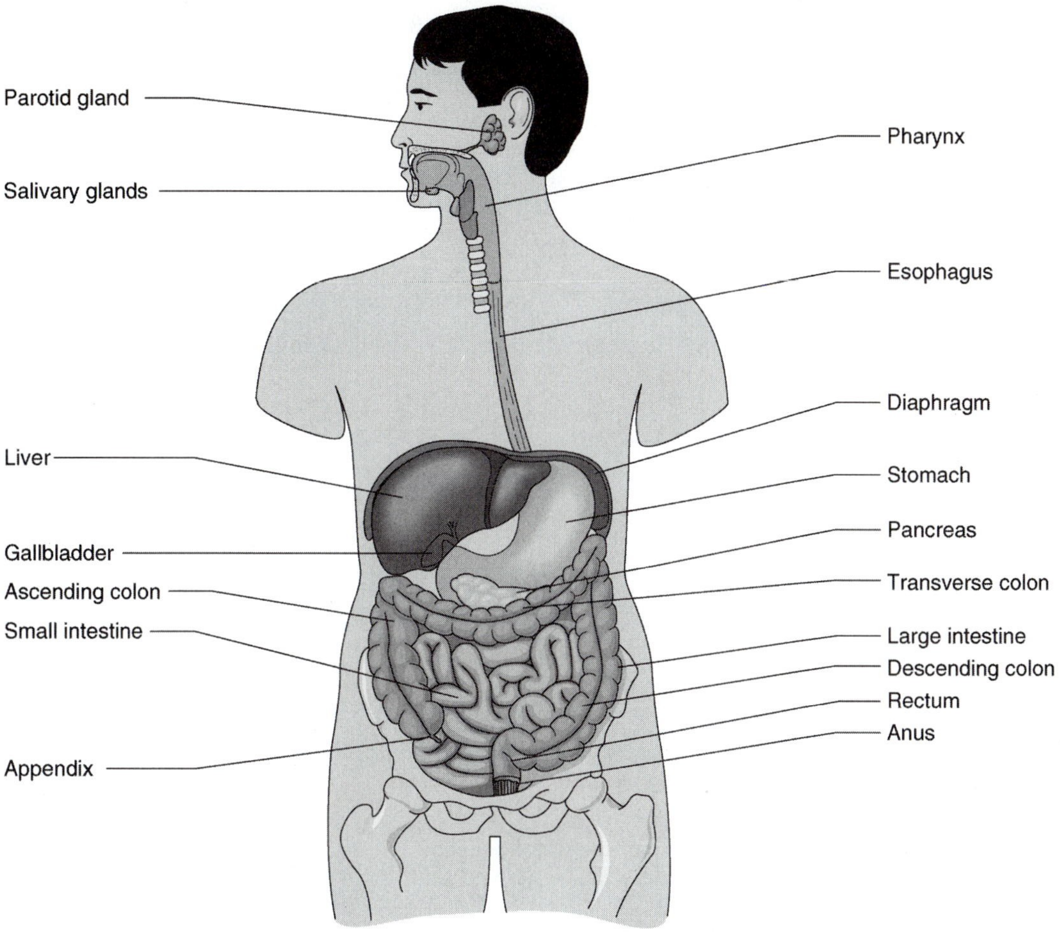

Figure 26–1 The gastrointestinal system

lifestyle. *Antacids* are drugs that neutralize hydrochloric acid in the stomach. They are used to relieve acid indigestion, gas, heartburn, and in the treatment of peptic ulcers. Ideally, an antacid should neutralize large amounts of acid with a small dose; should have a long-lasting effect; should not interfere with electrolyte balance; and should not cause a secondary increase in gastric acidity. The majority of antacids are classified as non-systemic agents because they remain largely in the gastrointestinal tract. See Table 26–1. These agents are useful for long-term treatment of ulcers and for occasional relief of gas, indigestion, and other complaints.

Sodium bicarbonate is a systemic antacid. It is readily absorbed, has a rapid onset, and a short duration of action. For these and other reasons, this antacid is not indicated for use in long-term therapy.

Table 26–1 Non-Systemic Antacids

Medication	Usual Dosage	Adverse Reactions
basic aluminum carbonate gel (Basaljel)	Oral: 10 ml of regular suspension, or 5 ml of extra strength, or 2 tablets or capsules every 2 hours, if necessary.	constipation, fecal impaction
aluminum hydroxide (Amphojel)	Oral: 5–10 ml (1–2 tsp), or 1–2 tablets or capsules, 4–6 times/day, if needed.	constipation, nausea, phosphorus deficiency syndrome
aluminum phosphate (Phosphaljel)	Oral: 15–30 ml every 2 hours	constipation
calcium carbonate, precipitated chalk (Tums)	Oral: 0.5–2 Gm 4–6 times daily, if necessary	constipation, acid rebound, nausea, flatulence
dihydroxyaluminum sodium carbonate (Rolaids)	Oral: 1–2 tablets 4 or more times per day.	constipation, intestinal concentrations
magaldrate (Riopan)	Oral: 1–2 tablets, or 5–10 ml of suspension 4 times/day.	infrequent diarrhea or constipation
magnesium carbonate	Oral: 0.5–2 Gm between meals and at bedtime, if necessary.	diarrhea, distention, belching, flatulence
magnesium hydroxide (Milk of Magnesia)	Oral: 5–10 ml, or 1–2 tablets 1 to 3 hours after meals and at bedtime.	diarrhea, nausea, hypermagnesemia
magnesium oxide (Maox)	250–1500 mg with water or milk, 4 times/day after meals and at bedtime.	diarrhea, nausea, hypermagnesemia

Actions. Antacids act in a variety of ways. They may neutralize gastric acidity, cause hydrogen ion absorption, bind phosphates in the GI tract, buffer the acid, and/or reduce the surface tension of gas bubbles so that the gas may be more easily eliminated.

Uses. Relief of heartburn, acid indigestion, gas, and in the symptomatic relief of hyperacidity associated with peptic ulcer, gastritis, peptic esophagitis, gastric hyperacidity, hiatal hernia, and postoperative gas pain.

Contraindications. Contraindicated in patients with hypersensitivity to any of its ingredients.

Adverse Reactions. Adverse reactions may vary with the type of preparation. See Table 26–1 and Table 26–2.

Dosage and Route. The dosage and route of administration is determined by the patient and the physician.

Table 26–2 Common Antacid Mixtures

Medication	Ingredients	Usual Dosage	Warnings
Gaviscon	aluminum hydroxide, magnesium carbonate (liquid), magnesium trisilicate (tablet)	Oral: 1 or 2 tablespoons, or 2 tablets (chewed), 1 hour after meals and at bedtime.	contraindicated in those with kidney disease, and those taking any form of tetracycline
Gelusil	aluminum hydroxide, magnesium hydroxide, and simethicone	Oral: 2 or more teaspoons or tablets (chewed) after meals and at bedtime.	see above
Maalox Plus	aluminum hydroxide, magnesium hydroxide, and simethicone	Oral: 1 to 4 tablets chewed 4 times a day, 20–60 minutes after meals and at bedtime.	see above
Mylanta	aluminum hydroxide, magnesium hydroxide and simethicone	Oral: 2–4 teaspoons or tablets (chewed), every 2–4 hours between meals and at bedtime.	see above

Implications for Patient Care. The patient should not take antacids for more than two weeks without the permission of the physician. The patient should not exceed the maximum dosage of any antacid or antacid mixture.

Calcium carbonate and sodium bicarbonate may cause rebound hyperacidity. Patients with renal failure should not use large quantities of antacids containing magnesium. The magnesium cannot be excreted and may produce hypermagnesemia and toxicity.

Patient Teaching

Educate the patient:

- that aluminum based and calcium carbonate antacids may cause constipation.
- to increase his/her fluid intake to 2000 ml/day while taking an aluminum based antacid to help relieve constipation, unless contraindicated.
- that magnesium based antacids may cause diarrhea.
- to notify the physician if there is any difficulty with constipation and/or diarrhea.
- that liquid suspensions must be shaken well before taking.
- to store suspensions in a cool place.
- that chewable tablets should be chewed thoroughly before swallowing and then followed with 8 ounces of water.

Special Considerations

- Antacids should not be used in patients who are taking any form of tetracycline.
- Antacids should be used with caution in geriatric patients, those who have de-

creased GI motility, bowel obstruction, dehydration, renal disease, sodium-restricted diets, and pregnancy.

- May decrease absorption of cimetidine, iron, benzodiazepines, corticosteroids, anticholinergics, digitalis, and phenytoin (Dilantin).
- Levodopa absorption is increased by antacids.

Antacid Mixtures

Products that combine aluminum and/or calcium compounds with magnesium salts often prove more useful than the single-entity antacids listed in Table 26–1. These agents are commonly used in the treatment of peptic ulcers, acid indigestion, and heartburn. By combining the antacid properties of two single-entity agents, products have been created that provide the antacid action of both, yet tend to counter the adverse effects of each ingredient. For example, a product containing aluminum hydroxide (a cause of constipation) and magnesium hydroxide (a cause of diarrhea) will minimize these effects while offering the sum of the antacid actions of both ingredients. Table 26–2 lists some common antacid mixtures.

Histamine H_2-Receptor Antagonist

Histamine H_2-receptor antagonist inhibits both daytime and nocturnal basal gastric acid secretion and inhibits gastric acid stimulated by food, histamines, caffeine, insulin, and pentagastrin. There are four drugs of this type (cimetidine, ranitidine, famotidine, and nizatidine) that have been approved for the treatment of active duodenal ulcer, and for pathological hypersecretory conditions (Zollinger-Ellison Syndrome). See Table 26–3.

Actions. Reduce gastric acid secretion by occupying H_2-receptor sites on parietal cells.

Uses. Active duodenal ulcer, and for pathological hypersecretory conditions (Zollinger-Ellison Syndrome). Short-term treatment of duodenal and gastric ulcers and maintenance therapy.

Contraindications. Contraindicated in patients with known hypersensitivity to any of its ingredients.

> **CAUTION:** Should not be used during pregnancy, breastfeeding, and in children under 16 years of age. Cautious use in patients with hepatic disease, and/or renal disease.

Adverse Reactions. Histamine H_2-receptor antagonist is generally well tolerated. Adverse reactions vary with the specific drug and the length of use. See Table 26–3. Some adverse reactions that may occur are: confusion, headache, depression, dizziness, anxiety, weakness, psychosis, tremors, convulsions, diarrhea, constipation, abdominal cramps,

Table 26–3 Histamine H_2-Receptor Antagonist

Medication	Usual Dosage	Adverse Reactions
cimetidine (Tagamet)	Active duodenal ulcer: 800 mg at bedtime. Maintenance: 400 mg at bedtime. Active gastric ulcer: 800 mg at bedtime or 300 mg 4 times a day with meals and at bedtime.	diarrhea, dizziness, somnolence, rash, headache, myalgia, arthralgia, facial edema, bradycardia, constipation, tiredness, confusion, jaundice, gynecomastia, impotence
famotidine (Pepcid)	Acute therapy: 1 (40 mg) tablet at bedtime. Maintenance Therapy: 1 (20 mg) tablet at bedtime.	headache, dizziness, diarrhea, constipation
nizatidine (Axid)	Active duodenal ulcer: 300 mg at bedtime. Alternate dose: 150 mg bid Maintenance Therapy: 150 mg at bedtime.	somnolence, sweating, urticaria, confusion, tachycardia, impotence, decreased libido
ranitidine (Zantac)	Active duodenal ulcer: 150 mg bid or 300 mg at bedtime. Maintenance Therapy: 150 mg at bedtime.	headache, malaise, dizziness, constipation, abdominal pain, diarrhea, insomnia, vertigo, arrhythmias, hepatitis, rash, blood dyscrasia, gynecomastia, impotence.

paralytic ileus, jaundice, rash, bradycardia, tachycardia, facial edema, malaise, insomnia, vertigo, gynecomastia, impotence, decreased libido, and/or blood dyscrasia.

Dosage and Route. Dosage and route of administration is determined by the physician and individualized for each patient. See Table 26–3.

Implications for Patient Care. Observe for signs of improvement and/or hypersensitivity. Monitor gastric pH (should be below 5), I&O ratio, BUN, CBC, liver function tests, creatinine, and prothrombin time.

Patient Teaching

Cimetidine and ranitidine: Educate the patient:

- that gynecomastia and impotence may occur while using. Explain that both are reversible after discontinuance of the drug(s).
- that the medication may impair mental alertness; therefore, one should not operate machinery or drive a motor vehicle, until his/her response to the medication has been determined.

Famotidine: Educate the patient:

- to report any signs of blood dyscrasia (bleeding, bruising, fatigue, and malaise) to the physician.
- that decreased libido may occur while using, but it is reversible after discontinuance of the drug.

Nizatidine: Educate the patient:

- that false-positive tests for urobilinogen with Multistix may occur while taking this medication.
- that impotence and decreased libido may occur while using.

Explain that both are reversible after discontinuance of the drug.

Special Considerations

- Patients with duodenal and/or gastric ulcers should avoid substances that may irritate the mucous membrane of the duodenum or stomach such as caffeine, nicotine, black pepper, alcohol, harsh spices, liquids and foods that are very hot and/or very cold, over-the-counter medications, especially those that contain aspirin.
- The effect of the medication may be decreased with the use of antacids and ketoconazole (antifungal drug).
- Cimetidine has been reported to reduce the hepatic metabolism of certain drugs, thereby increasing their blood level and delaying their elimination. These drugs include the warfarin-type anticoagulants (Coumadin, Panwarfin), phenytoin (Dilantin), propranolol (Inderal), lidocaine, chlordiazepoxide (Librium), diazepam (Valium), certain tricyclic antidepressants, theophylline, and metronidazole (Flagyl).
- Inhibits the metabolism of calcium channel blocking agents (antianginals and/or antihypertensives) diltiazem, nifedipine, and verapamil.

Other Ulcer Medications

sucralfate (Carafate)

Sucralfate (Carafate) is a cytoprotective agent that is used to prevent further damage by ulcers and to promote the healing process by coating the surface of the damaged mucosa. It exerts its effect through a local, rather than systemic action. Following administration, this agent mixes with gastric acid to form a paste-like coating that prevents further damage by ulcerogenic secretions.

Uses. Short-term treatment (up to 8 weeks) of active duodenal ulcer and for maintenance therapy.

Contraindications. No known contraindications.

Adverse Reactions. Constipation, diarrhea, nausea, vomiting, gastric discomfort, indigestion, flatulence, dry mouth, pruritus, rash, dizziness, sleepiness, vertigo, back pain, headache.

Dosage and Route. *Adult dose:* 1 gm four times a day on an empty stomach. *Maintenance therapy:* 1 gm twice a day. Do not crush to dissolve. Allow to form a slurry (a thin, watery mixture) by adding water.

Interactions. Avoid antacids within 30 minutes of dosing. May reduce absorption of tetracyclines, phenytoin, cimetidine, digoxin, ciprofloxacin, norfloxacin, ranitidine, theophylline. When prescribed, these medications should be given separately and in two hour intervals of dosing with sucralfate.

misoprostol (Cytotec)

Misoprostol (Cytotec) is an antiulcer agent that is used to prevent NSAID (nonsteroidal anti-inflammatory drugs) induced gastric ulcers. It has not been shown to prevent duodenal ulcers in patients taking NSAIDs. It is contraindicated during pregnancy and childbearing potential because of its abortifacient property. Adverse reactions include diarrhea, abdominal pain, flatulence, headache and nausea. Dosage for adults is 200 mcg four times a day with food. If not tolerated, 100 mcg can be used. One should avoid magnesium-containing antacids while taking this medication.

SPOTLIGHT

Ulcers and *Helicobacter pylori* Bacteria

In 1981, Doctor Barry Marshall and Doctor Robin Warren of the Royal Perth Hospital in Western Australia noticed a bacterial infection in the stomach linings of patients in the hospital. Out of 100 patients with various diseases, 65 percent were tested and found to have the infection, and half of these were found to have ulcers.

In 1986, in a treatment study among 100 patients whose ulcers would not go away, Doctor Marshall gave half of them Tagamet and the other half received an antibiotic (Flagyl) and an antacid bismuth. According to the study, the ulcers returned in 95 percent of the patients not treated with an antibiotic. Among those treated with Flagyl and bismuth the ulcers returned in only 20 percent.

Because it was hard for many doctors to believe that bacteria could live in an acid (stomach) and also to believe in Doctor Marshall's findings, he put himself at some risk to prove his hypothesis. He infected himself by swallowing a teaspoonful of culture containing the *Helicobacter pylori* bacteria. He came down with gastritis. As further proof

(continued)

of his theory, Doctor Marshall said, the antibiotic cured him. He added that not all ulcer patients are cured. One reason is that the bacteria sometimes develops resistance to the antibiotic.

There is now scientific proof showing that approximately 90 percent of duodenal ulcers and 70 percent of gastric ulcers are associated with *Helicobacter pylori* bacteria. The bacteria settle in the lining of the duodenum or stomach, opening a wound that is then made worse by digestive juices and stomach acids. The wound is said to resemble a flattened volcano or a white-centered, red-rimmed, painful canker sore. By killing the bacteria with antibiotics, it is estimated that 90 percent of the ulcers caused by *H. pylori* could be cured.

The National Institutes of Health (NIH) recommends a three-drug treatment regimen with two antibiotics: metronidazole (Flagyl) and either tetracycline or amoxicillin and Pepto Bismol. The reported problems associated with this drug regimen is that the patient has to complete the full treatment program that involves taking 15 pills a day for a total of at least two weeks and many of the patients quit prematurely. If the treatment isn't completed, it is believed that only the weakest of the bacteria are killed, leaving the more resistant ones to cause further damage. The patients also complained of side effects that included changes in taste, a metallic taste in the mouth, nausea, vomiting, diarrhea, and skin rash.

Ulcers have afflicted one in ten adult Americans at some point. There are about 500,000 new cases of peptic ulcer disease in the United States each year. A peptic ulcer is defined as an ulcer occurring in the lower end of the esophagus; in the stomach usually along the lesser curvature; in the duodenum; or on the jejunal side of a gastrojejunostomy.

The traditional medical treatment of ulcers involves giving agents that reduce the levels of acid and pepsin in the stomach. These agents include histamine-blocking agents, antacids, and coating agents. If hemorrhage, perforation, or intractable bleeding occurs surgery is usually indicated and this may include a vagotomy and subtotal gastric resection.

With the breakthrough discovery that some ulcers are caused by *Helicobacter pylori*, the treatment regimen of antibiotics and an antacid is now becoming a standard part of treatment for ulcers. Before the National Institutes of Health's consensus panel, the *H. pylori* issue had some believers and some nonbelievers. Since that time, the issue has been resolved and the number of physicians treating *H. pylori* as part of ulcer therapy has been growing.

There are studies being conducted to evaluate the feasibility of a two-drug regimen of the antibiotic clarithromycin (Biaxin) and omeprazole (Prilosec) for the treatment of ulcers caused by *H. pylori*. Omeprazole (Prilosec) has similar antisecretory effects to Pepto Bismol and may also work against the *H. pylori* bacteria itself.

The symptoms of a peptic ulcer include:

- pain usually described as "gnawing"
- dyspepsia
- heartburn
- acid eructations
- nausea
- vomiting
- anorexia

Special Considerations: The Older Adult

With aging there are certain changes that occur in gastrointestinal functioning. The digestive system motion slows as muscle contractions become weaker. Glandular secretions decrease, causing a drier mouth and a lower volume of gastric juices. Atrophy of the mucosal lining may reduce the rate of nutrient absorption. Other changes that generally occur are:

- deterioration of the teeth.
- decrease in functional taste buds.
- muscles associated with chewing weaken.
- difficulty in swallowing.
- peristalsis becomes slower.
- gastric emptying becomes slower.
- bile may become thicker, thereby the emptying of the gallbladder may be slower.
- decreased liver size.
- reduced blood flow through the liver.
- reduced liver enzyme activity.

The changes in the gastrointestinal system caused by aging generally increase the older person's risk for anorexia, bloating, indigestion, flatulence, diarrhea, and constipation. Constipation is one of the most frequent gastrointestinal complaints of the older adult. Constipation may result from intestinal immotility, a diet low in bulk and roughage, lack of physical exercise, and an altered bacteria flora. In addition to the changes given, age-related and disease-related changes contribute to decreased ability

(continued)

of the older adult to clear drugs through the liver and the renal system. Serum albumin concentration is lower, which tends to make available more free drug to tissues or to make available more drug to be eliminated from the body. A gradual decrease in blood flow to the internal organs in the abdomen reduces drug clearance through the liver or kidneys.

The older adult should be carefully evaluated before the initiation of any type of drug therapy. Reduced dosage and less frequent doses may be given to the older adult to help avoid drug accumulation and adverse effects.

Special Considerations: The Child

The gastrointestinal system of the child differs from that of the adult. The child who is not developing normally according to established growth parameters, such as height, weight, and head circumference should be evaluated for gastrointestinal disorders. Signs and/or symptoms such as constipation, rectal bleeding, hematemesis, jaundice, nausea, and vomiting usually indicate GI disorders.

The child with nausea and vomiting will dehydrate more quickly than an adult. Fluid imbalances can quickly develop in infants and young children. It is important to accurately assess fluid intake and output and to seek medical attention if dehydration is suspected.

Signs of Dehydration:

- Loss of body weight: mild dehydration up to 5 percent; moderate dehydration 5 to 10 percent; severe dehydration over 10 percent
- Irritability and lethargy
- Skin turgor—loss of elasticity
- Dry mucous membranes
- Sunken eyeballs and fontanels
- Absent or decreased tearing and salivation
- Abnormal thirst
- Decreased urine output; specific gravity elevated
- Subnormal to elevated body temperature
- Rapid respirations
- Normal to low blood pressure
- Rapid pulse

Critical Thinking Questions/Activities

There is now scientific proof showing that approximately 90 percent of duodenal ulcers and 70 percent of gastric ulcers are associated with *Helicobacter pylori* bacteria.

Your patient is a 66-year-old male who has a history of dyspepsia, heartburn, nausea, vomiting, anorexia, and a "gnawing" pain in the epigastric region. His diagnosis is peptic ulcer disease. He states that he has taken Tagamet, Pepcid, Zantac, and numerous antacids, but none of these have seemed to cure his ulcer.

Ask Yourself:

- Could this patient have an ulcer caused by *Helicobacter pylori* bacteria?
- What does the *H. pylori* bacteria do to the lining of the stomach?
- Since the traditional medical treatment for an ulcer was not successful in this patient, what other treatment regimen could be prescribed?
- What are the reported problems associated with the drug regimen for ulcers caused by *Helicobacter pylori* bacteria?
- What are some of the side effects associated with the drug regimen that is used to treat ulcers caused by *Helicobacter pylori* bacteria?

Antispasmodics/Anticholinergics

Actions. Natural and synthetic antispasmodic drugs reduce gastric motility by antagonizing the action of acetylcholine at the postganglionic receptors in the parasympathetic nervous system. These drugs are generally referred to as anticholinergics.

Uses. (**Please Note:** The efficacy of anticholinergics in the treatment of gastric ulcer has not been proven conclusively. It is not known whether they aid in the healing or decrease the rate of recurrence or prevent complication of peptic ulcers.) For use as adjunctive therapy in the treatment of peptic ulcer. Useful in the management of dyspepsia, irritable colon, mild diarrhea, pylorospasm, biliary colic, hypermotility, and acute pancreatitis.

Contraindications. Contraindicated in patients with known hypersensitivity to any of its ingredients, glaucoma, obstructive uropathy, prostatic hypertrophy, GI obstruction, paralytic ileus, intestinal atony of the elderly or debilitated patient, unstable cardiovascular state in acute hemorrhage, severe ulcerative colitis, toxic megacolon complicating ulcerative colitis, myasthenia gravis.

Warnings:

1. Safety of anticholinergic preparations during pregnancy, lactation, and child-bearing age has not been established.
2. Diarrhea may be a sign of incomplete intestinal obstruction and the use of these medications could be harmful.

Adverse Reactions. Xerostomia, blurred vision, tachycardia, headache, drowsiness, dizziness, urticaria, nausea, vomiting, urinary hesitancy, confusion and excitement, palpitations, constipation, impotence, insomnia, nervousness, photophobia, loss of taste, and/or dysphagia.

Dosage and Route. The dosage and route of administration is determined by the physician and is individualized for each patient. See Table 26–4.

Implications for Patient Care. Observe for signs of improvement and/or hypersensitivity. Assess vital signs, urinary output, and bowel movements. Monitor patient for any signs of dysrhythmia, palpitations, increased pulse rate and flushing. Administer medication $\frac{1}{2}$–1 hour before meals for better absorption. A geriatric patient usually needs a smaller dose of medication. With the average adult dose, they may experience excitement, confusion, agitation or drowsiness.

Patient Teaching Educate the patient:

- to the fact that anticholinergics may impair mental alertness; therefore, one should not operate machinery or drive a motor vehicle, until his/her response to the medication has been determined.
- to the fact that alcohol or other sedative drugs may enhance the drowsiness caused by anticholinergics.
- to avoid hot environments, as perspiration is suppressed by anticholinergics.
- to wear sunglasses when outside (helps protect the eyes from ultraviolet rays).
- that if dryness of the mouth occurs to suck on ice chips, hard candy, and increase fluid intake.

Special Considerations

- Caution patient not to chew or crush time-release tablets.
- Patients who experience blurred vision, headache, palpitations, urinary difficulty, constipation, and signs of glaucoma (halos around lights) should notify their physician immediately.
- The effect of the medication may be increased with the use of antihistamines, MAO inhibitors, tricyclic antidepressants, amantadine and/or other anticholinergic agents.
- The effect of the medication may be decreased with the use of antacids.

Laxatives

Laxatives are commonly used to relieve constipation and to facilitate the passage of feces through the lower gastrointestinal tract. Normally, an active, healthy person who eats a balanced diet does not suffer from constipation. Occasionally, this condition results from travel, emotional stress, and other factors. More often, constipation results from decreased fluid intake, poor diet, lack of physical activity, eating constipating foods, and as a result of certain drugs.

Table 26–4 Antispasmodics/Anticholinergics

Medication	Type	Usual Dosage	Adverse Reactions
atropine sulfate	belladona alkaloid	Oral, SC, IM, IV: (Adult): 0.4–0.6 mg, may be repeated every 4–6 hrs (Child): 0.01 mg/kg every 4–6 hrs.	headache, drowsiness, dizziness, mental depression, blurred vision, dry mouth
anisotropine methylbromide (Valpin 50)	synthetic anticholinergic	Oral: 50 mg 3 times daily	urticaria, skin rashes, dry mouth, nausea, dizziness, drowsiness, headache, blurred vision, urinary hesitancy
dicyclomine HCl (Bentyl)	synthetic anticholinergic	Oral, (Adult): 10–20 mg 3–4 times daily Oral, (Child): 10 mg 3–4 times daily.	transient dizziness, brief euphoria, headache, fever, confusion and excitement, palpitation, dry mouth
glycopyrrolate (Robinul)	synthetic anticholinergic	Oral: 1–2 mg 2–3 times/day. IM, IV: 0.1–0.2 mg as single dose.	xerostomia, blurred vision, decreased sweating, constipation, tachycardia
hyoscyamine sulfate (Levsin)	belladonna alkaloid	Oral, (Adult): 0.125–0.25 mg 3–4 times daily as needed. SC, IM, IV, (Adult): 1–2 ml every 6 hours. Oral (Child): one-half of adult dose.	confusion, excitement in elderly patients, blurred vision, constipation, xerostomia, paralytic ileus, urinary retention
methantheline bromide (Banthine)	synthetic anticholinergic	Oral, (Adult): 50–100 mg 4 times daily at 6 hour intervals. Oral, (Child): 12.5–50 mg 4 times daily.	urinary retention, blurred vision, dry mouth, constipation, mydriasis, impotence
methscopolamine bromide (Pamine)	synthetic anticholinergic	Oral: 2.5–5 mg before meals and at bedtime.	dry mouth, blurred vision, dizziness, drowsiness, flushing of skin
Oxyphencyclimine HCl (Daricon)	synthetic anticholinergic	Oral: 5–10 mg twice daily.	headache, drowsiness, dry mouth, mental depression, blurred vision, dizziness
propantheline bromide (Pro-Banthine)	synthetic anticholinergic	Oral: 15 mg with meals and 30 mg at bedtime. ocular pressure, mydriasis	constipation, blurred vision, dry mouth, increased intra-
tridihexethyl chloride (Pathilon)	synthetic anticholinergic	Oral: 25 mg 3 times/day and 50 mg at bedtime, then dosage adjusted to patient's needs.	xerostomia, nausea, urinary retention, impotence, loss of taste, blurred vision

Although relief of constipation is the leading reason for using a laxative, the agents are also used to prepare the bowel prior to surgery and before x-ray or proctoscopic examination of the lower GI tract. Laxatives are used after anthelmintic therapy to speed elimination of parasites, and as a means of reducing the strain of defecation in those with cardiovascular weaknesses.

Several types of laxatives are in general use. See Table 26–5. These agents have been grouped into the following classifications: *bulk-forming* agents, that absorb water,

Table 26–5 Various Types of Laxative Agents

Medication	Type	Usual Dosage	Onset of Action
bisacodyl (Dulcolax)	stimulant laxative	Oral, (Adult): 10–15 mg Oral, (Child): 5–10 mg Rectal: 10 mg if over 2 years of age; 5 mg if under 2 years old	acts within 5–12 hours of oral administration; acts 15–60 minutes after rectal suppository insertion
docusate calcium (Surfak)	wetting agent	Oral, (Adults): 50–200 mg/day. Oral, (Child 6–12 years): 40–120 mg, (Child 3–6 years): 20–60 mg, (Child under 3): 10–40 mg.	acts within 1–3 days after first administration
docusate sodium (Colace)	wetting agent	Oral: same as docusate calcium.	same as docusate calcium
magnesium hydroxide (Milk of Magnesia)	saline laxative	Oral, (Adult): 15–30 ml. Oral (Child 2–6 years): 5–15 ml. Oral, (Child under 2 yrs): 5 ml.	acts within 4–8 hours, depending upon dosage
methylcellulose (Cologel)	bulk-forming	Oral, (Adult): 5–20 ml 3 times/day. Oral, (Child): one-half the adult dosage.	acts within 12–24 hours in most patients
mineral oil (Liquid Petrolatum)	lubricant laxative	Oral: 15–30 ml, usually in the evening.	acts within 6–12 hours
phenolphthalein (Ex-Lax)	stimulant laxative	Oral: 30–200 mg	acts in 6–8 hours
psyllium hydrophilic muciloid (Metamucil)	bulk-forming	Oral, (Adult): 1–2 rounded teaspoons, or 1 packet 1–3 times/day. Oral, (Child): 1 rounded teaspoon in one-half glass/liquid 1–2 times/day.	acts within 12–72 hours

expand, and thereby stimulate peristaltic action; *stimulants*, that act by irritating the intestinal mucosa or nerves in the intestinal wall; *saline laxatives*, that are salts that draw water into the intestinal lumen osmotically to mix with the stool and stimulate motility; *lubricants*, that are various oils that soften the fecal mass and facilitate penetration of the fecal mass by intestinal fluids, thereby softening the mass and aiding defecation. Wetting agents are easily administered and are especially useful with infants, children, and certain elderly patients. See Table 26–6.

Special Considerations

- Contraindicated in patients with hypersensitivity to any of the ingredients used in laxative preparations.
- Laxatives are contraindicated in patients with abdominal pain, nausea, vomiting, fecal impaction, intestinal obstruction, appendicitis, biliary tract obstructions and/or acute hepatitis.
- Side effects may include nausea, vomiting, diarrhea, anorexia, abdominal cramps, electrolyte imbalance.

Table 26–6 Classification, Example, and Patient Teaching

Classification	Example	Patient Teaching
Bulk-forming	Metamucil	Do not take dry. Take with 8 ounces of water and follow with 8 ounces of water. If abdominal distention or unusual amount of flatulence occurs notify your physician. Do not take within 1 hour of antacids, milk or cimetidine. Report muscle cramps, pain, weakness, dizziness, or excessive thirst to your physician.
Stimulants	Dulcolax	Tablets should be swallowed. Do not crush or chew. Avoid milk or antacids within 1 hour of taking because the enteric coating may dissolve prematurely.
Saline	Milk of Magnesia	Magnesium laxatives should not be taken by patients who have renal insufficiency. Only short-term use is recommended because of possibility of CNS or neuromuscular depression, and/or electrolyte imbalance. Medicine should be followed by 8 ounces of water. Chilling helps taste.
Lubricant	Mineral oil	Mineral oil may impair the absorption of fat-soluble vitamins (A, D, E, K). May increase effect of oral anticoagulants. Swallow carefully as access of oil into the pharynx, bronchi, and lung may produce a lipid pneumonia.
Wetting agent	Colace	May be taken alone or with 8 ounces of water. Store in cool environment, but do not freeze. Swallow tablets whole, do not chew. May be used safely by patients who should avoid straining.

- It is stated that approximately $400 million a year is spent on laxatives. Many patients abuse laxatives so you should evaluate each patient for signs of abuse. Laxative abuse causes the colon to become lazy and it stops responding to the defecation reflex, causing true constipation. If the patient is abusing laxatives he/she should gradually reduce the dose or use a milder preparation, at the same time slowly increasing fiber and fluid intake until the defecation reflex returns to a normal state.
- Stimulant laxatives discolor alkaline urine red-pink; acid urine yellow-brown and they may give a reddish color to feces.
- Administration of laxatives should be such that results will not interfere with a patient's daily activities.

Antidiarrheal Agents

Diarrhea is characterized by frequent defecation of loose, watery stools. It is not a disease; rather, it is a symptom that has been associated with numerous medical conditions. Diarrhea may be caused by infection, intoxication, allergy, malabsorption, inflammation, tumors of the GI tract, food poisoning, and by certain medications.

Diarrhea may be described as *acute* when it has a sudden and severe onset, or *chronic* when it is of long-term duration. Acute diarrhea can cause water and salt depletion resulting in dehydration and electrolyte imbalance.

Since diarrhea is a symptom of an underlying disorder, it is often more important to determine and treat its specific cause than it is to alleviate the diarrhea.

When the specific cause of diarrhea can be diagnosed, therapy may involve the use of an antiprotozoal agent, an antibacterial drug, or an adrenal corticosteroid. Should it become necessary, certain nonspecific *antidiarrheal* agents may be used to treat severe acute diarrhea when its cause is unknown. Table 26–7 lists some of these agents.

Special Considerations

Special considerations related to drug therapy include:

- When diarrhea is severe or prolonged the patient can become dehydrated and experience electrolyte imbalance. Monitor potassium, sodium, and chloride levels. Increase fluids if not contraindicated. Monitor bowel pattern.
- Patients using antidiarrheal agents should avoid over-the-counter products unless prescribed by their physician.
- Pepto-Bismol tablets should be chewed or allowed to dissolve in the mouth; do not swallow them. While taking this medicine patient should avoid salicylates.
- Lomotil is contraindicated in patients with known hypersensitivity, severe liver disease, pseudomembranous enterocolitis, glaucoma, electrolyte imbalance, and by children under 2 years of age. Precautions in patients with hepatic disease, renal disease, ulcerative colitis, and during pregnancy and lactation. Lo-

Table 26–7 Nonspecific Antidiarrheal Agents

Medication	Usual Antidiarrheal Dosage	Adverse Reactions
bismuth subsalicylate (Pepto-Bismol)	Oral, (Adult): 30 ml or 2 tablets, (maximum of 8 doses/day at 30–60 minute intervals). (Child 10–14 years): 20 ml as above. (Child 6–10 years): 10 ml or 1 tablet. (Child 3–6 years): 5 ml or one-half tablet.	temporary darkening of stool and tongue
diphenoxylate HCl with atropine sulfate (Lomotil)	Oral, (Adult): 5 mg 3–4 times/day as needed. Oral, (Child 2–12 years): 0.3–0.4 mg/kg/day of liquid in divided doses.	headache, sedation, dizziness, flushing nausea, dry mouth, blurred vision
kaolin mixture with pectin (Kaopectate)	Oral, (Adults): 4 to 8 tablespoons Oral, (Children): Over 12 years: 4 tablespoons. 6–12 years: 2 to 4 tablespoons. 3–6 years: 1 to 2 tablespoons.	few adverse reactions. in the elderly and debilitated patients, constipation may occur
loperamide HCl (Imodium)	Oral: 4 mg initially, then 2 mg after each unformed stool, maintenance dose: 4–8 mg/day.	drowsiness, abdominal discomfort or pain, nausea
paregoric (in Parepectolin)	Oral, (Adult): 5–10 ml after bowel movement (maximum of 4 doses at 2 hour intervals). Oral, (Child): 0.25–0.5 ml/kg 1–4 times/day	anorexia, nausea, constipation, vomiting, abdominal pain

motil is a Schedule V controlled substance. This medication should not be used with MAO inhibitors as hypertensive crisis may occur.

- Imodium is contraindicated in patients with known hypersensitivity, severe ulcerative colitis, and pseudomembranous enterocolitis. Precautions in patients with liver disease, dehydration, bacterial disease, during pregnancy and lactation, and children under 2 years of age.
- Paregoric is contraindicated in patients with known hypersensitivity. Precautions in patients with liver disease, addiction-prone individuals, prostatic hypertrophy, during pregnancy and lactation. Paregoric is a controlled substance and depending upon the amount of opium may be a Schedule II or III drug. The patient should not take other CNS depressants while taking this medication.

Antiemetics

Antiemetics are agents that prevent or arrest vomiting. These drugs are the same as those listed in Chapter 30, Table 30–11 for the treatment of vertigo, motion sickness, and the nausea associated with the use of antineoplastic agents and radiation.

For information on route, dosage, and adverse reactions of the various antiemetic agents, see Table 30–11.

Emetics

Emetics are used to induce vomiting in people who have taken an overdose of oral drugs or who have ingested certain poisons. An emetic agent should not be given to a patient who is unconscious, in shock, or in a semicomatose state. Emetics are also contraindicated in individuals who have ingested strongly caustic substances, such as lye or acid, since their use could result in additional injury to the patient's esophagus.

Apomorphine hydrochloride acts on the chemoreceptor trigger zone of the medulla and causes vomiting in adults in 2 to 10 minutes. This emetic is more effective when the stomach is full; therefore, 200–300 ml of water should be given prior to its injection. The usual adult dose is 5 mg by the subcutaneous route. Apomorphine HCl is available as a hypodermic tablet which must be dissolved to facilitate ingestion. The drug is not stable and should be protected from light during storage. Apomorphine HCl should not be used if the solution is green or brown in color.

Ipecac syrup is available without a prescription from local pharmacies in amounts up to 30 ml. Some physicians advise parents of young children to keep a small amount of this emetic on hand for use in an emergency. Ipecac syrup causes less CNS depression than apomorphine HCl, especially in young patients. It acts directly on the chemoreceptor trigger zone of the medulla and reflexly on the gastric mucosa to cause vomiting. The usual dose for adults is 20 ml followed by 1–2 full glasses of water. For children between 1 and 12 years of age, the usual dose is 15 ml (one tablespoon) followed by $1–1\frac{1}{2}$ full glasses of water. The usual dose for infants 9–12 months of age is 2 teaspoonsful followed by $\frac{1}{2}$ to 1 full glass of water. Ipecac syrup will usually cause vomiting within 20 minutes of administration and the dosage can be repeated should vomiting not occur within this time. Activated charcoal may be used *after* vomiting has subsided to absorb the remaining poison.

Spot Check

There are several medications that may be used to treat ulcers. For each of the selected drugs listed, give the usual dosage and several adverse reactions.

Drug	Usual Dosage	Adverse Reactions
Tagamet		

Pepcid		
Axid		
Zantac		
Carafate		
Cytotec		

Review Questions

Directions: Select the best answer to each multiple choice question. Circle the letter of your choice.

1. During the digestive process a partially digested mass, known as __________, leaves the stomach and passes into the small intestine.
   a. bolus
   b. chyme
   c. bile
   d. chole
2. Typical complaints and disorders of the gastrointestinal system include dyspepsia, __________.
   a. dysphagia, and pyrosis
   b. pyrosis, and nausea
   c. dysphonia, and pyrosis
   d. dysphasia, and pyrosis
3. __________ are drugs that neutralize hydrochloric acid in the stomach.
   a. Antispasmodics
   b. Antagonist
   c. Antacids
   d. Agonists
4. The usual oral dosage of Milk of Magnesia is __________.
   a. 0.5–2 Gm between meals and at bedtime
   b. 250–1500 mg with water or milk, 4 times/day
   c. 5–10 ml, or 1–2 tablets 1 to 3 hours after meals and at bedtime
   d. 15–30 ml every 2 hours
5. The generic name of Amphojel is __________.
   a. basic aluminum carbonate gel
   b. aluminum phosphate
   c. magaldrate
   d. aluminum hydroxide
6. Constipation and fecal impaction are adverse reactions of __________.
   a. Basaljel
   b. Amphojel
   c. Phosphajel
   d. Tums
7. Antacid mixtures are commonly used in the treatment of __________.
   a. peptic ulcers
   b. acid indigestion
   c. heartburn
   d. all of these
8. Products that contain magnesium hydroxide frequently cause __________.
   a. constipation
   b. diarrhea
   c. belching
   d. vomiting
9. Gelusil is a combination of __________.
   a. aluminum hydroxide
   b. magnesium hydroxide
   c. simethicone
   d. all of these

10. The usual oral dosage of Mylanta is __________ .
    a. 2–4 teaspoons or tablets (chewed), every 2–4 hours
    b. 1–2 tablespoons or tablets (chewed), every 2–4 hours
    c. 1–2 ounces or tablets (chewed), every 2–4 hours
    d. 2–4 teaspoons every 6 hours
11. The generic name of Tagamet is __________ .
    a. cimetidine
    b. ranitidine
    c. sucralfate
    d. ciemtidine
12. Tagamet and Zantac are __________ .
    a. histamine agonist
    b. histamine H_2-receptor antagonists
    c. antispasmodics
    d. antacids
13. For an active gastric ulcer the usual oral dosage of Tagamet is __________ .
    a. 150 mg twice daily
    b. 1 Gm 4 times a day
    c. 800 mg at bedtime or 300 mg 4 times a day, with meals and at bedtime
    d. 300 mg every 6 hours
14. __________ mixes with gastric acid to form a paste-like coating that prevents further damage by ulcerogenic secretions.
    a. Tagamet
    b. Zantac
    c. Carafate
    d. cimetidine
15. Antispasmodics are useful in the management of dyspepsia, __________ .
    a. peptic ulcer, mild diarrhea
    b. irritable colon, mild diarrhea
    c. dysphagia, mild diarrhea
    d. peptic ulcers, severe diarrhea
16. The generic name of Pro-Banthine is __________ .
    a. hyoscyamine sulfate
    b. methantheline bromide
    c. propantheline bromide
    d. dicyclomine HCl
17. The usual oral adult dosage of atropine sulfate is __________ .
    a. 0.4–0.5 mg
    b. 0.4–0.6 mg
    c. 1–2 mg
    d. 2.5–5 mg
18. Dry mouth, blurred vision, dizziness, drowsiness, and flushing of skin are adverse reactions of __________ .
    a. Daricon
    b. Bentyl
    c. Pamine
    d. Bathine

19. __________ are various oils that soften the fecal mass and facilitate its passage through the colon.

a. Stimulants
b. Bulk-forming agents
c. Wetting agents
d. Lubricants

20. The generic name of Dulcolax is __________ .

a. bisacodyl
b. phenolphthalcin
c. docusate
d. magnesium hydroxide

21. The onset of action of Surfak is __________ .

a. 5–12 hours
b. 6–12 hours
c. 1–3 days
d. 3–6 days

22. Docusate sodium (Colace) is a __________ .

a. stimulant laxative
b. saline laxative
c. bulk-forming laxative
d. wetting agent

23. The usual oral adult dosage of Metamucil is __________ .

a. 10–15 mg
b. 1–2 rounded teaspoons, or 1 packet 1–3 times/day
c. 50–200 mg/day
d. 15–30 ml

24. __________ is characterized by frequent defecation of loose, watery stools.

a. Constipation
b. Diarrhea
c. Dehydration
d. all of these

25. Temporary darkening of the stool and tongue is an adverse reaction of __________ .

a. Pepto-Bismol
b. Lomotil
c. Imodium
d. Laudanum

26. The usual antidiarrheal dosage of paregoric is __________ .

a. 30 ml
b. 0.3–1 ml
c. 5–10 ml
d. 4 mg

27. __________ are agents that prevent or arrest vomiting.

a. Emetics
b. Antacids
c. Antiemetics
d. Antidiarrheals

28. An emetic agent should not be given to a patient who is __________ .

a. unconscious
b. in shock
c. in a semicomatose state
d. all of these

29. Apomorphine HCl and Ipecac syrup are __________ .

a. antiemetics
b. emetics
c. antispasmodics
d. antacids

Case Study: Mr. Raymond Bryant, a 58-year-old school principal is returning to the office for a follow-up visit. He has been diagnosed as having a duodenal ulcer. Today his chief complaints consist of recurrent pains in his stomach, indigestion, and heartburn. He has been taking Mylanta 2–4 tabs every 2–4 hours between meals and at bedtime. He states that the medication is no longer relieving his symptoms. After careful evaluation, the physician orders ranitidine (Zantac) 300 mg at bedtime and continued use of the antacid. The patient is to return in one week.

30. Mylanta is a common antacid mixture that is contraindicated in patients __________.
    a. with kidney disease
    b. taking any form of an antibiotic
    c. taking any form of a tetracycline
    d. a and c
31. The nurse should know that ranitidine (Zantac) is a/an __________.
    a. antispasmodic
    b. anticholinergic
    c. histamine H_2-receptor antagonist
    d. antacid
32. While taking ranitidine the patient should be taught that __________.
    a. gynecomastia and impotence may occur
    b. impaired mental alertness may occur
    c. increased mental alertness may occur
    d. a and b
33. Patients with duodenal ulcers should avoid certain substances such as __________.
    a. aspirin, alcohol, nicotine, caffeine
    b. spices, alcohol, breads, cereals
    c. aspirin, rice, nicotine
    d. caffeine, potatoes, fish

Case Study: While taking a medication history on a 72-year-old female patient who has been diagnosed as having renal insufficiency, you find out that she has been taking Milk of Magnesia for the past two months for constipation.

34. As a nurse you should know that Milk of Magnesia is classified as a __________ laxative.
    a. bulk-forming
    b. stimulant
    c. saline
    d. lubricant

35. You should report your finding to the physician because Milk of Magnesia __________ .

a. is a magnesium laxative

b. is relatively safe and can be taken over a long period of time

c. is contraindicated in patients with renal insufficiency

d. is a stimulant laxative

36. Once laxative abuse has been determined, the patient should __________ .

a. decrease fluid and fiber intake

b. increase fluid and fiber intake slowly

c. increase fluid and fiber intake quickly

d. discontinue taking any laxative

CHAPTER 27

Diuretics and Medications Used for Urinary System Disorders

OBJECTIVES

Upon completion of this chapter, you should be able to:

- Define the terms listed in the vocabulary.
- State two vital functions of the kidneys.
- State the actions, uses, contraindications, adverse reactions, dosage and route, implications for patient care, patient teaching, and special considerations for thiazide, loop, potassium-sparing, osmotic, and carbonic anhydrase diuretics, sulfonamides, and urinary tract antiseptics.
- Define cystitis.
- Describe the symptoms of cystitis.
- Explain the diagnosis for cystitis.
- Give the treatment regimen for cystitis.
- Describe interstitial cystitis.
- Describe the process of aging on the kidneys.
- List some causes of stressful situations that may cause the kidneys of the older adult to respond more slowly and contribute to fluid and electrolyte imbalance.
- Explain why it is important to assess an older adult's voiding history and medication history.
- State the signs of nephrotoxicity.
- Describe the signs and symptoms of urinary tract infection in the child.
- Explain the treatment regimen for a child with a urinary tract infection.
- Complete the critical thinking questions/activities presented in this chapter.
- Complete the Spot Check on selected drugs used to treat urinary tract infections.
- State the action, usual dosage, and adverse reactions of selected drugs used for urologic disorders.
- Identify selected agents that discolor urine.
- Answer the review questions correctly.

Vocabulary

edema (e-de′ma). Swelling. A local or generalized collection of fluid in the body tissues.

excretion (eks-kre′shun). The process of eliminating waste products from the body.

escherichia coli (esh-er″ik′e-a ko′li). A type of bacteria that is commonly found in the alimentary canal of man and other animals.

proteus mirabilis (pro′te-us mi″ra-bi′lis). A species of enteric bacilli, that may cause urinary tract infections. It is found in the intestines of man and animals.

Synopsis: The Urinary System

The urinary system is composed of two kidneys, two ureters, one bladder, and one urethra, Figure 27–1. Within each kidney there are a million or more functional units called *nephrons* where the filtration and reabsorption process occurs, Figure 27–2.

Blood undergoes a process of filtration and reabsorption as it passes through the kidneys. During this process, two vital functions are performed: (1) urine is produced for excretion, and (2) the amount of water, electrolytes, and other substances in the blood is regulated.

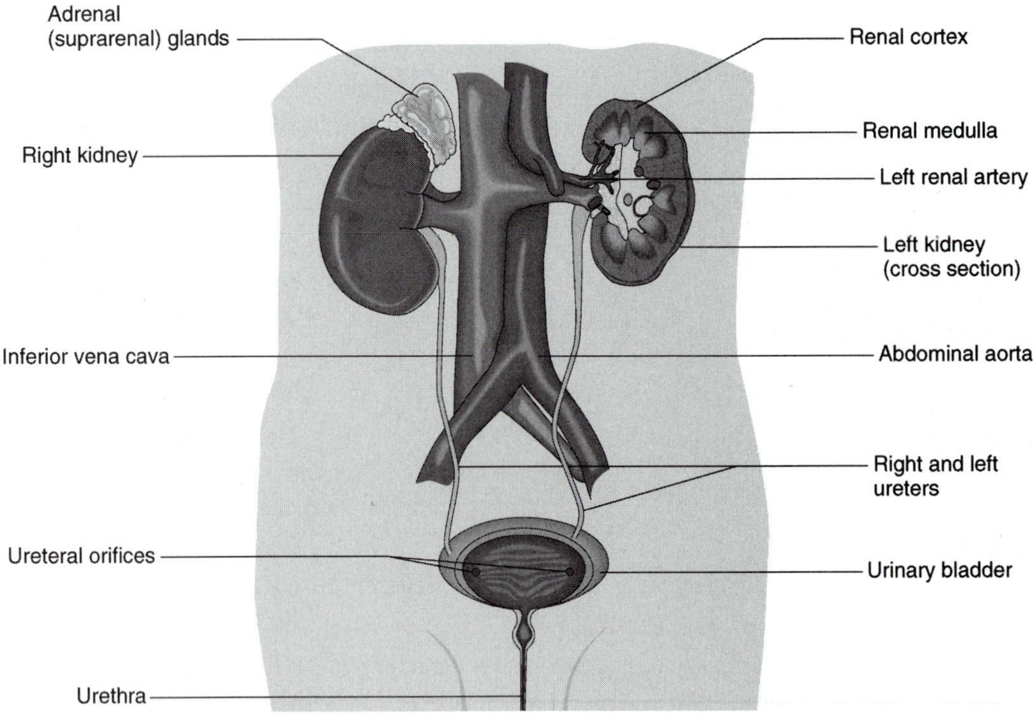

Figure 27–1 Structures of the urinary system

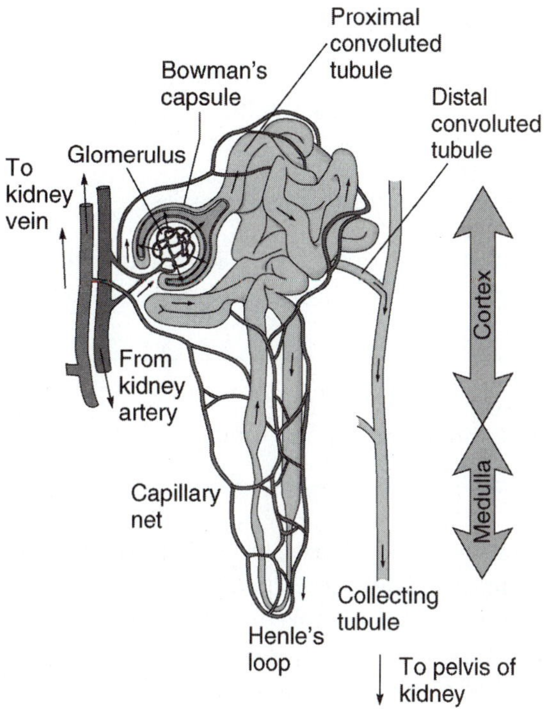

Figure 27–2 Nephron

Disorders of the urinary system can be attributed to a variety of causes, including infection, or damage or dysfunction of the kidneys, bladder, or other organs in the system.

Diuretics

Diuretics decrease reabsorption of sodium chloride by the kidneys, thereby increasing the amount of salt and water excreted in the urine. This action reduces the amount of fluid retained in the body and prevents edema. Diuretics are classified according to site and mechanism of action.

- *Thiazide diuretics* appear to act by inhibiting sodium and chloride reabsorption in the early portion of the distal tubule. They may also block chloride reabsorption in the ascending loop of Henle.
- *Loop diuretics* act by inhibiting the reabsorption of sodium and chloride in the ascending loop of Henle.
- *Potassium-sparing diuretics* exert their action in the distal tubule. They inhibit potassium excretion.
- *Osmotic diuretics* are agents that are capable of being filtered by the glomerulus but have a limited capability of being reabsorbed into the bloodstream.
- *Carbonic anhydrase diuretics* act to promote the reabsorption of sodium and bicarbonate from the proximal tubule.

Thiazide Diuretics

Thiazide diuretics appear to act by inhibiting sodium and chloride reabsorption in the early portion of the distal tubule. They may also block chloride reabsorption in the ascending loop of Henle.

Uses. Edema, hypertension, diuresis.

Contraindications. Contraindicated in patients who are known to be hypersensitive to any of its ingredients. They should not be used in anuria, and/or renal decompensation.

> **Warning:** Should be used with caution in patients with severe renal disease, impaired hepatic function or progressive liver disease.

Adverse Reactions. Weakness, hypotension, orthostatic hypotension, pancreatitis, jaundice, diarrhea, vomiting, constipation, nausea, anorexia, aplastic anemia, agranulocytosis, leukopenia, hemolytic anemia, thrombocytopenia, electrolyte imbalance, hyperglycemia, glycosuria, hyperuricemia, muscle spasm, vertigo, dizziness, headache, restlessness, renal failure, blurred vision, xanthopsia, anaphylactic reactions, rash, urticaria, photosensitivity fever.

Dosage and Route. The dosage and route of administration is determined by the physician and individualized for each patient. See Table 27–1.

Implications for Patient Care. Observe patient for evidence of fluid or electrolyte imbalance. **Warning signs:** dryness of mouth, thirst, weakness, lethargy, drowsiness, restlessness, muscle pains or cramps, muscular fatigue, hypotension, oliguria, tachycardia, nausea and vomiting. Monitor weight, intake and output ratio, blood pressure, respirations, and serum electrolytes.

Patient Teaching

Educate the patient:

- to increase fluid intake to 2–3 liters per day unless contraindicated and to eat potassium-rich foods such as bananas, oranges, prunes, raisins, dried peas and beans, fresh vegetables, nuts, meats, and cereals.
- about warning signs of fluid or electrolyte imbalance.
- to contact the physician without delay if warning signs occur.
- that the medication should be taken in the morning to avoid nocturia.

Special Considerations

- Thiazide diuretics may increase blood sugar in the diabetic patient. Dosage adjustment of oral hypoglycemic agents and insulin may be required.

Table 27–1 Diuretics

Medication	Classification	Usual Dosage	Adverse Reactions
acetazolamide (Diamox)	carbonic anhydrace inhibitor	Oral, IV: 250–375 mg once daily.	tingling in the extremities, loss of appetite, polyuria
bendroflumethiazide (Naturetin)	thiazide diuretic	Oral: 2.5–5 mg/day following an initial dose of up to 20 mg.	anorexia, nausea, vomiting, dizziness
chlorothiazide (Diuril)	thiazide diuretic	Oral, IV: 500 mg to 1 Gm 1–2 times/day.	weakness, anorexia, gastric irritation, hyperglycemia, purpura, muscle spasm
furosemide (Lasix)	loop diuretic	Oral, (Adult): 20–80 mg as a single dose. Oral, (Child): 1–2 mg/kg 1–2 times/day.	anorexia, vertigo, purpura, hyperglycemia, anemia
hydrochlorothiazide (Esidrix) (HydroDIURIL)	thiazide diuretic	Oral, (Adult): 50 mg–100 mg 1–2 times/day. Oral, (Child): 1 mg/lb daily in 2 doses.	orthostatic hypotension, muscle spasm, pancreatitis, vertigo, aplastic anemia
mannitol (Osmitrol)	osmotic diuretic	IV, (Adult): 300–400 mg/kg of a 20–25% solution in 1 dose.	headache, nausea, dizziness, polydipsia, chills, feeling of constriction or pain in the chest
methyclothiazide (Enduron)	thiazide diuretic	Oral, (Adult): 2.5–10 mg once daily. Oral, (Child): 0.05–0.2 mg/kg daily.	anorexia, nausea, vomiting, dizziness, headache, rash, leukopenia, hyperglycemia
polythiazide (Renese)	thiazide diuretic	Oral, (Adult): 1–4 mg daily.	anorexia, dizziness, purpura, leukopenia, hypoglycemia
spironolactone (Aldactone)	potassium-sparing diuretic	Oral, (Adult): 50–100 mg daily. Oral, (Child): 3.3 mg/kg in divided doses.	gynecomastia, cramping and diarrhea, drowsiness, rash, irregular menses
triamterene (Dyrenium)	potassium-sparing diuretic	Oral, (Adult): 100–300 mg daily in divided doses. Oral, (Child): 2–4 mg/kg daily in divided doses.	diarrhea, nausea, vomiting, weakness, headache, rash, dry mouth, anaphylaxis

- Use in pregnancy is not recommended.
- Alcohol, barbiturates, and narcotics may potentiate the occurrence of orthostatic hypotension.
- There may be an additive effect when taken with other antihypertensive agents.
- Electrolyte depletion may be intensified when taken with corticosteroids.
- Patients taking lithium should not take diuretics as they reduce the renal clearance of lithium and add a high risk of lithium toxicity.

Loop Diuretics

Loop diuretics act by inhibiting reabsorption of sodium and chloride in the proximal and distal tubules and in the ascending loop of Henle.

Uses. Edema, hypertension, as adjunctive therapy in acute pulmonary embolism.

Contraindications. Contraindicated in patients who are known to be hypersensitive to any of its ingredients. They should not be used in patients with anuria, electrolyte depletion, hypovolemia, by infants, or during lactation.

> **Warnings:**
>
> 1. Lasix (furosemide) is a potent loop diuretic and if given in excessive amounts, can lead to profound diuresis with water and electrolyte depletion. Careful medical supervision is required.
> 2. In patients with hepatic cirrhosis and ascites, drug therapy should be initiated in the hospital, after the basic condition is improved.
> 3. Ototoxicity has been reported and is usually associated with rapid injection, severe renal impairment, doses higher than recommended, and when given with other agents that cause ototoxicity.

Adverse Reactions. Anorexia, jaundice, pancreatitis, diarrhea, cramping, constipation, nausea, vomiting, tinnitus, hearing loss, paresthesia, vertigo, dizziness, headache, blurred vision, xanthopsia, aplastic anemia, thrombocytopenia, leukopenia, purpura, photosensitivity, urticaria, rash, pruritus, orthostatic hypotension, hyperglycemia, glycosuria, muscle spasm, weakness, restlessness, thrombophlebitis, fever, necrotizing angiitis.

Dosage and Route. The dosage and route of administration is determined by the physician and individualized for each patient. See Table 27–1.

Implications for Patient Care. Observe patient for evidence of fluid or electrolyte imbalance. Monitor weight, intake and output ratio, blood pressure, respirations, and serum electrolytes.

Patient Teaching

Educate the patient:

- to increase fluid intake to 2–3 liters per day unless contraindicated and to eat potassium-rich foods.
- that potassium supplements may be prescribed by the physician.
- about warning signs of fluid and electrolyte imbalance.
- to contact the physician without delay if warning signs occur.
- that the medication should be taken in the morning to avoid nocturia.

Special Considerations

- Loop diuretics may increase blood sugar in the diabetic patient. Dosage adjustment of oral hypoglycemic agents and insulin may be required.
- Some patients may be more sensitive to sunlight while taking loop diuretics.
- Use in pregnancy is not recommended.
- May increase ototoxicity effect of aminoglycosides.
- Patients taking lithium should not take loop diuretics as they reduce the renal clearance of lithium and add a higher risk of lithium toxicity.
- There may be an additive effect when taken with other antihypertensive agents.
- Alcohol, barbiturates and narcotics may potentiate the occurrence of orthostatic hypotension.

Potassium-Sparing Diuretics

Potassium-sparing diuretics exert their action in the distal tubule. They cause increased amounts of sodium and water to be excreted, while potassium is retained.

Uses. Edema, primary hyperaldosteronism, congestive heart failure, cirrhosis of the liver, essential hypertension, hypokalemia.

Contraindications. Contraindicated in patients who are known to be hypersensitive to any of its ingredients. They should not be used in anuria, acute renal disease, hyperkalemia, and during pregnancy or lactation.

> **Warning:** Potassium supplements and foods rich in potassium should not generally be given with potassium-sparing diuretics. Hyperkalemia could occur. Also, most salt substitutes contain potassium salts, therefore cautious use should be followed.

Adverse Reactions. Gynecomastia, agranulocytosis, cramping, diarrhea, drowsiness, lethargy, headache, urticaria, rash, pruritus, mental confusion, drug fever, ataxia, impotence, irregular menses or amenorrhea, postmenopausal bleeding, hirsutism, gastritis, vomiting.

Dosage and Route. The dosage and route of administration is determined by the physician and individualized for each patient. See Table 27–1.

Implications for Patient Care. Observe patient for evidence of fluid and electrolyte imbalance. Monitor cardiac function and be alert for signs of hyperkalemia: nausea, diarrhea, muscle weakness, marked ECG changes (elevated T waves, depressed P waves), atrial systole, slow irregular pulse, ventricular fibrillation, cardiac arrest. Treatment of hyperkalemia-IV administration of 20 percent to 50 percent glucose and 0.25–0.5 units of regular insulin per gram of glucose. Assess weight, intake and output ratio, vital signs, serum electrolytes, and mental status.

Patient Teaching

Educate the patient:

- not to take potassium supplements or eat foods rich in potassium.
- that the medication may cause drowsiness, mental confusion, gynecomastia, and menstrual irregularities.
- about the warning signs of fluid and electrolyte imbalance.
- to contact the physician without delay if warning signs occur.

Special Considerations

- Excessive potassium intake may cause hyperkalemia in patients taking potassium-sparing diuretics.
- When used in combination with other diuretics or antihypertensive agents potassium-sparing diuretics potentiate their effects. Dosage of such drugs, particularly the ganglionic blocking agents should be reduced by 50 percent.
- Severe hyperkalemia may occur when ACE inhibitors or indomethacin are administered concurrently with potassium-sparing diuretics.
- Reduces the vascular response to norepinephrine, therefore cautious use in patients undergoing regional or general anesthesia should be the rule.
- Increases the half-life of digoxin, therefore patients receiving any form of digitalis should be monitored very carefully while taking any potassium-sparing diuretic.

Osmotic Diuretics

Osmotic diuretics are agents that are capable of being filtered by the glomerulus, but have a limited capability of being reabsorbed into the bloodstream. They act by increasing the osmolality of the plasma, glomerular filtrate, and tubular fluid thereby increasing the excretion of water, chloride, sodium, and potassium.

Uses. To prevent acute renal failure during trauma or prolonged surgery, to prevent increased cerebral, cerebrospinal or intraocular pressures during trauma or surgery or disease, and to reduce intraocular pressure in acute glaucoma.

Contraindications. Contraindicated in patients who are known to be hypersensitive to any of its ingredients. They should not be used in anuria, diagnosed acute renal failure, cardiac dysfunction, congestive heart failure, active intracranial hemorrhage, severe dehydration, and/or severe pulmonary congestion.

Adverse Reactions. Marked diuresis, urinary retention, thirst, dizziness, headache, convulsions, nausea, vomiting, dry mouth, diarrhea, thrombophlebitis, hypotension, hypertension, tachycardia, angina-like chest pains, fever, chills, pulmonary congestion, fluid, electrolyte imbalance, dehydration, loss of hearing, blurred vision, nasal congestion, decreased intraocular pressure.

Dosage and Route. The dosage and route of administration is determined by the physician and individualized for each patient. See Table 27–1.

Implications for Patient Care. Observe patient for evidence of fluid or electrolyte imbalance and signs of circulatory overload. Monitor weight, intake and output ratio, vital signs, and serum electrolytes. Observe IV administration sites for signs of local irritation, extravasation, and/or thrombophlebitis.

Patient Teaching

Educate the patient:

- to increase fluid intake to 2–3 liters per day unless contraindicated.
- that sucking on ice chips and/or hard candy will help relieve his/her thirst.

Special Considerations

- Parenteral mannitol crystallizes at low temperatures. Store at 59° to 89°F, unless otherwise ordered. Do not allow it to freeze. If the medication crystallizes, warm it in a hot-water bath and shake container vigorously, then allow the solution to return to room temperature before administration.
- Do not add whole blood to IV lines used for mannitol.
- Do not mix this medication with any other drug or solution.

Carbonic Anhydrase Diuretics

Carbonic anhydrase diuretics act to promote the reabsorption of sodium and bicarbonate from the proximal tubules. They block the action of the enzyme carbonic anhydrase (found in the kidneys, eyes, and other organs), thereby reversing the hydration of carbon dioxide and producing a bicarbonate diuresis that promotes the excretion of water, sodium, and potassium. These effects also decrease the formation of aqueous humor, thus reducing intraocular pressure.

Uses. For adjunctive therapy of chronic simple (open-angle), glaucoma, secondary glaucoma, and preoperatively in acute angle-closure glaucoma where delay of surgery is desired in order to lower intraocular pressure.

Contraindications. Contraindicated in patients who are known to be hypersensitive to any of its ingredients. Should not be used in hepatic insufficiency, renal failure, adrenocortical insufficiency, hyperchloremic acidosis, or in conditions where serum levels of sodium and potassium are depressed, and/or severe pulmonary obstruction.

Adverse Reactions. Anorexia, nausea, vomiting, drowsiness, paresthesia, ataxia, tremor, tinnitus, headache, weakness, nervousness, depression, confusion, dizziness, constipation, hepatic insufficiency, loss of weight, electrolyte imbalance, metabolic acidosis, skin eruptions, pruritus, fever, agranulocytosis, thrombocytopenia, frequency of urination, renal colic, renal calculi, phosphaturia.

Dosage and Route. The dosage and route of administration is determined by the physician and individualized for each patient. See Table 27–1.

Implications for Patient Care. Observe patient for evidence of fluid or electrolyte imbalance. Monitor weight, intake and output ratio, vital signs, and serum electrolytes. Administer medication by mouth or IV if possible, because administration by IM injcction is painful. Monitor patient for signs of metabolic acidosis.

Patient Teaching

Educate the patient:

- to increase fluid intake to 2–3 liters per day unless contraindicated.
- to eat potassium-rich foods.
- to avoid hazardous activities if drowsiness or dizziness occurs.
- about warning signs of fluid or electrolyte imbalance.
- to contact the physician without delay if warning signs occur.
- that the medication should be taken in the morning to avoid nocturia.
- that any eye pain should be reported to the physician without delay.

Special Considerations

- If serum potassium is below 3.0, potassium supplements are needed.
- Cautious use in patients receiving high doses of aspirin, and during pregnancy and lactation.
- Metabolic acidosis signs and symptoms: headache, fatigue, hypotension, anorexia, nausea, vomiting, dysrhythmia, drowsiness, confusion, seizures, coma, Kussmaul's respirations.

SPOTLIGHT

Urinary Tract Infections (UTI): Cystitis

Cystitis is an inflammation of the urinary bladder. The urinary bladder is a muscular, membranous sac that serves as a reservoir for urine. It is located in the anterior portion of the pelvic cavity and consists of a lower portion, the neck, which is continuous with the urethra, and an upper portion, the apex, which is connected to the umbilicus by the median umbilical ligament. The urethra is the musculomembranous tube extending from the bladder to the outside of the body. The external urinary opening is the urinary meatus. The male urethra is approximately 8 inches long and the female urethra is approximately 1.5 inches long.

Each year, in the United States, approximately 10 million patients seek treatment for urinary tract infections, with cystitis being the most common. Cystitis is most often caused by an ascending infection from the urethra and it is more common in the female, because of the short length of the urethra that promotes the transmission of bacteria from the skin and genitals to the internal bladder. The most common type of bacteria that causes cystitis in the female is *Escherichia coli* (E. coli), the colon bacillus. This bacillus is constantly present in the alimentary canal and is normally nonpathogenic, but when it enters the urinary tract and is transmitted to the bladder, it can cause infection. Cystitis in men is usually secondary to some other type of infection such as epididymitis, prostatitis, gonorrhea, syphilis, and/or kidney stones.

Symptoms

Urgency
Pyuria
Chills and fever
Burning sensation and pain during urination
Frequency
Hematuria
Pain or spasm in the region of the bladder bladder and pelvic area

Diagnosis

History of symptoms
Microscopic urinalysis
Dipstick
Gram stain
Urine culture

Treatment

Treatment of cystitis usually consists of taking an antibiotic or antibacterial agent for a specified number of times and days, depending of the type of infection and its severity. The sulfonamides and antibiotics such as penicillins, cephalosporins, tetracyclines, and aminoglycosides are generally the drugs of first choice. Always ask the patient if he/she is

(continued)

allergic to any medication before the initiation of drug therapy. Note: if there is any question about a person's hypersensitivity to an antibiotic and/or sulfa drugs, an appropriate skin test should be performed before the initiation of drug therapy.

The patient should be informed about possible adverse reactions to the prescribed medication and be instructed to report any signs to his/her physician. Advise the patient to take the medication as prescribed until all of the drug has been taken.

Interstitial Cystitis

Interstitial cystitis (IC) is a painful inflammation of the bladder wall. Approximately 450,000 people suffer from this condition and 90 percent are women. Research showed that the median age of onset was 40, with many women experiencing symptoms as early as their twenties and thirties.

Symptoms can vary from mild to severe and are similar to a urinary tract infection (cystitis). There is usually pelvic pain and pressure, frequent urination, sometimes as often as 50 times a day. Diagnosis is difficult because the standard blood tests, urine tests, and x-rays come up negative. The cause is unknown and IC does not respond to antibiotic therapy. Women with IC often live in chronic pain. They are always tired, because they are going to the bathroom often and their sexual, social, and work life are affected.

FYI: For a referral to a data base center, send a self-addressed, stamped, business-size envelope to the Interstitial Cystitis Association, P.O. Box 1553, Madison Square Station, New York, NY 10159.

Guidelines to Help Avoid Cystitis (Female)

- Drink plenty of fluids (8 glasses or more) a day.
- To avoid contaminating the urinary meatus, females should wipe themselves from front to back.
- Females who have repeated infections (cystitis) should drink a glass of water before engaging in sexual intercourse, and then urinate right after intercourse. This helps flush out any bacteria that could have entered the urethra.
- Have your sexual partner wear a condom.
- Do not use vaginal deodorants, bubble baths, colored toilet paper, and other substances that could cause irritation to the urinary meatus.
- Wear cotton underclothes and keep the genital area dry.

Special Considerations: The Older Adult

As aging occurs, the kidneys may lose mass as blood vessels degenerate. The loss of glomerular capillaries causes a decrease in glomerular filtration and the kidneys lose their ability to conserve water and sodium. Additionally, the tubules of the aging kidneys diminish their capacity for conserving base and ridding the body of excess hydrogen ions. Because the renal system helps to regulate acid-base balance, fluid and electrolyte imbalance may occur quickly in the older adult.

During the fourth decade the kidneys begin to decrease in size and function. By the eighth decade the kidneys have generally shrunk 30 percent and have lost a proportionate amount of function. If stressed, kidneys respond more slowly to changes in one's internal environment. Some causes of stressful situations that may cause the kidneys to respond more slowly and contribute to fluid and electrolyte imbalance are:

- vomiting and diarrhea
- fever
- diuretics
- decreased fluid intake
- surgery
- renal damage from medications

When assessing urinary system disorders and/or diseases in the older adult, it is important to assess the patient's voiding history and medication history. Fluid intake and output should be carefully monitored, because the older adult who is having urinary problems, such as dribbling urine or losing urine when coughing or sneezing, may be limiting his/her fluid intake in an attempt to control the symptoms. This self-imposed fluid restriction can cause dehydration, and water and electrolyte imbalance.

The older adult who takes many medications (polypharmacy) may be at a higher risk in developing nephrotoxicity. **Signs of Nephrotoxicity:** oliguria and proteinuria.

Since many medications are metabolized by the liver and then excreted via the kidneys it is important that the older adult be aware of possible signs of nephrotoxicity and have renal function tests performed on a regular basis.

Special Considerations: The Child

In the child the kidneys are more susceptible to trauma, because they usually do not have as much fat padding as the adult. The child of one to two years has a lower glomerular filtration and absorption rate than the older child and/or adult. Infants are more prone to fluid volume changes, excess and/or dehydration. Additionally infants do not concentrate urine.

Urinary tract infections (UTIs) are common in children. The microorganisms *Escherichia coli, Klebsiella*, and *Proteus* cause most urinary tract infections seen in children. *Escherichia coli* is the most common cause, contributing to 75 to 90 percent of

(continued)

the infections. Except during the neonatal period, girls are more prone to UTIs than boys. This is because of the shorter urethra of the female, and the location of the urethra near the anus.

The signs and symptoms of urinary tract infection are age related.

- **Infants**—fever, loss of weight, nausea, vomiting, increased urination, foul-smelling urine, persistent diaper rash, failure to thrive.
- **Older Child**—increased urination (frequency), pain during urination, abdominal pain, hematuria.
- **Other indications** of infection are: bedwetting in a "trained child" and when the kidneys are involved—fever, chills, and flank pain may be present.
- Some children do not exhibit any symptoms.

Diagnosis is based upon a urine culture and the presence of bacteria in the urine. When a urinary tract infection is diagnosed, treatment should begin immediately to prevent the possible development of pyelonephritis. Treatment of cystitis usually consists of taking an antibiotic or antibacterial agent for a specified number of times and days, depending on the type of infection and its severity. A careful assessment of the child's allergies and body weight and/or body surface area are essential before the initiation of drug therapy. The dosage prescribed must be individualized for each child. The parent should be informed of possible adverse reactions to the prescribed medication and report any signs to the physician. Advise the parent to be sure to give the medication as ordered and to complete the drug regimen for the specified number of days.

Critical Thinking Questions/Activities

Your patient is a 30-year-old female who complains of urinary frequency and urgency. She states that she has pain in her pelvic area and that it burns and "hurts" when she uses the bathroom.

Ask yourself:

- What do these symptoms indicate?
- What diagnostic test might the physician order to determine the cause of the patient's symptoms?
- After the diagnosis is determined, what treatment regimen will the patient most likely be placed on?
- With regard to a medication history, what questions should be asked of this patient?
- What information should you give the patient about a prescribed medication regimen?
- What are some guidelines that you could use to explain ways this patient could possibly help avoid the cause(s) of her symptoms?

Spot Check

There are several medications that may be used to treat urinary tract infections. For each of the selected drugs, list several aspects of patient teaching, the contraindications, and several adverse reactions.

Drug	Usual Dosage	Adverse Reactions
Gantrisin		
Furadantin		
Hiprex		
Cipro		
Pyridium		

Urinary Tract Antibacterials

Sulfonamides are among the drugs of choice for treating acute, uncomplicated urinary tract infections; especially those caused by *Escherichia coli* and *Proteus mirabilis* bacterial strains. The sulfonamides may be classified according to the length of time they remain in the body. Using this criterion, these drugs can be separated into three groupings: short-, intermediate-, and long-acting sulfonamides. The short-acting sulfonamides are used in the treatment of urinary infections because they are rapidly absorbed, can be terminated quickly if adverse reactions occur, and produce high levels of the drug in urine.

Sulfonamides

Actions. Sulfonamides exert a bacteriostatic effect against a wide range of gram-positive and gram-negative microorganisms. They prevent the growth of microorganisms by inhibiting the production of dihydrofolic acid in the bacterial cells by competing with para aminobenzoic acid (PABA).

Uses. Acute, recurrent, or chronic urinary tract infections due to susceptible organisms (*Escherichia coli, Klebsiella-Enterobacter, staphylococcus, Proteus mirabilis,* and *Proteus vulgaris.*) Also used in meningococcal meningitis, acute otitis media, trachoma, inclusion conjunctivitis, nocardiosis, and/or chancroid.

Contraindications. Contraindicated in patients who are known to be hypersensitive to any of its ingredients. They should not be used in infants less than 2 months of age, pregnancy and lactation.

> **Warning:** Should not be used for the treatment of group A beta-hemolytic streptococcal infections.

Adverse Reactions. Agranulocytosis, aplastic anemia, myocarditis, serum sickness, hemolytic anemia, purpura, anaphylaxis, hepatitis, pancreatitis, nausea, vomiting, abdominal pain, diarrhea, anorexia, convulsions, peripheral neuritis, ataxia, vertigo, headache, tinnitus, depression, apathy, arthralgia, myalgia, edema, fever, chills, weakness, fatigue, insomnia, photosensitivity.

Dosage and Route. The dosage and route of administration is determined by the physician and individualized for each patient. See Table 27–2.

Implications for Patient Care. Before initiation of drug therapy make sure that the patient is not allergic to sulfonamides. Monitor the patient for any adverse reactions, especially for signs that may indicate serious reactions and/or blood dyscrasia (fever, sore throat, arthral-

Table 27–2 Selected Sulfonamides

Medication	Usual Dosage	Adverse Reactions
sulfamethizole (Thiosulfil)	Oral, (Adults, children over 34 kg): 500 mg–1 Gm 3–4 times daily.	hematologic changes, Stevens-Johnson syndrome, nausea, vomiting, diarrhea, head-, ache, chills, fever
sulfisoxazole (Gantrisin)	Oral, (Adult): 2–4 Gm initially, then 1–2 Gm every 4–6 hours. Oral, (Child): 75 mg/kg initially, then 150 mg/kg/day in divided doses every 4 hours (maximum, 6 Gm daily).	agranulocytosis, erythema multiform, nausea, emesis, headache, drug fever, chills
sulfamethoxazole (Gantanol)	Oral, (Adult): 1–2 Gm initially, then 1 Gm two times a day. Oral, (Child—over 2 months): 50–60 mg/kg initially, then 25–30 mg/kg two times a day (maximum 75 mg/kg/day).	blood dyscrasias, hemolysis, drug fever, rash, nausea, vomiting, headache
sulfadiazine (Microsulfon)	Oral, (Adult): 2–4 Gm initially, then 0.5–1 Gm every 6 hours times 10 days Oral, (Child): 74 mg/kg initially, then 150 mg/kg in 4–6 divided doses.	nausea, vomiting, headache, confusion, drug fever, head-, ache, blood dyscrasias
MIXTURES		
trimethoprim and sulfamethoxazole (Bactrim) (Septra)	Oral, (Adult): 2 tablets or 4 teaspoons (20 ml) of suspension every 12 hours for 10–14 days. Oral, (Child): 8 mg/kg of trimethoprim and 40 mg/kg of sulfamethoxazole daily in 2 divided doses every 12 hours for 10 days.	blood dyscrasias, nausea, vomiting, anorexia, rash, urticaria

gia, cough, shortness of breath, pallor, purpura, jaundice). Monitor intake and output ratio, kidney function studies, and note the color, character and pH of the patient's urine.

Patient Teaching

Educate the patient:

- to drink plenty of fluids.
- to take the medication with 8 ounces of water.
- to take the medication as ordered and for the full time period to prevent superimposed infection.
- to avoid direct sunlight, as one may be more sensitive to burns and photosensitivity while taking sulfonamides.
- not to take over-the-counter medications that contain aspirin and vitamin C unless prescribed by physician.
- about signs of serious adverse reactions.
- to contact physician without delay if signs of serious adverse reactions occur.

Special Considerations

- Sulfonamides may decrease the effectiveness of oral contraceptives. Therefore one may choose to use additional methods of birth control.
- Some sulfonamide preparations may produce orange-yellow discoloration of the urine.
- May decrease the absorption of digoxin; therefore serum digoxin levels should be carefully monitored and dosage adjustment made as necessary.
- Can potentiate the blood sugar lowering activity of sulfonylurea. Blood glucose levels should be monitored and dosage adjustment made as necessary.
- May increase anticoagulant effect of warfarin agents. Coagulation time should be monitored and dosage adjustment made as necessary.
- Can displace methotrexate from plasma protein-binding sites, thereby increasing free methotrexate concentrations.

Urinary Tract Antiseptics

The urinary antiseptics, although used against urinary tract infections, are not usually drugs of first choice in such treatments. The sulfonamides and antibiotics such as penicillins, cephalosporins, tetracyclines, and aminoglycosides are generally the drugs of first choice that are used to treat urinary tract infections.

Urinary antiseptics are most often used in patients who are either intolerant of or unresponsive to one of the first choice antibiotics. They are also used for the control of chronic urinary infections due to microorganisms that have developed resistance to other drugs.

Actions. Urinary antiseptics may inhibit the growth of microorganisms by bactericidal, bacteriostatic, anti-infective and/or antibaterial action.

Uses. Treatment of acute and chronic upper and lower urinary tract infections, asymptomatic bacteriuria caused by susceptible strains of *Escherichia coli, Proteus mirabilis, Morganella morganii, Providencia rettgeri, Proteus vulgaris, Pseudomonas, Enterobacter*, and *Enterococci.*

Contraindications. Contraindicated in patients who are known to be hypersensitive to any of its ingredients. They should not be used in anuria, renal insufficiency, severe dehydration, pregnancy and lactation. Certain urinary tract antiseptics are contraindicated in children, patients with convulsive disorders, anemia, diabetes, and/or chronic lung disease.

Adverse Reactions. The adverse reactions of urinary antiseptics are listed according to the drug.

Dosage and Route. The dosage and route of administration is determined by the physician and individualized for each patient. See Table 27–3.

Table 27–3 Urinary Antiseptics

Medication	Usual Dosage	Adverse Reactions
nalidixic acid (NegGram)	Oral, (Adult): 4 Gm/day in 4 divided doses for 2 weeks, reduced to 2 Gm per day for long-term therapy. Oral, (Child under 12): 55 mg/kg/day in 4 divided doses.	headache, malaise, weakness, convulsions, photosensitivity, nausea, vomiting
nitrofurantoin (Furadantin) (Macrodantin)	Oral, (Adult): 50–100 mg 4 times/day. Oral, (Child): 5–7 mg/kg/24 hours in 4 divided doses (dose reduced by half if continued past 10 days).	nausea, vomiting, diarrhea, fever, rash, urticaria
methenamine (Mandelamine) (Hiprex)	Oral, (Adult): 1 Gm 4 times/day after meals and at bedtime. Oral, (Child 6–12): one half the adult dose as shown above.	mild gastric irritation, rash, headache, nausea, vomiting
ciprofloxacin (Cipro)	Oral, (Adult): 250–500 mg every 12 hours.	CNA stimulation, superinfection, nausea, diarrhea, vomiting, GI discomfort, headache, restlessness, rash, crystalluria
cinoxacin (Cinobac)	Oral, (Adult): 1 Gm daily in 2–4 divided doses for 7–14 days.	nausea, headache, dizziness, rash, pruritus, edema, anorexia, in-, somnia, photophobia, perineal burning
norfloxacin (Noroxin)	Oral, (Adult): 400 mg twice a day for 7–10 days. Take 1 hr before or 2 hrs after meals with 8 ounces of water.	crystalluria, dizziness, nausea, headache
trimethoprim (Trimpex)	Oral, (Adult): 100–200 mg every 24 hours for 10 days.	rash, pruritus, GI discomfort, blood dyscrasias, drug fever, liver and renal disorders, exfoliative dermatitis

Implications for Patient Care. Observe the patient for signs of improvement and/or adverse reactions. Monitor intake and output ratio, vital signs, culture and sensitivity tests. Methenamine yields formaldehyde in the presence of an acidic urine, which helps suppress the growth and multiplication of bacteria. This may cause recurrent infection.

Ascorbic acid may be prescribed to help maintain the acidity of urine. Ascorbic acid tablets should not be crushed as they allow the formation of formaldehyde in the stomach, resulting in nausea and belching.

Patient Teaching

Educate the patient:

- to increase fluid intake to 2–3 liters per day unless contraindicated.
- to report any signs of adverse reactions.
- to take his/her medication as prescribed until all of the drug has been taken. (It is most important that the patient understands this, as many times once the patient

starts to feel better he or she may discontinue taking the drug, and a relapse can occur.)

- about proper personal hygienic practices.

Special Considerations

- A culture and sensitivity test should be performed prior to the initiation of drug therapy to determine the causative type of microorganism.
- A culture and sensitivity test should be performed after the completion of drug therapy to determine the effectiveness of therapy.
- Medication must be taken in equal intervals, day and night, to maintain proper blood levels.

Treatment of Urologic Disorders

Disorders of the lower urinary tract are treated with drugs that either stimulate or inhibit smooth muscle activity, thereby improving the functions of the urinary bladder. These functions consist of the storage of urine and its subsequent excretion from the body. See Table 27–4 for selected drugs used for urologic disorders.

Table 27–4 Drugs Used for Urologic Disorders

Medication	Action	Usual Dosage	Adverse Reactions
hyoscyamine sulfate (Cystospaz-M) (Levsin)	relaxes smooth muscle bladder spasm	Oral, (Adult): 1 capsule every 12 hours.	dryness of the mouth, photophobia, constipation
flavoxate HCl (Urispas)	reduces dysuria, nocturia, and urinary frequency	Oral, (Adult): 100–200 mg 3–4 times/day.	nausea, vomiting, dryness of the mouth, nervousness, blurred vision, vertigo
imipramine HCl (Tofranil)	treatment of nocturnal enuresis in children	Oral, (Child): 10 mg nightly for 1 week or as needed.	drowsiness, dryness of the mouth, constipation, nausea, blurred vision
bethanechol chloride (Duvoid) (Myotonachol) (Urecholine)	facilitates bladder emptying	Oral, (Adult): 25 mg every 6 hours.	flushing, headache, nausea, vomiting, diarrhea, sweating, salivation
dimethyl sulfoxide (Rimso-50)	treatment of interstitial cystitis	Intravesical instillation: 50 ml of a 50% solution into the bladder.	garlic-like taste and odor
*phenazopyridine HCl (Pyridium)	analgesic, anesthetic action on the urinary tract mucosa	Oral, (Adult): 200 mg three times a day after meals. Stains urine and fabric red-orange.	headache, rash, GI discomfort, hemolytic anemia, renal and hepatic toxicity

*Phenazopyridine may cause the sclera to turn yellow—this may indicate an accumulation of the drug due to decreased renal function

Table 27–5 Selected Agents That Discolor Urine

Agent	Color
Aldomet (methyldopa)	red to black
Aralen (chloroquine)	rust-yellow to brown
Atabrine (quinacrine HCl)	yellow
Azulfidine (sulfasalazine)	orange-yellow
Coumadin sodium (warfarin sodium)	orange
Desferal (deferoxamine mesylate)	red
Dilantin (phenytoin)	pink or red to red-brown
Dopar (levodopa)	darkening of urine upon standing
Dyrenium (triamterene)	pale blue fluorescence
Elavil (amitriptyline HCl)	blue-green
Flagyl (metronidazole)	darkened urine
Furadantin (nitrofurantoin)	rust-yellow or brownish
Furoxone (furazolidone)	brown, orange-brown
Indocin (indomethacin)	green
Iron (IV)	blackening
Macrodantin (nitrofurantoin)	rust-yellow or brownish
Pyridium (phenazopyridine HCl)	red or orange
quinine	brown-black
Rifadin (rifampin)	bright red-orange
Robaxin (methocarbamol)	brown to black to green upon standing
sulfonamides	rust-yellow or brownish
Vitamin B_2 (riboflavin)	yellow

◆ Review Questions

Directions: Select the best answer to each multiple choice question. Circle the letter of your choice:

1. A local or generalized collection of fluid in the body tissues is known as _______.
   a. excretion   b. emia   c. edema   d. secretion
2. Diuretics are agents that __________ .
   a. increase reabsorption of sodium chloride in the kidneys
   b. decrease reabsorption of sodium chloride in the kidneys
   c. increase the amount of fluid retained in the body
   d. decrease the amount of salt and water excreted in the urine
3. Potassium-sparing diuretics exert their action in the __________.
   a. distal tubule   c. proximal tubule
   b. loop of Henle   d. glomerulus

4. The usual oral adult dosage of hydrochlorothiazide (HydroDIURIL) is ________.
   a. 300–400 mg/kg/day
   b. 50–100 mg daily
   c. 100–300 mg daily
   d. 50–100 mg 1–2 times a day
5. Adverse reactions to furosemide (Lasix) are ________.
   a. hypoglycemia, headache, rash
   b. anorexia, vertigo, purpura, hyperglycemia, anemia
   c. dry mouth, gynecomastia, diarrhea
   d. polydipsia, chills, fever
6. ________ are among the drugs of choice for treating acute, uncomplicated urinary tract infection:
   a. Urinary antiseptics
   b. Diuretics
   c. Sulfonamides
   d. none of these
7. The usual adult dosage of nitrofurantoin (Furadantin) is ________.
   a. 50–100 mg qid
   b. 1 Gm qid
   c. 4 Gm/day
   d. 5–7 mg/kg/day
8. Phenazopyridine (Pyridium) has a/an ________ effect upon the urinary tract mucosa.
   a. antibacterial
   b. analgesic
   c. antipyretic
   d. soothing
9. Pyridium stains urine and fabric ________.
   a. rust-yellow
   b. brownish
   c. red-orange
   d. black
10. Two vital functions of the kidneys are ________.
    a. production of urine
    b. regulation of water, electrolytes, and substances
    c. excretion of waste
    d. a and b
11. Individuals who take diuretics should include foods that are rich in ________ in their diet.
    a. sodium
    b. potassium
    c. chloride
    d. iron
12. The functional units of the kidneys are called ________.
    a. neurons
    b. nephrons
    c. glomerulus
    d. Bowman's capsule

13. Disorders of the urinary system may be caused by __________.
    a. infection
    b. damage
    c. dysfunction
    d. all of these
14. Blood undergoes a process of __________ and __________ as it passes through the kidneys.
    a. dilution, absorption
    b. filtration, absorption
    c. filtration, reabsorption
    d. none of these
15. Thiazide diuretics appear to act by inhibiting __________ and __________ reabsorption in the early portion of the distal tubule.
    a. potassium, chloride
    b. potassium, sodium
    c. sodium, chloride
    d. calcium, sodium
16. Osmotic diuretics are agents that are capable of being filtered by the __________.
    a. distal tubule
    b. loop of Henle
    c. glomerulus
    d. proximal tubule
17. Carbonic anhydrase diuretics act to promote the reabsorption of __________ and __________ from the proximal tubule.
    a. potassium, chloride
    b. potassium, sodium
    c. sodium, chloride
    d. sodium, bicarbonate
18. Diuretics may be used in the treatment of __________.
    a. congestive heart failure
    b. hypertension
    c. edema
    d. all of these
19. Foods rich in potassium include __________.
    a. bananas, prunes, raisins, oranges, and fresh vegetables
    b. milk, cheese, and other dairy products
    c. butter, breads, and nuts
    d. none of these

Case Study: Mrs. Katherine Thomas, a 64-year-old retired social worker, is admitted with a diagnosis of essential hypertension, edema, and diabetes mellitus. Her vital signs are: T 99, P 88, R 22, and B/P 172/100. The physician has ordered chlorothiazide 500 mg IV. The patient is on Humulin R and Ultralente.

20. The trade name for chlorothiazide is __________.
    a. Osmitrol
    b. Diamox
    c. Aldactone
    d. Diuril

21. The nurse should know that chlorothiazide is a __________ diuretic.
    a. thiazide
    b. loop
    c. potassium-sparing
    d. osmotic
22. It is important to observe the patient for signs of fluid or electrolyte imbalance. These signs may include __________.
    a. thirst, weakness, muscle pains
    b. hypertension, constipation
    c. urinary frequency, nocturia
    d. irritability, hyperactivity
23. The nurse should teach Mrs. Thomas to include which of the following foods in her diet?
    a. milk, bread, and cheese
    b. bananas, fresh vegetables, cereals
    c. eggs, bacon, potatoes
    d. fish, liver, beans
24. While Mrs. Thomas is on diuretic therapy, you must carefully monitor her blood sugar level because it may __________.
    a. decrease
    b. increase
    c. alter the effectiveness of the drug
    d. not change

Matching: Place the correct letter from Column II on the appropriate line of Column I.

Column I

25. __________ Edema
26. __________ Excretion
27. __________ *Escherichia coli*
28. __________ Sulfonamides
29. __________ *Proteus mirabilis*
30. __________ Lasix

Column II

A. A species of enteric bacilli that may cause urinary tract infections.
B. Discolors urine rust-yellow.
C. Swelling.
D. The process of eliminating waste products from the body.
E. A type of bacteria that is commonly found in the alimentary canal of man and other animals.
F. Antibacterial.
G. Diuretic.

CHAPTER 28

Medications Used in Treatment of Endocrine Disorders

OBJECTIVES

Upon completion of this chapter, you should be able to:

- Define the terms listed in the vocabulary.
- Name the primary glands of the endocrine system.
- Give the location and functions of the primary endocrine glands.
- State the actions, uses, contraindications, adverse reactions, dosage and route, implications for patient care, patient teaching, and special considerations for thyroid hormones, antithyroid hormones, insulin, and oral hypoglycemic agents.
- Describe diabetes mellitus.
- List the warning signs and symptoms of diabetes.
- Categorize diabetes mellitus according to the National Diabetes Data Group of the National Institutes of Health.
- Describe how you would teach a patient self-monitoring of his/her blood glucose level.
- List the signs and symptoms of hypoglycemia and it's treatment.
- List the signs and symptoms of hyperglycemia and it's treatment.
- List some drugs that cause hypoglycemia and some that cause hyperglycemia.
- Describe some risk factors associated with an older adult developing diabetes.
- Explain why drug therapy may present special problems for the older adult.
- Explain why the management of diabetes mellitus during childhood is most difficult.
- Describe some of the factors associated with the management of diabetes in the child.
- Complete the critical thinking questions/activities presented in the chapter.
- List the types of insulin preparations according to rapid-acting, intermediate-acting, and long-acting.

- State the onset of action, peak action, and duration of action, and give the appearance of selected insulin preparations.
- Complete the Spot Check on insulin.
- Answer the review questions correctly.

Vocabulary

gigantism (ji-gan′tizm). A condition in which there is excessive development of the body or of a body part.

acromegaly (ak″ro-meg′a-le). A condition in which there is enlargement of the extremities and certain head bones, accompanied by enlargement of the nose and lips.

dwarfism (dwar′fizm). A condition of being abnormally small.

diabetes insipidus (di″a-be′tez in-sip′e-dus). A condition caused by inadequate secretion of vasopressin. Classic symptoms are: polyuria and polydipsia.

cretinism (kre′tin-izm). A congenital condition that is due to a deficiency in the secretion of thyroid hormones in which there is arrested physical and mental development.

myxedema (miks″e-de′ma). An acquired condition (in older children and adults) that is due to a deficiency in the secretion of thyroid hormones.

diabetes mellitus (di″a-be′tez mel-i′tus). A disorder of carbohydrate metabolism. Classic symptoms are: polyuria, polydipsia, and polyphagia. Also glycosuria and hyperglycemia.

sulfonylurea (sul″fo-nil-u′re-ah). A class of chemical compounds that includes oral hypoglycemic agents.

Synopsis: The Endocrine System

The primary glands of the endocrine system are the pituitary, the thyroid, the parathyroids, the islets of Langerhans in the pancreas, the adrenals, the testes, and the ovaries, Figure 28–1. This chapter covers each of these glands, with the exception of the testes and ovaries which are discussed as part of the reproductive system in Chapter 31.

The ductless glands of the endocrine system secrete chemical substances, known as *hormones*, directly into the bloodstream. Each of the endocrine glands performs an important part in growth, development, and maintenance of normal body functions. The hormones secreted by these glands act as chemical transmitters that either stimulate or inhibit specific organs of the body. When abnormal production of hormones occurs (too little or too much), the resultant disorders can be life threatening.

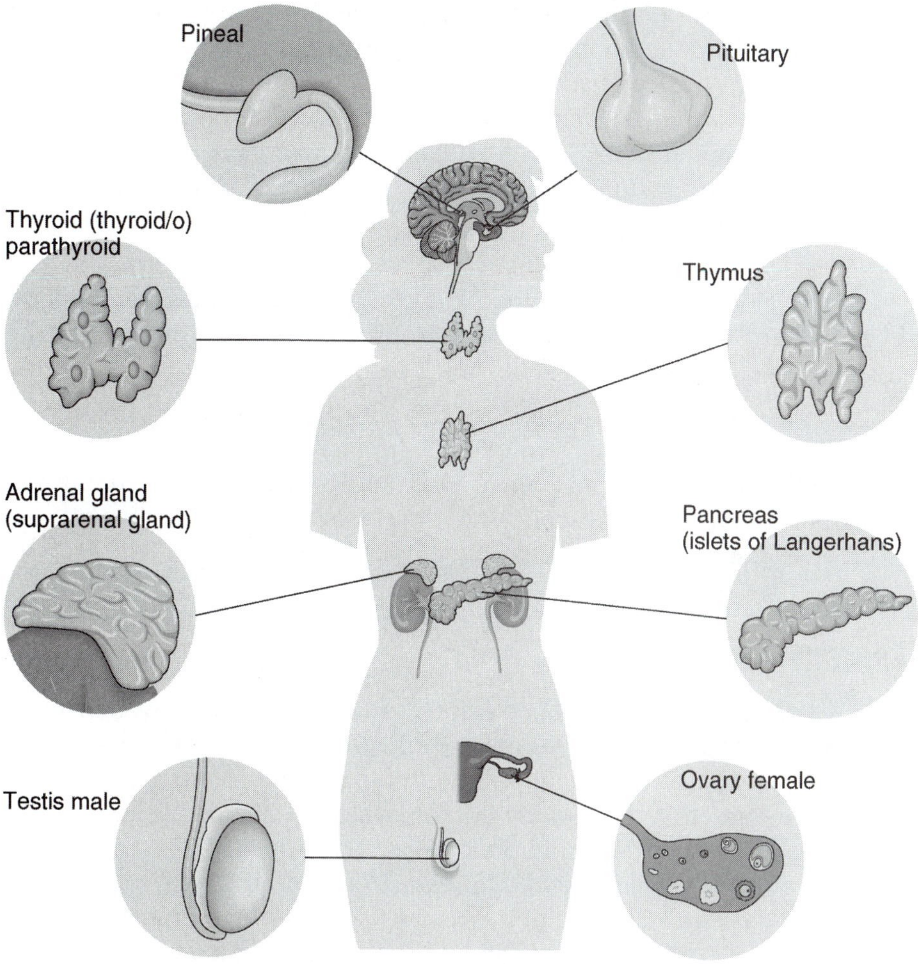

Figure 28–1 Location of the endocrine glands

The Pituitary

The *pituitary* is a small gland located at the base of the brain. Sometimes called the *master gland*, the pituitary secretes hormones that are essential for the body's growth and development and the regulation of actions by other endocrine glands. Pituitary hormones are grouped according to the lobe of the gland in which they originate.

An improperly functioning pituitary gland can be caused by a genetic condition or it may be the result of injury, surgery, tumors, or radiation. Disorders of the pituitary relate to the overproduction or underproduction of certain hormones.

- Hyperpituitarism occurs with the *overproduction* of hormones and can cause *gigantism* if the condition is present prior to puberty. If hyperpituitarism occurs after puberty, the feet, hands, and face show overgrowth and the resultant condition is known as *acromegaly*. The overproduction of pituitary hormones is often associated with the presence of a tumor. Treatment may involve radiation, chemotherapy, or surgery.
- Hypopituitarism occurs with the *underproduction* of hormones by the gland. An inadequate supply of pituitary hormones can cause *dwarfism* in the developing child as well as poor growth and function of the thyroid gland, the sex glands, and the adrenal cortex. Somatropin (Asellacrin) is administered to individuals with this condition following careful screening.
- Diabetes Insipidus occurs with the underproduction or absence of the hormone *vasopressin*, also known as antidiuretic hormone (ADH). This condition should not be confused with diabetes mellitus, and is treated by the administration of natural and synthetic substances (Vasopressin, Lypressin) that produce antidiuretic hormone activity.

The Thyroid

The thyroid gland is large, bilobed gland located in the neck. Two hormones, thyroxine (T_4) and triiodothyronine (T_3) are stored and secreted by the thyroid. When released into the bloodstream, these hormones influence the metabolic rate (the rate at which foods are burned in the tissues). Iodine, which is obtained from the diet, is essential for the production of thyroid hormones.

The amount of hormone produced is also important. If the thyroid produces too much hormone, the resulting condition is known as *hyperthyroidism* and is characterized by a high basal metabolism rate. Should the gland produce too little hormone, a condition known as *hypothyroidism* results and is characterized by a low metabolic rate. The thyroid stimulating hormone, thyrotropin (TSH) from the anterior lobe of the pituitary gland regulates the activity of the thyroid and must be present along with an adequate iodine intake for it to function properly. Cretinism in children and myxedema in adults are conditions resulting from untreated hypothyroidism. Graves' disease, characterized by bulging eyeballs and other symptoms, is the most common form of hyperthyroidism. Early detection and appropriate replacement therapy with thyroid preparations is necessary in treating hypothyroidism. Antithyroid drugs, radiation, or surgery are used in the treatment of hyperthyroidism.

Thyroid Hormones

Actions. Thyroid hormones increase metabolic rate, cardiac output, oxygen consumption, body temperature, respiratory rate, blood volume, carbohydrate, fat, and protein metabolism, and influence growth and development at cellular level.

Uses. Thyroid hormones are used as supplements or replacement therapy in hypothyroidism, myxedema, and cretinism.

Contraindications. Thyroid hormones are contraindicated in patients with adrenal insufficiency, myocardial infarction, and thyrotoxicosis.

Adverse Reactions. Sweating, alopecia, anxiety, insomnia, tremors, headache, heat intolerance, fever, tachycardia, palpitations, angina, dysrhythmia, hypertension, nausea, diarrhea, increased or decreased appctite.

Dosage and Route. The dosage and route of administration is determined by the physician and individualized for each patient. See Table 28–1 for selected drugs used to treat hypothyroidism.

Implications for Patient Care. Assess blood pressure and pulse before each dose. If pulse is above 100 beats per minute in adults and in excess of the normal range in children, withhold the medication and notify the physician. Monitor weight gain and/or loss, intake and output ratio, and the child's height and growth rate. Report any signs of hyperthyroidism (loss of weight, palpitations, diaphoresis, tachycardia, and insomnia) to the patient's physician. Administer medication at the same time each day, preferably before breakfast, to maintain drug level and help reduce the possibility of insomnia.

Patient Teaching

Educate the patient:

- to take the medication as prescribed (best to take before breakfast).
- to avoid foods and over-the-counter medications that contain iodine.
- to report any signs of excitability, irritability, and anxiety to the physician.
- that if loss of hair occurs it is generally temporary.
- that the child on thyroid hormone therapy will show almost immediate personality and behavior changes.

Special Considerations

- When a patient's medication regimen includes anticoagulants, the pro-time should be monitored carefully, as the dosage of the anticoagulant may have to be *decreased.*
- When a patient's medication regimen includes insulin, blood glucose level should be monitored carefully, as the dosage of insulin may have to be *increased.*
- Medication is generally not taken one to several weeks before thyroid function studies.
- To prevent binding of thyroid hormones by cholestyramine, administer at least four hours apart.

Table 28–1 Drugs Used in Thyroid Disorders

Medication	Usual Dosage	Adverse Reactions
HYPERTHYROIDISM		
methimazole Tapazole)	Oral, (Adult): Initial: 15–60 mg in divided doses every 6 hours, then 5–15 mg daily. Oral, (Child): 0.4 mg/kg/day in 3 doses every 8 hours initially, then 0.2 mg/kg/day.	pruritus, rash, abdominal discomfort, nausea, headache, agranulocytosis
potassium iodide solution	Oral: 0.3 ml 3 times daily.	brassy taste, burning in the mouth, hypersalivation, rash, productive cough, diarrhea
propylthiouracil (PTU)	Oral, (Adult): 300 mg/day divided into 3 doses at 8-hour intervals, maintenance dosage 100–150 mg/day.	pruritus, nausea, headache, agranulocytosis, abdominal discomfort, rash
propranolol HCl (Inderal)	Oral, 10–30 mg 3–4 times daily.	bradycardia, bronchospasm, nausea, abdominal cramping, hypotension
strong iodine solution (Lugol's solution)	Oral: 0.3 ml 3 times daily.	brassy taste, diarrhea, rash, hypersalivation, burning in the mouth, cough
sodium iodide I 131 (Iodotope I–131)	Dosage varies with use.	permanent hypothyroidism **Note:** One should wear latex gloves whenever administering radioactive iodine or disposing of patient's excreta.
HYPOTHYROIDISM		
levothyroxine sodium (Levothroid) (Synthroid)	Oral: 50–100 mcg/day, increased by increments of 50–100 mcg/day at 2–3 week intervals until the desired response is maintained.	symptoms of hyperthyroidism may occur with overdose
liothyronine sodium (Cytomel)	Oral: 25 mcg/day, increased by increments of 12.5–25 mcg/day at 1–2 week intervals until the desired response is maintained.	symptoms of hyperthyroidism may occur with overdose
liotrix (Euthroid) (Thyrolar)	Oral: initially 1 tablet daily, increased by 1 tablet every 2 weeks until the desired response is maintained.	symptoms of hyperthyroidism may occur with overdose
thyroid, USP	Oral: initially 15–30 mg/daily, increased by increments of 15–30 mg/day at 2 week intervals until the desired response is obtained. Usual maintenance dose is 60–120 mg in a single dose.	symptoms of hyperthyroidism may occur with overdose
thyroglobulin (Proloid)	Oral: Same as for thyroid, USP.	same as for thyroid, USP

Antithyroid Hormones

Actions. Inhibits the synthesis of thyroid hormones by decreasing iodine use in manufacture of thyroglobin and iodothyronine. Does not inactivate or inhibit thyroxine or triiodothyronine.

Uses. Antithyroid hormones are used to treat hyperthyroidism, in preparation for thyroidectomy, in thyrotoxic crisis and thyroid storm.

Contraindications. Antithyroid hormones are contraindicated in patients who are hypersensitive to any of the ingredients, during pregnancy (3rd trimester) and lactation.

Adverse Reactions. Rash, urticaria, pruritus, alopecia, hyperpigmentation, irregular menses, drowsiness, headache, vertigo, fever, paresthesia, neuritis, nausea, diarrhea, vomiting, jaundice, loss of taste, myalgia, arthralgia, nocturnal muscle cramps, agranulocytosis, leukopenia, thrombocytopenia.

Dosage and Route. The dosage and route of administration is determined by the physician and individualized for each patient. See Table 28–1 for selected drugs used to treat hyperthyroidism.

Implications for Patient Care. Assess blood pressure, pulse, temperature, intake and output ratio, and weight. Observe for signs of improvement and/or hypersensitivity, also edema, bleeding, petechiae, ecchymosis. Evaluate blood work, especially CBC for blood dyscrasia: leukopenia, agranulocytosis, thrombocytopenia. Unless contraindicated encourage patient to drink plenty of fluids (3–4 liters/day).

Patient Teaching

Educate the patient:

- to follow the prescribed medication regimen.
- that the medicine should be stored in a light-resistant container.
- to dilute liquid iodine preparation and take through a straw to minimize unpleasant taste.
- to report any signs of blood dyscrasia (redness, swelling, sore throat, mouth lesions); signs of overdose (periorbital edema, cold intolerance, mental depression); signs of inadequate dose (tachycardia, diarrhea, fever, irritability) to the physician.
- to take his/her pulse daily, measure weight, and be aware of mood changes.
- to avoid foods and over-the-counter medications that contain iodine.

Special Considerations

- Medication may increase effect of anticoagulants. Pro-time should be monitored carefully.
- Best to administer with meals to decrease gastrointestinal upset and at the same time each day to maintain proper drug level.

- Liquid preparations should be diluted and given through a straw to minimize unpleasant taste.
- Medication should be stored in a light-resistant container.

The Parathyroids

The parathyroid glands are about the size of a pinhead and can be found on either side of the thyroid gland. They secrete *parathormone* in response to lowered serum calcium levels. Parathormone (or PTH) acts in several ways to increase levels of calcium and phosphorus in the body.

A deficiency of parathormone may occur as a consequence of surgery or due to a genetic defect. Symptoms of parathormone deficiency include increased neuromuscular irritability and psychiatric disorders.

The Adrenals

Located atop each kidney are the triangular-shaped adrenal glands, each with a tough outer cortex and an inner medulla that secrete hormones. Adrenocorticotropic hormone (ACTH) from the pituitary gland stimulates the adrenals to produce a number of important hormones that regulate fat, salt, and water metabolism; are essential to the development of male secondary sex characteristics; and that assist in the regulation of the sympathetic branch of the autonomic nervous system. The adrenal cortex secretes three groups of hormones: the glucocortocoids, the mineralocorticoids, and the androgens. The adrenal medulla synthesizes, stores, and secretes dopamine, epinephrine, and norepinephrine.

Primary adrenocortical insufficiency (Addison's disease) is a progressive condition associated with adrenal atrophy. Symptoms of this disease include hyperpigmentation (copper colored skin), nausea, vomiting, weight loss, anorexia, weakness, hypotension, and a danger of dehydration. Cortisone and cortisol are the agents most often used in replacement therapy for primary adrenal insufficiency.

The Islets of Langerhans

The word insulin comes from the Latin *insula* which means island. Therefore, it is not surprising that the source of the hormone insulin is the beta cells of the islets of Langerhans. These endocrine glands are masses of cells scattered throughout the pancreas.

Insulin is essential for the proper metabolism of carbohydrates, fats, and proteins. Normally, insulin is released following the rise in blood glucose level that accompanies the ingestion of food. As with other endocrine glands, the oversecretion or undersecretion of hormone results in specific disorders.

When too much insulin is present in the blood, an abnormally low level of blood sugar (glucose) is the result. This condition, known as *hypoglycemia*, is characterized by acute fatigue, marked irritability, and weakness. An overdose of insulin can produce a condition known as insulin shock.

When too little insulin is present in the blood, an abnormally high level of blood sugar is the result. This condition, known as *hyperglycemia*, increases the body's susceptibility to infection and produces symptoms of the disease diabetes mellitus.

SPOTLIGHT

Diabetes Mellitus

Diabetes mellitus is a complex metabolic disorder that disrupts the body's ability to produce or use insulin. Insulin is a hormone secreted by the beta cells of the islets of Langerhans. It is essential for the metabolism of carbohydrates, fats, and proteins. Insulin helps convert food into the vital energy source that is needed by the body to help make it function properly. The insulin in the body must be maintained at a certain level, usually between 70 and 110 mg/dL of blood. When the level of insulin is too high, hypoglycemia (low blood sugar) can occur. When the level of insulin is too low, hyperglycemia (high blood sugar) can occur.

Diabetes affects 14 million Americans, with care and treatment costing $20 billion annually. The National Institute of Diabetes and Digestive and Kidney Diseases conducted a ten-year Diabetes Control and Complications Trial on how best to control the complications of insulin-dependent diabetes mellitus (IDDM) and found that those in the intensive-control group who tested their blood sugar four or more times a day and injected insulin three or more times a day, or who used an insulin pump and followed a special diet showed reductions in complications.

The American Diabetes Association estimates that 7 million Americans have diabetes and don't know it. Are you at risk for diabetes? Do you have any, some, or many of the signs and symptoms of diabetes? If your answer is yes, you should see a physician and be carefully evaluated and tested for diabetes. For more information on diabetes you may call 1-800-DIABETES.

Warning Signs and Symptoms of Diabetes

- Frequent urination (polyuria)
- Excessive thirst (polydipsia)
- Extreme hunger (polyphagia)
- Unexplained weight loss
- Extreme fatigue
- Blurred vision
- Slow healing wounds
- Tingling or numbing in your feet and/or hands
- Frequent vaginal (female) or skin infections
- Itchy skin
- Irritability
- Drowsiness

(continued)

The National Diabetes Data Group of the National Institutes of Health has categorized the various forms of diabetes mellitus as: Type I—insulin-dependent diabetes mellitus (IDDM); Type II—noninsulin-dependent diabetes mellitus (NIDDM); Type III—women who have developed glucose intolerance in association with pregnancy; and Type IV—diabetes associated with pancreatic disease, hormonal changes, the adverse effects of drugs, and other anomalies.

One in ten people who have diabetes are Type I diabetics and must take insulin on a regular basis. Insulin was discovered in 1921 by Sir F. G. Banting. The individual with Type I diabetes is faced with a lifetime commitment of trying to "juggle and balance" insulin, diet, exercise, other disease processes, stress, and all the other factors that are involved in one's life. Without proper treatment and control diabetes can lead to cardiovascular disease, nephropathy, neuropathy, retinopathy, and death.

Understanding diabetes is the best method for controlling the disease. Through knowledge, self-regulation, discipline, and following the proper medication regimen, diet, exercise program, and weight control one may be successful in living a full life. Self-monitoring of blood glucose is an important part of managing diabetes. To teach self-monitoring to a patient you must consider the person's age, cognitive level of understanding, physical ability, and desire to learn the skill. The following are suggestions you may use as you teach a patient self-monitoring of his/her blood glucose level.

Show and instruct the patient:

- on how to use the blood glucose monitoring equipment/instrument that the physician has recommended.
- on how to use a prepackaged sterile alcohol swab to cleanse the finger before performing a skin puncture.
- that if recommended, how to wipe off the first drop of blood with a sterile cotton ball.
- on how to place a drop of blood onto the test strip and how to place the strip onto/into the monitor.
- on how to read the test results,
- on how to record the results and the importance of keeping a daily log, with time (s) and date.
- on how to determine the dosage of insulin based upon the physician's ordered sliding scale.
- on how to properly dispose of used materials.

The patient should be instructed on when and how many times a day to check his/her blood glucose level. Usually, this is before meals and when one "feels" different than normal. The patient should report a high blood glucose level to his/her physician and take insulin as instructed. When the blood glucose level is low, the patient should eat some "quick sugar." For example: 1/2 cup of orange juice, milk, or soda; several hard candies, and/or take three glucose tablets.

Signs and Symptoms of Hypoglycemia

- tremors (shaking)
- fast heart beat (palpitations)
- blurred vision
- sweating
- hunger
- irritability
- headache
- weakness
- confusion
- loss of consciousness
- convulsions
- blood sugar subnormal: 20–50 mg/dL

Signs and Symptoms of Hyperglycemia

- skin is flushed, hot, and dry
- pulse rapid and weak
- drowsiness, loss of consciousness
- low blood pressure
- rapid, deep respirations
- breath-sweet, fruity odor
- thirsty
- blood sugar above 200 mg/dL

Drugs and Blood Glucose Levels

There are many medications that can affect blood glucose levels. The diabetic patient needs to know of these medications and the physician should be informed about all drugs that his/her diabetic patient takes. The following are some drugs with examples that can affect blood glucose levels.

Drugs That Can Cause Hypoglycemia

- Alcohol
- Allopurinol (Lopurin, Zyloprim)
- Chloramphenicol (Chloromycetin)
- Clofibrate (Abitrate, Atromid-S)
- Fenfluramine (Pondimin)
- Monoamine oxidase inhibitors (MAOIs)
- Phenylbutazone (Butatab, Butazolidin)
- Salicylates
- Sulfonamides

Drugs That Can Cause Hyperglycemia

- Calcium-channel blockers
- Corticosteroids
- Diazoxide (Proglycem)
- Isoniazid (Laniazid, Nydrazid)
- Levothyroxine (Levoxine, Synthroid)
- Oral contraceptives
- Phenytoin (Dilantin)
- Rifampin (Rifadin, Rimactane)
- Thiazide diuretics

Special Considerations: The Older Adult

Diabetes mellitus may develop at any age, but generally insulin-dependent diabetes (Type I diabetes) appears before age 30 and non-insulin-dependent diabetes (Type II diabetes) develops in mid-life or later. Because the onset of Type II diabetes is gradual and symptoms may be vague, it can go undiagnosed and untreated for years. More than 90% of diabetics have Type II diabetes and it is this type that will most likely affect the older adult. An older adult may not be diagnosed with diabetes until he/she

(continued)

goes in for a regular eye exam and the ophthalmologist discovers a problem, and/or one goes in for a physical exam and the blood tests indicate an elevated blood glucose level. There are multiple risk factors associated with the older adult and the development of diabetes.

Risk Factors Associated with Developing Type II Diabetes

- Heredity
- Decreased activity
- New stressors in life
- Age-related insulin resistance
- Obesity
- Multiple diseases
- Polypharmacy
- Age-related decreased insulin production

Treatment

The treatment regimen of medication, diet, exercise, self-monitoring, and weight control are aimed at keeping the older adult's blood glucose level at acceptable levels and preventing complications from occurring. This is generally a complex process and must be individualized for each patient. The older adult may have more difficulty managing his/her diabetes than a younger person, because of physical and psychosocial limitations. In addition, drug therapy may present special problems for the older adult because of multiple illnesses, polypharmacy, and/or poor nutrition.

Drug Therapy and Some Other Special Problems

- Certain medications may cause hypoglycemia and/or hyperglycemia. See Spotlight on Diabetes.
- The older adult may have reduced blood flow to the liver and kidneys causing a slowing of drug clearance, thereby increasing the concentration in his/her blood which could cause lactic acidosis or hypoglycemia.
- Cost of medication (s) may be more than the person can afford, causing the person not to adhere to a medication regimen.
- Impaired vision and/or loss of physical ability (dexterity) may interfere with the person following the treatment regimen.

Special Considerations: The Child

Type I insulin-dependent diabetes mellitus (IDDM) is the most common endocrine system disorder of childhood. The rate of occurrence is highest among the 5 to 7 year-old and the 11 to 13 year-old. Annually in the United States there are 12–15 new cases per 100,000 children. The classic symptoms of diabetes mellitus: polyuria, polydipsia, and polyphagia appear more rapidly in children. The child will excrete a large amount of urine (polyuria), complain of thirst (polydipsia), and be constantly hungry (polyphagia). Other symptoms seen during childhood are weakness, loss of weight, lethargy, anorexia, irritability, dry skin, vaginal yeast infections in the female child and/or recurrent infections, and abdominal cramps.

The management of diabetes mellitus during childhood is most difficult, because diet, exercise, and medication has to be adjusted and regulated according to the various stages of growth and development of the child. Other factors that should be considered are: age, cognitive level of understanding, financial, social, cultural, and religious belief. Because children are growing and developing, special considerations must be provided for each stage of development.

Infants and Toddlers

- During illness infants and toddlers are more prone to hydration problems.

Preschool Children

- Have irregular activity and eating patterns.

School-Age Children

- May use their disease as a method of escape from responsibility or to gain attention.

Adolescence

- Onset of puberty will generally require adjustments in diet and insulin.
- Disease adds an additional stressor to a normally stressful growth period.

Some other factors involved with management are:

- The child expends a great deal of energy, thereby,
- nutritional needs vary with growth and development.
- The normal stresses of childhood are increased by this disease process.
- Management of diabetes becomes a lifetime commitment.

Critical Thinking Questions/Activities

Diabetes mellitus is a complex metabolic disorder that disrupts the body's ability to produce or use insulin. In this chapter some basic facts about diabetes mellitus are presented. Your patient is a 67-year-old female who has been diagnosed with non-insulin-dependent diabetes. She states that she is having some problems managing her diabetes. Ask yourself:

- What factors are involved in the "juggling and balancing" of diabetes?
- What are some special problems that an older adult may have with drug therapy?
- How can I explain to my patient about certain medications that cause hypoglycemia and those that can cause hyperglycemia?
- How can I be sure that my patient knows the signs and symptoms of hypoglycemia and its treatment?

(continued)

- How can I be sure that my patient knows the signs and symptoms of hyperglycemia and its treatment?
- What 1-800 number should I provide for my patient, so that she can find out more about diabetes?

Insulin

Actions. Insulin stimulates carbohydrate metabolism by increasing the movement of glucose and other monosaccharides into cells. It also influences fat and carbohydrate metabolism in the liver and adipose cells. It decreases blood sugar, phosphate, and potassium, and increases blood pyruvate and lactate.

Uses. Insulin is used in insulin-dependent diabetes mellitus (Type I IDDM), non-insulin-dependent diabetes mellitus (Type II NIDDM) when other treatment regimens are not effective, and to treat ketoacidosis.

Contraindications. Insulin is essential for life and if the patient becomes hypersensitive to one type of insulin, another type is prescribed by the physician.

Adverse Reactions. Headache, lethargy, tremors, weakness, fatigue, delirium, sweating, tachycardia, palpitations, blurred vision, hunger, nausea, hypoglycemia, flushing, rash, urticaria, and anaphylaxis.

Dosage and Route. The dosage is individualized for each patient and depends upon the patient's blood glucose level. The route of administration is parenteral. It cannot be given orally because peptidases in the digestive juices destroy the protein molecule.

Implications for Patient Care. To provide essential care to a diabetic patient, the nurse must be familiar with the various types of insulin preparations and their onset of action, peak action, duration of action, and appearance. See Table 28–2.

Patient Teaching. Patient teaching involves a wide scope of activities and the involvement of numerous health professionals.

Educate the patient:

- and his/her family about the patient's specific type of diabetes.
- about the treatment regimen (medication, diet, exercise, weight control/reduction/management, rest, stress management, and life style modification).
- about how to properly test blood sugar and/or urine glucose levels.
- about how to store and handle insulin.
- about the symptoms and treatment for hypoglycemia and hyperglycemia.
- about when to seek medical attention.

Table 28–2 Insulin Preparations

Type of Insulin (Trade Name)	Onset of Action	Peak Action	Duration of Action	Appearance
RAPID-ACTING				
insulin injection				
(Regular Iletin I)	0.5 hr	2–3 hrs	6–8 hrs	clear
(Regular Insulin)	0.5 hr	2.5–5 hrs	6–8 hrs	clear
(Novolin R)	0.5 hr	2.5–5 hrs	6–8 hrs	clear
(Humulin R)	0.5 hr	1–3 hrs	6–8 hrs	clear
(Velosulin)	0.5 hr	1–3 hrs	6–8 hrs	clear
prompt insulin zinc suspension				
(Semilente Iletin I)	1–1.5 hrs	5–10 hrs	12–16 hrs	cloudy
(Semilente Insulin)	1–1.5 hrs	5–10 hrs	12–16 hrs	cloudy
INTERMEDIATE-ACTING				
isophane insulin suspension				
(NPH Iletin I)	1–1.5 hrs	4–12 hrs	18–24 hrs	cloudy
(NPH Insulin)	1–1.5 hrs	4–12 hrs	18–24 hrs	cloudy
(Insulatard NPH)	1–1.5 hrs	4–12 hrs	18–24 hrs	cloudy
(Novolin N)	1–1.5 hrs	4–12 hrs	18–24 hrs	cloudy
(Humulin N)	1–1.5 hrs	4–12 hrs	18–24 hrs	cloudy
insulin zinc suspension				
(Lente Iletin I)	1–1.5 hrs	8–12 hrs	18–24 hrs	cloudy
(Lente Insulin)	2–2.5 hrs	7–15 hrs	18–24 hrs	cloudy
(Novolin L)	2–2.5 hrs	7–15 hrs	18–24 hrs	cloudy
LONG-ACTING				
protamine zinc insulin suspension				
(Protamine, Zinc and Iletin I)	4–8 hrs	16–18 hrs	36 hrs	cloudy
extended insulin zinc suspension				
(Ultralente)	4–6 hrs	10–30 hrs	36 hrs	cloudy
(Ultralente Iletin I)	4–6 hrs	10–30 hrs	36 hrs	cloudy

- about how to properly administer insulin. (To teach a patient and/or a family member how to administer insulin, you should use the information on subcutaneous injection provided in Chapter 17, Administration of Parenteral Medications.)

To teach other aspects of diabetic care, one should use an appropriate source and seek the assistance of other health professionals. It is not possible to include all the information a nurse needs to know about diabetes and its management in this text, but the following is basic information a nurse should know and be able to teach to the patient and his/her family.

- Insulin is given subcutaneously, using a site rotation system.
- While using, most insulin preparations may be stored at room temperature. Other insulin should be stored in a refrigerator, and then warmed to room temperature before use. Always check the expiration date before use. Insulin should be gently rotated in the palms of the hands to mix, and it should never be shaken.
- The patient needs to know that with the initiation of insulin therapy, blurred vision may occur and that usually vision is stabilized in 1–2 months. One should not change contact lenses or eye glasses without the advice of the physician.
- The patient needs to know that with unusual stress, infection, and/or other health related conditions, the need to increase his or her dosage of insulin may be necessary.
- One should monitor blood glucose levels very carefully and use the correct dose of insulin to maintain proper blood glucose level during times of stress and/or disease.
- The patient should always wear or carry a Medic Alert ID. The patient should always have the appropriate equipment, medication (Insulin), and candy or lump sugar in his/her possession.
- The patient should not use over-the-counter medications without the physician's permission.
- The patient should not smoke or drink alcoholic beverages while taking insulin.
- The patient needs to know that insulin is a life-time drug and that its proper use is essential in helping to prevent complicating conditions/diseases from occurring.

Special Considerations

- The patient needs special care and consideration for the prescribed treatment regimen to be an effective life-time mode of life.
- Hypoglycemia may be increased with the use of MAO inhibitors, alcohol, beta-blockers, anabolic steroids, guanethidine, salicylate, fenfluramine, tetracycline, clofibrate and oral hypoglycemics.
- Hyperglycemia may be increased with the use of oral contraceptives, corticosteroids, estrogens, lithium, thiazides, thyroid hormones, triamterene, phenothiazines, and phenytoin.

Oral Hypoglycemic Agents

Oral hypoglycemics, agents of the sulfonylurea class of chemical compounds, are used to stimulate insulin secretion from pancreatic islet cells in non-insulin-dependent diabetics with some pancreatic function.

Actions. Sulfonylureas stimulate functioning beta cells in the pancreas to release insulin, thereby lowering blood glucose levels. These agents are not effective if the patient lacks functioning beta cells.

Uses. Sulfonylureas are used in non-insulin-dependent (NIDDM) Type II stable adult-onset diabetes mellitus.

Contraindications. Sulfonylureas are contraindicated in patients who are hypersensitive to any of its ingredients, juvenile or brittle diabetes, severe renal disease, and severe hepatic disease.

Adverse Reactions. Headache, weakness, paresthesia, nausea, heartburn, vomiting, abdominal pain, diarrhea, hepatotoxicity, cholestatic jaundice, leukopenia, thrombocytopenia, agranulocytosis, aplastic anemia, rash, allergic reaction, pruritus, urticaria, eczema, photosensitivity, erythema, hypoglycemia, and joint pains.

Dosage and Route. The dosage is determined by the physician and individualized for each patient. The route of administration is oral. See Table 28–3 for selected oral hypoglycemic agents.

Table 28–3 Oral Hypoglycemics

Medications	Usual Dosage	Duration	Adverse Reactions
acetohexamide (Dymelor)	Oral: 250 mg to 1.5 Gm daily in single or divided doses.	8–10 hours	hypoglycemia, nausea, heartburn, epigastric fullness
chlorpropamide (Diabinese)	Oral: 100–500 mg once daily.	72 hours	hypoglycemia, nausea, vomiting, diarrhea, pruritus
glipizide (Glucotrol)	Oral: 5 mg initially, then increased by 2.5–5 mg/day until blood glucose level is satisfactory. (Maximum dose is 40 mg daily.)	10–24 hours	hypoglycemia, nausea and diarrhea, constipation and gastralgia
glyburide (DiaBeta) (Micronase)	Oral: 2.5–5 mg/day initially, maintenance dose ranges from 1.25 to 20 mg/daily.	24 hours	hypoglycemia, nausea, heartburn, epigastric fullness, allergic skin reactions
tolazamide (Tolinase)	Oral: 100–1000 mg/day in single or divided doses.	10–14 hours	hypoglycemia, nausea, heartburn, epigastric fullness
tolbutamide (Orinase)	Oral: 1–2 Gm/day initially, maintenance dose ranges from 0.25 to 3 Gm/daily.	6–12 hours	hypoglycemia, nausea, heartburn, epigastric fullness, allergic skin reactions

Implications for Patient Care. Monitor the patient's blood glucose level and urine test to determine glucose balance. Observe the patient for signs of improvement and any adverse reactions.

Patient Teaching

Educate the patient:

- and his/her family about the patient's specific type of diabetes.
- about the treatment regimen (medication, diet, exercise, weight control/reduction/management, rest, stress management, and life style modification).
- about how to properly test blood sugar and/or urine glucose levels.
- about the symptoms and treatment for hypoglycemia and hyperglycemia.
- about when to seek medical attention.
- to take the medication in the morning to prevent hypoglycemic reactions at night.
- to be alert for signs of cholestatic jaundice (dark urine, pruritus [severe itching], and yellow sclera). (The physician should be notified immediately if any of these signs occur.)
- to wear a Medic Alert ID.
- not to use over-the-counter medications without the physician's permission.
- not smoke or drink alcoholic beverages while taking oral hypoglycemic agents.

Special Considerations

- The patient needs special care and consideration for the prescribed treatment regimen to be an effective life-time mode of life.
- The effect of oral hypoglycemic agents may be increased with the use of insulin, MAO inhibitors, and cimetidine.
- The effect of oral hypoglycemic agents may be decreased with the use of calcium channel blockers, corticosteroids, oral contraceptives, estrogens, thiazide diuretics, thyroid preparations, phenothiazines, phenytoin, rifampin, and isoniazid.

metformin hydrochloride (Glucophage)

Glucophage is an oral hypoglycemic agent in the chemical group known as biguanides. It can be either used alone or in combination with sulfonylurea agents, when glycemia control is inadequate with a sulfonylurea or the patient suffers too many adverse reactions.

Actions. Decreases hepatic glucose production, decreases intestinal absorption of glucose, and improves insulin sensitivity (increases peripheral glucose uptake and utilization).

Uses. In the management of non-insulin-dependent diabetes mellitus (NIDM).

Contraindications

- Renal disease or renal dysfunction.
- It should be temporarily withheld in patients undergoing radiologic studies involving parenteral administration of iodinated contrast materials, because use of such products may result in acute alteration of renal function.
- Known hypersensitivity to metformin hydrochloride.
- Acute or chronic metabolic acidosis, including diabetic ketoacidosis, with or without coma. Diabetic ketoacidosis should be treated with insulin.
- Not recommended for use in pregnancy or for use in children.

Warnings:

Lactic acidosis is a rare, but serious, metabolic complication that can occur due to metformin accumulation during treatment with Glucophage; when it occurs, it is fatal in approximately 50% of cases. Lactic acidosis is characterized by elevated blood lactate levels (>5 mmol/L), decreased blood pH, electrolyte disturbances with an increased anion gap, and an increased lactate/pyruvate ratio. When metformin is implicated as the cause of lactic acidosis, metformin levels >5 microgram/mL are generally found.

Adverse Reactions. Lactic acidosis, diarrhea, nausea, vomiting, abdominal bloating, flatulence, anorexia, unpleasant or metallic taste, rash, dermatitis.

Dosage and Route. Dosage is individualized for each patient. The usual starting dose is 500 mg tablets, one tablet twice a day with the morning and evening meals. Dosage increases should be made in increments of one tablet every week, given in divided doses, up to a maximum of 2500 mg per day.

Implications for Patient Care. Monitor the patient's blood glucose level and urine test to determine glucose balance. Observe the patient for signs of improvement and any adverse reactions.

troglitazone (Rezulin)

Rezulin is an oral antihyperglycemic agent that acts primarily by decreasing insulin resistance. It improves sensitivity to insulin in muscle and adipose tissue and inhibits hepatic gluconeogenesis.

Actions. Lowers blood glucose by improving target cell response to insulin. Troglitazone has a unique mechanism of action that is dependent on the presence of insulin for activity. It decreases hepatic glucose output and increases insulin-dependent glucose disposal in skeletal muscle.

Uses. Indicated for use in patients with type II diabetes currently on insulin therapy whose hyperglycemia is inadequately controlled despite insulin therapy of over 30 units per day given as multiple injections.

Contraindications. Rezulin is contraindicated in patients with known hypersensitivity or allergy to Rezulin or any of its components.

Precautions. Because of its mechanism of action, Rezulin is active only in the presence of insulin. Therefore, Rezulin should not be used in type I diabetes or for the treatment of diabetic keto-acidosis. Liver function abnormalities may occur and the patient has to be withdrawn from Rezulin. Patients receiving Rezulin in combination with insulin may be at risk for hypoglycemia and a reduction in the dose of insulin may be necessary. In premenopausal anovulatory patients with insulin resistance, Rezulin treatment may result in resumption of ovulation. These patients may be at risk for pregnancy.

Adverse Reactions. Reversible jaundice, infection, headache, ashenia, pain, dizziness, back pain, nausea, diarrhea, rhinitis, peripheral edema, pharyngitis, and urinary tract infection.

Dosage and Route. The current insulin dose should be continued upon initiation of Rezulin therapy. Rezulin therapy should be initiated at 200 mg once daily in patients on insulin therapy. For patients not responding adequately, the dose should be increased after approximately 2 to 4 weeks. The usual dose of Rezulin is 400 mg once daily. The maximum recommended daily dose is 600 mg. Rezulin is available in 200 and 400 mg tablets.

Information for Patients. Rezulin should be taken with meals. If the dose is missed at the usual meal, it may be taken at the next meal. If the dose is missed on one day, the dose should not be doubled the following day. It is important to adhere to dietary instructions and to regularly have blood glucose and glycosylated hemoglobin tested. During periods of stress such as fever, trauma, infection, or surgery, insulin requirements may change and patients should seek the advice of their physician. When using combination therapy with insulin, the risks of hypoglycemia, its symptoms and treatment, and conditions that predispose to its development should be explained to patients and their family members.

Spot Check

There are many types of insulin preparations. For each of the following types, give the onset of action, peak of action, duration of action, and the normal appearance.

Type of Insulin	Onset	Peak	Duration	Appearance
Regular Insulin				
Semilente Insulin				
NPH Insulin				
Lente Insulin				
Protamine Zinc Insulin Suspension				

◆ Review Questions

Directions: Select the best answer to each multiple choice question. Circle the letter of your choice.

1. An acquired condition (in older children and adults) that is due to a deficiency in the secretion of thyroid hormones is called __________ .
   a. gigantism
   b. cretinism
   c. myxedema
   d. acromegaly
2. The pituitary secretes hormones that are essential for __________ .
   a. body growth
   b. body development
   c. regulation of actions by other endocrine glands
   d. all of these
3. Diabetes insipidus occurs with the underproduction or absence of the hormone __________ .
   a. thyroxine
   b. vasopressin
   c. parathormone
   d. adrenocorticotropic

4. Two hormones stored and secreted by the thyroid gland are __________ .
   a. thyroxine
   b. triiodothyronine
   c. vasopressin and thyroxine
   d. a and b
5. The usual oral adult dosage of methimazole (Tapazole) is __________ .
   a. 300 mg/day
   b. 50–100 mcg/day
   c. 15–30 mg daily
   d. 15–60 mg in divided doses every 6 hours, then 5–15 mg daily
6. Parathormone increases the levels of __________ and __________ in the body.
   a. sodium, chloride
   b. calcium, phosphorus
   c. magnesium, phosphorus
   d. calcium, sodium
7. The adrenal medulla synthesizes, stores, and secretes __________ .
   a. dopamine, epinephrine, and norepinephrine
   b. glucocorticoids, mineralocorticoids, and androgens
   c. parathormone
   d. thyroxine
8. __________ __________ is a complex disorder of carbohydrate metabolism.
   a. Diabetes insipidus
   b. Diabetes mellitus
   c. Grave's disease
   d. Addison's disease
9. Regular insulin's onset of action is ____ hours.
   a. 1–1.5
   b. 2–2.5
   c. 4–8
   d. 0.5
10. The appearance of protamine zinc insulin suspension is __________ .
    a. clear
    b. cloudy
    c. bright
    d. transparent
11. The usual dosage of chlorpropamide (Diabinese) is __________ .
    a. 250 mg to 1.5 Gm daily
    b. 100–1000 mg/day
    c. 100–500 mg once daily
    d. 1–2 Gm/day
12. The symptoms of hypoglycemia include __________ .
    a. tremors
    b. sweating
    c. irritability
    d. all of these
13. The symptoms of hyperglycemia include __________ .
    a. flushed, hot, and dry skin
    b. fruity breath odor
    c. pulse rapid and weak
    d. all of these

14. The ductless glands of the endocrine system secrete chemical substances known as __________ directly into the bloodstream.
   a. enzymes
   b. catecholamines
   c. hormones
   d. neurotransmitters

15. The __________ is sometimes called the master gland of the body.
   a. pineal
   b. pituitary
   c. thyroid
   d. pancreas

16. All of the following are intermediate-acting insulins except __________.
   a. NPH Iletin 1
   c. Novolin N
   b. Humulin N
   d. Ultralente

> **Case Study:** Mrs. Anna Mathis, a 56-year-old housewife is admitted with a diagnosis insulin-dependent-diabetes mellitus and peripheral vascular disease. Admitting vital signs are: BP 146/94, P 86, T 99, R 16. The admitting orders are: 30 units of NPH Iletin I (isophane insulin suspension) daily; 1500-calorie diet; warm, moist packs to left leg ulcer.

17. The nurse should know that NPH Iletin I is a/an __________ insulin preparation.
   a. rapid-acting
   b. intermediate-acting
   c. long-acting
   d. slow-acting

18. This type of insulin preparation will have a peak action in __________ hours.
   a. 2–3
   b. 5–10
   c. 4–12
   d. 10–30

19. To evaluate the effectiveness of the medication the nurse should monitor __________.
   a. the vital signs
   b. blood glucose level
   c. blood urea level
   d. urine urea level

20. The nurse should know the symptoms of hyperglycemia, which include __________.
   a. cool and moist skin
   b. flushed, hot, and dry skin
   c. drowsiness, thirst
   d. b and c

21. The nurse should know the symptoms of hypoglycemia, which include __________.
   a. flushed, hot, and dry skin
   b. tremors
   c. sweating
   d. b and c

22. Insulin is a life-time drug and its proper use is essential in helping to prevent complicating conditions from occurring. Mrs. Mathis may not have understood this because of the development of which of her conditions?
   a. hypertension
   b. left leg ulcer
   c. fever
   d. hypotension

23. Mrs. Mathis asks the nurse not to give her any more injections. "I have a friend that takes a pill. I am so tired of these shots. Please just give me a pill." Which of the following responses would be best for you to give?
    a. "Your friend could have a different type of diabetes, and it is treated differently than yours."
    b. "I know that you are tired of shots, but oral hypoglycemic agents are not effective in your type of diabetes."
    c. "I will chart that you don't like to take shots."
    d. "Ask your doctor if you can take pills instead of shots."

Matching: Place the correct letter from Column II on the appropriate line of Column I.

Column I

24. ________ Acromegaly
25. ________ Cretinism
26. ________ Diabetes insipidus
27. ________ Diabetes mellitus
28. ________ Dwarfism
29. ________ Gigantism
30. ________ Myxedema
31. ________ Sulfonylurea
32. ________ Hyperthyroidism

Column II

A. A class of chemical compounds that includes oral hypoglycemic agents.
B. A condition of being abnormally small.
C. A condition in which there is excessive development of the body or a body part.
D. A condition in which there is enlargement of the extremities and certain head bones.
E. A congenital condition that is due to a deficiency in the secretion of thyroid hormones.
F. An acquired condition that is due to a deficiency in the secretion of thyroid hormones.
G. A disorder of carbohydrate metabolism that is a result of inadequate production or utilization of insulin.
H. A condition caused by inadequate secretion of vasopressin.
I. Characterized by a low basal metabolism rate.
J. Characterized by a high basal metabolism rate.

CHAPTER 29

Medications Used for Musculoskeletal System Disorders

OBJECTIVES

Upon completion of this chapter, you should be able to:

- Define the terms listed in the vocabulary.
- Describe the musculoskeletal system.
- Describe the benefits and injuries associated with exercise.
- List the normal aging changes that can predispose an older adult to falls.
- List ways an older adult may use to help prevent falls.
- Explain why musculoskeletal injuries can be common in childhood.
- List ways that may be used to help prevent sports injuries during childhood.
- Complete the critical thinking question/activities presented in this chapter.
- State the actions, uses, contraindications, warnings, adverse reactions, dosage and route, implications for patient care, patient teaching, and special considerations for corticosteroids.
- State the usual anti-inflammatory dose and adverse reactions of selected nonsteroidal anti-inflammatory agents.
- State the usual anti-inflammatory dose and adverse reactions of selected antirheumatic agents.
- Describe Rheumatrex and give the dosage, adverse reactions, contraindications, patient teaching, and special considerations.
- Describe agents that are used to treat gout.
- State the actions, uses, types, usual dosage, adverse reactions, implications for patient care, patient teaching, and special considerations for selected skeletal muscle relaxants.
- State the actions, uses, type, usual dosage, and adverse reactions of selected neuromuscular blocking agents.

- State the actions, uses, usual dosage, adverse reactions, implications for patient care, patient teaching, and special considerations for selected muscle stimulants.
- Complete the Spot Check on selected nonsteroidal anti-inflammatory drugs.
- Answer the review questions correctly.

Vocabulary

acetylcholine (as″e-til-ko′len). A neurotransmitter (ester of choline) that occurs in various tissues and organs of the body. It is thought to play an important role in the transmission of nerve impulses at synapses and myoneural junctions.

acetylcholinesterase (as″e-til-ko″lin-es′ter-as). An enzyme that inactivates the neurotransmitter acetylcholine. It catalyzes the breakdown of acetylcholine to acetic acid and choline.

anticholinesterase (an″ti-ko′lin-es′ter-as). A substance that inactivates the action of cholinesterase.

cholinesterase (ko″lin-es′ter-as). An enzyme that acts as a catalyst in the hydrolysis of acetylcholine.

chrysotherapy (kris″o-ther′a-pe). The use of gold compounds as treatment; especially for rheumatoid arthritis.

corticosteroid (kor″ti-ko′ster′oyd). Any of a number of hormonal steroid substances (glucocorticoids, mineralocorticoids, and androgens) that are secreted by the adrenal cortex.

prostaglandins (pros′ta-gland-ins). A group of hormone-like unsaturated fatty acids that are present in many body tissues (brain, kidney, thymus, prostate gland, menstrual fluid, lung, seminal fluid, and pancreas). They are secreted in small amounts and effect changes in vasomotor tone, capillary permeability, smooth muscle tone, autonomic, and central nervous system.

receptor (re-sep′tor). A receiver—a cell component that combines with a drug or hormone to alter the function of the cell.

Synopsis: The Musculoskeletal System

The musculoskeletal system is made up of muscles, bones, ligaments, and tendons. The skeleton consists of 206 interconnected bones that give the body its unique shape and provide support for its organs and tissues. There are more than 650 muscles in the body. Those that attach to the skeleton are known as *skeletal muscles.* The maintenance of normal body posture and the production of movement in response to voluntary control are basic functions of these muscles.

Each skeletal muscle is activated by a motor nerve that has its origin at the spinal cord and which terminates in fibers connected to muscle cells. The point at which a motor nerve fiber connects to a muscle cell is known as a *neuromuscular junction.* When an electrical impulse of sufficient strength passes from the spinal cord, over the motor nerve, to this junction, it causes the release of the cholinergic neurotransmitter *acetylcholine.* This substance passes across the neuromuscular junction and binds to specialized receptor sites on that part of the muscle opposite the nerve ending. The presence of acetylcholine sends electrical stimulation throughout the muscle, causing it to contract. This action is countered by the presence of *acetylcholinesterase,* an enzyme that destroys acetylcholine and readies muscle fibers for the next nerve impulse.

Because the musculoskeletal system is made up of living tissues and depends upon neuromuscular activity to function, this chapter will cover medications for the relief of pain and inflammation as well as drugs used to relax or stimulate skeletal muscles. See Chapter 30 for drugs used as analgesics.

SPOTLIGHT

Exercise—Benefits and Injuries

Each year, more and more evidence indicates that regular physical activity can help the human body maintain, repair, and improve itself. Regular aerobic and weight-bearing exercises, such as aerobic dance, brisk walking, weight-lifting, and bicycling, improve heart and lung function and muscle tone. To maintain aerobic fitness one needs to exercise three times a week for 20–30 minutes at his/her target heart rate.

Although there are many benefits of exercise, it carries a number of risks due to the stresses placed on joints, muscles, tendons, and connective tissue. Injuries caused by sports and/or exercise are very common. Some of the most common types of injuries are bone bruise, bursitis, tendonitis, muscle cramps, sprains, stress fractures, strains, bone spurs, and pulled muscles.

In basketball, tennis, track, running, and brisk walking, the Achilles' tendon is most commonly injured. This tendon can become inflamed and/or torn. In baseball and swimming, the tendons of the shoulder are commonly injured. In tennis, players are susceptible to tennis elbow, as are politicians who shake the hands of many people. Knee injuries account for many sports injuries, as well as presenting problems for many patients who engage in strenuous physical activity.

The best way to prevent injuries due to exercise and/or sports is to build muscle strength gradually. Muscles respond to increased use by becoming larger and stronger. Warm-up exercises are very important in conditioning the body and preparing it for exercise. Stretching exercises stimulate muscle circulation, and help keep joints and tendons flexible.

The Aerobics and Fitness Association of America recommends the following guidelines for stretching your workout:

(continued)

1. A warm-up should include a balanced combination of static stretching and rhythmic limbering.
2. End a workout with static stretching.
3. Follow aerobic workouts with a sufficient cool-down period including hamstring and calf stretches.
4. After completing exercises for a specific muscle group, always stretch those muscles.

When there is a minor musculoskeletal injury, the First Aid treatment is RICE (rest, ice, compression, and elevation). If the injury is severe, medical and/or surgical treatment should begin as soon as possible. Medical treatment may involve the use of anti-inflammatory drugs, analgesics, and skeletal muscle relaxants.

It is wise to know one's body and to recognize any warning signs that could indicate injury. It is best to always seek advice from your physician before beginning any exercise program.

Some benefits of exercise are:

- It reduces the risk for heart disease.
- It may slow down the progression of osteoporosis.
- It reduces the levels of triglycerides and raises the "good" cholesterol (high density lipoproteins).
- It can lower systolic and diastolic blood pressure.
- It may improve blood glucose levels in the diabetic patient.
- Combined with a low-fat, low-calorie diet, it is effective in preventing obesity and helping individuals maintain a proper body weight.
- It strengthens muscles and keeps joints, tendons, and ligaments more flexible.
- It can elevate one's mood and reduce anxiety and tension.
- Vigorous exercise in youth reduces the risk of coronary heart disease, hypertension, and stroke.
- People who improve aerobic fitness also boost their ability to recall names and perform other mental tasks. Researchers have found that fit older people are better at solving arithmetic problems than out-of-shape seniors.
- When older people improve their aerobic fitness, reaction times quicken. This may allow an older person to stop a car 15 to 20 feet earlier than an older person who is not fit.
- Women who walk 45 minutes a day are half as likely as sedentary women to come down with colds or the flu. Researchers found that exceptionally active women in their seventies had immune systems that were just as robust as in those women half their age, and were almost twice as strong as those of most sedentary seniors.

- Women who keep up aerobic exercise during pregnancy are less troubled by backaches, headaches, hot flashes, shortness of breath, and fatigue than sedentary mothers-to-be.
- Researchers found that as fitness levels improve, so does sex life.
- According to a theoretical model developed by the RAND Corporation, every mile that you cover—walking or running—saves society an average of 24 cents in medical and other costs.

Special Considerations: The Older Adult

It has been estimated that approximately 50 percent of all accidental deaths in persons over 65 years of age are a result of falls. Studies show that underlying medical problems and hazards in the environment cause about half of the falls, thereby only half of the falls are truly accidental.

As the body ages, there are certain normal changes that can predispose an older adult to falls.

Normal Aging Changes That Predispose to Falls:

- Poor vision.
- Bones lose strength, becoming more brittle. Such changes make the bones easier to break.
- Muscles, if not exercised, lose strength.
- Collagen and elastic fibers of tendons and ligaments degenerate, lose flexibility, and affect muscle activity. This can also cause a decrease in range of motion and make joints more painful.
- Decreased reaction time.
- Fall in blood pressure on sitting or standing.
- Decreased ability to judge exact height or depth of a surface.
- Medical problems such as osteoporosis, vertigo, mental confusion, heart valve or rhythm abnormalities.
- Polypharmacy.

Education is a key concept in helping the older adult prevent falls. The older adult should be taught to eat properly, to exercise, and to see a physician on a regular basis. In addition, the older adult should:

- Use a non-skid mat in the bathtub.
- Use wall-mounted rails in the shower or tub when getting into and out of the bath.

(continued)

- Use nightlights in the bedroom and bathroom.
- Use non-skid rugs on the floor. Do not use throw rugs.
- Not wear shoes with slick bottoms.
- Keep house and walkways free of objects, in good repair, and well-lighted.
- Not rearrange furniture. Keep familiar patterns in place.
- Be very careful if going out in the snow and/or ice.

Special Considerations: The Child

Injury to the musculoskeletal system can be common in childhood. Approximately 200,000 children are admitted to hospitals each year with head injuries. Head injuries occur more frequently in males than in females and are prevalent during adolescence. The toddler can also be prone to head injuries. The major complications of head injury are hemorrhage, swelling of the brain, compression of the brain stem, and infection.

The school-age child is generally more prone to fractures because of bicycle accidents, falls on the playground, and sports injuries. Sports injuries are also common in the adolescent. Concussion, injured ligaments, fractures, sprains, strains, muscle cramps, shin splints, and neck injury are some of the common sports injuries seen during adolescence. There are various ways to help prevent sports injuries and the following are some suggestions.

Prevention of Sports Injuries

- Before and after sports activity allow for adequate warm-up and cool-down periods.
- Year-round conditioning of the body through a regular exercise program, is very important.
- Choose sports activities according to physical and mental ability.
- Sports activities should be supervised by a qualified adult.
- Safe and well-fitting athletic gear and/or equipment should be worn by all participants.
- Safety rules and regulations of the sports activity should be followed by all participants.
- Proper nutrition and adequate fluids are necessary for the child to perform at his/her best.
- Emergency services should be readily available in case of injury.
- Each child should have a physical examination before beginning any athletic activity.
- Male athletes should wear proper supportive gear and female athletes should wear proper supportive bras.

Critical Thinking Questions/Activities

Regular physical activity can help the human body maintain, repair, and improve itself. Although there are many benefits of exercise, it carries a number of risks due to stresses placed on joints, muscles, tendons, and connective tissue.

Ask yourself:

- What are some of the common injuries due to exercise?
- What is the best way to prevent injuries due to exercise?
- What is the first aid treatment for a minor musculoskeletal injury?
- What is the medical treatment for a musculoskeletal injury?

Anti-Inflammatory Drugs

Inflammation is a normal response to injury, infection, or irritation of living tissue. Redness, tenderness, pain, and swelling of the affected area are characteristics of the inflammatory process. Minor inflammations may occur as the result of a break in the skin or casual contact with a caustic substance. The more severe forms of inflammation are usually associated with rheumatic disorders such as arthritis.

Drugs that relieve the swelling, tenderness, redness, and pain of inflammation are known as anti-inflammatory agents. All but a few of these agents provide only symptomatic relief of pain and inflammation and do not treat its cause.

Steroidal anti-inflammatory agents are those that are chemically related to the naturally occurring hormone cortisone which is secreted by the adrenal cortex. These agents are most often used in the treatment of local inflammatory disorders. Corticosteroids may be injected into a joint, bursa, or skin lesion to reduce the effects of inflammation (Table 29–1), or may be applied to the skin for topical treatment of dermatological conditions (Table 29–2). The use of steroidal agents to treat systemic inflammatory disorders is limited by the array of serious side effects caused by these drugs.

Corticosteroids

Actions. Corticosteroids have potent anti-inflammatory effects in disorders of many organ systems. They also cause varied metabolic effects and modify the body's immune responses to assorted stimuli.

Uses. Primary or secondary adrenocortical insufficiency, congenital adrenal hyperplasia, nonsuppurative thyroiditis, hypercalcemia associated with cancer, as adjunctive therapy in psoriatic arthritis, rheumatoid arthritis, ankylosing spondylitis, acute and subacute bursitis, acute nonspecific tenosynovitis, acute gouty arthritis, post-traumatic osteoarthritis, synovitis of osteoarthritis, epicondylitis, and in the treatment of certain collagen, dermatologic, ophthalmic, respiratory, hematologic, gastrointestinal, and neoplastic diseases, during allergic states, edematous states, and cerebral edema.

Table 29–1 Corticosteroids for Oral and Parenteral Use

Medication	Oral Dose	Parenteral Dose	Local Injection
betamethasone (Celestone)	0.6–7.2 mg/day	IM, IV: 0.5–9 mg/day	—
cortisone acetate (Cortone)	25–300 mg/day	IM: 20–300 mg/day	—
dexamethasone (Decadron)	0.75–9 mg/day	IM, IV: 0.5–9 mg/day	—
dexamethasone acetate (Decadron-LA)	—	—	0.8–16 mg, rapid onset/ long duration
dexamethasone sodium phosphate (Decadron Phosphate)	—	—	0.4–6 mg, rapid onset/ short duration
hydrocortisone (Cortef)	20–240 mg/day	IM: 10–150 mg every 12 hours	—
hydrocortisone acetate (Cortef Acetate)	—	Intra-articular: 10–50 mg/dose	25–50 mg, slow onset/ long duration
hydrocortisone cypionate (Cortef fluids)	20–240 mg/day	—	—
hydrocortisonc sodium phosphate (Hydrocortone Phosphate)	—	IM, IV: 15–240 mg/day	—
hydrocortisone sodium (Solu-Cortef)	—	IM, IV: 100–500 mg/day	—
methylprednisolone (Medrol)	4–48 mg/day	—	—
methylprednisolone acetate (Depo-Medrol)	—	IM: 40–120 mg every 1–4 weeks	4–80 mg, slow onset/ long duration
methylprednisolone sodium succinate (Solu-Medrol)	—	IM, IV: 10–40 mg, may be repeated every 6 hours	—
paramethasone acetate (Haldron)	2–24 mg/day	—	—
prednisolone (Delta-Cortef)	5–60 mg/day	—	—
prednisolone acetate (Meticortelone)	—	IM: 4–60 mg/day	5–100 mg, slow onset/ long duration
prednisolone sodium phosphate (Hydeltrasol)	—	IM, IV: 4–60 mg/day	2–30 mg, rapid onset/ short duration
prednisolone tebutate (Hydeltra-TBA)	—	—	8–30 mg, slow onset/ long duration
prednisone (Deltasone)	5–60 mg/day	—	—
triamcinolone (Aristocort)	4–40 mg/day	IM: 40 mg once a week	—
triamcinolone acetonide (Kenalog)	—	—	2.5–15 mg, slow onset/ long duration
triamcinolone diacetate (Amcort)	—	—	5–40 mg, intermediate onset and duration
triamcinolone hexacetonide (Aristospan)	—	—	2–20 mg, slow onset/ long duration

Table 29–2 Corticosteroids for Topical Use

Medication	Usual Strength	Medication	Usual Strength
amcinonide (Cyclocort)	0.1% cream	diflorasone diacetate (Florone)	0.05% cream, ointment
betamethasone (Celestone)	0.2% cream	fluocinolone acetonide (Fluonid)	0.01–0.2% cream, ointment, solution
betamethasone benzoate (Uticort)	0.025% cream, gel, lotion, ointment	fluocinonide (Lidex)	0.05% cream, ointment
betamethasone dipropionate (Diprosone)	0.05–0.1% aerosol, cream, lotion, ointment	flurandrenolide (Cordran)	0.025–0.05% lotion, cream, ointment, tape
betamethasone valerate (Valisone)	0.1–0.15% aerosol, cream, ointment	halcinonide (Halog)	0.025–0.1% cream, ointment, solution
clocortolone pivalate (Cloderm)	0.1% cream	hydrocortisone (Cort-Dome)	0.125–2.5% aerosol, cream, gel, ointment
desonide (Tridesilon)	0.05% cream, ointment	hydrocortisone acetate (Cortaid)	0.5–2.5% aerosol, cream, ointment
desoximetasone (Topicort)	0.25% cream	methylprednisolone acetate (Medrol Acetate)	0.25–1% ointment
dexamethasone (Decaderm)	0.01–0.1% aerosol, cream, gel	triamcinolone acetonide (Aristocort)	0.025–0.5% aerosol, cream, gel, lotion, ointment

Contraindications. Contraindicated in patients with known hypersensitivity to any of its ingredients. They should not be used in patients with systemic fungal infections, idiopathic thrombocytopenia purpura, acute glomerulonephritis, amebiasis, nonasthmatic bronchial disease, and by children under two years of age.

Warnings:

1. Corticosteroids may mask some signs of infection and new infections may appear during their use.
2. Prolonged use may produce posterior subcapsular cataracts, glaucoma with possible damage of the optic nerves, and may enhance the establishment of secondary ocular infections due to fungi or viruses.
3. Cautious use during pregnancy, lactation, active tuberculosis, and myocardial infarction.
4. Average and large doses of the drug(s) can cause elevation of blood pressure, salt and water retention, and increased excretion of potassium.
5. All corticosteroids increase calcium secretion.
6. Administration of live virus vaccines are contraindicated in patients receiving immunosuppressive doses of corticosteroids.
7. There are many precautions associated with corticosteroids. Please refer to current edition of a *Physicians' Desk Reference* for information on precautions.

Adverse Reactions. Sodium and fluid retention, congestive heart failure, potassium loss, hypokalemic alkalosis, hypertension, muscle weakness, steroid myopathy, loss of muscle mass, osteoporosis, peptic ulcer, pancreatitis, abdominal distention, poor wound healing, acne, ecchymosis, petechiae, depression, flushing, headache, mood changes, tachycardia, diarrhea, nausea, vertigo, convulsions, menstrual irregularities, development of cushingoid state, hirsutism, glaucoma, weight gain, increased appetite, malaise, hiccups.

Dosage and Route. The dosage and route of administration is determined by the physician and individualized for each patient. (See Tables 29–1 and 29–2.)

Implications for Patient Care. Observe patient for evidence of fluid or electrolyte imbalance and any signs of adverse reactions. Monitor weight, intake and output ratio, vital signs, serum electrolytes, and during long-term therapy monitor blood sugar, urine glucose, and plasma cortisol levels. Protect the patient from infection.

Patient Teaching

Educate the patient:

- to take the medication as prescribed.
- to be alert for signs of adverse reactions.
- to avoid the use of tobacco, alcohol, aspirin, caffeine and over-the-counter medications unless he/she has the permission of the physician.
- to wear or carry a Medic Alert ID stating that he/she is on corticosteroid therapy.
- to avoid individuals who have respiratory infections and guard against other types of infection.
- to weigh weekly and report weight gain of 5 pounds or more to the physician.
- to include foods high in potassium, low in sodium, and to take in an adequate amount of proteins, vitamins, and calcium in his/her diet.

Special Considerations

- Prolonged corticosteroid therapy may result in a cushingoid state. Signs and symptoms include: acne, moon face, hirsutism, Buffalo hump, hypertension, protruding abdomen, girdle obesity, amenorrhea, glycosuria, purplish abdominal striae, edema, thinning and atrophy of extremities.
- The effect of corticosteroids may be decreased by barbiturates, rifampin, ephedrine, and/or phenytoin.
- Corticosteroids may decrease the effect of anticoagulants, anticonvulsants, hypoglycemic agents, insulin, isoniazid, and/or neostigmine.
- Corticosteroids may increase digitalis toxicity as a result of increased potassium loss.
- The effect of corticosteroids may be increased by estrogens, salicylates, and/or indomethacin.

Nonsteroidal anti-inflammatory drugs (NSAIDs) are synthetic products that are unrelated to substances produced by the body. See Table 29–3. These agents are widely used in the treatment of inflammation, arthritis, and related disorders. Although the exact mechanism by which these agents act is not fully understood, their anti-inflammatory action is believed to result from inhibition of prostaglandins synthesis.

Table 29–3 Nonsteroidal Anti-Inflammatory Agents

Medication	Usual Anti-Inflammatory Dose	Adverse Reactions
acetylsalicylic acid (aspirin)	Oral: 3.6–5.4 Gm/day in divided doses.	GI distress, tinnitus, rapid pulse, pulmonary edema
choline salicylate (Arthropan)	Oral: 1–2 tsp up to 4 times/day.	see aspirin
diflunisal (Dolobid)	Oral: 500–1000 mg/day in 2 divided doses.	GI distress, dizziness, skin rash, headache, tinnitus
fenoprofen calcium (Nalfon)	Oral: 300–600 mg 3–4 times/day.	GI distress, dizziness, headache, drowsiness, tinnitus
ibuprofen (Motrin, Advil)	Oral: 300–600 mg 3–4 times/day.	GI distress, dizziness, headache, drowsiness, tinnitus
indomethacin (Indocin)	Oral, Rectal: 25–50 mg 2–3 times/day. Sustained Release: 75 mg once/day.	GI distress, dizziness, headache, drowsiness
meclofenamate sodium (Meclomen)	Oral: 50–100 mg 3–4 times/day.	GI distress
mefenamic acid (Ponstel)	Oral: 500 mg, then 250 mg every 6 hours for no more than 1 week.	GI distress, skin rash
naproxen (Naprosyn)	Oral: 250–375 mg 2 times/day.	GI distress, dizziness, headache, drowsiness, tinnitus
phenylbutazone (Butazolidin)	Oral: 300–600 mg 3–4 times/day.	GI distress, edema, dizziness, rapid pulse
piroxicam (Feldene)	Oral: 20 mg/day as a single or divided dose.	GI distress, dizziness, rash, rapid pulse
salsalate (Disalcid)	Oral: 325–1000 mg 2–3 times/day.	GI distress, tinnitus, rapid pulse, pulmonary edema
sodium salicylate (Uracel-5)	Oral: 3.6–5.4 Gm/day in divided doses.	GI distress, tinnitus, rapid pulse
sulindac (Clinoril)	Oral: 150–200 mg 2 times/day.	GI distress, dizziness, skin rash
tolmetin sodium (Tolectin)	Oral: 600–1800 mg/day in divided doses.	GI distress, light-headedness, dizziness
etodolac (Lodine)	Oral: Initially 800–1200 mg/day in divided doses. Then 600–1200 mg/day in divided doses. For acute pain: 200–400 mg every 6–8 hours, not to exceed 1200 mg/day.	dyspepsia, GI ulceration, GI bleeding, GI perforation, chills, fever, dizziness, malaise
ketorolac (Toradol)	IM: Loading dose: 30–60 mg. Maintenance: 15–30 mg.	drowsiness, nausea, gastrointestinal pain, GI bleeding, GI ulceration

The most common adverse reactions associated with NSAIDs are nausea, vomiting, abdominal discomfort, diarrhea, constipation, gastric or duodenal ulcer formation, and gastrointestinal bleeding. Hematologic changes can occur and other adverse reactions that may occur are: jaundice, toxic hepatitis, visual disturbances, rash, dermatitis, and hypersensitivity reactions. Usually, these adverse reactions are associated with high doses and prolonged drug therapy.

Gastrointestinal disturbances may occur with the use of NSAIDs and can be severe and even fatal, especially in patients with a history of gastric or duodenal ulcers. For the diabetic patient, these agents can affect the blood glucose level, thereby insulin dosage may require adjustment. For the patient taking warfarin, these drugs may potentiate the anticoagulant effect and increase the risk of bleeding. According to research it is recommended that patients taking warfarin should avoid NSAIDs. If given, these drugs should be introduced slowly and given in lower dosages where feasible. Prothrombin time should be monitored closely, especially during the first two weeks. When NSAIDs are stopped, there may be a loss of anticoagulant control.

Other Antirheumatic Agents

Gold preparations are used in the long-term treatment of rheumatoid arthritis. These agents have been shown to be effective in reducing the progression of the disease as well as relieving inflammation. The usefulness of gold therapy (*chrysotherapy*) is limited by the toxicity of these drugs. The adverse effects of gold compounds may occur shortly after administration, at anytime during the course of therapy, or even after therapy has been discontinued. Other antirheumatic agents are described in Table 29–4.

The *antimalarial* drug *hydroxychloroquine sulfate* has been used as a second-line therapeutic agent for the treatment of rheumatoid arthritis. Treatment with this agent usually requires six to twelve months, and is complicated by its potential toxicity and the variability of beneficial effects produced. Ocular toxicity is the most serious complication and regular ophthalmologic examinations should accompany therapy with this drug.

Penicillamine, a chelating agent, has been shown to be effective in long-term treatment of rheumatoid arthritis. Its mechanism of action is not fully understood. Because penicillamine causes potentially serious adverse reactions, its use is recommended for those with long-standing progressive disease that has not responded to other agents.

methotrexate (Rheumatrex)

Rheumatrex is a low-dose form of methotrexate approved for adult rheumatoid arthritis. It reduces inflammation, pain, swelling, and stiffness in adult rheumatoid arthritis and is recommended for selected adults with severe, active, classical, or definite rheumatoid arthritis who have had insufficient response to other forms of treatment. The patient may see improvement within three to six weeks.

Dosage. Can be given as a single, oral dose of 7.5 mg, once weekly, or in divided doses of 2.5 mg at 12 hour intervals for three doses. Dosage may be adjusted gradually for opti-

Table 29–4 Other Antirheumatic Agents

Medication	Usual Anti-Inflammatory Dose	Adverse Reactions
auranofin (Ridaura)	Oral: 3 mg twice/day or 6 mg once/day.	loose stools or diarrhea, nausea, rash, pruritus, stomatitis, proteinuria
aurothioglucose (Solganal)	IM: 10 mg the 1st week, 25 mg the 2nd and third week, then 50 mg thereafter until a total of 800–1000 mg has been given.	pruritus, "gold dermatitis," ulcerative stomatitis, hypersensitivity reactions, nephrotic syndrome with proteinuria, conjunctivitis
gold sodium thiomalate (Myochrysine)	IM, (Weekly): 1st injection 10 mg; 2nd injection 25 mg; then 25–50 mg weekly until a cumulative dose of 1000 mg has been given.	hypersensitivity reactions, nephrotic syndrome, stomatitis, dermatitis, colitis
hydroxychloroquine sulfate (Plaquenil Sulfate)	Oral: 200–600 mg daily.	GI distress, visual disturbances, retinopathy, vertigo, tinnitus, nerve deafness, dermatologic reactions
penicillamine (Cuprimine)	Oral: initially 125–250 mg/day. Dosage increases of 125–250 mg/day at 1 to 3 month intervals, if necessary	dermatologic reactions, GI distress, thrombocytopenia, cholestatic jaundice, membraneous glomerulopathy
ketoprofen (Orudis)	Oral: 150–300 mg, divided in 3 or 4 doses.	peptic ulcer, GI bleeding, nausea, malaise, diarrhea, anorexia, headache, dizziness, rash, tinnitus
tolmetin sodium (Tolectin)	Oral: 1200 mg daily, divided in 3 doses.	nausea, dyspepsia, GI distress, diarrhea, peptic ulcer, headache, dizziness

mal response, ordinarily not to exceed a weekly dose of 20 mg. Dosage should be reduced to the least possible amount of drug once response is achieved.

Adverse Reactions. Nausea, mucositis, GI discomfort, rash, diarrhea, headache. Severe toxic reactions possible are: hepatotoxic effects, elevation of liver enzymes, cirrhosis, bone marrow depression with anemia, leukopenia, and/or thrombocytopenia, potentially dangerous lung disease may occur, diarrhea and ulcerative stomatitis.

Contraindications. Contraindicated in pregnancy, lactation, alcoholism, alcoholic liver disease, chronic liver disease, preexisting blood dyscrasias, immunodeficiency syndromes, and patients with known hypersensitivity.

Patient Teaching

Educate the patient:

- to read the patient package insert inside the Rheumatrex dose pack.
- to take the medication as prescribed
- to contact physician without delay if any adverse reactions occur.

Special Considerations

- The patient should be monitored carefully while on this medication, especially the geriatric patient.
- Complete blood counts should be monitored on a monthly basis. Renal and liver function studies should be performed every one to three months. A chest x-ray should be taken if symptoms of lung disease occur.
- There is an increased risk of toxicity when this medication is taken with aspirin, other non-steroidal anti-inflammatory drugs, certain oral antibiotics, or phenytoin (Dilantin).

Agents Used to Treat Gout

Gout is a hereditary metabolic disease that is a form of acute arthritis. It is marked by inflammation of the joints and can affect any joint, but usually begins in the knee or foot. It is believed to be caused by excessive uric acid in the blood (hyperuricemia) and deposits of urates of sodium in and around the joints.

Acute attacks of gout are extremely painful and may persist for several days to several weeks. Acute attacks should be treated as soon as possible and *colchicine*, a drug used for gout may be administered either orally or intravenously. When given orally, an initial dose of 0.5 to 1.2 mg is administered. This dose may be given every 1 to 2 hours until pain is relieved or until nausea, vomiting, and/or diarrhea occur. The total dosage during a 24-hour-period should not exceed 4–8 mg. When administered intravenously, an initial dose of 1–2 mg is usually given. This may be followed by doses of 0.5 mg every 6 hours until a satisfactory response is achieved. The total dosage during a 24 hour period should not exceed 4 mg. The major adverse reactions of *colchicine* are nausea, vomiting, and diarrhea. Other adverse reactions are gastrointestinal bleeding, neuritis, myopathy, alopecia, and bone marrow depression.

Once the acute attack of gout has been controlled, drug therapy to control hyperuricemia can be initiated. The aim of treatment is to reduce the serum urate levels to below 6 mg/dL. Two types of drug therapy may be employed to reduce serum urate levels. Uricosuric agents, such as *probenecid* (Benemid) and *sulfinpyrazone* (Anturane) that increase the urinary excretion of uric acid, and *allopurinol* (Zyloprim) that prevents the formation of uric acid in the body.

Probenecid and *sulfinpyrazone* increase uric acid excretion by preventing the reabsorption of uric acid in the renal tubules. Because of this, urate stones may form in the kidneys and the patient is advised to drink 10 to 12 eight-ounce glasses of water per day to ensure a urine output of more than 1 liter per day. Adverse reactions of probenecid are headache, anorexia, nausea, vomiting, urinary frequency, flushing, and dizziness. Adverse reactions of sulfinpyrazone are nausea and vomiting.

Allopurinol, unlike the uricosuric agents, interferes with the conversion of purines to uric acid by inhibiting the enzyme xanthine oxidase. Two drugs, *6-mercaptopurine* (Purinethol) and *azathioprine* (Imuran) are normally metabolized by the enzyme xanthine oxidase and their use must be avoided or dosage reduced when allopurinol is prescribed. The major adverse reactions of allopurinol are skin rashes and hepatotoxicity. Other adverse reaction are nausea, vomiting, abdominal pain, and hematologic changes.

Skeletal Muscle Relaxants

Skeletal muscle relaxants, Table 29–5, are used to treat painful muscle spasms that may result from musculoskeletal strains, sprains, trauma, or disease. A muscle spasm is an involuntary contraction of one or more muscles and is usually accompanied by pain and the limitation of function.

Centrally acting muscle relaxants depress the central nervous system and can be administered either orally or by injection. Individuals taking centrally acting muscle relaxants should be aware of the sedative effect produced by most of these drugs. Drowsiness, dizziness, and blurred vision may diminish the patient's ability to drive a vehicle, operate equipment, or climb stairs. The use of these agents in combination with other CNS depressants (alcohol, narcotic analgesics) may produce an additive effect; therefore, such use must be with caution.

Implications for Patient Care. Observe patient for signs of improvement and adverse reactions. Monitor blood studies (CBC, WBC, differential), liver function tests, and ECG in epileptic patients. Administer with meals to decrease GI distress.

Patient Teaching

Educate the patient:

- to take the medication as prescribed.
- that the drug should be tapered off over 1–2 weeks.
- that sudden discontinuance of the medication may cause insomnia, nausea, headache, spasticity, and/or tachycardia.
- not to use alcohol or other CNS depressants while on skeletal muscle relaxants.
- to avoid hazardous activities if drowsiness or dizziness occurs.
- not to use over-the-counter medication such as antihistamines, decongestants, and cough preparations unless prescribed by the physician.

Special Considerations

- Motor skill impairment, increased sedative effect, and respiratory depression may occur if taken with other CNS depressants (alcohol, narcotics, barbiturates, tricyclic antidepressants, antianxiety agents, and/or anticonvulsants).
- Cyclobenzaprine (Flexeril), may cause hyperpyrexia, excitation, and convulsions if taken with MAO inhibitors.
- May decrease the antihypertensive effect of guanethidine (Ismelin) and clonidine (Catapres).
- May increase anticholinergic effects, including confusion and hallucinations if taken with cholinergic blocking agents.

Table 29–5 Skeletal Muscle Relaxants

Medication	Type	Usual Dosage	Adverse Reactions
baclofen (Lioresal)	centrally acting agent	Oral: 5 mg 3 times/day; increased by 5 mg/dose every 3 days until optimum response is obtained (maximum, 80 mg/day).	hypotension, tinnitus, nasal congestion, blurred vision, nausea, dry mouth, dizziness, drowsiness, weakness
chlorzoxazone (Paraflex)	centrally acting agent	Oral (Adult): 250–500 mg 3–4 times/day. Oral (Child): 20 mg/kg in 3–4 divided doses.	drowsiness, dizziness, rash, erythema, nausea, anorexia, jaundice, liver damage
cyclobenzaprine HCl (Flexeril)	centrally acting agent	Oral: 20–40 mg/day in 2–4 divided doses (maximum, 60 mg/day).	edema of the face and tongue, pruritus, tachycardia, dry mouth, fatigue, blurred vision
dantrolene sodium (Dantrium)	peripherally acting agent	Oral (Adult): initial 25 mg/day; increased to 25 mg 2–4 times/day, then, by increments, to 50–100 mg 4 times/day. Oral (Child): 0.5 mg/kg twice/day; then, by increments of 0.5 mg to a maximum of 3 mg/kg 2–4 times/day.	drowsiness, muscle weakness, speech disturbances, tachycardia, diarrhea, nausea, anorexia, abdominal cramps, bloody or dark urine, burning with urination, blurred vision, pruritus, jaundice
diazepam (Valium)	centrally acting agent	Oral (Adult): 2–10 mg 2–4 times daily. IM, IV (Adult): 2–10 mg as needed. Oral (Child): 1–2.5 mg 3–4 times daily. IM, IV (Child): 1–2 mg as needed.	drowsiness, slurred speech, muscle weakness, vertigo, hypotension, tachycardia, urinary retention, nausea, xerostomia, blurred vision, hiccups, coughing, hepatic dysfunction, jaundice
metaxalone (Skelaxin)	centrally acting agent	Oral (Adult, child over 12): 800 mg 3–4 times daily	nausea, vomiting, gastrointestinal upset, drowsiness, headache, irritability, rash
methocarbamol (Robaxin)	centrally acting agent	Oral (Adult): 1.5 Gm 4 times/day; then 1 to 1.5 Gm 4 times daily. IM (Adult): 0.5 to 1 Gm at 8-hour intervals as necessary. IV (Adult): 1 to 3 Gm daily.	urticaria, pruritus, nasal congestion, rash, blurred vision, drowsiness, dizziness, headache, nausea
orphenadrine citrate (Norflex)	centrally acting agent	Oral: 100 mg 2 times daily. IM, IV: 60 mg (may be repeated every 12 hours as needed).	drowsiness, weakness, headache, dry mouth, nausea, urinary retention, blurred vision, dilated pupils

Neuromuscular Blocking Agents

Neuromuscular blocking agents are used to provide muscle relaxation and to reduce the need for deep general anesthesia in patients undergoing surgery. These drugs are also used to facilitate endotracheal intubation, to relieve laryngospasm, and to provide muscle relaxation in patients undergoing electroconvulsive therapy.

Neuromuscular blocking agents are of two types: competitive and depolarizing. The *competitive* drugs compete with the neurotransmitter acetylcholine for cholinergic receptor sites at the neuromuscular junction. These drugs act by occupying the receptor sites, thereby preventing the stimulation of muscle fibers by acetylcholine and causing paralysis of the affected muscle fibers. The *depolarizing* drugs are believed to mimic the action of acetylcholine in depolarizing muscle fibers but, because they are not readily destroyed by the enzyme cholinesterase, their prolonged action results in a persistent depolarization block and paralysis of muscle fibers. See Table 29–6.

Table 29–6 Neuromuscular Blocking Agents

Medication	Type	Usual Dosage	Adverse Reactions
atracurium besylate (Tracrium)	competitive (non-depolarizing)	IV: 0.4–0.5 mg/kg; then 0.08 to 0.1 mg/kg after 20–45 minutes if needed for maintenance.	increased bronchial secretions, bronchospasm, cyanosis, respiratory depression
gallamine triethiodide (Flaxedil)	competitive (non-depolarizing)	IV: 1 mg/kg (single dose not to exceed 100 mg), additional dose of 0.5–1 mg/kg after 30 minutes if needed.	tachycardia, hypertension, increased cardiac output
metocurine iodide (Metubine)	competitive (non-depolarizing)	IV: 1.5–7 mg depending upon the type of anesthetic used: followed by additional 0.5–1 mg if needed.	hypotension, dizziness, increased salivation, respiratory depression
pancuronium bromide (Pavulon)	competitive (non-depolarizing)	IV: 0.04–0.1 mg/kg followed by an additional 0.01 mg/kg dose at 30–60 minute intervals, if necessary.	increased pulse rate and blood pressure, respiratory, depression, salivation
succinylcholine chloride (Anectine)	depolarizing	IV: 0.6 mg/kg over 10–30 seconds. IM: 2.5 mg/kg (maximum, 150 mg).	arrhythmias, sinus arrest, muscle fasciculations, respiratory depression
tubocurarine chloride (Tubarine)	competitive (non-depolarizing)	IV: 40–60 units at beginning of surgery; then 20–30 units in 3–5 minutes, if required.	slight dizziness, respiratory depression, increased salivation, bronchospasm
vecuronium (Norcuron)	competitive (non-depolarizing)	IV: (Adults, older children): 0.04–0.1 mg/kg initially; then 0.010 to 0.015 mg/kg after 20–40 minutes, if needed.	generally well tolerated, rarely: respiratory depression, hyperthermia

Skeletal Muscle Stimulants

Impaired neuromuscular transmission, thought to result from an autoimmune disorder, produces the condition known as *myasthenia gravis.* This disease, characterized by progressive weakness of skeletal muscles and their rapid fatiguing, is treated by the use of *anticholinesterase* muscle stimulants.

Skeletal muscle stimulant drugs, Table 29–7, act by inhibiting the action of acetylcholinesterase, the enzyme that halts the action of acetylcholine at the neuromuscular junction. By slowing the destruction of acetylcholine, these drugs foster accumulation of higher concentrations of this neurotransmitter and increase the number of interactions between acetylcholine and the available receptors on muscle fibers. The increase in the number of transmitter/receptor interactions improves muscle strength but has no curative effect on the cause of the disease.

Table 29–7 Skeletal Muscle Stimulants

Medication	Action	Usual Dosage	Adverse Reactions
ambenonium chloride (Mytelase)	cholinesterase inhibitor	Oral (Adult): 2.5–5 mg 3–4 times daily, increased every few days as needed. Oral (Child): 0.3 mg/kg/day in 3–4 divided doses, then 1.5 mg/kg/day in 3–4 divided doses.	headache, incoordination, dizziness, fasciculations, respiratory depression, bradycardia, hypotension, nausea, diarrhea, blurred vision, urinary frequency
edrophonium chloride (Tensilon)	cholinesterase inhibitor used in diagnosis of myasthenia gravis	IV (Adult): 2–10 mg IM (Adult): 10 mg IV (Child): 1–5 mg IM (Child): 2–5 mg	uncommon with usual doses; can cause weakness, muscle tension, nausea, diarrhea, respiratory paralysis
neostigmine bromide (Prostigmin Bromide)	cholinesterase inhibitor	Oral: 15–30 mg 2–4 times/day, increased until maximum benefit is obtained (15–375 mg/day).	fear, agitation, restlessness, nausea, epigastric discomfort, muscle cramps, fasciculations, pallor
neostigmine methylsulfate (Prostigmin Methylsulfate)	cholinesterase inhibitor	IM, SC: 0.5 mg with subsequent dose based on individua response.	see neostigmine bromide
pyridostigmine bromide (Mestinon)	cholinesterase inhibitor	Oral: 60–600 mg/day in divided doses. IM, IV: 1/30 of oral dose.	acneiform rash, nausea, vomiting, diarrhea, miosis, bronchoconstriction, bradycardia, fasciculation

Implications for Patient Care. Observe patient for signs of improvement and adverse reactions. Monitor intake and output ratio and vital signs. Atropine sulfate must be available before administration of a skeletal muscle stimulant because of the possibility of a cholinergic crisis (pronounced muscular weakness and respiratory paralysis caused by excessive acetylcholine). May be given with food to decrease GI distress, but better absorption takes place when given on an empty stomach. Discontinue drug if bradycardia, hypotension, bronchospasm, headache, dizziness, convulsions, and/or respiratory depression occurs.

Patient Teaching

Educate the patient:

- to take the medication as prescribed.
- to report any signs of cholinergic crisis to the physician without delay.
- that skeletal muscle stimulants are used to relieve symptoms and are not a cure for his/her disease.

Special Considerations

- These medications should not be given with other cholinergic agents.
- Because of the possibility of cholinergic crisis, emergency equipment and supplies should be available.
- Positive response to the medication includes increased muscle strength, hand grasp, improved gait, and absence of labored breathing.
- The effect of skeletal muscle stimulants may be decreased by aminoglycosides, anesthetics, procainamide (Procan SR), and/or quinidine.
- Skeletal muscle stimulants may decrease the effects of gallamine (Flaxedil), metocurine (Metubine Iodide), pancuronium (Pavulon), tubocurarine (Tubarine), and/or atropine.
- Skeletal muscle stimulants may increase the effects of succinylcholine (Anectine, Quelicin).

Spot Check

There are many nonsteroidal anti-inflammatory drugs that are used to treat the symptoms of inflammation. For each of the following drugs, give the usual anti-inflammatory dose and several adverse reactions.

Drug(s)	Usual Anti-inflammatory Dose	Adverse Reactions
Acetylsalicylic Acid		
Ibuprofen		
Naproxen		
Piroxicam		
Ketorolac		

◆ Review Questions

Directions. Select the best answer to each multiple choice question. Circle the letter of your choice.

1. __________ is a neurotransmitter that is thought to play an important role in the transmission of nerve impulses at synapses and myoneural junctions.

   a. Cholinesterase
   b. Prostaglandin
   c. Acetylcholine
   d. Acetylcholinesterase

2. __________ is an enzyme that destroys acetylcholine and readies muscle fibers for the next nerve impulse.

   a. Cholinesterase
   b. Prostaglandin
   c. Anticholinesterase
   d. Acetylcholinesterase

3. Drugs that relieve the swelling, tenderness, redness, and pain of inflammation are known as __________.
   a. analgesics
   b. anti-inflammatory agents
   c. antipyretics
   d. antibiotics
4. The generic name of Depo-Medrol is __________.
   a. methylprednisolone acetate
   b. methylprednisolone sodium
   c. betamethasone
   d. triamcinolone
5. The oral dose of hydrocortisone (Cortef fluids) is __________ mg/day.
   a. 20–30
   b. 5–60
   c. 20–240
   d. 4–40
6. The adverse reactions of aspirin include __________.
   a. GI distress
   b. tinnitus
   c. rapid pulse
   d. all of these
7. The generic name of Motrin is __________.
   a. indomethacin
   b. ibuprofen
   c. naproxen
   d. salsalate
8. The anti-inflammatory oral dose of Motrin is __________.
   a. 300–600 mg 3–4 times/day
   b. 250–375 mg 2 times/day
   c. 150–200 mg 2 times/day
   d. 600–1800 mg/day in divided doses
9. Antirheumatic agents that may be used in the treatment of rheumatoid arthritis include __________.
   a. gold preparations
   b. hydroxychloroquine sulfate
   c. penicillamine
   d. all of these
10. The usual anti-inflammatory oral dose of auranofin (Ridaura) is __________.
    a. 200–600 mg daily
    b. 125–250 mg/day
    c. 3 mg twice/day
    d. 25–50 mg weekly
11. Individuals taking centrally acting muscle relaxants should be advised that these agents may __________.
    a. cause drowsiness, dizziness, and blurred vision
    b. produce an additive effect when taken in combination with other CNS depressants
    c. impair their ability to drive a vehicle
    d. all of these
12. The generic name of Robaxin is __________.
    a. baclofen
    b. chlorzoxazone
    c. methocarbamol
    d. metaxalone
13. The generic name of Valium is __________.
    a. diazepam
    b. dantrolene
    c. chlorzoxazone
    d. baclofen

14. Drowsiness, dizziness, rash, erythemia, nausea, anorexia, jaundice, and liver damage are adverse reactions of __________.
    a. Valium
    b. Robaxin
    c. Paraflex
    d. Norflex
15. The usual oral dosage of Norflex is __________.
    a. 5 mg 3 times/day
    b. 250–500 mg 3–4 times/day
    c. 100 mg 2 times daily
    d. 25 mg/day
16. Neuromuscular blocking agents may be used to __________.
    a. provide muscle stimulation
    b. relieve laryngospasm
    c. facilitate endotracheal intubation
    d. b and c
17. Tachycardia, hypertension, and increased cardiac output are adverse reactions of __________.
    a. Tracrium
    b. Flaxedil
    c. Metubine
    d. Pavulon
18. The usual oral dosage of Prostigmin Bromide is __________.
    a. 2.5–5 mg 3–4 times daily
    b. 15–30 mg 3–4 times/day
    c. 60–600 mg/day in divided doses
    d. 50–100 mg/day
19. Skeletal muscle stimulants act by inhibiting __________.
    a. the action of acetylcholinesterase
    b. the action of cholinesterase
    c. the action of prostaglandin
    d. none of these
20. Fear, agitation, restlessness, nausea, epigastric discomfort, muscle cramps, fasciculations, and pallor are adverse reactions of __________.
    a. Mytelase
    b. Tensilon
    c. Postigmin Bromide
    d. Mestinon

Case Study: Mr. Bart Namath, a 24-year-old quarterback for the Chicago Bears is seeing his orthopedic surgeon with complaints of pain, burning, and limitation of motion of his right shoulder. He states that he was "sacked" several times during the game and hurt his shoulder again. The physician asks you to draw up 50 mg of triamcinolone diacetate for local injection. After cleansing the injection site with Betadine, the physician slowly injects the medication into the bursa.

21. The nurse should know that triamcinolone diacetate is a/an __________.
    a. skeletal muscle stimulant
    b. skeletal muscle relaxant
    c. corticosteroid
    d. non-steroidal agent
22. The trade name for triamcinolone diacetate is __________.
    a. Aristocort
    b. Kenalog
    c. Haldron
    d. Amcort

23. Prolonged use of this type of medication may result in cushingoid state. Signs and symptoms include ________.
    a. acne, moon face, Buffalo hump
    b. diarrhea, nausea, vomiting
    c. hypotension, hyperglycemia, urticaria
    d. purpura, petechiae, hypertension
24. In teaching Mr. Namath about the medication, it is important to advise him to avoid the use of ________.
    a. foods high in fats, proteins, carbohydrates
    b. alcohol, tobacco, caffeine, over-the-counter drugs
    c. alcohol, foods high in potassium
    d. alcohol, foods low in sodium
25. The physician tells Bart to stay away from people with colds and respiratory infections. This is because triamcinolone diacetate and this drug classification ________.
    a. decreases the effects of antibiotics
    b. increases the effects of antibiotics
    c. can mask some signs of infection
    d. can make the signs of infection more noticeable

Matching: Place the correct letter from Column II on the appropriate line of Column I.

Column I

26. ________ Chrysotherapy
27. ________ Corticosteroid
28. ________ Prostaglandins
29. ________ Cholinesterase
30. ________ Receptor

Column II

A. Any number of hormonal steroid substances that are secreted by the adrenal cortex.
B. A group of hormone-like unsaturated fatty acids that are present in many body tissues.
C. The use of gold compounds as treatment, especially for rheumatoid arthritis.
D. A receiver; a cell component that combines with a drug or hormone to alter the function of the cell.
E. An enzyme that acts as a catalyst in the hydrolysis of acetylcholine.
F. An enzyme that inactivates the neurotransmitter acetylcholine.

CHAPTER 30

Medications That Affect the Nervous System

OBJECTIVES

Upon completion of this chapter, you should be able to:

- Define the terms listed in the vocabulary.
- Describe the nervous system.
- Define pain.
- Describe acute pain and chronic pain.
- State the treatment for acute pain and for chronic pain.
- List some alternative methods that may be used for relief of pain.
- To assess a patient's pain.
- State the Standards developed by the American Pain Society for Relief of Acute Pain and Cancer Pain.
- Explain the special considerations for the older adult with pain.
- Give some indications of pain in the neonate, infant, toddler, and the older child.
- Explain various techniques for assessing pain in a child.
- Complete the critical thinking questions/activities presented in this chapter.
- State the actions, uses, contraindications, warnings, adverse reactions, dosage and route, implications for patient care, patient teaching, and special considerations for narcotic analgesics, barbiturates, anti-parkinsonian drugs, and anticonvulsants.
- State the actions, usual dosage, and adverse reactions of selected analgesic-antipyretics and a narcotic antagonist (Narcan).
- Complete the Spot Check on selected medications used to treat pain.
- Describe the characteristics of a good hypnotic.
- State the schedule, duration, usual sedative dose, and usual hypnotic dose of selected barbiturates.

- List the three benzodiazepines that are effective sedative-hypnotics.
- State the schedule, usual sedative dose, and usual hypnotic dose of selected non-barbiturate sedative-hypnotic drugs.
- Describe the characteristic symptoms of Parkinson's disease.
- Describe epilepsy.
- Describe anesthetic drugs as local or general acting.
- Identify selected local anesthetic drugs.
- Identify selected general anesthetic drugs.
- State three uses of ophthalmic drugs.
- State the classification, usual dosage, and adverse reactions of selected drugs used to treat glaucoma.
- State four uses of mydriatic drugs.
- State the classification, usual dosage, and adverse reactions of selected mydriatic drugs.
- Describe vertigo, motion sickness, and vomiting.
- State the uses, usual dosage, and adverse reactions of selected drugs used in the treatment of vertigo, motion sickness, and vomiting.
- Answer the review questions correctly.

Vocabulary

agonist (ag′on-ist). A drug that has affinity for the cellular receptors of another drug or natural substance and produces a physiological effect.

anhydrase (an″hi′dras). An enzyme that promotes the removal of water from a chemical compound.

antagonist (an-tag′o-nist). A drug that binds to a cellular receptor for a hormone, neurotransmitter, or another drug, blocking the action of that substance without producing any physiologic effect itself.

aqueous humor (a′kwe-us hu′mor). The transparent liquid contained in the anterior and posterior chambers of the eye.

carbonic (kar-bon′ik). Pertaining to carbon.

carbonic anhydrase (kar′bon-ik an″hi′dras). An enzyme that catalyzes union of water and carbon dioxide to form carbonic acid. Present in red blood cells.

dopamine (do′pa-men). A catecholamine synthesized by the adrenal gland. It is the immediate precursor in the synthesis of norepinephrine. It increases blood pressure and urinary output.

inhibitor (in″hib′i-tor). That which inhibits; a chemical substance that stops enzyme activity.

sympathomimetic (sim″pa-tho-mim-et′ik). That which imitates the sympathetic nervous system; adrenergic.

Synopsis: The Nervous System

The nervous system is comprised of the brain and spinal cord (the central nervous system or CNS) plus the network of nerves and neural tissues throughout the body (the peripheral nervous system or PNS), Figure 30–1. The peripheral system connects to

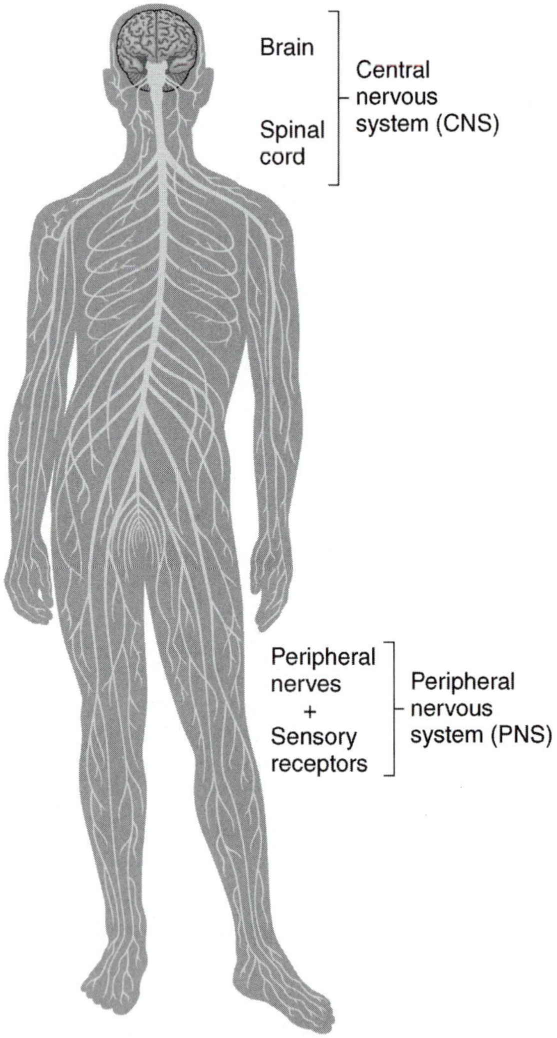

Figure 30–1 Central and peripheral nervous systems

the brain and spinal cord by way of 12 pairs of cranial nerves and 31 pairs of spinal nerves. These two systems, functioning as a unit, regulate body functions in relationship to the environment.

Our sense of hearing, taste, equilibrium, touch, smell, and sight all rely on nerves to function properly. Pain receptors alert us to danger from inflammation or hot surfaces. Muscular activity is dependent upon proper stimulation by nerve impulses. Our ability to think, reason, feel emotions, and interact with others is directly related to our neurological processes.

Disorders that interfere with central or peripheral nervous system function are treated with a variety of drugs, some of which are discussed in this chapter. Separate chapters are provided for drugs used primarily with the musculoskeletal system and for mental disorders. (See Chapters 22 and 29.)

SPOTLIGHT

Pain

Pain is a symptom of a physical or emotional condition. The International Association for the Study of Pain defines pain as the sensory and emotional experience associated with actual or potential tissue damage.

A person's pain may be measured by its threshold and its intensity. Pain threshold is the level of stimulus that results in the perception of pain. How one responds to pain is an individual process. Some factors associated with how a person perceives pain are age, gender, and the physical, mental, social, cultural and emotional makeup of the individual. Pain tolerance is the amount of pain a person can manage without disrupting normal functioning and without requiring pain medication. Intensity is the degree of pain felt by the individual.

In the United States approximately 155 million persons experience an episode of acute pain each year. Annually, an estimated 700 million workdays are lost each year because of pain, with a cost of 60 billion dollars. Acute pain may be described as one that comes on suddenly, is severe, and is a warning that something is wrong. Some signs of acute pain are increased heart rate and respiratory rate, increased blood pressure, dilated pupils, sweating (many times profuse), nausea, vomiting, anxiety, and fear. The treatment of acute pain depends upon the cause, but generally it is treated with nonnarcotic analgesics and/or narcotic analgesics.

Chronic pain is one that last for a long time. It is a pain that persists beyond the expected time required for the healing of an injury or expected course of recovery. Some signs of chronic pain include disturbances in sleep and eating patterns, irritability, constipation, depression, fatigue, and withdrawal from social activities. Chronic pain is generally managed with analgesics, but the patient may wish to try alternative methods for relief.

(continued)

Some Alternative Methods for Relief of Pain

- Behavior modification—relaxation training, biofeedback, and hypnosis.
- Surgery—destroying nerves responsible for pain.
- Electrostimulation—implanting electrodes at certain sites in the body and then stimulating them to prevent pain messages.
- Acupuncture.
- Exercise—aerobic exercise increases the secretion of endorphins (natural painkillers).
- Ice—useful for headaches, and in the first 48 hours of an injury (sprains, strains, bumps), because it reduces swelling.
- Heat—useful for cramps and muscle aches, and after swelling of an injury has subsided.

Chronic intractable pain may be caused by cancer, mental illness, neurologic disorders such as neuralgias, phantom limb pain, nerve entrapment syndromes, spinal cord damage, myofascial syndromes, or thalamic syndrome pain. New federal guidelines urge doctors to aggressively attack cancer pain, which a study showed, severely afflicts one-third of Americans with spreading cancer. The guidelines issued by the Agency for Health Care Policy and Research urge doctors to start patients on mild painkillers, then work up to more potent medicines. The next step is codeine and other weak opiates, followed by morphine and similar powerful drugs. The guidelines say there is no limit on the maximum dose of morphine. Very large doses, several hundred milligrams every four hours may be needed for some patients with extreme pain.

Usual Doses and Intervals of Selected Drugs Used for Relief of Pain

Drug	Dose and Route	Interval
Acetylsalicylic acid	650 mg (oral)	4 hr
Acetaminophen	650 mg (oral)	4 hr
Ibuprofen	400 mg (oral)	4–6 hr
Naproxen	250–500 mg (oral)	12 hr
Codeine	15–60 mg (oral)	4 hr
Hydromorphone	2 mg (oral)	4 hr
Meperidine	50–150 mg (SC, IM, IV)	3–4 hr
Methadone	2.5–10 mg (SC, IM, IV)	6–8 hr
Morphine	10–20 mg (SC, IM)	4 hr

Assessment of Pain

It is important to obtain an accurate assessment of a patient's pain. Because pain is subjective, the patient needs to describe in detail the location, intensity, quality, onset, duration, variations, what relieves the pain, and what causes or increases the pain.

- **History of the Pain**—questions to ask the patient: when did the pain start, how long does the pain last, what increases or decreases the pain, what methods are used to relieve the pain, how effective are these methods?
- **Physical Signs and Symptoms**—increased heart rate and respiratory rate, increased blood pressure, dilated pupils, sweating, nausea, vomiting, anxiety, fear.
- **Facial Expressions**—strained look, clenched teeth, tightly shut lips, tightening of the jaw muscles, furrowed brow, tears.
- **Body Movements**—protective or guarding movements toward a specific area of the body, limping, clenched fist, hunched shoulders, doubling-over.
- **Quality and/or Character**—verbal description (aching, burning, prickling, sharp, cutting, throbbing, intense, pressure, mild, moderate, severe, local, deep).

Effectiveness of Treatment

Two methods that are used to monitor treatment effectiveness for pain management are questionnaires and rating scales. The McGill-Melzack Pain Questionnaire measures both sensory and affective dimensions of pain. Ratings scales may use numbers, drawings, and/or lines. The number scale may be 0–5 or 0–10 with zero indicating no pain and the upper number signifying the most intense pain. The Wong-Baker face rating scale shows five faces with the numbers 0–5 beneath the picture, and zero indicating no pain with five signifying the most intense pain. This is useful for children and for patients who cannot speak English.

Standards for Pain Relief

In 1991 the American Pain Society developed Standards for the Relief Acute Pain and Cancer Pain. Following are these standards summarized:

1. Acute pain and cancer pain are recognized and effectively treated. Essential to this process is the development of a clinically useful and easy to use scale for rating pain and its relief. Patients will be evaluated according to the scales and the results recorded as frequently as needed.
2. Information about analgesics is readily available. This includes data concerning the effectiveness of various agents in controlling pain and the availability of equianalgesic charts wherever drugs are used for pain.
3. Patients are informed on admission of the availability of methods of relieving pain, and that they must communicate the presence and persistence of pain to the health care staff.

(continued)

4. Explicit policies for use of advanced analgesic technologies are defined. These advances include patient-control analgesia, epidural analgesia, and regional analgesia. Specific instructions concerning use of these techniques need to be available for the medical care staff.
5. Adherence to standards is monitored by an interdisciplinary committee. The committee is responsible for overseeing the activities related to implementing and evaluating the effectiveness of these pain standards.

Special Considerations: The Older Adult

By the year 2000 there will be more than 35 million adults over 65 years of age. Eighty-five percent of these adults are expected to function independently and to maintain a sense of well-being. Only approximately 15 percent are expected to be unable to function independently and fail to maintain or sustain a sense of well-being.

According to an article in the *American Journal of Nursing*, February 1996, Vol. 96, No. 2, as many as 80 percent of nursing home residents have pain that impairs their quality of life. But pain remains unrelieved in many, due to clinical myths and lack of data. The effects of unrelieved pain go far beyond the pain itself. Depression, sleep disturbance, slow rehabilitation, malnutrition, and cognitive dysfunction may all be worsened.

Pain is not a normal part of the aging process. An older adult may believe that his/her pain is just a part of "growing old" and be reluctant in reporting pain, therefore pain goes untreated and unrelieved. It is true that an older adult may be more vulnerable to adverse drug reactions, may have multiple disease processes, and often take multiple medications, but an older adult's pain should be properly treated. Most older adults can generally take nosteroidal anti-inflammatory drugs (NSAIDs) and analgesics for pain. There are precautions and warnings associated with these drugs, and some of the special considerations for the older adult are:

- Long-term use of acetaminophen can cause end-stage renal disease and liver damage when combined with fasting. A study found that those who took 105 to 365 acetaminophen pills per year had a 40 percent increased risk of kidney failure. The risk was double in people who took more that 366 pills per year—at least one per day. Researchers also found that moderate to heavy doses of acetaminophen taken on an empty stomach can change the way the body metabolizes the analgesic. Alcohol also alters the way acetaminophen is metabolized. There is evidence that alcohol leads to liver damage if acetaminophen is taken within the recommended dose. Alcoholics may be at a higher risk than nonalcoholics for liver damage because it is believed that they are more likely to exceed the recommended dose.
- Nonsteroidal anti-inflammatory drugs may cause peptic ulcer disease, bleeding, and among the frail elderly, constipation, cognitive, impairment, and headaches.

- Opiates have a long serum half-life in the older adult, therefore relatively small doses may provide long-lasting pain relief. Meperidine can cause delirium and seizures. Methadone should be used with caution because it accumulates and its analgesic effect may be shorter than its serum half-life, which heightens the potential for accumulation or overdosing.

Assessment of Pain

It is important to obtain an accurate assessment of an older adult's pain. You may use the same assessment tools as used for any adult, but realize that as a person ages there are certain normal aging processes that occur and these processes may affect the way a person perceives pain and responds to questions about pain.

Some of these process are:

- Decreasing levels of neurotransmitter or chemicals communicating in synapses between nerve cells affect short-term memory and motor coordination and control.
- Loss of cells in the brainstem changes sleep patterns. Individual variation and response to these changes are great.
- Sensory decline alters one's perception of the world. Hearing loss is common, especially at high frequencies. Smells become harder to distinguish and detect. Eyes may need corrective lenses to adjust for decreasing ability to focus. As the ciliary muscles weaken, pupil size is decreased, reducing light to the retina. The lens becomes stiff, thicker, and more opaque and begins to yellow.

Special Considerations: The Child

The mechanism for pain perception is fully developed and functioning by the time the fetus is born. Some indications of pain in the neonate are crying, eye rolling, breath holding with cyanosis, seizures, slow heart rate and vomiting. Infants through twelve months of age show pain through body language, crying, coughing and withdrawing the area of the body where the pain is felt. Toddlers from one to three years may indicate pain by aggressive behavior such as biting and pinching, by quiet withdrawal, and by regression. A toddler does not understand the concept of pain and is often afraid and fearful. Children who communicate verbally can usually use words to express their pain. Hurt is a common expression said by children who are in pain. This one word can say it all, "Mommy, I hurt."

Common Causes and Indications of Pain in Children

- Earache—pulling on the ear, crying, rubbing on the ear.
- Stomachache—does not want to eat, rubs the area, may wake up in the middle of the night crying.
- Headache—rubbing the head, crying, may wake up in the middle of the night.

(continued)

Assessment of Pain in an Older Child

There are various techniques that you may use to assess pain in an older child. Some of these are:

- **Visual Analog Scale**—child points to the number from 1 to 10, with 1 being no hurt and 10 being the most hurt ever felt.
- **Faces (Oucher) Scale**—child tells which face represents the pain at the moment.
- **Descriptive Word Scale**—child chooses the word that describes the pain (no pain, mild, moderate, quite a lot, very bad, worst).
- **Poker Chip**—use four poker chips, place horizontally in front of the child, tell the child "These are pieces of hurt"—one piece is a little, and four pieces are a lot. Ask the child "How many pieces of hurt do you have right now?" Record the number—(no pain equals zero chips).

Critical Thinking Questions/Activities

It is important to obtain an accurate assessment of a patient's pain. Ask yourself:

- What questions must I ask the patient to obtain an accurate history of pain?
- What are the physical signs and symptoms of pain—in an adult, in a child?
- What facial expressions should I be aware of that would indicate pain?
- What body movements should I be aware of that would indicate pain?
- What are some of the verbal descriptions that a patient may use to relate the quality and/or character of his/her pain?

Analgesics

Analgesic agents are used to relieve pain caused by disease or other conditions without causing the patient to lose consciousness. Morphine, a narcotic derivative of opium, was the forerunner of many natural and synthetic analgesics used today. Because they trace their origin back to opium, the natural and synthetic drugs derived from morphine are known as *opiates*. Other synthetic drugs, not chemically related to morphine, have been developed because they mimic the action of morphine. These drugs, called *opioids*, are also classified as narcotics because they can cause dependency. Table 30–1 lists opiate and opioid narcotic analgesics.

Table 30–1 Opiate and Opioid Analgesics

Medication	Class/Use	Usual Dosage	Adverse Reactions
OPIATES & OPIOIDS			
codeine phosphate, codeine sulfate	C II analgesic	Oral, SC, IM, (Adult): 15–60 mg 4–6 times/day as necessary. Oral, SC, IM, (Child): 0.5 mg/kg every 4–6 hours as necessary.	dizziness, drowsiness, palpitations, bradycardia, urinary retention, nausea, vomiting, constipation
hydromorphone HCl (Dilaudid)	C II analgesic	Oral, SC, IM, IV (slow): 2 mg every 4–6 hours.	respiratory depression, nausea, hypotension
levorphanol tartrate (Levo-Dromoran)	C II analgesic	Oral, SC: 2–3 mg repeated in 4–6 hours as necessary.	as above
meperidine HCl (Demerol)	C II analgesic	Oral, SC, IM, IV, (Adult): 50–150 mg every 3–4 hours. SC, IM, (Child): 1 mg/kg every 4 hours as necessary.	dizziness, weakness, dry mouth, nausea, vomiting, respiratory, depression, palpitations, bradycardia
methadone HCl (Dolophine)	C II analgesic	Oral, SC, IM, (Adult): 2.5–10 mg every 3–4 hours, if necessary.	drowsiness, nausea, dry mouth, constipation
morphine sulfate	C II analgesic	Oral: 10–20 mg every 4 hours. SC, IM: 5–20 mg every 4 hours. SC, IM, (Child): 0.05–0.2 mg/kg per dose.	deep sleep, respiratory depression, nausea, urinary retention, pruritus, edema, bradycardia, sweating
oxymorphone HCl (Numorphan)	C II analgesic	SC, IM (Adult): 0.5–1.5 mg every 4–6 hours as needed.	nausea, vomiting, euphoria, dizziness
pentazocine HCl (Talwin)	C IV analgesic	Oral: 50 mg every 3–4 hours. SC, IM. IV: 30 mg every 3–4 hours.	drowsiness, sweating, dry mouth, nausea, vomiting
propoxyphene HCl, propoxyphene napsylate (Darvon, Darvon-N)	C IV analgesic	Oral (HCl): 65 mg every 4 hours as needed. Oral (napsylate): 100 mg every 4 hours as needed.	dizziness, weakness, headache, nausea, vomiting, constipation, abdominal pain

Narcotic Analgesics

Actions. Analgesics inhibit ascending pain pathways in the central nervous system. They increase pain threshold and alter pain perception.

Uses. For the relief of moderate to severe pain, as a preoperative medication, and as support of anesthesia.

Contraindications. Contraindicated in patients with known hypersensitivity to any of its ingredients and those with addiction, also in patients taking MAO inhibitors.

Warnings:

1. Narcotic analgesics can produce drug dependence and have the potential for being abused.
2. Must be used with great caution and in reduced dosage in patients who are concurrently taking other narcotic analgesics, general anesthetics, phenothiazines, other tranquilizers, sedative-hypnotics, tricyclic antidepressants, and alcohol. Respiratory depression, hypotension and profound sedation or coma may result.
3. Must be used with extreme caution in patients with head injury, increased intracranial pressure, asthma and other respiratory conditions, acute myocardial infarction, severe heart disease, hepatic disease, and renal disease.
4. Safe use in pregnancy prior to labor has not been established. Medication will cross the placental barrier and can produce depression of respiration and psychophysiologic functions in the newborn.

Adverse Reactions. Respiratory depression, circulatory depression, lightheadedness, dizziness, sedation, hallucinations, nausea, vomiting, sweating, euphoria, dysphoria, weakness, headache, agitation, tremor, convulsions, dry mouth, constipation, biliary tract spasm, flushing of the face, tachycardia, bradycardia, palpitation, hypotension, syncope, urinary retention, pruritus, urticaria, rash, pain at injection site, visual disturbances.

Dosage and Route. The dosage and route of administration is determined by the physician and individualized for each patient. (See Table 30–1.)

Implications for Patient Care. Observe patient for evidence of respiratory depression (respirations below 12), urinary retention (decreased output), central nervous system changes (dizziness, drowsiness, hallucinations, euphoria), allergic reactions (rash, urticaria), cardiac dysfunction (tachycardia, bradycardia, palpitation) and constipation. Monitor intake and output ratio, respirations, therapeutic response, need for pain medication, and signs of physical dependence. Protect the patient from possible injury. After administration, patient should be properly positioned in bed, with siderails up and call bell within easy reach.

Patient Teaching

Educate the patient:

- about possible adverse reactions.
- to report any symptoms of CNS changes, and/or allergic reactions to the physician.
- not to operate machinery or drive a motor vehicle while taking narcotic/analgesics.
- to avoid the use of alcohol and other CNS depressants that can enhance the drowsiness caused by analgesics.

Special Considerations

- Always assess the patient's respiratory rate before administration. Withhold medication and notify the physician if respiratory rate is 12 or below.
- Physical dependency may occur with the long-term use of narcotic analgesics. Withdrawal symptoms include nausea, vomiting, anorexia abdominal cramps, fever, and faintness.
- Federal law requires that all controlled substances be kept separate from other drugs. They are to be stored in a substantially constructed metal box or compartment that is equipped with a double lock. The nurse who is responsible for administering narcotics must keep the narcotic's key protected from possible misuse. A separate record book is required for information concerning the administration of controlled substances. This data system must be maintained on a daily basis and kept for a minimum of two years (three years in some states). Narcotics are counted at the end of each shift, and the inventory of controlled drugs must be recorded on an audit sheet. This sheet must be signed for correctness of count by two individuals.
- The patient who is receiving a narcotic analgesic via a PCA (patient-controlled analgesia) should be properly instructed in its use and monitored on a regular basis. See Figure 30–2.

Several non narcotic analgesic drugs have been developed in an effort to provide alternative agents with less potential for abuse. Like the opiates, these drugs act on the central nervous system. They include *butorphanol tartrate* (Stadol), *methotrimeprazine* (Levoprome), and *nalbuphine HCl* (Nubain). They produce adverse reactions similar to those listed in Table 30–1. The use of methotrimeprazine is somewhat limited by its tendency to cause orthostatic hypotension with fainting, weakness, and dizziness in a significant number of those taking the drug.

Narcotic Antagonist

naloxone hydrochloride (Narcan)

Narcan (naloxone hydrochloride) is a narcotic antagonist that prevents or reverses the effects of opioids including respiratory depression, sedation and hypotension.

Warning:

Should be administered cautiously to persons including newborns of mothers who are known or suspected to be physically dependent on opioids.

Dosage, May be given intravenously, muscularly, and subcutaneously. Narcotic Overdose: initial dose of 0.4 mg to 2 mg IV. Intravenous onset of action is generally apparent within 2 minutes.

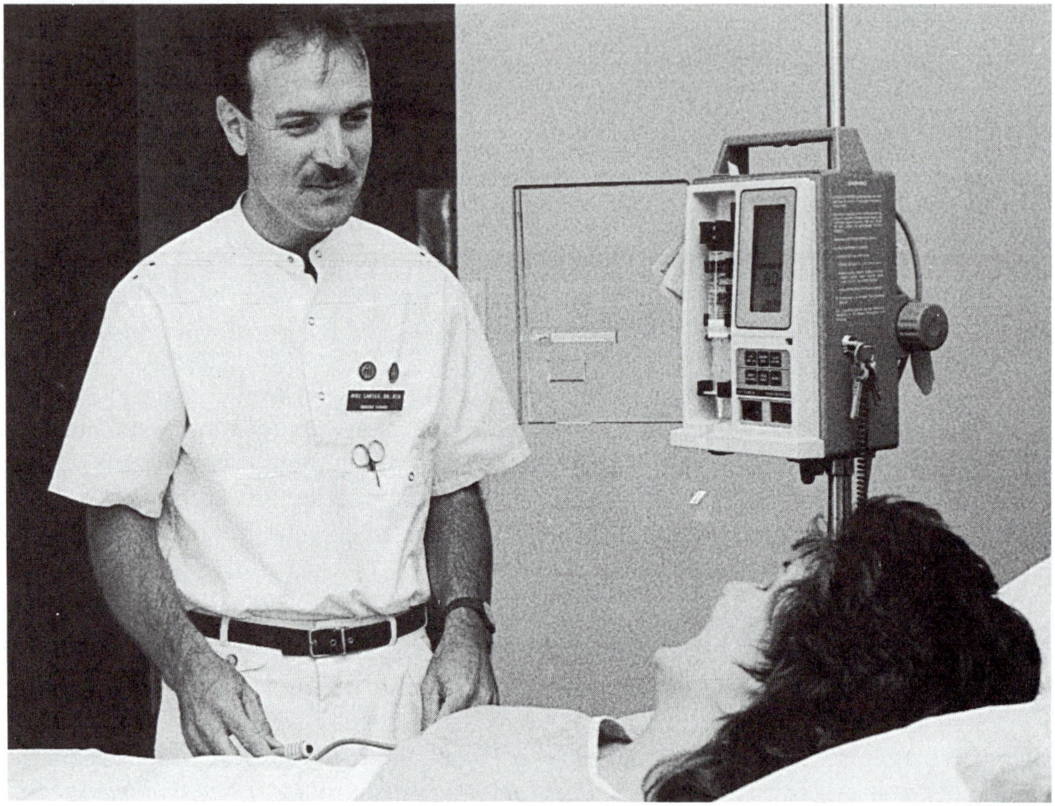

Figure 30–2 An RN instructing a patient in the use of the PCA (patient-controlled analgesia) intravenous system. The system is a portable, computerized pump that is programmed for the exact amount of medication prescribed by the physician. The system is equipped with a safeguard mechanism that prevents a patient from receiving more than the prescribed amount of drug. It also has a locking door on the pump that guards against unauthorized tampering with the dose settings and the prefilled syringe. Note the keys hanging in the lock. These are removed when the unit is set and functioning. To receive the medicine, the patient presses a button (held in the nurse's right hand) that is attached to the cord of the pump. When the patient presses this button, the syringe dispenses a prescribed dose of drug into the patient's IV line. Studies show that less analgesic is required when the patient has control over his or her own pain medications.

Adverse Reactions. Abrupt reversal of narcotic depression may result in nausea, vomiting, sweating, tachycardia, increased blood pressure, tremulousness, seizures and cardiac arrest.

Analgesic-Antipyretics

Certain medications act to relieve pain (analgesic effect) and reduce fever (antipyretic effect). Although the exact mechanism by which these drugs act is not completely understood, they appear to act peripherally by blocking pain impulse generation. Their antipyretic effect results from direct action on the heat-regulating center in the hypo-

Table 30–2 Analgesic-Antipyretics

Medication	Actions	Usual Dosage	Adverse Reactions
acetaminophen (Tylenol)	analgesic/ antipyretic	Oral (Adult): 325–650 mg at 4 hour intervals. Oral (Child): 160–480 mg at 4–6 hour intervals.	nausea, vomiting, rash, urticaria, anemia, liver damage
aspirin (Bayer)	analgesic/ antipyretic, anti-inflammatory antirheumatic	Oral (Adult): 325–650 mg at 4–6 hour intervals. Oral (Child): 160–480 mg at 4–6 hour intervals.	gastric irritation, easy bruising, hypersensitivity reactions such as tight-such as tightness in the chest, bronchospasm, Reyes Syndrome
ibuprofen (Advil) (Motrin) (Nuprin)	anti-inflammatory antirheumatic analgesic/ antipyetic	Oral: 200–800 mg 3–4 times per day (maximum, 2400 mg per day).	headache, dizziness, nausea, vomiting, dyspepsia, leukopenia, flatulence
naproxen (Naprosyn)	anti-inflammatory, analgesic/ antipyretic	Oral: 250–500 mg 2 times daily (maximum, 1000 mg/ day).	headache, blurred vision, indigestion, anorexia, agranulocytosis, pruritus

thalamus. In addition to their analgesic-antipyretic properties, all except acetaminophen produce significant anti-inflammatory action. See Table 30–2.

Aspirin or acetaminophen in combination with codeine phosphate or another narcotic analgesic is sometimes prescribed to provide greater relief from pain than is available from aspirin alone. Examples of such combination products include Empirin with Codeine, Percodan, Percodan-Demi, Percocet-5, Tylenol with Codeine, and Phenaphen with Codeine. Tablets and capsules containing these preparations are included in Schedule III of the Controlled Substance Act.

Spot Check

There are many medications that are used to help relieve pain. For each of the following drugs, give the usual dose, route, and the time interval for administration.

Drugs(s)	Dose and Route	Interval
Acetaminophen		
Ibuprofen		

(continued)

Naproxen		
Codeine		
Meperidine		
Methadone		
Morphine		

Sedatives and Hypnotics

Anxiety and insomnia are conditions that often interfere with job performance and one's ability to interact with others. Sedatives and hypnotics are frequently used in the overall treatment of these disorders. These drugs depress the central nervous system by interfering with the transmission of nerve impulses. Depending upon the dosage, barbiturates, benzodiazepines, and certain other drugs can produce either a sedative or a hypnotic effect. When used as a sedative, the dosage is designed to produce a calming effect without causing sleep. Used as a hypnotic, the dosage is sufficient to cause sleep. A good hypnotic should have fairly rapid action, produce near normal sleep, and not give the patient a delayed effect on the next day.

Barbiturates

The action of barbiturate drugs affects the entire central nervous system. Their use may produce a state ranging from mild sedation to deep sleep and anesthesia, depending upon the drug, the dosage prescribed, and the individual reaction of the patient. Large doses of barbiturates depress the respiratory vasomotor centers in the medulla and can lead to respiratory arrest and death.

Continued use of barbiturates over an extended period of time diminishes their effectiveness. Depending upon the drug, tolerance can develop as soon as a week after first administration, thereby requiring an increase in dosage to sustain the same effect. Psychological and physical dependency can result from the use of these drugs; therefore, they are subject to control under the Federal Controlled Substances Act. The adverse effects commonly associated with barbiturates include residual sedation, vertigo, nausea, and vomiting. Barbiturates used as sedatives and hypnotics are listed in Table 30–3.

Table 30–3 Barbiturates Used as Sedatives and Hypnotics

Medication	Schedule	Duration	Usual Sedative Dose	Usual Hypnotic Dose
amobarbital (Amytal)	C II	intermediate-acting	Oral: 30–50 mg 2–3 times daily.	Oral: 65–200 mg.
aprobarbital (Alurate)	C III	intermediate-acting	Oral: 20–40 mg 3 times daily.	Oral: 40–60 mg.
butabarbital sodium (Buticaps)	C III	intermediate-acting	Oral: 15–30 mg 3–4 times daily.	Oral: 50–100 mg.
mephobarbital (Mebaral)	C IV	long-acting	Oral: 32–100 mg 3–4 times daily.	no listing
pentobarbital (Nembutal)	C II	short-acting	Oral: 20–30 mg 2–4 times daily.	Oral: 100 mg. Rectal: 120–200 mg. IM, IV: 100–200 mg.
phenobarbital (Luminal)	C IV	long-acting	Oral: 15–32 mg 2–4 times daily.	Oral: 50–100 mg. SC, IM, IV: 100–300 mg daily.
secobarbital (Seconal)	C II	short-acting	Oral: 30–50 mg 3 times daily.	Oral, IM: 100–200 mg.
talbutal (Lotusate)	C III	short- to intermediate-acting	Oral: 30–60 mg 2–3 times daily.	Oral: 120 mg.

Barbiturates differ widely in the duration of their action which may range from a few seconds (ultra-short-acting) to several days (long-acting). They also differ in onset of action which can be as little as 30 seconds or as long as 20 to 60 minutes. Short- and intermediate-acting agents are often used in the treatment of insomnia because of their rapid onset and the fact that their use rarely produces a "hangover" effect. Long-acting barbiturates are used as anticonvulsants in patients with epilepsy and as sedatives for a variety of anxiety/tension states.

Actions. As sedatives and hypnotics, barbiturates depress the sensory cortex, decrease motor activity, alter cerebral function, and produce drowsiness, sedation, and hypnosis. They depress activity in brain cells, primarily in the reticular activating system in the brainstem, thus interfering with the transmission of impulses to the cortex.

Uses. Short-term treatment of insomnia, for sedation, as a preoperative medication, and as adjuncts to cancer chemotherapy.

Contraindications. Contraindicated in patients with known hypersensitivity to any of its ingredients. They should not be used in patients with a history of manifest or latent prophyria, respiratory depression, and severe liver impairment.

Warnings:

1. Barbiturates may be habit forming. Tolerance, psychological and physical dependence may occur with continued use.
2. Cautious use in acute and chronic pain.
3. Barbiturates can cause fetal damage when administered to a pregnant woman.
4. Alcohol and other CNS depressants may produce additive CNS depressant effects.
5. There are many precautions associated with the use of barbiturates. Please refer to a current edition of a *Physicians' Desk Reference* for information on precautions.

Adverse Reactions. Somnolence, agitation, confusion, hyperkinesia, ataxia, CNS depression, nightmares, nervousness, hallucinations, insomnia, anxiety, dizziness, hypoventilation, apnea, bradycardia, hypotension, syncope, nausea, vomiting, constipation, headache, angioedema, rash, exfoliative dermatitis, fever, liver damage, megaloblastic anemia.

Dosage and Route. The dosage and route of administration is determined by the physician and individualized for each patient. (See Table 30–3.)

Implications for Patient Care. Observe patient for evidence of CNS depression and any signs of adverse reactions. Monitor vital signs, blood and hepatic tests, and therapeutic effects. Be alert for signs of drug dependency. Protect the patient from possible injury. Remove tobacco products that are smoked from the reach of the patient. After administration, the patient should be properly positioned in bed, with siderails up and call bell within easy reach. The nurse should be alert for signs of *barbiturate toxicity, respiratory dysfunction*, and *blood dyscrasias.*

Signs of:

1. *Barbiturate toxicity:* hypotension, cold and clammy skin, cyanosis of lips, insomnia, nausea, vomiting, hallucinations, delirium, and/or weakness
2. *Respiratory dysfunction:* respirations below 10/minute in the adult and pupils dilated
3. *Blood dyscrasias:* fever, rash, sore throat, bruising, jaundice, and/or epistaxis

Patient Teaching

Educate the patient:

- to take the medication as prescribed.
- to be alert for signs of adverse reactions.
- to avoid the use of alcohol and other CNS depressants.

- not to smoke, operate machinery or drive a motor vehicle after taking the medication.
- that physical dependency may occur if medication is used for an extended period (45–90 days, depending on dose).
- about alternate methods of relaxation to improve sleep (exercise, reading, warm bath/shower, music, deep breathing, biofeedback, and so forth).

Special Considerations

- Barbiturates are subject to control by the Federal Controlled Substances Act under DEA schedule II. They may be habit forming and are often abused.
- Emergency supplies and equipment should be readily available for use when administering barbiturates to a patient in a hospital setting, long-term care facility, or other health related facility.
- Barbiturates may decrease the effect of corticosteroids, oral anticoagulants, griseofulvin, and quinidine.
- The effects of barbiturates may be increased by alcohol, MAO inhibitors, other sedatives, and narcotics.
- Barbiturates should not be mixed with other drugs in solution or syringe.
- Barbiturates should not be used for more than 14 days for insomnia, since they are not effective after that time and tolerance may develop.
- Barbiturates that are used for long-term therapy should not be discontinued quickly as symptoms of withdrawal can be severe and may cause death. Drug must be tapered-off over 1–2 weeks.

Benzodiazepines

Although many of the drugs in this chemical class are best known for their use in the relief of anxiety, three of the benzodiazepines are also recognized as effective sedative hypnotics. *Flurazepam HCl, temazepam*, and *triazolam* reduce incidents of night and early morning awakening, increase the duration of total sleep time, and do not produce rebound sleep disturbances. The onset of action for these drugs is between 15 and 40 minutes and their effect has a duration of 6 to 8 hours.

Other Sedative-Hypnotics

Chloral hydrate is one of the oldest hypnotics and is regarded as a relatively safe, inexpensive agent for the management of insomnia or for preoperative and postoperative sedation. *Ethchlorvynol* is rapidly absorbed from the GI tract and is used for short-term treatment of insomnia. *Ethinamate* is rapidly absorbed, produces sleep in about 20 minutes, and is effective for 3 to 5 hours. It is used primarily as a rapid-acting hypnotic for insomnia. *Glutethimide* produces actions similar to barbiturates but with less

Table 30–4 Nonbarbiturate Sedative-Hypnotic Drugs

Medication	Schedule	Usual Sedative Dose	Usual Hypnotic Dose
chloral hydrate (Noctec)	C IV	Oral, Rectal (Adult): 250 mg 3 times a day after meals. Oral (Child): 8–25 mg/kg/24 hours divided into 2–3 doses.	Oral, Rectal (Adult): 500 mg to 1 Gm before bedtime. Oral (Child): 50 mg/kg to a maximum of 1 Gm.
ethchlorvynol (Placidyl)	C IV	Oral: 100–200 mg 2–3 times a day.	Oral: 500–1000 mg at bedtime.
flurazepam HCl (Dalmane)	C IV	No listing.	Oral: 15–30 mg at bedtime.
glutethimide (Doriden)	C III	Oral (Preoperative): 500 mg the night before, and 500–1000 mg before anesthesia.	Oral: 250–500 mg at bedtime.
temazepam (Restoril)	C IV	No listing.	Oral (Adult): 15–30 mg at bedtime. Oral (Elderly): 15 mg as an initial dose.
triazolam (Halcion)	C IV	No listing.	Oral (Adult): 0.25–0.5 mg Oral (Elderly): 0.125–0.25 mg.

respiratory depression. Used preoperatively and during the first stages of labor. *Methyprylon* produces effects that are similar to the short-acting barbiturates and is used in the treatment of simple insomnia. See Table 30–4.

Antiparkinsonian Drugs

Named for British physician James Parkinson, Parkinson's disease is a neurologic disorder characterized by the development of a fine, slowly spreading tremor, muscular weakness and rigidity, and the development of disturbances in posture and equilibrium. The cause of the disease is not fully understood, but it is believed to be associated with an imbalance of the neurotransmitters *acetylcholine* and *dopamine* in the brain.

Antiparkinsonian drugs are used for palliative relief from such major symptoms as bradykinesia, rigidity, tremor, and disorders of equilibrium and posture. The drug of choice depends upon the severity of the disease at the time of diagnosis and is subject to change with the continuation of the disease. Therapy involves an attempt to replenish dopamine levels and/or inhibit the effects of the neurotransmitter acetylcholine. See Table 30–5.

Actions. Exerts an inhibitory effect upon the parasympathetic nervous system. They prolong the action of dopamine by blocking its uptake into presynaptic neurons in the central nervous system.

Uses. Treatment of all forms of parkinsonism.

Contraindications. Contraindicated in patients with known hypersensitivity to any of its ingredients. They should not be used in patients with narrow-angle glaucoma, myas-

Table 30–5 Antiparkinsonian Drugs

Medication	Drug Action	Usual Dosage	Adverse Reactions
amantadine HCl (Symmetrel)	anticholinergic	Oral: 100 mg twice daily.	dizziness, light-headedness, irritability, hypotension, edema, anorexia, nausea
benztropine mesylate (Cogentin)	anticholinergic	Oral: 0.5–6 mg/day if required and tolerated.	sedation, dizziness, tachycardia, nausea, vomiting, urinary retention, dysuria
biperiden HCl (Akineton)	anticholinergic	Oral: 2 mg 1–4 times daily.	dry mouth, blurred vision, constipation, dizziness
bromocriptine mesylate (Parlodel)	dopamine receptor agonist	Oral: 10–40 mg daily in divided doses.	orthostatic hypotension, rash, shock, nausea, dizziness, epigastric pain, blurred vision
carbidopa/levodopa (Sinemet)	anticholinergic	Oral: 1–6 tablets 3 times daily (tablets contain 10 mg carbidopa and 100 mg levodopa).	no reactions for carbidopa; for levodopa: involuntary movements, nausea, anorexia, urinary retention, dry mouth
ethopropazine HCl (Parsidol)	anticholinergic	Oral: 50–400 mg daily in divided doses.	drowsiness, headache, forgetfulness, hypotension, nausea, constipation, blurred vision
levodopa (Dopar)	metabolic precursor of dopamine	Oral: 0.5–8 Gm daily divided into 2 or more equal doses.	orthostatic hypotension, anorexia, nausea, abdominal distress, increased hand tremor, grinding of the teeth
procyclidine HCl (Kemadrin)	anticholinergic	Oral: 2–5 mg 3 times daily after meals.	dry mouth, blurred vision, palpitations, tachycardia, nausea, epigastric distress
trihexyphenidyl HCl (Artane)	anticholinergic	Oral: 1–10 mg daily in 3 or more divided doses.	dry mouth, dizziness, nausea, blurred vision, nervousness

thenia gravis, gastrointestinal and/or genitourinary obstructions, and children under 3 years of age.

Warnings:

1. Before initiation of drug therapy, patient should have a gonioscope evaluation, and close monitoring of intraocular pressure at regular periodic intervals.
2. Cautious use during pregnancy, lactation, and in the geriatric patient.
3. Patients with cardiac, liver, or kidney disorders, and/or hypertension should be carefully monitored while on an antiparkinsonian drug.

Adverse Reactions. Dryness of the mouth, blurring of vision, dizziness, mild nausea, nervousness, suppurative parotitis, skin rash, dilatation of the colon, paralytic ileus, delusions, hallucinations, paranoia, constipation, drowsiness, urinary hesitancy or retention, tachycardia, dilation of the pupil, increased intraocular tension, weakness, vomiting, headache, angle-closure glaucoma.

Dosage and Route. The dosage and route of administration is determined by the physician and individualized for each patient. (See Table 30–5.)

Implications for Patient Care. Observe the patient for evidence of improvement and signs of adverse reactions. Monitor vital signs, intake and output ratio, gastrointestinal function, and mental status of the patient.

Patient Teaching

Educate the patient:

- to take the medication as prescribed.
- to be alert for signs of adverse reactions.
- to avoid the use of alcohol and over-the-counter medications.
- to not operate machinery or drive a motor vehicle after taking the medication.

Special Considerations

- Medication should not be discontinued abruptly. Should be tapered-off over 1–2 weeks. Sudden withdrawal of medication may precipitate a parkinsonian crisis characterized by anxiety, sweating, and tachycardia, and an exacerbation of tremors, rigidity, and dyskinesia.
- Administer with or after meals to help prevent gastrointestinal upset.
- Anticholinergic effects may be increased by alcohol, narcotics, barbiturates, antihistamines, MAO inhibitors, phenothiazines, and/or amantadine.
- Pyridoxine will reduce the therapeutic effect of levodopa, therefore only pyridoxine-free multivitamins should be taken when taking levodopa. Larobec is a vitamin supplement made specifically for patients taking levodopa.
- When taking levodopa, adequate fluid intake and eating bulk forming foods should be encouraged to minimize the possibility of constipation.
- When taking levodopa, the urine may turn red to black on exposure to air or alkaline substances (toilet-bowl cleansers). The patient needs to be informed of this, so that he/she will not be alarmed.

Anticonvulsants

Epilepsy is the most common of the seizure disorders and affects approximately 1 percent of the population. It is characterized by recurrent abnormal electrical discharges within the brain. An epileptic convulsion may be characterized by sudden, brief episodes of altered consciousness, abnormal motor function, and/or sensory function interference. The disorder may be classified as *idiopathic* or *symptomatic* in origin, depending upon whether or not the cause of the condition is known. The majority of cases are idiopathic (cause is not identified) and symptoms begin during childhood or early adolescence. Tiny lesions in the brain at birth, metabolic disease, and developmental defects are possible causes. When developed in adulthood, epilepsy can usually be identified with such causes as trauma, tumors, strokes, and other disease processes affecting the brain.

Further classification has been applied to the types of seizures that are experienced by those with epilepsy. They have been divided into four main categories, some of which have subtypes. The four main categories are:

1. *Partial seizures* (focal seizures) are those in which electrical disturbance is localized to areas of the brain near the source or focal point of the seizure.
2. *Generalized seizures* (bilateral, symmetrical) are those without local onset that involve both the right and left hemispheres of the brain.
3. *Unilateral seizures are* those in which the electrical discharge is predominately confined to one of the two hemispheres of the brain.
4. *Unclassified epileptic seizures* are those that cannot be placed into the other three categories because of incomplete data.

With all types of epilepsy, the objective of drug therapy is to obtain the greatest degree of control over seizures without causing intolerable side effects. Selection of the most appropriate drug for a patient with epilepsy depends upon proper diagnosis and classification. The appropriate dosage must be individualized and is related to the size, age, and condition of the patient; how the patient responds to treatment, and whether or not the patient is taking other medication. See Table 30–6.

Actions. Inhibits spread of seizure activity in the motor cortex.

Uses. Indicated for the control of tonic-clonic and psychomotor (grand mal and temporal lobe) seizures, and prevention and treatment of seizures occurring during or following neurosurgery.

Contraindications. Contraindicated in patients with known hypersensitivity to any of its ingredients. They should not be used in patients with psychiatric disease and during pregnancy/lactation.

Warnings:

1. Abrupt withdrawal of medication in epileptic patients may precipitate status epilepticus.
2. There may be a relationship between anticonvulsants and the development of lymphadenopathy.
3. Acute alcohol intake may increase anticonvulsant drugs serum levels while chronic alcohol use may decrease serum levels.
4. There are many precautions associated with anticonvulsants. Please refer to a current edition of a *Physicians' Desk Reference* for information on precautions.

Table 30–6 Anticonvulsants

Medication	Usual Dosage	Adverse Reactions
acetazolamide (Diamox)	Oral: 375–1000 mg daily in divided doses.	drowsiness, rash, nausea, thirst, weakness, paresthesias of tongue
carbamazepine (Tegretol)	Oral (Adult): 200 mg twice/day, increased to a maximum of 120 mg/day in 3–4 doses. Oral (Child): 100 mg twice/day, increased to a maximum of 1000 mg/day in 3–4 doses.	dizziness, vertigo, drowsiness, edema, arrhythmias, skin rashes, nausea, vomiting, abdominal pain, aplastic anemia, blurred vision
clonazepam (Klonopin)	Oral (Adult): 1.5 mg/day divided into 3 doses, increased by 0.5–1 mg every 3 days until seizures are controlled. Oral (Child): 0.01–0.03 mg/kg/day not to exceed 0.05 mg/day in 3 divided doses.	palpitations, bradycardia, hair loss, hirsutism, skin rash, sore gums, drowsiness, ataxia, dysuria
diazepam (Valium)	Oral (Adult): 2–10 mg 2–4 times daily. IM, IV (Adult): 2–10 mg repeated in 3–4 hours if necessary. Oral (Child): 1 to 2.5 mg 3–4 times/day. IM, IV (Child): 0.2 to 1 mg every 2–5 minutes (maximum, 5 mg under age 5).	drowsiness, fatigue, hypotension, ataxia, vivid dreams, tachycardia, urinary retention, blurred vision, hiccups, throat and chest pain, hepatic dysfunction including jaundice
ethosuximide (Zarontin)	Oral: 250 mg twice/day, increased by 250 mg every 4–7 hours until controlled. Oral (Child under 6): 250 mg daily.	hiccups, ataxia, dizziness, hyperactivity, anxiety, epigastric distress, nausea, leukopenia
mephenytoin (Mesantoin)	Oral: 50–100 mg/day for first week, then increase weekly by same amount (maintenance dose 200–600 mg/day in 3 equal doses.	drowsiness, dizziness, skin rashes, blood dyscrasias, hepatic damage
mephobarbital (Mebaral)	Oral (Adult): 400–600 mg daily. Oral (Child under 5): 16–32 mg 4 times/day. Oral (Child over 5): 32–64 mg 4 times/day.	drowsiness, dizziness, hangover, paradoxical excitement, nausea, vomiting, respiratory depression
phenobarbital sodium (Luminal)	Oral (Adult): 50–100 mg. IV (Adult): 100–320 mg/day. Oral (Child): 16–50 mg 2–3 times daily.	nightmares, insomnia, hangover, dizziness, bradycardia, nausea, coughing, hiccups, liver damage
phenytoin, phenytoin sodium (Dilantin)	Oral (Adult): 100 mg 3 times/day, then gradual increase up to 600 mg/day. Parenteral (Adult): 300–400 mg/daily. Oral (Child): 4–8 mg/kg/day in 1–3 doses. Parenteral (Child): 5 mg/kg in 1–2 doses.	nystagmus, diplopia, blurred or dimmed vision, drowsiness, ataxia, slurred speech, hypotension, nausea, epigastric pain, pruritus, acute renal failure, hyperglycemia, gingival hyperplasia, hirsutism
primidone (Mysoline)	Oral: 250 mg/day, increased by 250 mg weekly (maximum 2 Gm/day in 2–4 doses). Oral (Child under 8): half of adult dose.	drowsiness, sedation, vertigo, nausea, anorexia, nystagmus, swelling of eyelids, alopecia
trimethadione (Tridione)	Oral (Adult): 0.9–2.4 Gm/day in 3–4 equally divided doses. Oral (Child): 0.3–0.9 Gm/day in 3–4 equally divided doses.	hemeralopia, photophobia, ataxia, exfoliative dermatitis, hiccups, nausea, gastric distress
valproic acid (Depakene)	Oral: 15 mg/kg/day, increased at 1 week intervals by 5–10 mg/kg/day (maximum recommended dose 60 mg/kg/day).	breakthrough seizures, sedation, drowsiness, dizziness, ataxia, nausea, hypersalivation, hepatic failure, depression, skin rash
felbamate (Felbatol)	Oral (Adult): 1200 mg/day in 3–4 divided doses gradually increase to 3600 mg/day. Oral (Children): With Lennox-Gastaut syndrome: 15 mg/kg/day. Maximum 45 mg/kg/day.	vomiting, constipation, insomnia, headache, fatigue, nausea, dizziness, anorexia, fever

Adverse Reactions. Nystagmus, ataxia, slurred speech, mental confusion, dizziness, insomnia, transient nervousness, motor twitching, headache, drug induced dyskinesias similar to those induced by phenothiazines and other neuroleptic agents, nausea, vomiting, constipation, toxic hepatitis, liver damage, fever, measles-like rash, thrombocytopenia, leukopenia, granulocytopenia, agranulocytosis, pancytopenia, lymphadenopathy, coarsening of facial features, enlargement of the lips, liver dysfunction.

Dosage and Route. The dosage and route of administration is determined by the physician and individualized for each patient. See Table 30–6.

Implications for Patient Care. Observe patient for signs of improvement and adverse reactions. Monitor vital signs, weight, blood and liver function studies, intake and output ratio, and drug serum levels.

Patient Teaching

Educate the patient:

- to take the medication as prescribed.
- to be alert for signs of adverse reactions.
- to avoid the use of alcohol and over-the-counter medications.
- to not operate machinery or drive a motor vehicle while taking medication.
- to wear a Medic Alert ID stating that he/she is an epileptic and on medication.
- to see his/her physician on a regular basis.
- about support groups and self-help/management programs that can assist in his/her treatment regimen.

> Teach the patient's family how to care for the patient during a seizure.

Special Considerations

- Some anticonvulsant agents may discolor the urine pink.
- Anticonvulsant medication should not be abruptly discontinued as seizures can occur.
- Drug therapy is individualized for each patient and it may involve trying several different drugs and dosages before therapeutic response is reached.
- The effects of anticonvulsants may be decreased by alcohol, antihistamines, antacids, antineoplastics, CNS depressants, rifampin, and/or folic acid.

Anesthetics

Anesthetics are drugs that interfere with the conduction of nerve impulses and are used to produce loss of sensation, muscle relaxation, and/or complete loss of consciousness. *Local anesthetics* block nerve transmission in the area to which they are applied. They produce loss of sensation and motor activity, but do not cause loss of consciousness. See Table 30–7. *General anesthetics* affect the central nervous system and produce either partial or complete loss of consciousness. They also cause varying degrees of analgesia, skeletal muscle relaxation, and reduction of reflex activity.

General anesthetics should be given only by those who have received adequate training. General anesthetics are of two types: *inhalation* and *injection.* Inhalation anesthetics can be further classified as gases or volatile liquids. Table 30–8 is a list of general anesthetic agents.

Table 30–7 Local (Regional) Anesthetic Drugs

Medication	Route(s)	Usual Strength of Dosage	Adverse Reactions
benzocaine (Solarcaine)	topical	0.5–20%, ointment, lotion, cream, aerosol spray, liquid.	contact urticaria, erythemia, contact dermatitis, swelling
bupivacaine HCl (Marcaine HCl)	injection	0.25–0.75% solution.	usually dose related: apnea, hypotension, heart block
chloroprocaine HCl (Nesacaine)	injection	1–3% solution.	usually does related: hypotension, ventricular arrhythmias, bradycardia
cocaine, cocaine HCl	topical	1–2% solution applied as a spray or on a tampon.	euphoria, excitement, chills, nausea, fever, respiratory and circulatory failure
cyclomethycaine sulfate (Surfacaine)	topical	0.5% cream, 1% ointment, 0.75% jelly.	stinging, burning sensation, pruritus, papules, vesicles, anaphylactoid reaction
dibucaine, dibucaine HCl (Nupercaine)	topical, injection	0.5% cream, 1% ointment. 0.25–0.5% solution.	hypotension, meningitis, nausea, vomiting, respiratory arrest
dyclonine HCl (Dyclone)	topical	0.5–1% solution.	urticaria, edema, burning, hypotension, blurred vision
etidocaine HCl (Duranest)	injection	1.0–1.5% solution.	nervousness, blurred vision, dizziness, hypotension
lidocaine HCl. (Xylocaine HCl)	topical, injection	2.5–5% cream, ointment, jelly. 0.5–4% solution.	drowsiness, light-headedness, euphoria, tinnitus, blurred vision, numbness of lips
pramoxine HCl (Tronothane)	topical	1% cream.	local stinging and burning
procaine HCl (Novocain)	injection	1–10% solution.	nervousness, dizziness, hypotension, postspinal headache
tetracaine HCl	topical, injection	0.5–2% ointment, cream. 1% solution.	nervousness, blurred vision, drowsiness, nausea, vomiting, chills, hypotension, edema

Table 30–8 General Anesthetics

Medication	Brand Name	Route(s)	Remarks
cyclopropane	—	inhalation	gas, pleasant odor
enflurane	Ethrane	inhalation	volatile liquid, pleasant odor
etomidate	Amidate	IV injection	nonbarbiturate hypnotic, rapid onset
fentanyl citrate and droperidol	Innovar	IV injection	combination drug containing a narcotic analgesic and a major tranquilizer
halothane	Fluothane	inhalation	volatile liquid, nonflammable
isoflurane	Forane	inhalation	volatile liquid, nonflammable
ketamine	Ketalar	IM, IV injection	rapid acting, stimulates muscle tone
methohexital sodium	Brevital	IV injection	ultra-short-acting barbiturate used for brief operative procedures
methoxyflurane	Penthrane	inhalation	volatile liquid, fruity odor
nitrous oxide	—	inhalation	"laughing gas," popular anesthetic gas
thiamylal sodium	Surital	IV injection	rapid-acting barbiturate
thiopental sodium	Pentothal Sodium	IV injection	ultra-short-acting barbiturate

Ophthalmic Drugs

Medications are used in the eye for the treatment of glaucoma, during diagnostic examination of the eye, and in intraocular surgery. Glaucoma is an eye disease characterized by increased intraocular pressure which, if not treated, causes atrophy of the optic nerve and blindness. The disease occurs when there is a failure to remove *aqueous humor* at a rate equal to its production. Drugs used to treat glaucoma either increase the outflow of aqueous humor, decrease its production, or produce both of these actions.

Drugs used to treat glaucoma are listed in Table 30–9.

Mydriatic Drugs

Anticholinergic agents produce dilation of the pupil (mydriasis) and interfere with the ability of the eye to focus properly (paralysis of accommodation or cycloplegia). Mydriatic drugs are used primarily as an aid in refraction, during internal examination of the eye, in intraocular surgery, and in the treatment of anterior uveitis and secondary glaucomas.

Sympathomimetic mydriatics produce mydriasis without cycloplegia. Pupil dilation is obtained as the drug causes contraction of the dilator muscle of the iris. These drugs also affect intraocular pressure by decreasing production of aqueous humor while increasing its outflow from the eyes. Mydriatic agents are listed in Table 30–10.

Table 30–9 Drugs Used to Treat Glaucoma

Medication	Classification	Usual Dosage	Adverse Reactions
acetazolamide (Diamox)	carbonic anhydrase inhibitor, diuretic	Oral: 250 mg every 6 hours. IM, IV: 500 mg repeated in 2–4 hours, if necessary.	paresthesias, drowsiness, tinnitus, nausea, rash, bone marrow depression
acetylcholine chloride (Miochol)	cholinergic (direct-acting), miotic	Intraocular: 0.5–2 ml of 1% solution instilled into the anterior chamber of the eye.	with systemic absorption: bradycardia, flushing, sweating, bronchospasm
carbachol (Carbacel)	cholinergic (direct-acting), miotic	Topical: 1–2 drops of 0.75–3% solution 3–4 times daily. Intraocular: 0.5 ml of 0.01% solution in anterior chamber.	headache, brow and eye pain, conjunctival hyperemia, ciliary spasm, iritis
demecarium bromide (Humorsol)	cholinesterase inhibitor, miotic	Topical: 1–2 drops of 0.125 or 0.25% solution two times/week up to twice daily.	stinging, burning, ciliary spasm, lacrimation, brow and eye pain, headache
dichlorphenamide (Daranide)	carbonic anhydrase inhibitor, diuretic	Oral: 100–200 mg followed by 100 mg every 12 hours, then 25–50 mg 1–3 times daily.	paresthesis, drowsiness, headache, fatigue, visual disturbances, nausea
echothiophate iodide (Phospholine Iodide)	cholinesterase inhibitor, miotic	Topical: 1 drop of 0.03–0.25% solution 1–2 times daily.	browache, headache, stinging, blurring of vision, iris cysts, ciliary spasm
glycerin (Glycerol)	osmotic diuretic	Oral: 1–1.5 Gm/kg 1–1$\frac{1}{2}$ hours prior to ocular surgery.	headache, nausea, thirst, diarrhea, glycosuria
isoflurophate (Floropryl)	cholinesterase inhibitor, miotic	Topical: a $\frac{1}{4}$-inch strip of ointment in the eye every 8–72 hours.	development of cataracts with long-term administration
isosorbide (Ismotic)	osmotic diuretic	Oral: Initially 1.5 Gm/kg then 1–3 Gm/kg 2–4 times/day.	headache, lethargy, rash, thirst, nausea, diarrhea
mannitol (Osmitrol)	osmotic diuretic	IV infusion: 1.5–2 Gm/kg as a 15–25% solution over 30 to 60 minutes.	dry mouth, thirst, blurred vision, urinary retention, congestive heart failure
methazolamide (Neptazane)	carbonic anhydrase inhibitor	Oral: 50–100 mg every 8 hours	malaise, drowsiness, mild GI disturbances, vertigo
physostigmine sulfate (Eserine Sulfate)	cholinesterase inhibitor, miotic	Topical: 1 cm strip of 0.25% ointment 1–3 times daily. Ophthalmic: 1–2 drops 3 times daily of 0.25–0.5% solution.	headache, eye and brow pain, marked miosis, dimness and blurring of vision, lacrimation
urea (Ureaphil)	osmotic diuretic	IV infusion: 1–1.5 Gm/kg over 1–2.5 hours, not to exceed 120 Gm/day.	headache, acute psychosis, tachycardia, dehydration, nausea, thirst, pain

Table 30–10 Mydriatic Agents

Medication	Classification	Usual Dosage	Adverse Reactions
atropine sulfate (Atropisol)	anticholinergic mydriatic	Topical: 1–2 drops of 0.5–1% solution 1–3 times daily.	blurred vision, photophobia, increased intraocular pressure
cyclopentolate HCl (Cyclogyl)	anticholinergic mydriatic	Topical: 1 drop of 0.5% solution and, if needed, another drop after 5 minutes.	blurred vision, photophobia, increased intraocular pressure
dipivefrin (Propine)	sympathomimetic, adrenergic agonist	Topical: 1 drop of 0.1% solution in eye every 12 hours.	burning, stinging upon application, photophobia
epinephrine HCl (Glaucon)	sympathomimetic, adrenergic agonist	Topical: 1–2 drops of 0.1% solution in eye.	lacrimation, headache, stinging sensation
homatropine HBr (Homatrocel)	anticholinergic mydriatic	Topical: 1–2 drops of 1–5% solution every 3–4 hours.	increased intraocular pressure
hydroxyamphetamine HBr (Paredrine)	sympathomimetic, adrenergic agonist	Topical: 1–2 drops of 1% solution.	mydriasis, photophobia
naphazoline HCl (Naphcon)	sympathomimetic, adrenergic agonist	Topical: 1–2 drops of 1% solution every 3–4 hours.	increased intraocular pressure, mydriasis
phenylephrine HCl (Neo-Synephrine)	sympathomimetic, adrenergic agonist	Topical: 1 drop of 2.5–10% solution 3 times/day.	stinging, browache, sensitivity to light
scopolamine HBr (Hyoscine)	anticholinergic mydriatic	Topical: 1–2 drops of 0.5–1% solution.	follicular conjunctivitis, local irritation
tetrahydrozoline HCl (Murine, Visine)	sympathomimetic, adrenergic agonist	Topical: 1–2 drops of 0.05% solution 2–3 times daily.	transient stinging, irritation, headache
tropicamide (Mydriacyl)	anticholinergic mydriatic	Topical: 1–2 drops of 1% solution, repeat in 5 minutes.	photophobia, transient stinging, blurred vision

Drugs Used in Vertigo, Motion Sickness, and Vomiting

Vertigo is a term used to describe an illusion of movement. Individuals experiencing vertigo may have the sensation of moving around in space, or know that they are stationary but sense that objects are in motion. Vertigo may be caused by a lesion or other process affecting the brain, the eighth cranial nerve, or the labyrinthine system of the ear. The result is a disturbance of equilibrium wherein the person experiences dizziness, light-headedness, and possible nausea and vomiting.

Motion sickness is usually associated with travel. Sometimes called seasickness, carsickness, or airsickness, this condition affects large numbers of people and causes nausea and vomiting. About one-third of the population is highly susceptible to motion and another third experiences symptoms when exposed to moderately rough travel conditions. Drugs are used for symptomatic relief rather than for treatment.

Vomiting is a complex reflex that may result from disease, drugs, radiation, toxins, and many other causes that serve to stimulate the vomiting center in the medulla. Since nausea and vomiting are symptoms of underlying causes, every effort should be made to identify and correct the causative condition.

Certain anticholinergic, antihistaminic, and antidopaminergic drugs have been identified as being effective in the treatment of vertigo, motion sickness, and vomiting; however not all of the drugs in these classifications are effective in these disorders. Those that are effective are listed in Table 30–11. See Figure 30–3 for an example of an transdermally provided drug used to treat motion sickness.

Table 30–11 Drugs Used in Vertigo, Motion Sickness, and Vomiting

Medication	Uses	Usual Dosage	Adverse Reactions
benzquinamide HCl (Emete-Con)	nausea, vomiting	IM: 50 mg (0.5–1 mg/kg).	drowsiness, insomnia, blurred vision, dry mouth
buclizine HCl (Bucladin-S Softabs)	nausea, vomiting, vertigo associated w/motion sickness	Oral: 25–50 mg 1–3 times daily at 4–6 hour intervals.	drowsiness, dizziness, headache, insomnia, dry mouth, anorexia, blurred vision
chlorpromazine (Thorazine)	nausea, vomiting	Oral: 10–25 mg every 4–6 hours as needed. IM: 25–50 mg every 3–4 hours as needed. Rectal: One 100 mg suppository every 6–8 hours.	sedation, depressed cough reflex, bizarre dreams, orthostatic hypotension, constipation, blurred vision, nasal congestion, respiratory depression

Table 30–11 *(Continued)*

Medication	Uses	Usual Dosage	Adverse Reactions
cyclizine HCl, cyclizine lactate (Marezine)	motion sickness, nausea, vomiting	Oral, IM: 50 mg every 4–6 hours as needed, not to exceed 200 mg/day.	hypotension, palpitations, drowsiness, vertigo, blurred vision, dry mouth, anorexia
dimenhydrinate (Dramamine)	motion sickness, nausea, vomiting, vertigo	Oral: 50–100 mg every 4–6 hours. IM, IV: 50 mg.	drowsiness, headache, dizziness, insomnia, hypotension, blurred vision, dry mouth
diphenhydramine HCl (Benadryl)	motion sickness, vertigo	Oral, IM, IV: 25–50 mg 3–4 times daily at 4–6 hours intervals.	drowsiness, dizziness, headache, fatigue, euphoria, dry mouth, blurred vision, dysuria
diphenidol HCl (Vontrol)	vertigo, nausea, vomiting	Oral: 25–50 mg every 4 hours as needed.	auditory and visual hallucinations, drowsiness
meclizine HCl (Antivert)	nausea, vomiting, motion sickness, vertigo	Oral: 25–100 mg daily in divided doses.	drowsiness, blurred vision, dry mouth, fatigue
promethazine HCl (Phenergan)	motion sickness, nausea, vomiting	Oral, IM, IV, Rectal suppository: 12.5–25 mg and again at 4–6 hour intervals as needed.	sedation, confusion, dizziness, tremors, anorexia, dry mouth, leukopenia, blurred vision, photosensitivity
scopolamine (Transderm-scop)	motion sickness, nausea, vomiting	Topical: transdermal delivery of 0.5 mg over 3 days.	fatigue, drowsiness, dry mouth, urinary retention, depressed respiration
thiethylperazine maleate (Torecan)	nausea, vomiting, vertigo	Oral, IM, Rectal suppository: 10 mg 1–3 times a day.	drowsiness, dizziness, dry mouth and nose, blurred vision, tinnitus, fever
triflupromazine HCl (Vesprin)	severe nausea and vomiting	Oral: 10–30 mg/day. IM: 5–60 mg/day. IV: 1–3 mg/day.	xerostomia, constipation, drowsiness, nasal congestion, urinary retention, hypotension
trimethobenzamide HCl (Tigan)	nausea, vomiting	Oral: 250 mg 3–4 times daily. Rectal: 200 mg 3–4 times daily. IM: 200 mg 3–4 times daily.	allergic skin eruptions, hypotension, blurred vision, headache, drowsiness, diarrhea, acute hepatitis, muscle cramps

Information for the Patient About —

Transderm® Scōp

Generic Name: scopolamine, pronounced skoe-POL-a-meen
(formerly Transderm-V)

Transdermal Therapeutic System

The Transderm Scōp system helps to prevent the nausea and vomiting of motion sickness for up to 3 days. It is an adhesive disc that you place behind your ear several hours before you travel. Wear only one disc at any time.

Be sure to wash your hands thoroughly with soap and water immediately after handling the disc, so that any drug that might get on your hands will not come into contact with your eyes.

Avoid drinking alcohol while using Transderm Scōp. Also, be careful about driving or operating any machinery while using the system because the drug might make you drowsy.

TRANSDERM SCŌP SHOULD NOT BE USED IN CHILDREN AND SHOULD BE USED WITH SPECIAL CAUTION IN THE ELDERLY.

How the Transderm Scōp System Works

A group of nerve fibers deep inside the ear helps people keep their balance. For some people, the motion of ships, airplanes, trains, automobiles, and buses increases the activity of these nerve fibers. This increased activity causes the *dizziness, nausea, and vomiting* of motion sickness. People may have one, some, or all of these symptoms.

Transderm Scōp contains the drug scopolamine, which helps reduce the activity of the nerve fibers in the inner ear. When a Transderm Scōp disc is placed on the skin behind one of the ears, scopolamine passes through the skin and into the bloodstream. One disc may be kept in place for 3 days if needed.

Precautions

Before using Transderm Scōp be sure to tell your doctor if you

- Are pregnant or nursing (or planning to become pregnant)
- Have glaucoma (increased pressure in the eyeball)
- Have (or have had) any metabolic, liver, or kidney disease
- Have any obstructions of the stomach or intestine
- Have trouble urinating or any bladder obstruction
- Have any skin allergy or have had a skin reaction such as a rash or redness to any drug, especially scopolamine, or chemical or food substance.

Any of these conditions could make Transderm Scōp unsuitable for you. Also tell your doctor if you are taking any other medicines.

Transderm Scōp should not be used in children. The safety of its use in children has not been determined. Children and the elderly may be particularly sensitive to the effects of scopolamine.

Side Effects

The most common side effect experienced by people using Transderm Scōp is dryness of the mouth. This occurs in about two thirds of the people. A less frequent side effect is drowsiness, which occurs in less than one sixth of the people. Temporary blurring of vision and dilation (widening) of the pupils may occur, especially if the drug is on your hands and comes in contact with the eyes. On infrequent occasions, disorientation, memory disturbances, dizziness, restlessness, hallucinations, confusion, difficulty urinating, skin rashes or redness, and dry, itchy, or red eyes have been reported. If these effects do occur, remove the disc and call your doctor. Since drowsiness, disorientation, and confusion may occur with the use of scopolamine, be careful driving or operating any dangerous machinery, especially when you first start using the drug system.

Figure 30–3 Scopolamine, a drug used to treat motion sickness, can be provided transdermally. *(Courtesy of CIBA-GEIGY Pharmaceuticals, Summit, NJ 07901)*

Drug Withdrawal: Symptoms including dizziness, nausea, vomiting, headache and disturbances of equilibrium have been reported in a few people following discontinuation of the Transderm Scōp System. These symptoms have occurred most often in people who have used the Systems for more than three days. We recommend that you consult your doctor if these symptoms occur.

How to Use Transderm Scōp

Transderm Scōp may be kept at room temperature until you are ready to use it.

1. Plan to apply one Transderm Scōp disc at least 4 hours before you need it. **Wear only one disc at any time.**
2. Select a hairless area of skin behind one ear, taking care to avoid any cuts or irritations. Wipe the area with a clean, dry tissue.
3. Peel the package open and remove the disc (Figure 1).

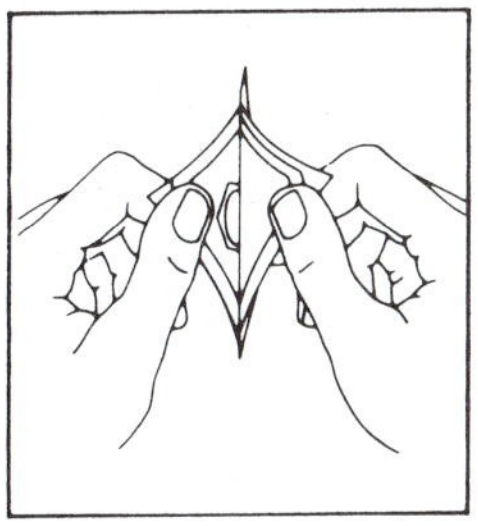

(Figure 1)

4. Remove the clear plastic six-sided backing from the round system. Try not to touch the adhesive surface on the disc with your hands (Figure 2).

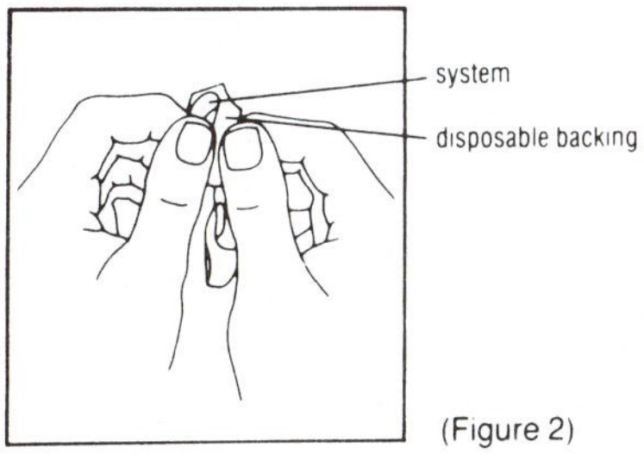

(Figure 2)

5. Firmly apply the adhesive surface (metallic side) to the dry area of skin behind the ear so that the tan-colored side is showing (Figure 3). Make good contact, especially around the edge. Once you have placed the disc behind your ear, do not move it for as long as you want to use it (up to 3 days).

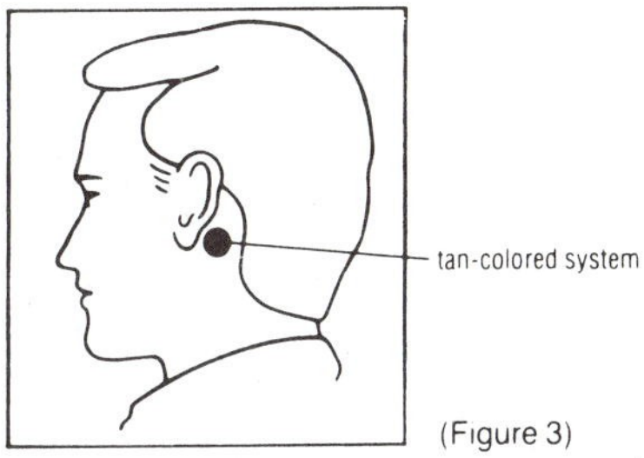

(Figure 3)

6. ***Important:* After the disc is in place, be sure to wash your hands thoroughly with soap and water to remove any scopolamine. If this drug were to contact your eyes, it could cause temporary blurring of vision and dilation (widening) of the pupils (the dark circles in the center of your eyes). This is not serious, and your pupils should return to normal.**
7. Remove the disc after 3 days and throw it away. (You may remove it sooner if you are no longer concerned about motion sickness.) After removing the disc, be sure to wash your hands and the area behind your ear thoroughly with soap and water.
8. If you wish to control nausea for longer than 3 days, *remove* the first disc after 3 days and place a new one *behind the other ear,* repeating instructions 2 to 7.
9. Keep the disc dry, if possible, to prevent it from falling off. Limited contact with water, however, as in bathing or swimming, will not affect the system. In the unlikely event that the disc falls off, throw it away and put a new one behind the other ear.

This leaflet presents a summary of information about Transderm Scōp. If you would like more information or if you have any questions, ask your doctor or pharmacist. A more technical leaflet is available, written for your doctor. If you would like to read the leaflet, ask your pharmacist to show you a copy. You may need the help of your doctor or pharmacist to understand some of the information.

Mfd. by:
ALZA Corporation
Palo Alto, CA 94304

Dist. by:
CIBA Consumer Pharmaceutical Co.
Division of CIBA-GEIGY Corp.
Summit, NJ 07901

Printed in U.S.A.

C84-19 (Rev. 7 84)
665954

Figure 30–3 *(Continued)*

◆ Review Questions

Directions: Select the best answer to each multiple choice question. Circle the letter of your choice.

1. __________ agents are used to relieve pain.
   a. Antipyretic
   b. Analgesic
   c. Anti-inflammatory
   d. Hypnotic
2. The peripheral nervous system is composed of __________ pairs of cranial nerves and __________ pairs of spinal nerves.
   a. 13 and 32
   b. 15 and 30
   c. 12 and 31
   d. 10 and 31
3. The natural and synthetic drugs derived from morphine are known as __________.
   a. opiates
   b. opioids
   c. opium
   d. opsin
4. The usual oral adult dosage of Demerol is __________.
   a. 50–150 mg every 3–4 hours
   b. 50–150 mg every hour
   c. 50–150 mg every 8 hours
   d. 50–150 mg once a day
5. Adverse reactions of Talwin are __________.
   a. edema, urinary retention, hypotension
   b. abdominal pain, pruritus, alopecia
   c. drowsiness, sweating, dry mouth, nausea, vomiting
   d. constipation, bradycardia, palpitations
6. Tylenol acts as __________.
   a an anti-inflammatory agent
   b. an analgesic/antipyretic
   c. an antirheumatic agent
   d. analgesic/anti-inflammatory
7. A good hypnotic should __________.
   a. have fairly rapid action
   b. produce near normal sleep
   c. not give the patient a delayed effect on the next day
   d. all of these
8. Psychological and physical dependency can result from the use of __________.
   a. analgesics
   b. barbiturates
   c. antipyretics
   d. anticonvulsants
9. Residual sedation, vertigo, nausea, and vomiting are commonly associated adverse effects of __________.
   a. analgesics
   b. barbiturates
   c. antipyretics
   d. anticonvulsants

10. The usual oral sedative dose of Seconal is __________ times daily.
    a. 15–32 mg 2–4
    b. 32–100 mg 3–4
    c. 30–50 mg 3
    d. 15–30 mg 3–4
11. Benzodiazepines that are recognized as effective sedative-hypnotics are __________.
    a. Dalmane, Restoril, and Halcion
    b. Flurazepam HCl, temazepam, and triazolam
    c. Noctec, Placidyl, and Valmid
    d. a and b
12. __________ is one of the oldest hypnotics and is regarded as a relatively safe, inexpensive agent for the management of insomnia.
    a. Methyprylon
    b. Ethinamate
    c. Chloral Hydrate
    d. Glutethimide
13. Antiparkinsonian drugs are used for the palliative relief of __________.
    a. tachykinesia, rigidity, tremor, and disorders of equilibrium
    b. bradykinesia, rigidity, tremor, and disorders of equilibrium
    c. bradycardia, rigidity, tremor, and disorders of equilibrium
    d. none of these
14. The usual oral dosage of Artane is __________.
    a. 1–10 mg daily in 3 or more divided doses
    b. 0.5–6 mg/day
    c. 0.5–8 Gm daily in 2 or more divided doses
    d. 2–5 mg 3 times daily after meals
15. The usual oral adult dosage of Dilantin is __________.
    a. 250 mg/day
    b. 15 mg/kg/day
    c. 2–10 mg 2–4 times daily
    d. 100 mg 3 times/day
16. The usual oral child's dosage of Dilantin is __________.
    a. 4–8 mg/kg/day in 1–3 divided doses
    b. 16–50 mg 2–3 times daily
    c. 16–32 mg 4 times/day
    d. 100 mg/kg/day
17. __________ are drugs that interfere with the conduction of nerve impulses and are used to produce loss of sensation, muscle relaxation, and/or complete loss of consciousness.
    a. Barbiturates
    b. Hypnotics
    c. Anesthetics
    d. Analgesics

18. The usual strength of procaine HCl (Novocain) is __________ .

a. 2.5–5% b. 1–19% c. 0.25–0.5% d. 1–2%

19. A popular general anesthetic that is known as "laughing gas" is __________.

a. nitrous oxide b. ether c. thiopental sodium d. ketamine

20. Ophthalmic drugs are used __________.

a. in the treatment of glaucoma

b. during diagnostic examination of the eye

c. in intraocular surgery

d. all of these

21. The usual oral dosage of Diamox that is used in the treatment of Glaucoma is __________.

a. 1.5 Gm/kg

b. 50–100 mg every 8 hours

c. 250 mg every 6 hours

d. 1–1.5 Gm/kg

22. Adverse reactions of mannitol include __________.

a. dry mouth, thirst

b. blurred vision, urinary retention

c. congestive heart failure

d. all of these

23. Mydriatic drugs are used primarily __________.

a. as an aid in refraction

b. during internal examination of the eye

c. in intraocular surgery and in the treatment of anterior uveitis and secondary glaucomas

d. all of these

24. Adverse reactions of Neo-Synephrine include __________.

a. stinging

b. brow ache

c. sensitivity to light

d. all of these

25. The usual dosage of tetrahydrozoline (Murine, Visine) is __________ solution 2–3 times daily.

a. 1–2 drops of 0.5%

b. 3–4 drops of 0.5%

c. 5–6 drops of 0.5%

d. none of these

26. __________ is a term used to describe an illusion of movement.

a. Motion sickness

b. Vomiting

c. Vertigo

d. Dizziness

27. All of the following classifications of drugs are used to treat vertigo, motion sickness, and vomiting except __________.

a. anticholinergic

b. antihistaminic

c. antidopaminergic

d. antipyretic

28. The usual adult oral dosage of promethazine HCl used in the treatment of motion sickness, nausea, and vomiting is __________.

    a. 25–50 mg 3–4 times daily
    b. 12.5–25 mg every 4–6 hours
    c. 10 mg 1–3 times daily
    d. 250 mg 3–4 times daily

29. Drowsiness, blurred vision, dry mouth, and fatigue are adverse reactions of __________.

    a. Tigan
    b. Vesprin
    c. Marezine
    d. Antivert

30. The generic name of Benadryl is __________.

    a. chlorpromazine
    b. dimenhydrinate
    c. diphenhydramine
    d. scopolamine

31. The generic name of Dramamine is __________.

    a. chlorpromazine
    b. dimenhydrinate
    c. diphenhydramine
    d. scopolamine

Case Study: A 22-year-old construction worker is admitted with a compound fracture of the left femur. His vital signs are T 99, P 86, R 22, B/P 126/76. The physician has ordered 100 mg of meperidine hydrochloride IM.

32. The trade name for meperidine hydrochloride is __________.

    a. Dolophine
    b. Dilaudid
    c. Demerol
    d. Pantopon

33. Before giving the medication, it would be *most* important for the nurse to assess which of the following? __________

    a. pupillary responses
    b. respirations
    c. blood pressure
    d. pulse count for one minute

34. To protect the patient from possible injury following the administration of the medication the nurse should __________.

    a. make sure that the siderails are up
    b. place the call bell within easy reach
    c. turn the patient on his right side
    d. a and b

35. Meperidine hydrochloride is classified as a Class __________ narcotic analgesic.

    a. I
    b. II
    c. III
    d. IV

36. In assessing the patient for possible allergic reactions it is most important to be aware of which signs? __________

    a. respiratory rate below 12
    b. dizziness, drowsiness
    c. rash, urticaria
    d. tachycardia, palpitations

37. The *most* important therapeutic response to meperidine hydrochloride includes a/an __________.
    a. elevation of pain perception
    b. increase in pain perception
    c. noted unaltered pain perception
    d. alteration of pain perception

Matching: Place the correct letter from Column II on the appropriate line of Column I.

Column I

38. __________ Agonist
39. __________ Analgesic
40. __________ Anhydrase
41. __________ Aqueous humor
42. __________ Carbonic
43. __________ Carbaric anhydrase
44. __________ Dopamine
45. __________ Inhibitor
46. __________ Sympathomimetic

Column II

A. That which inhibits; a chemical substance that stops enzyme activity.
B. That which imitates the sympathetic nervous system; adrenergic.
C. A drug that has affinity for the cellular receptors of another drug or natural substance and produces a physiological effect.
D. An enzyme that catalyzes union of water and carbon dioxide to form carbonic acid.
E. A catecholamine synthesized by the adrenal gland.
F. Agents used to relieve pain.
G. The transparent liquid contained in the anterior and posterior chambers of the eye.
H. Pertaining to carbon.
I. An enzyme that promotes the removal of water from a chemical compound.
J. That which stimulates enzyme activity.

CHAPTER 31

Medications That Affect the Reproductive System

OBJECTIVES

Upon completion of this chapter, you should be able to:

- Define the terms listed in the vocabulary.
- State two functions of the ovaries.
- State two functions of the testes.
- State the actions, uses, contraindications, warnings, adverse reactions, dosage and route, implications for patient care, patient teaching, and special considerations for estrogens.
- State the actions, uses, contraindications, adverse reactions, dosage and route, implications for patient care, patient teaching, and special considerations for progesterones.
- Describe ESTRADERM®.
- Describe how oral contraceptives, when used as directed, prevent the occurrence of pregnancy.
- List the adverse reactions of oral contraceptives.
- Describe monophasic, biphasic, and triphasic oral contraceptive preparations.
- List the conditions in which taking an oral contraceptive could be dangerous.
- Identify selected oral contraceptives as monophasic, biphasic, triphasic, and progesterone-only preparations.
- State the actions, uses, contraindications, adverse reactions, dosage and route, implications for patient care, patient teaching, and special considerations for testosterones.
- Describe the drugs that may be used during labor and delivery.
- State the uses, usual dosage, and adverse reactions of selected uterine stimulants and relaxants.
- List several findings that relate to the older adult and sexual activity.
- State the main cause of sexual difficulties in the older adult.

- Give the signs and symptoms of selected sexually transmitted diseases.
- State the prevalence of sexually transmitted diseases in children.
- Explain how sexually transmitted diseases are diagnosed.
- Complete the critical thinking questions/activities presented in this chapter.
- Complete the Spot Check on sexually transmitted diseases (STDs).
- Answer the review questions correctly.

Vocabulary

amenorrhea (a-men″o-re′a). Without or lack of the monthly menstrual flow.

hirsutism (hur′sut-izm). A condition characterized by excessive growth of hair, especially in women.

menopause (men′o-pawz). Climacteric. The time when there is a naturally occurring pause and/or stoppage of the monthly menstrual flow.

osteoporosis (os″te-o-por-o′sis). A softening of bones or increased porosity of bones seen most often in aging women.

hypogonadism (hi″po-go′nad-izm). A condition of defective secretion of the gonads.

cryptorchidism (kript-or′kid-izm). Failure of the testicles to descend into the scrotum.

progestin (pro-jes′tin). A term used to refer to a large group of drugs that have a progesterone effect on the uterus. SYN: progesterone.

progestogen (pro-jes′to-jen). Any natural or synthetic hormonal substance that produces progesterone-like effects.

Synopsis: The Reproductive System

The ovaries in the female (Figure 31–1) and the testes in the male (Figure 31–2) are the primary organs of sexual reproduction. With the onset of puberty (ages 9–16 in females, 13–15 in males), the pituitary gland secretes increased amounts of two gonad-stimulating hormones that cause the reproductive organs to mature and begin the production of ova and sperm. Known as *follicle-stimulating hormone* (FSH) and *luteinizing hormone* (LH), these secretions continue to exert control over the functions of the reproductive organs after maturation.

The functions of the ovaries are (1) production of ova, and (2) secretion of the female sex hormones estrogen and progesterone. The functions of the testes are (1) production of sperm, and (2) secretion of the male sex hormone testosterone. The female sex hormones are instrumental in the development of breast tissue, pubic and axillary hair growth, and the preparation of the uterus for pregnancy. In the male, testosterone is essential for the growth and development of male accessory sexual organs, the deep-

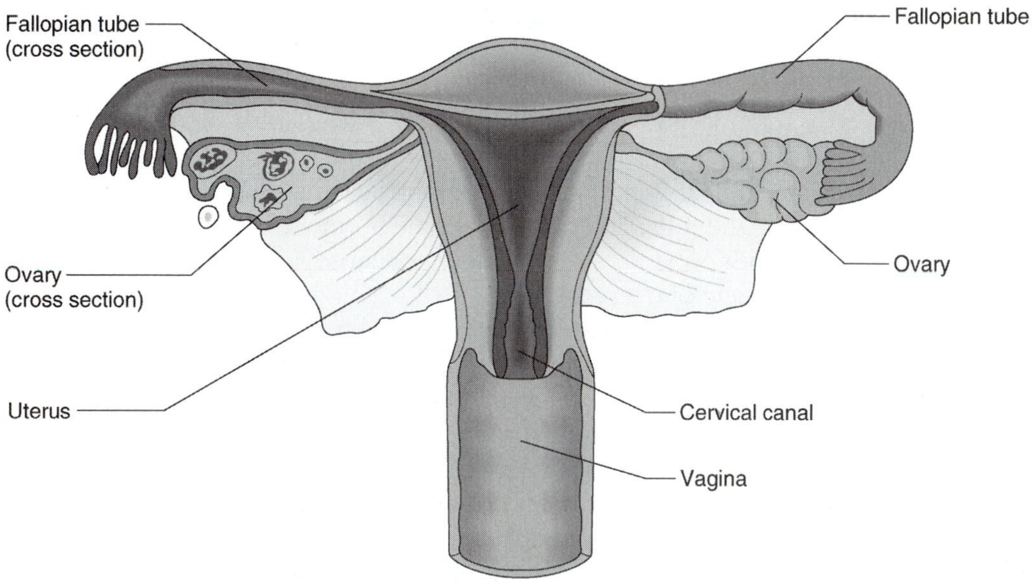

Figure 31–1 Female reproductive organs

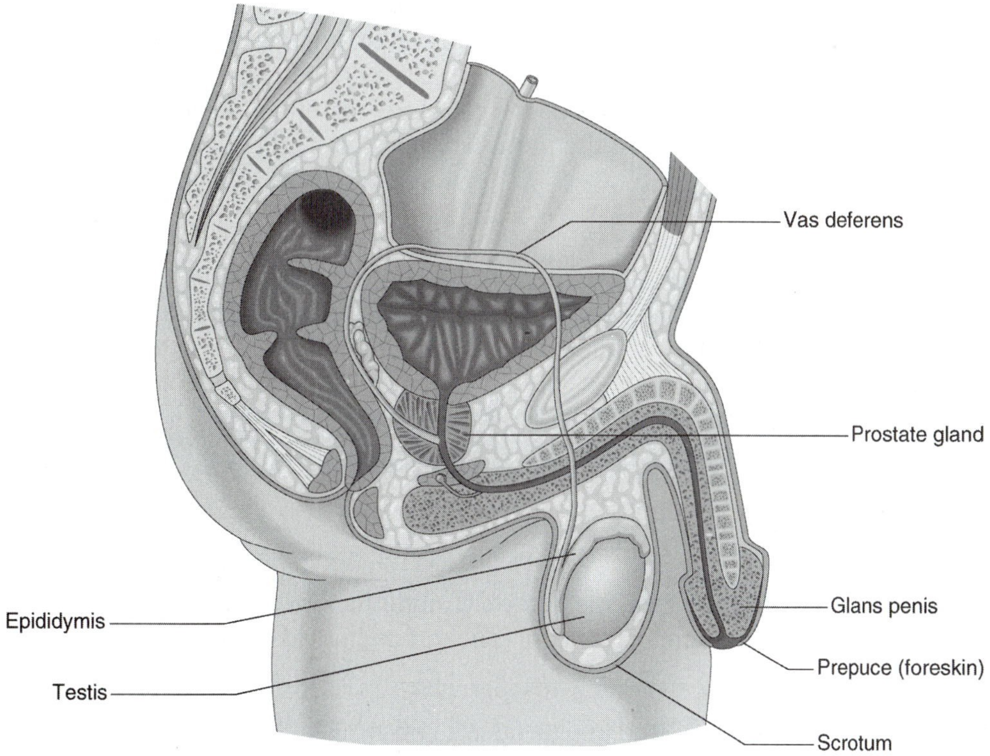

Figure 31–2 Male reproductive organs

ening of the voice, muscular development, the growth of facial, pubic, and axillary hair, and the occurrence of penile erection.

Female Hormones

One needs to be familiar with the interrelated processes of the menstrual cycle in order to fully appreciate the role played by the female hormones. The onset of the menstrual cycle coincides with puberty, ends during menopause, and in human females occurs monthly on an average of every 28 days.

The menstrual cycle can be divided into four distinct phases. During the *proliferation phase*, the ovarian (graafian follicle) undergoes maturation, secretes estrogen, and thickening and vascularization of the endometrium occurs. This phase ends when the ovarian follicle ruptures, expelling the ovum into the fallopian tube. Estrogen, due to the source of its secretion, is sometimes referred to as the *follicular hormone*. The next phase in the cycle is the *luteal* or *secretory* phase which is characterized by continued thickening and vascularization of the endometrium and the secretion of progesterone by the corpus luteum, a small yellow body within the ruptured ovarian follicle. Because it is produced by the corpus luteum, progesterone is called the *luteal hormone*. At this point, the thick, spongy uterine lining is engorged with blood. If conception has not occurred, the cycle enters the *premenstrual phase* characterized by constriction of the coiled arteries within the uterine lining, shrinkage of the endometrium, and a decrease in hormonal secretion by the corpus luteum. This phase ends with the start of the menstrual flow. The fourth phase is known as *menstruation*. This is a period of uterine bleeding, containing endometrial cells, blood, and glandular secretions, lasting 4–5 days. After menstruation, the endometrium of the uterus is again thin and the cycle begins anew.

Estrogen

Estrogen preparations are used for a variety of conditions such as in the treatment of amenorrhea, dysfunctional bleeding, hirsutism, and in palliative therapy for breast cancer in women and prostatic cancer in men. They may also be used to relieve the uncomfortable symptoms of menopause. In this instance, estrogen replacement therapy is also useful in the prevention of osteoporosis. (See Figure 31–3.)

Actions. Estrogens promote growth, development, and maintenance of the female reproductive system and secondary sex characteristics. They also effect the release of pituitary gonadotropins.

Uses. Menopause, atrophic vaginitis, atrophic urethritis, osteoporosis, hypogonadism, castration, primary ovarian failure, breast cancer, and androgen-dependent carcinoma of the prostate.

Contraindications. Contraindicated in patients with known hypersensitivity to any of its ingredients, known or suspected pregnancy, breast cancer, estrogen-dependent neoplasia, undiagnosed abnormal genital bleeding, thrombophlebitis, thromboembolic disorders.

ESTRADERM®
Estradiol Transdermal System

What is ESTRADERM®?

Estraderm is an estrogen skin patch that relieves menopausal symptoms such as hot flashes, night sweats and vaginal dryness.

Less than two inches in diameter, the wafer-thin patch delivers estradiol, the same estrogen as that produced by a woman's ovaries prior to menopause, through the skin directly to the bloodstream, without first passing through the liver. This avoids changes in hepatic function that may be associated with other forms of estrogen therapy.

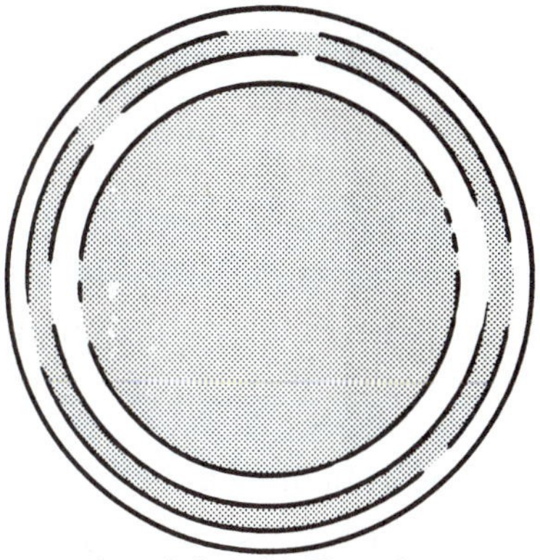

Actual size of 0.05 mg dosage

The ESTRADERM® skin patch is composed of five layers.

1. A sealed backing that holds the drug in the system.
2. A reservoir containing estradiol.
3. A membrane that controls the release of estradiol.
4. A non-allergenic adhesive that keeps the patch on the skin.
5. A protective peel strip.

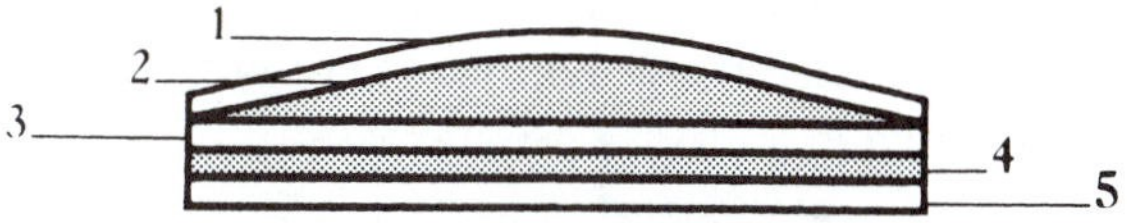

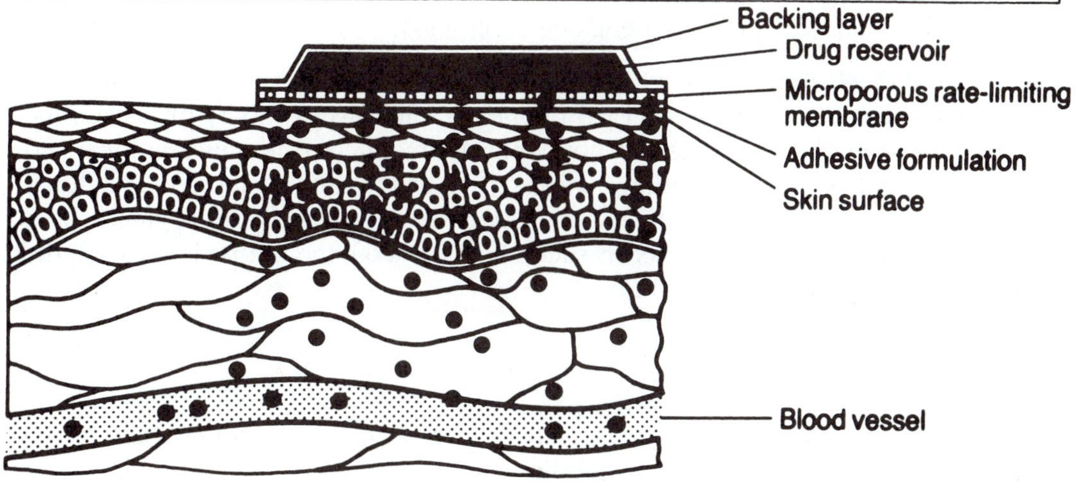

Four separate layers are inside the transdermal therapeutic system, a revolutionary way of delivering medicine to the body. Applied like an adhesive bandage, the system provides a consistent and controlled amount of medication through the skin, directly into the bloodstream over an extended period of time. The latest application of transdermal technology is Estraderm® (Estradiol Transdermal System), a low-dose estrogen skin patch available by prescription for the relief of such menopausal symptoms as hot flashes, night sweats and vaginal dryness.

Figure 31–3 Estrogen can be provided transdermally. *(Courtesy of CIBA-GEIGY Pharmaceuticals, Summit, NJ 07901)*

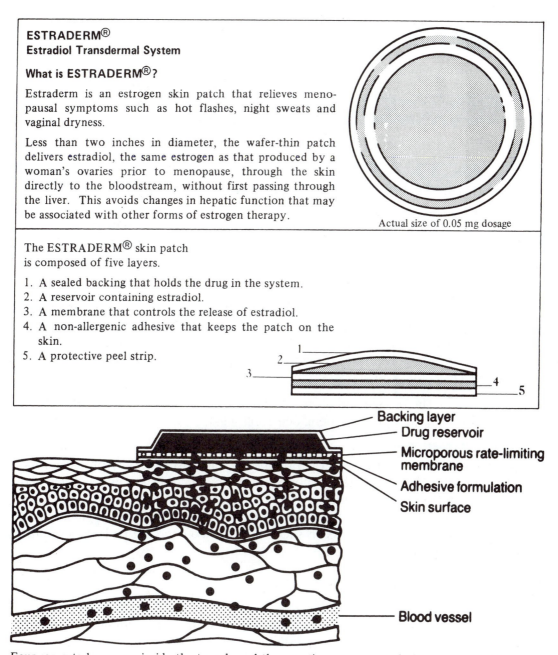

Warning:

1. Patients who take higher doses of estrogens for a long period of time (5 years or more) may have an increased risk of breast cancer.
2. There is a 2.5-fold increase in the risk of developing gallbladder disease in women receiving postmenopausal estrogens.
3. Large doses of estrogen (5 mg/day) may increase the risk of myocardial infarction in men. This dose is comparable to the dose used to treat cancer of the prostate and breast.
4. If higher doses of estrogen are used there may be an increase in the risk of developing hypertension.
5. In patients with breast cancer and bone metastases the administration of estrogen may lead to severe hypercalcemia. If this occurs, the drug should be stopped and appropriate action taken.

Adverse Reactions. Breakthrough bleeding, spotting, breast tenderness and enlargement, nausea, vomiting, abdominal cramps, bloating, cholestatic jaundice, chloasma or melasma, erythema, loss of scalp hair, hirsutism, headache, migraine, dizziness, mental depression, edema, hypertension, intolerance to contact lenses, vaginal candidiasis, changes in weight, hypercalcemia.

Dosage and Route. The dosage and route of administration is determined by the physician and individualized for each patient. See Table 31–1.

Implications for Patient Care. Observe for signs of improvement and adverse reactions. Weigh daily and if weight increases by 5 pounds within a week, notify physician. Assess blood pressure every 4 hours and notify physician if a consistent increase is noted in the systolic and/or diastolic readings. Monitor intake and output ratio and liver function studies. Be aware that a diabetic patient may have an increase in urine glucose and that the physician should be notified if such occurs. Encourage the patient to see the physician on a regular basis.

Patient Teaching

Educate the patient:

- to read the package insert (leaflet) that comes with the prescription and to call the physician if there are any questions.
- to weigh daily, at the same time of day and with the same amount of clothing on/off.
- to notify the physician if there is a weight gain of 5 pounds or more within a week.
- to be aware of possible adverse reactions and report any of the following to the physician without delay: abnormal vaginal bleeding, pains in the calves or chest, sudden shortness of breath, severe headache, dizziness, faintness, or changes in vision, breast lumps, jaundice, pain, swelling or tenderness in the abdomen.

Table 31–1 Estrogens

Medication	Usual Dosage
chlorotrianisene (TACE)	Oral: 12–25 mg daily.
conjugated estrogens, USP (Premarin)	Oral: 0.3–1.25 mg daily. Vaginal: 2–4 Gm daily.
dienestrol cream (DV)	Vaginal: 1 applicatorful 1–2 times daily for 1–2 weeks.
diethylstilbestrol (DES)	Oral: 0.2–0.5 mg daily. Vaginal: 0.1–0.5 mg daily for 10–14 days.
esterified estrogens (Menest)	Oral: 0.3–1.25 mg daily (cyclic regimen).
estradiol (Estrace)	Oral: 1–2 mg daily.
estradiol cypionate in oil (Depo-Estradiol)	IM: 1–5 mg every 3–4 weeks.
estradiol valerate in oil (Delestrogen)	IM: 10–20 mg every 4 weeks.
estrone (Theelin)	IM: 0.1–0.5 mg 2–3 times per week.
estropipate (Ogen)	Oral: one Ogen 0.625 tab to 2.5 mg per day. Vaginal: 2–4 Gm of cream daily.
ethinyl estradiol (Estinyl)	Oral: 0.02–0.05 mg daily.
quinestrol (Estrovis)	Oral: Initial: 100 mcg once daily for 7 days. Maintenance: 100 mcg tab weekly.

- to check with the physician before taking calcium supplements.
- about breast self-examination.
- to see the physician on a regular basis.

Special Considerations

- Estrogen replacement therapy is relatively well tolerated by most menopausal women who take the recommended lowest effective dose.
- Estrogens may decrease the action of anticoagulants and oral hypoglycemics.
- Estrogens may increase the action of corticosteroids.
- Anticonvulsants, barbiturates, phenylbutazone and rifampin may decrease the action of estrogen.
- Possible toxic effect if taken with tricyclic antidepressants.

Progesterone

Progesterone is produced by the ovaries and, to a lesser extent, by the adrenal cortex. The primary source of this hormone is the corpus luteum that forms monthly in the ruptured ovarian follicle. Progesterone prepares the uterus for the implantation of the fertilized ovum. It also suppresses ovulation during pregnancy and stimulates the breast to secrete milk following delivery. Natural progesterone, taken orally, is quickly inactivated by the liver; therefore, chemical modification of the progesterone molecule or the use of a synthetic preparation is necessary to provide a sustained effect. Synthetic preparations are called Progestogens/Progestins. See Table 31–2.

Progesterone is used to prevent uterine bleeding and is combined with estrogen for treatment of amenorrhea. It is also ordered in cases of infertility and threatened or habitual miscarriage.

Actions. Responsible for changes in the uterine endometrium during the second half of the menstrual cycle, development of maternal placenta after implantation, and development of mammary glands.

Uses. Secondary amenorrhea, abnormal uterine bleeding, infertility, threatened or habitual miscarriage.

Contraindications. Contraindicated in patients with known hypersensitivity to any of its ingredients, thrombophlebitis, thromboembolic disorders, cerebral apoplexy, liver disease, breast cancer, reproductive organ cancer(s), undiagnosed vaginal bleeding, missed abortion. Use during pregnancy and lactation is not recommended.

Adverse Reactions. Breast tenderness, galactorrhea, urticaria, pruritus, edema, rash, acne, alopecia, hirsutism, thrombophlebitis, pulmonary embolism, breakthrough bleeding, spotting, amenorrhea, changes in weight, changes in cervical erosion and cervical secretions, cholestatic jaundice, anaphylaxis, mental depression, insomnia, nausea, somnolence.

Dosage and Route. The dosage and route of administration is determined by the physician and individualized for each patient. See Table 31–2.

Table 31–2 Progestogens/Progestins

Medications	Usual Dosage
medroxyprogesterone acetate (Provera)	Oral: 5–10 mg daily.
norethindrone (Norlutin)	Oral: 5–30 mg daily.
norethindrone acetate (Norlutate)	Oral: 2.5–15 mg daily.
progesterone (Gesterol)	IM: 5–10 mg daily for 6–8 consecutive days.

Implications for Patient Care. Observe for signs of improvement and adverse reactions. Weigh daily and if weight increases by 5 pounds within a week, notify physician. Assess blood pressure every 4 hours and notify physician if a consistent increase is noted in the systolic and/or diastolic readings. Monitor intake and output ratio and liver function studies.

Patient Teaching

Educate the patient:

- to weigh daily, at the same time of day and with the same amount of clothing on/off.
- to notify the physician if there is a weight gain of 5 pounds or more within a week.
- to be aware of possible adverse reactions and report any of the following to the physician without delay: abnormal vaginal bleeding, pains in the calves or chest, jaundice, dark urine, clay colored stools, dyspnea, blurred vision.
- about breast self-examination.
- to see the physician on a regular basis.

Special Considerations

- Progestins may cause fluid retention. Used with caution in patients with epilepsy, migraine, asthma, cardiac disease, and renal dysfunction.
- Patients with mental depression should be carefully observed while using progestins. Discontinue drug if depressive state becomes severe.
- Diabetic patients should be carefully monitored while taking progestogens. A decrease in glucose tolerance may occur.

SPOTLIGHT

Birth Control

According to the Association of Reproductive Health Professional's survey, four out of five American women ages 18 to 50 are sexually active. Of these, nine out of ten, were interested in becoming more educated about various methods of birth control.

In the United States there are numerous methods that may be used for birth control and some of these are: birth control pills, condoms, a diaphragm, foams, jellies, natural planning, an IUD (intrauterine device), a cervical cap, a contraceptive sponge, a vasectomy and female sterilization. Other methods of birth control that have been approved by the Food and Drug Administration (FDA) include the Norplant System®, DEPO-PROVERA® contraceptive injection, and the female condom (Reality®).

(continued)

The Norplant System—The Norplant System consists of six thin capsules that contain levonorgestrel (a progestin). The capsules are made of a soft flexible material and are placed in a fan-like pattern just under the skin, on the inside surface of the upper arm.

Contraceptive action that is 99 percent effective begins within hours and lasts up to five years. The capsules must be removed at the end of five years and the contraceptive effect stops within 24 hours.

Prior to the placement of the Norplant System, a complete medical history and physical examination are performed. It is recommended that the capsules be inserted within seven days after the onset of menses, during menses, or immediately following an abortion. The patient who chooses this method should be carefully evaluated on a regular basis and the physician should inform her about warnings and possible side effects.

Reported side effects of the Norplant System include prolonged menstrual bleeding, unexpected bleeding, spotting between periods, no bleeding at all for several months, and/or a combination of these. There are other side effects that may occur and the patient should report any unusual symptoms to her physician.

DEPO-PROVERA—is a contraceptive injection (medroxyprogesterone acetate) and when administered at the recommended dose to women every 3 months, it inhibits the secretion of gonadotropins which, in turn, prevents follicular maturation and ovulation and results in endometrial thinning. These actions produce its contraceptive effect which is 99 percent effective. DEPO-PROVERA is given as an intramuscular injection in the dorsogluteal area or in the deltoid muscle.

Before the initiation of this type of contraception the patient should have a complete medical history and physical examination performed. The physician should inform the patient of precautions, warnings, adverse reactions, and possible side effects. Because DEPO-PROVERA is a long-acting birth control method, it takes some time after the last injection for its effect to wear off.

The Female Condom (Reality)—The FDA approved the use of Reality in 1993. It affords women some protection against sexually transmitted diseases, including AIDS, as well as pregnancy. The female condom in tests had a 26 percent failure rate in preventing pregnancy and the FDA stresses that male latex condoms are better safeguards against pregnancy and disease.

Reality is a pre-lubricated polyurethane sheath that has flexible polyurethane rings on each end, one of which is inserted into the vagina like a diaphragm. One of its two flexible rings holds the device in place, fitting over the cervix and the other ring forms the external edge and remains outside the vagina. It shields the entire vaginal and urethral area from the shaft and base of the penis. It provides women with an opportunity to protect themselves when their sexual partner refuses to use a male condom.

"Case-In-Point"

According to a national survey of men that was published in an issue of Family Planning Perspectives, nearly all men ages 20–39 in the United States are sexually experienced.

- Twenty-three percent have had 20 or more partners in their lifetimes, yet only 25 percent say they used a condom in the past four weeks.
- Single men (45 percent) are twice as likely as married men (18 percent) to use a condom.
- Twenty-seven percent of men say they are embarrassed to buy condoms.

Oral Contraceptives

Women who desire to prevent the occurrence of pregnancy may take oral contraceptive pills that are nearly 100 percent effective when used as directed. These pills contain mixtures of estrogen and progestin in various levels of strength. The estrogen in the pill inhibits ovulation by suppressing the normal secretion of FSH and LH from the anterior pituitary gland. The progestin inhibits pituitary secretion of LH, causes changes in the cervical mucus that renders it unfavorable to penetration by sperm, and alters the nature of the endometrium.

Most oral contraceptives are taken daily for 20 to 21 days, beginning with the 5th day after menstrual bleeding starts. This cycle is then followed by a week without medication to allow bleeding to occur. An exception to this regimen is a pill that contains only progestin. Called a *minipill*, this product is taken daily and continuously. It acts by interfering with sperm and ovum transport and by adversely affecting the suitability of the endometrium for ovum implant. Progestin-only minipills have been associated with menstrual irregularities (breakthough bleeding) and are slightly less effective than the combination products.

Combination products may contain estrogen and progestin in varying formulations; some having more estrogen, others more progestin. They are available in regular or low-dose strength, again based on the amounts of the two hormones in the product. See Figure 31–4.

Adverse reactions to oral contraceptives are related to their hormone content. Those with high estrogen content tend to cause estrogen-related reactions (nausea, weight gain, edema, swelling of the breast), and those with high progestin content cause progestin-related effects (headache, acne, fatigue). As a rule, those preparations containing the lowest hormone content, but which provide consistently effective contraceptive action, are likely to be preferred because of a lower incidence of adverse reaction.

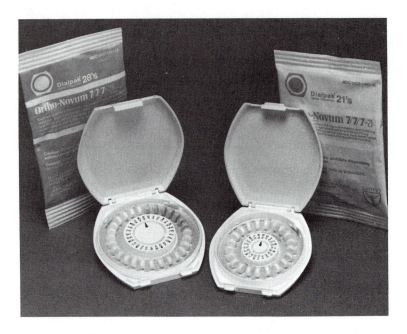

Figure 31–4 Dialpak® Ortho-Novum 7/7/7 *(Courtesy of Ortho Pharmaceutical Corporation)*

Oral contraceptive may be grouped according to the amount of hormone that is available at a given time during the 20–21 day cycle of administration. *Monophasic* preparations provide a fixed concentration of hormones throughout the entire cycle. With *biphasic* preparations, estrogen is available in fixed amounts for the duration of the cycle, but the progestin content is varied. Low levels of progestin are provided during the first half of the cycle and high amounts are included during the last half when endometrial secretions are desired. *Triphasic* preparations vary both the estrogen and progestin dosages within the cycle in an effort to mimic the normal hormonal fluctuation found in women of childbearing age. See Figure 31–5.

Patient literature accompanying oral contraceptive preparations usually cautions those who either have or once had any of the following conditions not to take an oral contraceptive:

1. Clots in the legs or lungs
2. Angina pectoris
3. Known or suspected cancer of the breast or sex organs
4. Unusual vaginal bleeding that has not yet been diagnosed
5. Heart attack or stroke
6. Known or suspected pregnancy

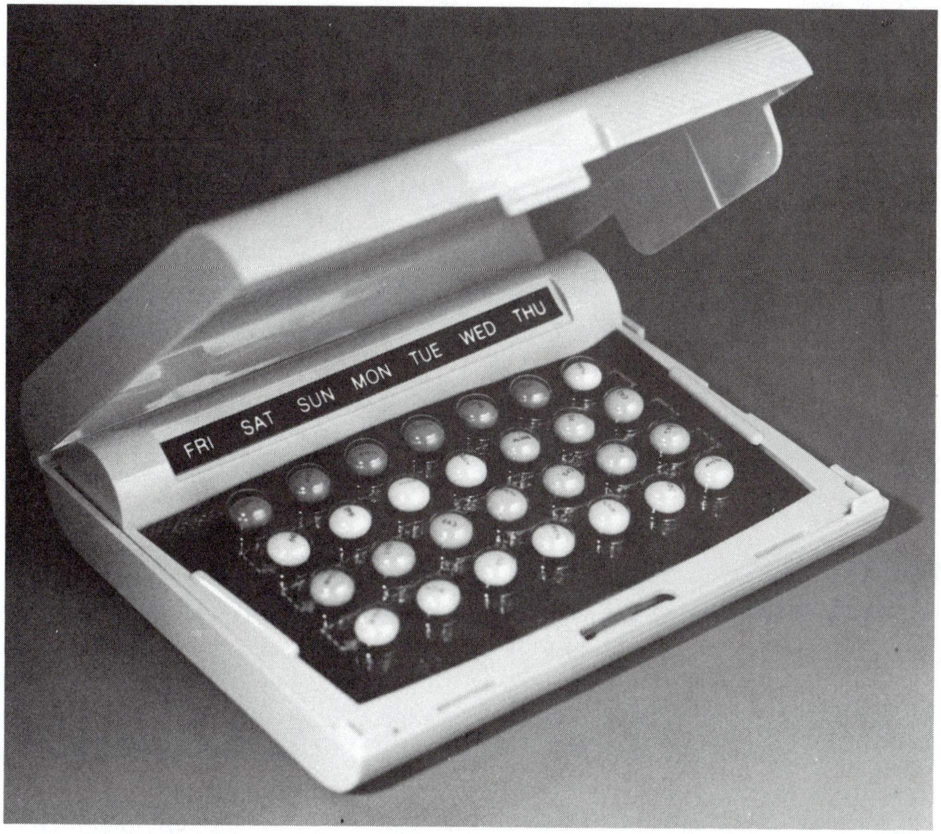

Figure 31–5 Triphasil® *(Courtesy of Wyeth Laboratories, Philadelphia, PA)*

Such literature will also include the following statement on cigarette smoking and the use of oral contraceptives:

> **CAUTION:** Cigarette smoking increases the risk of serious adverse effects on the heart and blood vessels from oral-contraceptive use. This risk increases with age and with heavy smoking (15 or more cigarettes per day) and is quite marked in women over 35 years of age. Women who use oral contraceptives should not smoke.

The choice of an oral contraceptive depends upon a number of factors, including sensitivities to hormones, how the preparation might interact with other drugs being taken, and other considerations. Table 31–3 lists selected oral contraceptive preparations currently in use.

Table 31–3 Selected Oral Contraceptives

Monophasic Preparations	Biphasic Preparations	Triphasic Preparations	Progesterone Only Preparation
Brevicon 21-day	Ortho-Novum 10/11-21	Ortho-Novum 7/7/7	Micronor
Demulen 1/50-21	Ortho-Novum 10/11-28	Tri-Norinyl	Nor-Q.D.
Enovid-E 21		Triphasil-21	Ovrette
Lo/Ovral-21			
Modicon 28			
Nordette 28			
Norinyl 1+35 21 day			
Norlestrin 28 1/50			
Ovcon-50			
Ovulen-28			

Male Hormones

Adequate secretions of androgenic hormones are necessary to maintain normal male sex characteristics, the male libido, and sexual potency.

Testosterone

Testosterone is the most important androgen and is secreted primarily by the Leydig cells located in the interstitial spaces of the testes. With the advent of puberty (ages 13–15), boys experience a dramatic increase in the amount of testosterone secreted. The increased levels of this hormone stimulate the development of male secondary sex characteristics, initiate the production of sperm, and enhance the functional capacity of the penis and the accessory sex organs in the male. Normal men produce 2.5 to 10 mg of testosterone per day. After the age of forty there is a gradual decline in the amount of testosterone produced, and by age eighty, output is approximately 20 percent of that produced during peak years.

Testosterone is rapidly inactivated by the liver; therefore, longer lasting testosterone derivatives and synthetic forms of the hormone are available for oral and parenteral administration. These agents are used for replacement therapy in androgen deficiency, for treatment of *hypogonadism, crytorchidism,* and for palliative treatment of certain metastatic breast carcinomas in women. See Table 31–4 for selected androgens.

Actions. Testosterone is responsible for growth, development, and maintenance of the male reproductive system and secondary sex characteristics.

Uses. As replacement therapy in primary hypogonadism, hypogonadotropic hypogonadism, to stimulate puberty in carefully selected males, and in impotence. It may be used in women with advanced inoperable metastatic breast cancer who are 1–5 years postmenopausal.

Table 31–4 Androgens

Medications	Usual Dosage
fluoxymesterone (Halotestin)	Oral: 5–20 mg/day for replacement therapy.
methyltestosterone (Metandren)	Oral: 10–40 mg/day for replacement therapy. Buccal: 5–20 mg/day.
testosterone (Andro 100)	IM: 10–25 mg 2–3 times/week for androgen deficiency.
testosterone cypionate in oil (Depo-Testosterone)	IM: 50–400 mg every 2–4 weeks for replacement therapy.
testosterone enanthate in oil (Delatestryl)	IM: 50–400 mg every 2–4 weeks for replacement therapy.
testosterone propionate in oil (Testex)	IM: 10–25 mg 2–3 times per week for replacement therapy.
testosterone transdermal systems (Testoderm® C-III) (Androderm® C-III)	Controlled delivery for once-daily application to the scrotum for replacement therapy.

Contraindications. Contraindicated in patients with known hypersensitivity to any of its ingredients, during pregnancy and lactation, in men with cancer of the breast or known or suspected cancer of the prostate, in patients with pituitary insufficiency, history of myocardial infarction, hypercalcemia, prostatic hypertrophy, hepatic dysfunction, nephrosis, and in infants and young children. There are many warnings associated with testosterone preparations. Please refer to a current *Physicians' Desk Reference* for information on warnings.

> **CAUTIOUS USE:** In geriatric patients, diabetic patients, and those with hypertension, coronary artery disease, renal disease, hypercholesterolemia, gynecomastia, and prepubertal males.

Adverse Reactions. *In males:* gynecomastia, excessive frequency and duration of penile erection, oligospermia, hirsutism, male-pattern baldness, acne, retention of sodium, chloride, water, potassium, calcium, and inorganic phosphates, nausea, cholestatic jaundice, alterations in liver function tests, hepatocellular neoplasms, peliosis hepatis (liver and spleen may become engorged with blood-filled cysts), suppression of clotting factors II, V, VII, and X, increased or decreased libido, headache, anxiety, depression, generalized paresthesia, increased serum cholesterol, and rarely anaphylactoid reactions. *In females:* amenorrhea, menstrual irregularities, inhibition of gonadotropin secretion, and virilization (deepening of the voice, clitoral enlargement, increased growth of facial and body hair, male-pattern baldness).

Dosage and Route. The dosage and route of administration is determined by the physician and individualized for each patient. (See Table 31–4.)

Implications for Patient Care. Observe for signs of improvement and adverse reactions. Weigh daily and if weight increases by 5 pounds within a week, notify physician. Assess blood pressure every 4 hours and notify physician if a consistent increase is noted in the systolic and/or diastolic readings. Monitor intake and output ratio, and liver function studies. Monitor electrolytes: sodium, chloride, calcium, potassium, and blood cholesterol level. When used in males to stimulate puberty, assess growth pattern.

Patient Teaching

Educate the patient:

- to weigh daily, at the same time of day and with the same amount of clothing on/off.
- to notify the physician if 5 pounds or more are gained within a week.
- to be aware of possible adverse reactions and report any of the following to the physician. All patients: nausea, vomiting, jaundice, edema. *Males:* frequent or persistent erections of the penis. *Adolescent Males:* signs of premature epiphyseal closure. Should have bone development checked every six months. *Females:* hoarseness, acne, changes in menstrual periods, growth of hair on face and/or body.
- that buccal tablets should be placed under the tongue or in the space between the cheek and gum; change the site of placement with each dose (rotate between the four locations in the mouth); the tablet should be completely dissolved before the patient engages in eating, drinking, or using any tobacco product.
- that oral tablets should be taken with food to minimize possible gastrointestinal distress.

Special Considerations

- In diabetic patients, the effects of testosterone may decrease blood glucose and insulin requirements.
- Testosterone may decrease the anticoagulant requirements of patients receiving oral anticoagulants. These patients require close monitoring when testosterone therapy is begun and then when it is stopped.

- Anabolic steroids (testosterone) may be abused by individuals who seek to increase muscle mass, strength, and overall athletic ability. This form of use is illegal and signs of abuse may include: flu-like symptoms, gastrointestinal distress, headaches, muscle aches, dizziness, bruises, needle marks, increased bleeding (nosebleeds, petechiae, gums, conjunctiva), enlarged spleen, liver, prostate, edema, and in the female increased facial hair, menstrual irregularities, and enlarged clitoris.

Drugs Used during Labor and Delivery

Drugs that selectively stimulate contraction of the myometrium are known as *oxytocic agents* because they act on smooth muscle much like the hormone *oxytocin* which is secreted by the posterior pituitary gland. They may be used in obstetrics to induce labor at term. They are also used to control postpartum hemorrhage and to induce therapeutic abortion. Three types of oxytocic drugs are in general use; they are synthetic oxytocin, the ergot derivatives, and the prostaglandins. These drugs are also known as *uterine stimulants.*

When labor begins before term, *uterine relaxants* may be administered to delay labor until the fetus has gained sufficient maturity as to be likely to survive. Agents used for this purpose are generally administered in cases where spontaneous labor begins after 20 weeks of gestation. The most commonly used uterine relaxants are Ethanol and ritodrine. See Table 31–5.

Table 31–5 Uterine Stimulants and Relaxants

Medications	Uses	Usual Dosages	Adverse Reactions
STIMULANTS			
carboprost tromethamine (Prostin/15 M)	used to induce abortion in weeks 13–20	IM: 250 mcg initially, then repeated at 1.5–3.5 hour intervals as indicated by uterine response.	nausea, diarrhea, vomiting, temperature increase more than, 2°F, flushing, cough, pain, hiccoughs, chills
dinoprost tromethamine (Prostin F_2 Alpha)	used to terminate pregnancy in weeks 16–20	Intra-amniotic instillation: 40 mg or 8 ml (5 mg/ml).	headache, dizziness, syncope, bradycardia, renal retention, bronchoconstriction, cough
dinoprostone (Prostin E_2)	used to terminate pregnancy in weeks 12–20	Intravaginal: 1 suppository (20 mg) inserted high into vagina; then another every 3–5 hours until abortion.	same as above
ergonovine maleate (Ergotate Maleate)	used to prevent postpartum and postabortal hemorrhage	IM: 0.2 mg every 2–4 hours up to maximum of 5 doses. Oral: 0.2–0.4 mg every 6–12 hours (usually for 48 hours).	nausea, vomiting, severe hypertensive episodes, bradycardia, allergic phenomena including shock, ergotism

(continued)

Table 31–5 Uterine Stimulants and Relaxants *(Continued)*

Medications	Uses	Usual Dosages	Adverse Reactions
methylergonovine maleate (Methergine)	used for routine management after delivery of placenta	Oral: 0.2 mg 3–4 times/day in puerperium for 1 week. IM: 1 ml every 2–4 hours as necessary after delivery of placenta.	anorexia, dizziness, headache, nervousness, insomnia, blood pressure and pulse changes, tachycardia, visual disturbances, abdominal pain
oxytocin (Pitocin) (Syntocinon)	used to initiate/improve uterine contraction at term	IV infusion (drip): 1–2 mU/minute (0.001–0.002 U/min) with gradual increase by 1–2 mU/minute until normal contraction pattern is established that stimulates normal labor.	Fetus: bradycardia, hypoxia, intracranial hemorrhage, neonatal jaundice, death Mother: hypersensitivity leading to uterine hypertonicity, uterine rupture
RELAXANTS			
ethyl alcohol (Ethanol)	used to suppress premature labor	IV: 1.25 Gm of absolute alcohol per kg/body weight.	depression of the central nervous system, inebriation
ritodrine HCl (Yutopar)	used to manage premature labor	IV: 50–100 mcg/minute administered by calibrated constant-rate infusion pump.	altered maternal and fetal heart rates, temporary hypoglycemia, nausea, anxiety

Special Considerations: The Older Adult

In 1996, a national survey of 1604 men and women ranging in age from 65 to 97, was conducted and reported in *Parade Magazine*. The following is a summary of portions of this survey.

Among the survey's key findings were:

- Men and women remain interested in and sexually active into their 60s, 70s, and beyond.
- Approximately 40 percent of the respondents, whose average age was 74, were sexually active.
- The older adults have sex an average of 2.5 times a month, compared to 7.1 times for the 18 to 65 year olds whom *Parade* surveyed in 1994. Both the younger and the older respondents said they would like to have sex more often. The seniors' ideal is 5.1 times a month, while the younger group's ideal is 12.9 times.

- At all ages, more men than women say sex is important.
- Sex is not the priority for older adults. When asked what matters most in an intimate relationship, only 5 percent of the survey respondents said sex. Nearly nine in ten said companionship was most important; 8 percent said romance.
- More older adults were happier with life in general. The happiest of all seniors were those who were sexually active.
- Approximately half of the respondents were satisfied with their quality of sexual activity.
- Among those surveyed, 60 percent said that they were "knowledgeable" about sex.
- More seniors than younger adults found it difficult to talk about sex with a partner.
- American's seniors tend to have sexually conservative values.
- The most common reasons reported for a decline in sexual satisfaction in later life were health or medical problems.
- Medications often are the culprit in sexual difficulties among the older adult. Two-thirds of the respondents (66 percent) reported taking medications. Half of the men and a fifth of the women on medications say that the drugs have affected their sex lives. The most common sexual side effects are lower sex drive/lack of interest, and impotence/inability to maintain an erection.

Special Considerations: The Child

It is reported that one in five persons with gonorrhea is under 20 years of age. Sexually transmitted diseases (STDs), syphilis, gonorrhea, chlamydia, genital herpes, hepatitis B, genital warts, and HIV are not just contracted by adults. These diseases are being seen in children ranging from 10 to 19 years of age. It is noted that young people are becoming sexually active at very early ages, therefore sex education courses should begin early. A person can have intercourse only once and contract a sexually transmitted disease. STDs can be passed on to sex partners and if left untreated can cause such medical problems as sterility, arthritis, pelvic inflammatory disease, and many other diseases and condition. Most STDs can be treated through the proper antibiotic therapy, except for those caused by viruses (hepatitis B, genital herpes, HIV). There is only one sure way to avoid STDs and that is through abstaining from sexual activity.

(continued)

Signs and Symptoms of Gonorrhea, Herpes Simplex II, Hepatitis B, and HIV (human immunodeficiency virus)

Gonorrhea	Herpes Simplex II	Hepatitis B	HIV
Genital discharge Genital swelling Burning sensation during urination Lower abdominal pain	Painful blisters Flu-like feeling Loss of appetite Burning sensation during urination	Abdominal discomfort Flu-like feeling Loss of appetite Yellowing of skin and eyes Itchy skin Dark urine and light stools	Swelling in the lymph glands Weight loss Night sweats Persistent cough

Diagnosis

Tests for the various diseases range from blood samples to genital exams and cultures. People as young as 12 may be tested at state health departments without parental consent.

National STD hotline: 1-800-277-8922

National AIDS hotline: 1-800-342-AIDS

Critical Thinking Questions/Activities

A 14-year-old boy has noticed a discharge from his penis, a burning sensation when he urinates, and an uncomfortable feeling in his lower abdominal area. Ask yourself:

- What disease does this boy possibly have?
- What should this boy do to find out what he has?
- What is the treatment for this disease?
- How is this disease contracted?
- What could happen if this disease was left untreated?

Spot Check

There are many sexually transmitted diseases (STDs) that one should be informed about. For the following selected diseases, give the signs and symptoms.

Disease	Signs and Symptoms
Gonorrhea	
Herpes Simplex II	
Hepatitis B	
HIV	

Review Questions

Directions: Select the best answer to each multiple choice question. Circle the letter of your choice.

1. A softening of bones or increased porosity of bones seen most often in aging women is called __________.
   a. osteoporosis b. menopause c. hirsutism d. amenorrhea
2. Estrogen preparations may be used for __________.
   a. amenorrhea
   b. dysfunctional bleeding
   c. hirsutism
   d. all of these
3. The usual oral dosage of Premarin is __________ mg daily.
   a. 0.2–0.5 b. 0.3–1.25 c. 1–2 d. 0.1–0.2
4. Adverse reactions to estrogens are __________.
   a. nausea
   b. fullness of the breasts
   c. edema
   d. all of these

5. Progesterone preparations may be used for __________.
   a. prevention of uterine bleeding
   b. infertility
   c. threatened or habitual miscarriage
   d. all of these
6. The usual IM dosage of Gesterol is __________.
   a. 5–10 mg daily
   b. 2.5–15 mg daily
   c. 5–30 mg daily
   d. 125–250 mg/cycle
7. __________ oral contraceptive preparations provide a fixed concentration of hormones throughout the entire cycle.
   a. Biphasic
   b. Monphasic
   c. Triphasic
   d. none of these
8. An example of a triphasic oral contraceptive is __________.
   a. Enovid-E 21
   b. Ortho-Novum 10/11-28
   c. Ortho-Novum 7/7/7
   d. Micronor
9. Testosterone preparations may be used for __________.
   a. replacement therapy
   b. hypogonadism
   c. cryptorchidism
   d. all of these
10. The usual IM dosage of Delatestryl is __________.
    a. 50–400 mg every 2–4 weeks
    b. 10–25 mg 2–3 times per week
    c. 10–40 mg/day
    d. 2–10 mg/day
11. Drugs that selectively stimulate contraction of the myometrium are known as __________.
    a. relaxants
    b. oxytocic agents
    c. androgens
    d. estrogens
12. A drug used to initiate and improve uterine contractions at term is __________.
    a. Pitocin
    b. Ethanol
    c. Yutopar
    d. Prostin
13. The __________ in the female and the __________ in the male are the primary organs of sexual reproduction.
    a. uterus, scrotum
    b. vagina, penis
    c. ovaries, testes
    d. breast, penis
14. The __________ secretes increased amounts of two gonad-stimulating hormones that cause the reproductive organs to mature and begin the production of ova and sperm.
    a. ovaries
    b. pituitary gland
    c. pineal gland
    d. testes
15. The functions of the ovaries are __________.
    a. the production of ova
    b. secretion of estrogen and progesterone
    c. secretion of luteinizing hormone
    d. a and b

16. The functions of the testes are ________.
    a. production of semen
    b. production of sperm
    c. secretion of testosterone
    d. b and c
17. Estrogen, due to the source of its secretion, is sometimes referred to as ________.
    a. luteinizing hormone
    b. follicular hormone
    c. premenstrual hormone
    d. all of these
18. ________ prepares the uterus for the implantation of the fertilized ovum.
    a. Estrogen
    b. Progesterone
    c. Testosterone
    d. Cortisone

Case Study: Mrs. Mary Parks, a 50-year-old real estate broker has an appointment for her annual physical. She states that she is bothered with hot flashes, night sweats, irritability, and vaginal dryness. She is very concerned about the hot flashes. "The heat radiates through my body and I feel like I am on fire. It is most embarrassing to be meeting with a client and all of a sudden, a hot flash overcomes me." You assess her vital signs and they are: T 98.6, P 76, R 18, B/P 134/78. After the complete physical and consultation, the physician orders ESTRADERM 0.05 mg for Mrs. Parks.

19. The symptoms described by Mrs. Parks indicate a/an ________.
    a. estrogen deficiency
    b. insulin deficiency
    c. electrolyte imbalance
    d. potassium deficiency
20. ESTRADERM delivers ________ through the skin directly into the bloodstream.
    a. progesterone
    b. progestin
    c. estradiol
    d. estardiol
21. Estrogen replacement therapy is contraindicated in patients with ________.
    a. breast cancer, thrombophlebitis
    b. hypertension, thrombophlebitis
    c. diabetes mellitus
    d. all of these
22. Some common adverse reactions to estrogens are ________.
    a. breakthrough bleeding, spotting
    b. breast tenderness
    c. edema
    d. all of these
23. In teaching Mrs. Parks to weigh daily, you should instruct her to ________.
    a. weigh at the same time of day
    b. report to her physician weight gain of 5 or more pounds/week
    c. report to her physician a weight loss of 5 or more pounds/week
    d. a and b

Case Study: A 20-year-old college student states that she and her fiance are sexually active. She states that she has been taking Triphasil for the past year. With her busy schedule she sometimes forgets to take her pills and she is concerned about getting pregnant. She is interested in the Norplant System.

24. The Norplant System consists of ________ thin capsules that contain _________.
    a. seven, estrogen
    b. six, estrogen
    c. six, levonorgestrel
    d. seven, levonorgestrel
25. The Norplant System is __________ percent effective and can stay in place for __________ years.
    a. 97, 5 b. 98, 5 c. 99, 5 d. 99,4
26. Side effects of the Norplant System are __________.
    a. irregular menstrual periods
    b. hypertension, weight loss
    c. osteoporosis, electrolyte imbalance
    d. weight loss, electrolyte imbalance
27. DEPO-PROVERA is a contraceptive injection containing __________.
    a. levonorgestrel
    b. delatestryl
    c. medroxyprogesterone acetate
    d. estradiol

Case Study: Mr. Thomas Barton, a 60-year-old insurance agent is returning to the office for a follow-up visit. He has been on Depo-Testosterone 100 mg, IM every two weeks for androgen deficiency. He states that he is concerned because his breasts have started to enlarge and he is gaining weight.

28. The symptoms describe by Mr. Barton may indicate which of the following adverse reactions to testosterone?
    a. hirsutism, hepatocellular neoplasms
    b. gynecomastia, retention of sodium and water
    c. increased serum cholesterol, peliosis hepatis
    d. cholestatic jaundice, oligospermia

29. The generic name for Depo-Testosterone is ________.
    a. fluoxymesterone
    b. methyltestosterone
    c. testosterone cypionate in oil
    d. testosterone enanthate in oil
30. The usual dosage of Depo-Testosterone is ________.
    a. 5–20 mg/day
    b. 10–25 mg 2–3 times/week
    c. 50–400 mg every 2–4 weeks
    d. 126–250 mg every 2–4 weeks

Matching: Place the correct letter from Column II on the appropriate line of Column I.

Column I

31. ________ Amenorrhea
32. ________ Cryptorchidism
33. ________ Hirsutism
34. ________ Menopause
35. ________ Osteoporosis
36. ________ Hypogonadism
37. ________ Testosterone

Column II

A. A condition of defective secretion of the gonads.
B. A softening of bone seen most often in aging women.
C. Literally means cessation of the monthly menstrual activity.
D. Without or lack of the monthly menstrual flow.
E. Failure of the testicles to descend into the scrotum.
F. A condition characterized by excessive growth of hair, especially in women.
G. The least important androgen.
H. The most important androgen.

APPENDIX

Answers to Practice Problems, Learning Exercises Self Assessment Tests, and Review Questions

Section 1 Basic Mathematics

Chapter 1 Introduction and Arithmetic Pretest

Arithmetic Pretest

1. a. XV b. XIX c. V d. IV
   e. XX f. I g. VIII h. VII
2. a. 10 b. 6 c. 9 d. 26
   e. 3 f. 24 g. 14 h. 13
3. a. one million, five thousand, two hundred and twenty-one
   b. one hundred twenty-five thousand, nine hundred and thirty-six
   c. forty-eight thousand, two hundred and twenty-four
   d. two thousand one and five-tenths
   e. one million, two hundred thousand
4. a. 2 b. $2\frac{1}{4}$ c. 4
   d. $5\frac{1}{3}$ e. 20 f. $4\frac{7}{15}$
5. a. 500 b. 2,598,000 c. 2,000,000
6. a. 0.216 b. 421.605 c. 1046.069
7. a. $\frac{19}{20}$ b. $\frac{31}{24}$ or $1\frac{7}{24}$ c. $11\frac{11}{8}$ or $12\frac{3}{8}$
8. a. $\frac{1}{6}$ b. $\frac{7}{15}$ c. $2\frac{1}{6}$ d. $3\frac{7}{8}$
9. a. 4 b. 1 c. 6 d. 26
10. a. 1.55 b. 3.50 c. 24.90 d. 89.80
11. a. 267.75 b. 27.505
    c. 589.0401 d. 67.2864
12. a. 2 b. 8 c. 4.071 d. 601
13. a. $\frac{5}{6}$ b. $\frac{3}{4}$ c. 0.75 d. 0.255
14. a. 45.5 b. 35.03
    c. 2.0005 d. 160.003
15. a. 0.7 b. 5.25 c. 2.5 d. 0.25
16. a. 50% b. 0.7% c. 75%
    d. 5% e. 25% f. 50%
17. a. 3.75 b. 2.50 c. 24
    d. 5.25 e. 50 f. 125
18. a. 4,280 b. 600,000
    c. 6,000,000 d. 40,208
    e. 200,020 f. 503.5 or $503\frac{5}{10}$

Chapter 2 Numerals and Fractions

Practice Problems

1. a. III b. V c. VIII
   d. X e. C f. VII
   g. L h. LX i. 24
   j. 4 k. 16 l. 19
   m. 9 n. 8 o. 20
2. a. $\frac{3}{4}$ b. $\frac{1}{3}$ c. $\frac{1}{4}$
   d. $\frac{1}{2}$ e. $\frac{1}{20}$ f. $\frac{1}{5}$
3. a. $1\frac{1}{3}$ b. $1\frac{1}{3}$ c. $1\frac{1}{2}$
   d. $1\frac{3}{5}$ e. $1\frac{1}{9}$ f. $1\frac{2}{13}$
4. a. $\frac{10}{3}$ b. $\frac{17}{4}$ c. $\frac{17}{3}$
   d. $\frac{67}{10}$ e. $\frac{50}{7}$ f. $\frac{82}{9}$
5.

	Largest	*Smallest*
a.	$\frac{1}{3}$	$\frac{1}{8}$
b.	$\frac{1}{4}$	$\frac{1}{150}$
c.	$\frac{1}{5}$	$\frac{1}{100}$
d.	$\frac{4}{5}$	$\frac{2}{5}$
e.	$\frac{10}{40}$	$\frac{2}{40}$
f.	$\frac{1}{100}$	$\frac{1}{150}$
g.	$\frac{3}{4}$	$\frac{1}{4}$
h.	$\frac{1}{2}$	$\frac{1}{5}$
i.	$\frac{75}{100}$	$\frac{25}{100}$
j.	$\frac{8}{10}$	$\frac{3}{10}$

6. a. $\frac{11}{12}$ b. $\frac{19}{21}$ c. $\frac{24}{16} = 1\frac{1}{2}$
   d. $\frac{28}{20} = 1\frac{2}{5}$ e. 99 f. $155\frac{6}{7}$
   g. 43 h. $29\frac{5}{6}$ i. $36\frac{29}{30}$
   j. $37\frac{1}{3}$ k. $\frac{49}{50}$ l. 1
7. a. $\frac{12}{16} = \frac{3}{4}$ b. $\frac{11}{45}$ c. $\frac{7}{32}$
   d. $33\frac{1}{3}$ e. $15\frac{7}{9}$ f. 9
   g. $7\frac{7}{10}$ h. $83\frac{4}{8} = 83\frac{1}{2}$ i. $49\frac{38}{25} = 50\frac{13}{25}$
   j. $\frac{34}{150}$ k. $\frac{1}{12}$ l. $2\frac{11}{24}$
8. a. $\frac{161}{144}$ b. $\frac{2}{15}$ c. $\frac{28}{32} = \frac{7}{8}$
   d. $\frac{410}{12} = 34\frac{1}{6}$ e. $61\frac{1}{9}$ f. $\frac{153}{40} = 3\frac{33}{40}$
   g. 21 h. $\frac{126}{5} = 25\frac{1}{5}$ i. 146
   j. 12 k. $\frac{1}{2}$ l. $\frac{1}{10}$
   m. $\frac{1}{6}$ n. $3\frac{3}{4}$ o. $\frac{95}{48} = 1\frac{47}{48}$
9. a. $\frac{368}{63} = 5\frac{53}{63}$ b. $\frac{6}{5} = 1\frac{1}{5}$ c. $\frac{7}{2} = 3\frac{1}{2}$
   d. $\frac{82}{60} = 1\frac{22}{60} = 1\frac{11}{30}$ e. $\frac{275}{2} = 137\frac{1}{2}$
   f. $\frac{15}{102} = \frac{5}{34}$ g. 84 h. $\frac{1120}{9} = 124\frac{4}{9}$
   i. $\frac{7}{6} = 1\frac{1}{6}$ j. 2 k. 2
   l. $\frac{2}{3}$ m. $\frac{3}{5}$ n. $\frac{9}{5} = 1\frac{4}{5}$
   o. $\frac{4}{33}$ p. $\frac{27}{32}$

Self Assessment Test

1. a. XV b. XXV c. L
   d. 4 e. 19 f. 16
2. a. $\frac{11}{2}$ b. $\frac{10}{3}$ c. $\frac{49}{6}$
   d. $\frac{55}{8}$ e. $\frac{14}{3}$ f. $\frac{5}{2}$
3. a. $1\frac{1}{2}$ b. $1\frac{2}{5}$ c. $1\frac{1}{2}$
   d. $7\frac{1}{2}$ e. $1\frac{1}{3}$ f. $1\frac{1}{2}$
4. a. $\frac{1}{2}$ b. $\frac{3}{4}$ c. $\frac{1}{2}$
   d. $\frac{3}{5}$ e. $\frac{1}{4}$ f. $\frac{1}{5}$
5. a. $\frac{7}{8}$ b. $25\frac{1}{3}$ c. $\frac{6}{21}$
   d. 41 e. $\frac{4}{9}$ f. $201\frac{1}{6}$
6. a. $\frac{5}{8}$ b. $15\frac{7}{9}$ c. $\frac{1}{12}$
   d. $22\frac{1}{3}$ e. $\frac{34}{150}$ f. 9
7. a. $\frac{1}{6}$ b. 146 c. 9 d. $16\frac{5}{36}$
8. a. $\frac{2}{3}$ b. $\frac{27}{32}$ c. $\frac{4}{33}$ d. $124\frac{4}{9}$

Chapter 3 Decimal Fractions and Percents

Learning Exercise

1. decimal
2. It is used for precise measurement.
3. whole

4. decimals or decimal fractions
5. place value
6. ten
7. one tenth
8. decimal fraction
9. to insure accuracy
10. powers of ten
11. a. one ten-thousandth
    b. two tenths
    c. six one-hundredths
    d. ten one hundred-thousandths
    e. twenty-five thousandths
12. a. twenty-five hundredths
    b. seven-tenths
    c. one hundred and fifty thousandths
    d. four thousand two hundred ten thousandths
    e. six hundrcd-thousandths
13. a. two and five-tenths (two point five)
    b. nine and twenty-five hundredths (nine point twenty five hundredths)
    c. one hundred twenty-five and forty thousandths (one hundred twenty-five point forty thousandths)
    d. fifteen and one hundred fifty ten-thousandths (fifteen point one hundred fifty ten-thousandths)
    e. four and five hundred thousandths (four point five hundred thousandths)

Practice Problems

1. a. 0.666 b. 0.25 c. 0.75
   d. 0.2 e. 0.875
2. a. $\frac{4}{10}$ b. $\frac{5}{100}$ c. $\frac{10}{1000}$
   d. $\frac{6}{10{,}000}$ e. $\frac{2}{1{,}000{,}000}$
3. a. 1 b. 1 c. 1.35
   d. 0.351 e. 134.26
4. a. 0.06 b. 0.5 c. 40.39
   d. 3.068 e. 0.444 f. 0.13
   g. 0.06 h. 0.21 i. 0.52
   j. 0.44
5. a. 13.175 b. 27.5625 c. 674.98312
   d. 221.9778 e. 0.317504 f. 250,000
   g. 104,000 h. 5200 i. 110
   j. 3
6. a. 7.2 b. 6.02 c. 5.02
   d. 8.02 e. 2.02 f. 0.002
   g. 0.005 h. 0.005 i. 0.004
   j. 3.443
7. a. 100 b. 2000 c. 200
   d. 1000 e. 100,000 f. 8000
   g. 1,000,000 h. 200 i. 5000
   j. 90
8. a. 0.08 b. 0.3 c. 0.1 d. 2
   e. 100 f. 3 g. 70 h. 0.9
   i. 0.03 j. 0.1
9. a. 0.000025 b. 0.00104 c. 0.0052
   d. 0.011 e. 0.03 f. 8.88
   g. 0.0015 h. 0.0000066 i. 0.00007
   j. 0.0001
10. a. 25% b. $33\frac{1}{3}\%$ c. 40%
    d. $66\frac{2}{3}\%$ e. 12%
11. a. 125% b. 70% c. 80%
    d. 495% e. 12.5%
12. a. $\frac{1}{50}$ and 0.02 b. $\frac{19}{400}$ and 0.0475
    c. $\frac{2}{5}$ and 0.4 d. $\frac{193}{1000}$ and 0.193
    e. $\frac{16}{25}$ and 0.64
13. a. 7.2 and $7\frac{1}{5}$ b. 4.8 and $4\frac{4}{5}$
    c. 3.75 and $3\frac{3}{4}$ d. 52.5 and $52\frac{1}{2}$
    e. 0.2 and $\frac{1}{5}$

Self Assessment Test

1. whole
2. decimals or decimal fractions
3. ten
4. $\frac{1}{10}$
5. a. five tenths
   b. ten one-thousandths
   c. five tenths
   d. five hundred-thousandths
   e. two and twenty-hundredths
   f. eight and seventy-five hundredths

6. a. 0.333 b. 0.25
7. a. $\frac{5}{10}$ b. $\frac{5}{100,000}$
8. a. 1 b. 1.74
9. a. 0.52 b. 3.068
10. a. 22.9778 b. 110
11. a. 0.002 b. 0.004 c. 200
    d. 5000 e. 0.1 f. 70
12. a. $33\frac{1}{3}$% b. 25% c. $66\frac{2}{3}$%

Chapter 4 Ratio and Proportion

Practice Problems

1. a. 1:25 b. 2:100 1:50
   c. 10:40 1:4 d. 25:75 1:3
   e. 8:64 1:8 f. 1:2
   g. 1:3 h. 1:250
   i. 3:500 j. 5:2
2. a. 24 ÷ 48 1 ÷ 2 b. 12 ÷ 6 2 ÷ 1
   c. 76 ÷ 304 1 ÷ 4 d. 5 ÷ 25 1 ÷ 5
   e. 2 ÷ 92 1 ÷ 46 f. 18 ÷ 108 1 ÷ 6
   g. 10 ÷ 50 1 ÷ 5 h. 17 ÷ 51 1 ÷ 3
   i. 11 ÷ 22 1 ÷ 2 j. 55 ÷ 165 1 ÷ 3
3. a. $\frac{33}{66}$ $\frac{1}{2}$ b. $\frac{4}{10}$ $\frac{2}{5}$
   c. $\frac{75}{100}$ $\frac{3}{4}$ d. $\frac{22}{88}$ $\frac{1}{4}$
   e. $\frac{43}{86}$ $\frac{1}{2}$ f. $\frac{2}{13}$
   g. $\frac{7}{49}$ $\frac{1}{7}$ h. $\frac{4}{100}$ $\frac{1}{25}$
   i. $\frac{1}{150}$ j. $\frac{12}{36}$ $\frac{1}{3}$
4. a. 0.02 b. 0.08 c. 0.006 d. 0.75
   e. 0.002 f. 0.08 g. 1.25 h. 0.001
   i. 0.005 j. 0.5
5. a. 8 b. 50 c. 2000 d. 24
   e. 8 f. 3 g. 2500 h. 12
   i. 540 j. 20
6. a. 46 b. 28 c. 46 d. 14
   e. 13,990 f. 18 g. 41 h. 85
   i. 15 j. 112
7. a. 4 b. 5 c. 20 d. 0.25
   e. $\frac{5}{9}$ f. 6 g. $\frac{1}{2}$ or 0.5
   h. 3 i. 200 j. $\frac{3}{4}$ or 0.75
8. a. 3 b. 500 c. 5 d. 2
   e. 1000 f. 10 g. $\frac{1}{2}$ or 0.5
   h. 30 i. 1000 j. 5

Self Assessment Test

1. a. 1:25, 1 ÷ 25, 0.04
   b. 12 ÷ 6, $\frac{12}{6}$, 2
   c. 33 ÷ 66, $\frac{33}{66}$ ($\frac{1}{2}$), 0.5
   d. 1 ÷ 50, $\frac{1}{50}$, 0.02
   e. 25:75, 25 ÷ 75, 0.333
2. a. X = 4 b. X = 540
   c. X = $\frac{6}{10}$ ($\frac{3}{5}$) d. X = $\frac{1}{2}$
   e. X = $\frac{1}{300}$ f. X = 3
   g. X = 20 h. X = 10
   i. X = 18 j. X = $\frac{1}{2}$

Chapter 5 Temperature Equivalents

Practice Problems

1. a. 104° b. 95° c. 35° d. 37.2°
2. a. 39° b. 36.5° or 36.6° c. 37.6°
   d. 39.4° e. 40° f. 96.8° g. 99°
   h. 100° i. 101° j. 102.2°

Self Assessment Test

1. 97 to 99; 36.1 to 37
2. 212
3. 0
4. a. 37.2 b. 37 c. 38.3
   d. 102.2 e. 96.8 f. 105.8

Section 2 Calculations of Doses and Solutions

Chapter 6 The Metric System

Learning Exercise

1. a. meter b. liter c. gram
2. a. kilo b. deci c. micro
   d. hecto e. milli f. deka
   g. centi
3. Decimal fractions
4. 0
5. 39.37

6. a. 0.001 meter b. 0.01 meter
   c. 0.1 meter d. 1 meter
   e. 10 meters f. 100 meters
   g. 1000 meters
7. $2\frac{1}{2}$
8. 1.056
9. 15 or 16
10. one cubic centimeter, one milliliter
11. a. 0.001 L b. 0.01 L c. 0.1 L
    d. 1 L e. 10 L f. 100 L
    g. 1000 L
12. 15 or 0.035
13. a. 0.000001 Gm b. 0.001 Gm
    c. 0.01 Gm d. 0.1 Gm
    e. 1 Gm f. 10 Gm
    g. 100 Gm h. 1000 Gm
14. *Volume* a. ml or cc b. L
    Weight a. mcg b. mg
    c. Gm d. kg
15. a. 1 Gm b. 0.25 L c. 200 mg
    d. 0.2 ml e. 12 kg
16. a. L b. Gm c. mg
    d. lb e. mg

Practice Problems

1. a. 0.25 b. 500 c. 2000 d. 0.5
   e. 30 f. 0.0005 g. 0.001 h. 2
   i. 1 j. 4.4
2. a. 0.06 b. 5 c. 0.2 d. 0.001
   e. 6.5 f. 0.0035 g. 4000 h. 0.001
   i. 100 j. 0.00005
3. a. 83.6 b. 95.5 c. 38.6 d. 24.5
4. a. 66 b. 99 c. 143 d. 165
5. 88 lb = 40 kg Dosage = 2000 mg

Self Assessment Test

1. a. meter b. liter c. gram
2. a. kilo b. deci c. micro d. hecto
   e. milli f. deka g. centi
3. $2\frac{1}{2}$
4. 1.056
5. 15 or 16
6. a. liter b. grams c. milligrams
   d. pounds e. milligrams
7. a. 0.001 b. 0.004 c. 5000
   d. 200 e. 0.001 f. 0.0035
8. a. 80 b. 45.45 c. 29.09

Chapter 7 Household Measures and Apothecaries' Measurements

Learning Exercise

1. a. gtt b. tsp c. T d. oz
   e. tcp f. C g. pt h. qt
   i. gal
2. a. 3 b. 6 c. 1 d. 4
   e. 8 f. 2 g. 5 h. 7
   i. 9
3. a. gtt b. gtt c. T d. oz
   e. oz f. oz g. C h. qt
   i. oz j. pt

Practice Problems

1. a. 150 b. $\frac{5}{8}$ c. 6 d. $7\frac{1}{2}$
   e. $\frac{5}{8}$ f. 160 g. 360 h. 3
   i. $\frac{3}{4}$ j. 80
2. a. 480 b. 45 c. 24 d. $\frac{3}{4}$
   e. $1\frac{1}{2}$ f. $\frac{1}{60}$ g. $\frac{1}{2}$ h. 6
   i. $\frac{3}{8}$ j. $\frac{1}{4}$

Self Assessment Test

1. a. gal b. qt c. pt d. C
   e. tcp f. oz g. T h. tsp
   i. gtt
2. a. gtt b. gtt c. oz d. C
   e. T f. T g. oz h. C
   i. pt
3. a. 10 b. 24 c. 15 d. 9
   e. $\frac{3}{4}$
4. a. gr b. dr c. oz
5. a. $\frac{1}{2}$ b. 45 c. $\frac{1}{60}$ d. 24
   e. $\frac{3}{4}$ f. $\frac{1}{4}$

Chapter 8 Calculating Adult Dosages: Oral Forms

Practice Problems

1. a. $\frac{1}{2}$ tab b. 2 caps c. 2 tabs
   d. 10 ml e. 2 tabs f. 2 tabs
   g. $\frac{1}{2}$ tab h. 2.5 ml i. $\frac{1}{2}$ tab
   j. 2 caps

2. a. 2 tabs b. $\frac{1}{2}$ tab c. $\frac{1}{2}$ tab
d. $1\frac{1}{2}$ tabs e. $\frac{1}{2}$ tab f. 2 tabs
g. 2 tabs h. 2 tabs i. 1 tab
j. $\frac{1}{2}$ tab

Self Assessment Test

1. $\frac{1}{2}$ tab
2. $\frac{1}{2}$ tab
3. 2 tabs
4. $\frac{1}{2}$ tab
5. $1\frac{1}{2}$ tabs
6. 1 tab
7. 2 caps
8. 3 ml

Chapter 9 Calculating Adult Dosages: Parenteral Forms

Practice Problems

1. a. 1.5 ml b. 0.2 ml c. 1.5 ml
d. 1 ml e. 1 ml
2. a. 1.5 ml b. 1 ml c. 0.7 ml
d. 0.5 ml e. 1.5 ml f. 0.5 ml
g. 2.5 ml h. 2 ml i. 0.5 ml
j. 1 ml
3. a. 0.5 ml b. 0.8 ml c. 1 ml
d. 32 units

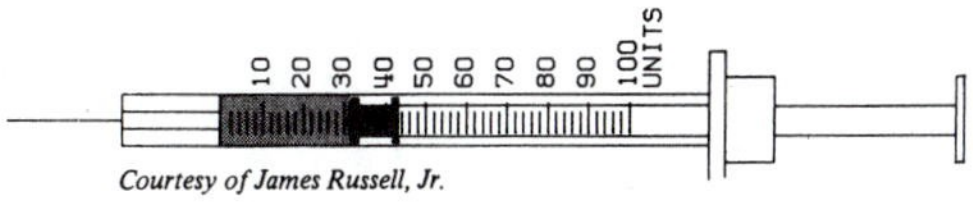

Courtesy of James Russell, Jr.

e. 64 units

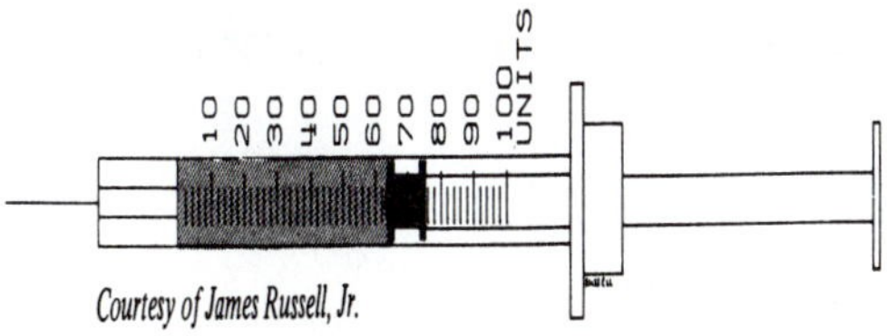

Courtesy of James Russell, Jr.

4. a. 41.6 = 42 gtt/min b. 83.3 = 83 gtt/min
c. 16.6 = 17 gtt/min d. 17.3 = 17 gtt/min
e. 18.7 = 19 gtt/min

Self Assessment Test

1. 1 ml
2. 1.5 ml
3. 20 minims
4. 2 ml
5. 12 minims
6. 41.4 = 42 gtt/ml
7. 16.6 = 17 gtt/ml

Chapter 10 Calculating Children's Dosages

Practice Problems

1. a. 300 mg q 12 h
b. 11 mg (22.72 kg) or 11.5 mg (23 kg)
c. 418 mg or 420 mg
d. 1145 mg (286 mg/daily)
e. 141.8 = 142 mg
2. a. 88 mg
b. 74 mg
c. 60.29 = 60 mg
d. 329.4 = 329 units
e. 147 units

Self Assessment Test

1. 20.5 = 21 mg
2. 900 mg
3. 300 mg
4. 88 mg

Section 3 Administration of Medications

Chapter 11 Drug Sources, Standards, and Dosages

Review Questions

1. c
2. b
3. c
4. c
5. b
6. d
7. c
8. d
9. c
10. b
11. d
12. b
13. d
14. a
15. d
16. c

17. F
18. I
19. G
20. H
21. B
22. A
23. C
24. E
25. D

Chapter 12 Forms of Drugs and How They Act

Review Questions

1. d
2. c
3. c
4. a
5. c
6. c
7. c
8. b
9. c
10. d
11. b
12. b
13. c
14. a
15. c
16. a
17. b
18. d
19. c
20. b
21. d
22. c
23. a
24. a
25. c
26. D
27. C
28. E
29. B
30. A

Chapter 13 The Medication Order

Review Questions

1. d
2. a
3. c
4. c
5. c
6. a
7. b
8. d
9. a
10. c
11. a
12. b
13. c
14. b
15. d
16. c
17. d
18. F
19. H
20. G
21. A
22. B
23. I
24. D
25. E

Chapter 14 Basic Principles for the Administration of Medications

Review Questions

1. b
2. a
3. c
4. c
5. d
6. d
7. b
8. d
9. b
10. b
11. c
12. b
13. d
14. d
15. a
16. b
17. b
18. c
19. a
20. a

Chapter 15 Administration of Nonparenteral Medications

Review Questions

1. a
2. c
3. d
4. d
5. d
6. d
7. b
8. b
9. c
10. d
11. a
12. b
13. d
14. b
15. a
16. b
17. d
18. c
19. b
20. d
21. d
22. a

Chapter 16 Parenteral Equipment and Supplies

Review Questions

1. d
2. c
3. c
4. c
5. c
6. b
7. c
8. b
9. c
10. d
11. c
12. b
13. a
14. a
15. c
16. d
17. b
18. c
19. d
20. d
21. E
22. C
23. A
24. D
25. B

Chapter 17 Administration of Parenteral Medications

Review Questions

1. b
2. d
3. d
4. c

5. b
6. b
7. c
8. d
9. d
10. d
11. a
12. d
13. d
14. d
15. d
16. c
17. d
18. b
19. d
20. C
21. D
22. A
23. B
24. E
25. F

Section 4 Drugs and Related Substances

Chapter 18 Drugs Used to Counteract Infections

Review Questions

1. b
2. c
3. c
4. c
5. a
6. c
7. b
8. d
9. d
10. b
11. b
12. a
13. d
14. c
15. d
16. c
17. c
18. c
19. c
20. c
21. d
22. b
23. d
24. b
25. c
26. b
27. c
28. b
29. D
30. E
31. F
32. G
33. A
34. C
35. H
36. B

Chapter 19 Antifungal, Antiviral, and Immunizing Agents

Review Questions

1. b
2. c
3. d
4. c
5. a
6. b
7. c
8. c
9. d
10. d
11. c
12. b
13. c
14. a
15. a
16. d
17. a
18. b
19. b
20. E
21. D
22. B
23. A
24. F
25. C
26. H
27. G
28. J

Chapter 20 Antineoplastic Agents

Review Questions

1. b
2. a
3. d
4. d
5. d
6. d
7. b
8. d
9. c
10. d
11. d
12. d
13. b
14. d
15. b
16. d
17. c
18. d
19. b
20. c
21. a
22. d
23. a
24. C
25. G
26. E
27. B
28. F
29. D
30. H

Chapter 21 Vitamins and Minerals

Review Questions

1. c
2. b
3. a
4. c
5. b
6. c
7. d
8. d
9. d
10. b
11. b
12. d
13. c
14. b
15. c
16. d
17. c
18. c
19. b
20. a
21. C
22. I
23. G
24. B
25. F
26. E
27. D
28. A
29. H

Chapter 22 Psychotropic Agents

Review Questions

1. d
2. b
3. a
4. d
5. d
6. a
7. a
8. d
9. c
10. c
11. b
12. d
13. d
14. d
15. c
16. d
17. b
18. d
19. b
20. a
21. b
22. d
23. c
24. c
25. a
26. c
27. d
28. B
29. C
30. A

Chapter 23 Substance Abuse

Review Questions

1. c
2. a
3. b
4. b
5. c
6. a
7. d
8. b
9. d
10. b
11. d
12. c
13. a
14. a
15. d
16. d
17. c
18. d
19. c
20. b
21. a
22. a
23. a
24. C
25. D
26. G
27. B
28. F
29. E
30. A

Section 5 Effects on Medications on Body Systems

Chapter 24 Medications Used for Circulatory System Disorders

Review Questions

1. c
2. d
3. b
4. d
5. c
6. b
7. d
8. b
9. c
10. d
11. a
12. d
13. d
14. d
15. b
16. c
17. a
18. b
19. c
20. b
21. c
22. a
23. c
24. a
25. D
26. E
27. B
28. F
29. G
30. C
31. A

Chapter 25 Medications That Affect the Respiratory System

Review Questions

1. c
2. b
3. d
4. a
5. c
6. a
7. c
8. a
9. d
10. b
11. a
12. b
13. c
14. a
15. d
16. d
17. a
18. a
19. c
20. b
21. a
22. c
23. b
24. a
25. c
26. b
27. a
28. C
29. G
30. F
31. B
32. D
33. A
34. E
35. I

Chapter 26 Medications Used for Gastrointestinal System Disorders

Review Questions

1. b
2. b
3. c
4. c
5. d
6. a
7. d
8. b
9. d
10. a

11. a
12. b
13. c
14. c
15. b
16. c
17. b
18. c
19. d
20. a
21. c
22. d
23. b
24. b
25. a
26. c
27. c
28. d
29. b
30. d
31. c
32. d
33. a
34. c
35. c
36. b

Chapter 27 Diuretics and Medications Used for Urinary System Disorders

Review Questions

1. c
2. b
3. a
4. d
5. b
6. c
7. a
8. b
9. c
10. d
11. b
12. b
13. d
14. c
15. c
16. c
17. d
18. d
19. a
20. d
21. a
22. a
23. b
24. b
25. C
26. D
27. E
28. B
29. A
30. G

Chapter 28 Medications Used in Treatment of Endocrine Disorders

Review Questions

1. c
2. d
3. b
4. d
5. d
6. b
7. a
8. b
9. d
10. b
11. c
12. d
13. d
14. c
15. b
16. d
17. b
18. c
19. b
20. d
21. d
22. b
23. b
24. D
25. E
26. H
27. G
28. B
29. C
30. F
31. A
32. J

Chapter 29 Medications Used for Musculoskeletal System Disorders

Review Questions

1. c
2. d
3. b
4. a
5. c
6. d
7. b
8. a
9. d
10. c
11. d
12. c
13. a
14. c
15. c
16. d
17. b
18. b
19. a
20. c
21. c
22. d
23. a
24. b
25. c
26. C
27. A
28. B
29. E
30. D

Chapter 30 Medications That Affect the Nervous System

Review Questions

1. b
2. c
3. a
4. a
5. c
6. b
7. d
8. b
9. b
10. c
11. b
12. c
13. b
14. a
15. d
16. a
17. c
18. b
19. a
20. d
21. c
22. d
23. d
24. d
25. a
26. c
27. d
28. b
29. d
30. d

31. b
32. c
33. b
34. d
35. b
36. c
37. d
38. C
39. F
40. I
41. G
42. H
43. D
44. E
45. A
46. B

Chapter 31 Medications That Affect the Reproductive System

Review Questions

1. a
2. d
3. b
4. d
5. d
6. a
7. b
8. c
9. d
10. a
11. b
12. a
13. c
14. b
15. d
16. d
17. b
18. b
19. a
20. c
21. a
22. d
23. d
24. c
25. c
26. a
27. c
28. b
29. c
30. c
31. D
32. E
33. F
34. C
35. B
36. A
37. H

DRUG INDEX

A

Abbokinase, **486**
(urokinase)

ABVD, **381**
(Adriamycin, Blenoxane,
Velban, and DTIC-Dome)

Achromycin, **306**
(tetracycline hydrochloride)

Activase, **487**
(alteplase)

Adapin, **419**
(doxepin hydrochloride)

Adrenalin, **512**
(epinephrine)

Adriamycin, **378**, **381**
(doxorubicin hydrochloride)

Advil, **611**, **637**
(ibuprofen)

Aerobid, **515**
(flunisolide)

Afrin, **506**
(oxymetazoline hydrochloride)

Akineton, **643**
(biperiden hydrochloride)

Aldactone, **479**, **557**
(spironolactone)

Aldomet, **479**
(methyldopa)

Aldoril, **479**
(methyldopa-
hydrochlorothiazide)

Alkeran, **377**
(melphalan)

Alupent, **512**
(metaproterenol sulfate)

Alurate, **639**
(aprobarbital)

Amcort, **608**
(triamcinolone diacetate)

Amgen, **491**
(epoetin alfa)

Amicar, **488**

Amidate, **649**
(etomidate)

Amikin, **308**
(amikacin sulfate)

aminophylline, **513**

Amoxil, **300**
(amoxicillin)

Amphojel, **530**
(aluminum hydroxide)

Amyl nitrate, **476**

Amytal, **639**
(amobarbital)

Ancef, **303**
(cefazolin sodium)

Ancobon, **329**
(flucytosine)

Andro 100, **675**
(testosterone)

Androderm, **675**
(testosterone transdermal
system)

Android, **379**
(methyltestosterone)

Android-F, **379**
(fluoxymesterone)

Anectine, **617**
(succinylcholine chloride)

Antepar, **315**
(piperazine citrate)

Antiminth, **315**
(pyrantel pamoate)

Antivert, **653**
(meclizine hydrochloride)

Anturane, **614**
(sulfinpyrazone)

Apogen, **308**
(gentamicin sulfate)

Apomorphine hydrochloride,
546

Apresoline, **479**
(hydralazine hydrochloride)

Aralen HCl, **317**
(chloroquine hydrochloride)

Aralen phosphate, **317**
(chloroquine phosphate)

Aramine, **474**
(metaraminol bitartrate)

Aristocort, **608**
(triamcinolone)

Cefadyl, **303**
(cephapirin sodium)

Cefizox, **303**
(ceftizoxime sodium)

Cefotan, **303**
(cefotetan)

Cefracycline, **306**
(tetracycline hydrochloride)

Ceftin, **304**
(cefuroxime)

Celestne, **608**, **609**
(betamethasone)

Ceporacin, **303**
(cephalothin sodium)

Cerespan, **477**
(papaverine hydrochloride)

Cerubidine, **378**
(daunorubicin hydrochloride)

Chloromycetin, **313**
(chloramphenicol)

Chlor-Trimeton, **504**
(chlorpheniramine maleate)

Choledyl, **513**
(oxtriphylline)

Cholybar, **493**
(cholestyramine)

Cibalith-S Syrup, **423**
(lithium)

Cinobac, **571**
(cinoxacin)

Cipro, **314**, **571**
(ciprofloxacin HCl)

Claforan, **303**
(cefotaxime)

Cleocin, **314**
(clindamycin hydrochloride)

Clinoril, **611**
(sulindac)

Cloderm, **609**
(clocortolone pivalate)

Cloxapen, **301**
(cloxacillin)

CMF, **381**
(Cytoxan, Mexate, and 5-FU)

CMFP, **381**
(Cytoxan Mexate, 5-FU, and prednisone)

Cocaine, **436**, **441**, **648**
(cocaine hydrochloride)

Codeine, **508**, **633**

Codone, **508**
(hydrocodone bitartrate)

Cogentin, **643**
(benztropine mesylate)

Colace, **542**
(docusate sodium)

colchicine, **614**

Colestid, **493**
(colestipol)

Cologel, **542**
(Methylcellulose)

Compazine, **426**
(prochlorperazine)

Coricidin, **506**
(phenylephrine hydrochloride)

Cortef, **608**
(hydrocortisone)

Cortef Acetate, **608**
(hydrocortisone acetate)

Cortef fluids, **608**
(hydrocortisone cypionate)

Cortone, **608**
(cortisone acetate)

Cosmegen, **378**
(dactinomycin)

Coumadin, **483**
(warfarin sodium)

Cozaar, **480**
(losartan)

Cromolyn sodium, **514**

Crystodigin, **465**
(digitoxin)

Cuprimine, **613**
(penicillamine)

Cyanocobalamin, **490**

Cyclocort, **609**
(amcinonide)

Cyclogyl, **651**
(cyclopentolate hydrochloride)

Cyclopropane, **649**

Cyclospasmol, **477**
(cyclandelate)

Cystospaz-M, **572**
(hyoscyamine sulfate)

Cytomel, **582**
(liothyronine sodium)

Cytosar, **378**
(cytarabine)

Cytotec, **535**
(misoprostol)

Cytoxan, **377**, **381**
(cyclophosphamide)

D

Dalmane, **642**
(flurazepam hydrochloride)

Dantrium, **616**
(dantrolene sodium)

Daranide, **650**
(dichlorphenamide)

Daraprim, **317**
(pyrimethamine)

MOPP, **381**
(Mustargen, Oncovin, Matulane, and prednisone)

Morphine sulfate, **633**

Motrin, **611**, **637**
(ibuprofen)

Mucomyst, **509**
(acetylcysteine)

Murine, **651**
(tetrahydrozoline hydrochloride)

Mustargen, **377**, **381**
(mechlorethamine hydrochloride)

Mutamycin, **378**
(mitomycin)

Myambutol, **520**
(ethambutol hydrochloride)

Mycostatin, **329**
(nystatin)

Mydriacyl, **651**
(tropicamide)

Mylanta, **531**

Myleran, **377**
(busulfan)

Myochrysine, **613**
(gold sodium thiomalate)

Myotonachol, **572**
(bethanechol chloride)

Mysoline, **646**
(primidone)

Mytelase, **618**
(ambenoium chloride)

N

Nalfon, **611**
(fenoprofen calcium)

Naphcon, **651**
(naphazoline hydrochloride)

Naprosyn, **611**, **637**
(naproxen)

Narcan, **635**
(naloxone hydrochloride)

Nardil, **420**
(phenelzine sulfate)

Naturetin, **479**, **557**
(bendroflumethiazide)

Navane, **427**
(thiothixene hydrochloride)

Nebcin, **308**
(tobramycin sulfate)

NegGram, **571**
(nalidixic acid)

Nembutal, **639**
(pentobarbital)

Neofer, **488**
(ferrous fumarate)

Neosporin, **313**
(polymyxin B-bacitracin neomycin)

Neo-Synephrine HCl, **506**, **651**
(phenylephrine hydrochloride)

Neo-Synephrine 1% injection, **474**
(phenylephrine hydrohloride)

Neptazane, **650**
(methazolamide)

Nesacaine, **648**
(chloroprocaine hydrochloride)

Netromycin, **308**
(netilmicin)

Neupogen, **383**
(filgrastin)

Niclocide, **315**
(niclosamide)

Nicobid, **493**
(niacin)

Nicolar, **493**
(niacin)

Nitro-Bid, **476**
(nitroglycerin)

Nitrogard, **476**
(nitroglycerin)

Nitroglyn, **476**
(nitroglycerin)

Nitrolingual Spray, **476**
(nitroglycerin)

Nitrospan, **476**
(nitroglycerin)

Nitrostat, **476**
(nitroglycerin)

nitrous oxide, **649**

Nizoral, **329**, **379**
(ketoconazole)

N-methylformamide, **382**

Noctec, **642**
(chloral hydrate)

Nolvadex, **379**, **384**
(tamoxifen citrate)

Norcuron, **617**
(vecuronium)

Nordette, **28**, **674**

Norflex, **616**
(orphenadrine citrate)

Norinyl 1 + 35 21 day, **674**

Norlestrin 28 1/50, **674**

GENERAL INDEX